FACTORS AFFECTING THE ACTION OF NARCOTICS

MONOGRAPHS OF
THE MARIO NEGRI INSTITUTE FOR
PHARMACOLOGICAL RESEARCH, MILAN

SERIES EDITOR: SILVIO GARATTINI

Amphetamines and Related Compounds
Edited by E. Costa and S. Garattini

Basic and Therapeutic Aspects of Perinatal Pharmacology
Edited by P. L. Morselli, S. Garattini, and F. Sereni

The Benzodiazepines
Edited by S. Garattini, E. Mussini, and L. O. Randall

Chemotherapy of Cancer Dissemination and Metastasis
Edited by S. Garattini and G. Franchi

Drug Interactions
Edited by P. L. Morselli, S. Garattini, and S. N. Cohen

Insolubilized Enzymes
Edited by M. Salmona, C. Saronio, and S. Garattini

Isolated Liver Perfusion and Its Applications
Edited by I. Bartošek, A. Guaitani, and L. L. Miller

Mass Spectrometry in Biochemistry and Medicine
Edited by A. Frigerio and N. Castagnoli, Jr.

Pharmacology of Steroid Contraceptive Drugs
Edited by S. Garattini and H. W. Berendes

Interactions Between Putative Neurotransmitters in the Brain
Edited by S. Garattini, J. F. Pujol, and R. Samanin

Central Mechanisms of Anorectic Drugs
Edited by S. Garattini and R. Samanin

Factors Affecting the Action of Narcotics
Edited by M. W. Adler, L. Manara, and R. Samanin

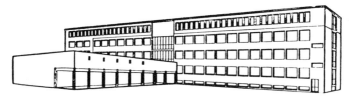

MONOGRAPHS OF
THE MARIO NEGRI INSTITUTE FOR
PHARMACOLOGICAL RESEARCH, MILAN

Factors Affecting the Action of Narcotics

Editors

Martin W. Adler, Ph.D.
Professor of Pharmacology
Temple University
School of Medicine
Philadelphia, Pennsylvania

Luciano Manara, M.D.
Head, Laboratory of Drug Metabolism
Mario Negri Institute for
  Pharmacological Research
Milan, Italy

Rosario Samanin, Pharm. D.
Head, Laboratory of Neuropharmacology
Mario Negri Institute for Pharmacological Research
Milan, Italy

Associate Editors

Judy D. Baggott
Biomedical Information Center
Mario Negri Institute for
  Pharmacological Research
Milan, Italy

Ellen B. Geller, M.A.
Research Assistant
Temple University School of Medicine
Philadelphia, Pennsylvania

Vanna Pistotti, Librarian
Gustavus A. Pfeiffer Memorial Library
Mario Negri Institute for Pharmacological Research
Milan, Italy

Raven Press ■ New York

Raven Press, 1140 Avenue of the Americas, New York, New York 10036

Made in the United States of America

Library of Congress Cataloging in Publication Data

Main entry under title

Factors affecting the action of narcotics

(A Monograph of the Mario Negri Institute for
Pharmacological Research)
'Proceedings of a meeting held at the Mario Negri
Institute for Pharmacological Research.'
    Includes bibliographical references and index.
    1. Narcotics-Physiological effect–Congresses.
I. Adler, Martin W   II. Manara, Luciano.
III. Samanin, R IV. Istituto di ricerche farma-
cologiche Mario Negri. Monographs.
RM328.F33   615'782   78-2999
ISBN 0-89004-272-1

Preface

Despite their serious drawbacks of tolerance and dependence, whose nature has still to be fully elucidated, and the allied problems of abuse, natural and synthetic drugs with morphine-like action, that is, narcotics, retain a very important place in therapy, especially in the treatment of pain.

Like the majority of drugs, narcotics elicit their pharmacological effects by interacting with specific receptors. Indeed one of the major recent efforts in narcotic research has been to characterize these receptors on the basis of the *in vitro* stereospecific binding of high specific activity labelled opiates. Even more recently this has progressed to the isolation of endogenous ligands, that is, physiologically occurring peptides with morphine-like action, a development that in turn has provided considerable openings, and is authoritatively reviewed in this volume.

Specific interaction at receptors may be considered the central event leading to the characteristic biological responses to administration of narcotics. Yet several other steps, either previous or subsequent to receptor activation, are likewise critical as regards the end results. The different levels and the various mechanisms involved are related in a complex cause-and-effect chain, each link potentially influencable by the experimental variables. Recognition and control of these factors, and awareness of the difficulty of varying only one of them at a time, are among the requisites of a scientifically correct approach to the question in laboratory investigations. Similarly, well controlled studies of the physiological and pathological entities modulating the effects of narcotics in man, as well as of drug interactions of clinical significance, are highly desirable.

This monograph contains the proceedings of a meeting held at the Mario Negri Institute for Pharmacological Research to review current information on the pharmacology of narcotics from a different perspective. The idea behind the organization of the meeting was in fact to provide a novel view of the considerable variety of modes of action of narcotic drugs, both in laboratory animals and at the clinical level, in order to better define the underlying factors.

The meeting represented a unique opportunity for discussion and exchange between scientists who take different but parallel approaches in their work on narcotics, and among whom there is limited cross-communication as a result of today's increasing tendency to narrow specialization.

Besides providing new insights and information, and — we hope — stimulating further research, this work should prove its worth as a lasting reference text.

Italy is now facing domestic escalation of the serious worldwide medical and social problem of opiate abuse: an estimate of ten thousand heroin addicts in the city of Milan, most of them under twenty years of age, speaks for itself. The gathering in our Institute of so many experts in the pharmacology of opiates, from different parts of the world, also bears witness to their belief that biomedical research plays a fundamental role in our endeavors to protect society from the modern epidemic represented by drug abuse.

On behalf of the Mario Negri Institute, it is my privilege to gratefully acknowledge the substantial contribution made by the authors, and the cooperation of all those who worked to render the meeting possible.

Luciano Manara

Acknowledgments

The Organizing Committee wishes to thank the Mario Negri Institute Foundation Inc., New York, Fondazione Lorenzini, Milano, and the following firms and organizations for their contributions to the success of the Symposium:

Alfa Farmaceutici, S.p.A., Bologna, Italy
Boehringer Biochemica s.r.l., Milano, Italy
Ciba-Geigy, S.p.A., Origgio, Italy
Clesa S.p.A., Bresso, Italy
Crinos S.p.A., Como, Italy
Cyanamid Italia S.p.A., Catania, Italy
Fondazione Hoechst, Milano, Italy
Hoffmann La Roche, Inc., Nutley, N.J., U.S.A.
Inverni Della Beffa, S.p.A., Milano, Italy
Istituto Biochimico Italiano, S.p.A., Milano, Italy
Laboratorio Guidotti, S.p.A., Pisa, Italy
Lederle, Pearl River, N.Y., U.S.A.
Lepetit, S.p.A., Milano, Italy
Merck Sharp & Dohme (Italia), S.p.A., Roma, Italy
Merck Sharp & Dohme, West Point P.A., U.S.A.
Midy Farmaceutici, S.p.A., Milano, Italy
Montedison, S.p.A., Milano, Italy
Reckitt & Colman, Kingston-upon-Hull, England
Roche, S.p.A., Milano, Italy
Schering, Kenilworth, N.J., U.S.A.
Selvi, S.p.A., Milano, Italy
Sigma Tau, S.p.A., Pomezia, Italy
Sigurtà Farmaceutici, S.p.A., Milano, Italy

Contents

ROUTE OF ADMINISTRATION, DRUG BINDING, DISTRIBUTION AND METABOLISM

BIOCHEMICAL CONSIDERATIONS

NEUROTRANSMITTER MODIFICATION OF OPIATE ACTIONS

ENVIRONMENTAL AND PATHOLOGICAL CONDITIONS, DRUG INTERACTIONS

PERSPECTIVES IN NARCOTIC RESEARCH

Contributors

M.W. Adler
Temple University School of Medicine
Department of Pharmacology
Philadelphia, Pennsylvania 19140

L. Ahtee
Department of Pharmacology,
School of Pharmacy
University of Helsinki
Kirkkokatu 20
SF-00170 Helsinki 17, Finland

A. Akil
Department of Psychiatry and
Behavioral Sciences
Stanford University School
of Medicine
Stanford, California 94305

C. Aldinio
Istituto di Ricerche Farmacologiche
"Mario Negri"
Via Eritrea, 62
20157 Milan, Italy

H.L. Altshuler
Department of Pharmacology
Baylor College of Medicine
Texas Medical Center
Houston, Texas 77025

H.S. Bachelard
Department of Biochemistry
University of Bath, United Kingdom

J.D. Barchas
Department of Psychiatry and
Behavioral Sciences
Stanford University School
of Medicine
Stanford, California 94305

G. Benelli
Zambon S.p.A.
Research Laboratories,
Bresso-Milan, Italy

B.A. Berkowitz
Roche Institute of Molecular Biology
Nutley, New Jersey 07110

J.M. Besson
INSERM
Unité 161, Groupe de Recherche
de Neurophysiologie
Pharmacologique,
2 rue d'Alésia,
75014 Paris, France

J. Bläsig
Max-Planck-Institut für Psychiatrie
Department of Neuropharmacology
Kraepelinstrasse 2
8000 Munich 40, West Germany

K.A. Bonnet
Department of Psychiatry
New York University Medical Center
New York, New York 10016

A. Carenzi
Zambon S.p.A.
Research Laboratories
Bresso-Milan, Italy

C. Castellano
Cattedra di Psicologia Fisiologica
della Facoltà di Magistero
dell'Università di Roma e
Laboratorio di Psicobiologia e
Psicofarmacologia, C.N.R.
Via Reno 1,
Roma, Italy

F. Cattabeni

Istituto di Farmacologia e
Farmacognosia
Università di Milano
Via A. Del Sarto, 21
Milan, Italy

C. Cerletti

Istituto di Ricerche Farmacologiche
"Mario Negri"
Via Eritrea, 62
20157 Milan, Italy

D.L. Cheney

Laboratory of Preclinical
Pharmacology
National Institute of Mental Health
Saint Elizabeths Hospital
Washington, D.C. 20032

D.H. Clouet

New York State Office of Drug
Abuse Services
Testing and Research Laboratory
Brooklyn, New York 11217

P. Coccia

Istituto di Ricerche Farmacologiche
"Mario Negri"
Via Eritrea, 62
20157 Milan, Italy

J. Cochin

Department of Pharmacology
Boston University School of Medicine
80 East Concord Street
Boston, Massachusetts 02118

E. Costa

Laboratory of Preclinical
Pharmacology
National Institute of Mental Health
Saint Elizabeths Hospital
Washington, D.C. 20032

A. Cowan

Department of Pharmacology
Temple University School of Medicine
Philadelphia, Pennsylvania

B.M. Cox

Addiction Research Foundation
and Stanford University
Palo Alto, California 94304

B.E. Dahlström

Department of Pharmacology
Pharmaceutical Faculty
Biomedical Center
University of Uppsala
Uppsala, Sweden

F.V. De Feudis

Departamento de Investigacion
Centro Nacional "Ramòn y Cajal"
and Facultad de Medicina
Universidad Autonoma
Madrid, Spain

P.A. De Feudis

Departamento de Investigacion
Centro Nacional "Ramòn y Cajal"
and Facultad de Medicina
Universidad Autonoma
Madrid, Spain

D. Della Bella

Zambon S.p.A.
Research Laboratories
Bresso-Milan, Italy

R. Drawbaugh

Department of Psychology
University of Rhode Island
Kingston, Rhode Island 02881

R. Eisenberg
Department of Pharmacology
University of Minnesota
Duluth, Minnesota 55812

W.B. Essman
Queens College of the City University
of New York
Flushing, New York 11367

L.A. Fisher
Department of Psychology
University of California
Santa Barbara, California 93106

J. Fishman
Institute for Steroid Research
Montefiore Hospital and Medical
Center
Albert Einstein College of Medicine
Bronx, New York 10467

V. Frigeni
Zambon, S.p.A.
Research Laboratories
Bresso-Milan, Italy

E.A.M. Frost
Department of Anesthesiology
Albert Einstein College of Medicine
Bronx, New York 10461

S. Garattini
Istituto di Ricerche Farmacologiche
"Mario Negri"
Via Eritrea 62
20157 Milan, Italy

E.B. Geller
Temple University School of Medicine
Department of Pharmacology
Philadelphia, Pennsylvania 19140

V.F. Gellert
Department of Pharmacology
Emory University
Atlanta, Georgia 30322

P.L. Gildenberg
Division of Neurosurgery
University of Texas Medical School
at Houston
Houston, Texas 77030

A. Goldstein
Addiction Research Foundation
and Stanford University
Palo Alto, California 94304

C. Gonzalez Portal
Departmento de Investigacion
Centro Nacional "Ramòn y Cajal"
and Facultad de Medicina
Universidad Autonoma
Madrid, Spain

Ch. Gramsch
Department of Neuropharmacology
Max-Planck-Institut für Psychiatrie
Kraepelinstrasse 2
800 München 40, West Germany

E.F. Hahn
Department of Biochemistry
Albert Einstein College of Medicine
Bronx, New York 10467

R.A. Harris
Department of Pharmacology
School of Medicine
University of California at
San Francisco
San Francisco, California 94143

J. Hempstead
*Roche Institute of Molecular Biology
Nutley, New Jersey
and Department of Anesthesiology and
   Pharmacology
Columbia University
College of Physicians and Surgeons
New York, New York 10032*

A. Herz
*Department of Neuropharmacology
Max-Planck-Institut für Psychiatrie
Kraepelinstrasse 2
8000 München 40, West Germany*

J.W. Holaday
*Department of Pharmacology
University of California
San Francisco, California 94143*

V. Höllt
*Department of Neuropharmacology
Max-Planck-Institut für Psychiatrie
Kraepelinstrasse 2
8000 München 40, West Germany*

R.B. Holman
*Department of Psychiatry and
   Behavioral Sciences
Stanford University
School of Medicine
Stanford, California 94305*

J.T. Huang
*New York State Research Institute for
   Neurochemistry and
   Drug Addiction
Ward's Island
New York, New York 10035*

J. Hughes
*Unit for Research on Addictive
   Drugs
University of Aberdeen
Aberdeen, AB9 1AS, Scotland*

A.E. Ibanez
*Departamento de Investigacion
Centro Nacional "Ramòn y Cajal"
and Facultad de Medicina
Universidad Autonoma
Madrid, Spain*

E.T. Iwamoto
*Department of Pharmacology
University of California
San Francisco, California 94143*

J.J.C. Jacob
*Laboratory of Pharmacology
Pasteur Institute
F 75724 Paris Cedex 15, France*

K. Jhamandas
*Department of Pharmacology
Faculty of Medicine
Queen's University
Kingston, Ontario, Canada*

H.W. Kosterlitz
*Unit for Research on Addictive
   Drugs
University of Aberdeen
Aberdeen, AB9 1AS, Scotland*

M.J. Kreek
*The Rockefeller University
1230 York Avenue
New York, New York 10021*

H. Lal
*Department of Pharmacology
   and Toxicology
University of Rhode Island
Kingston, Rhode Island 02881*

E. Laschka
*Department of Neuropharmacology
Max-Planck-Institut für Psychiatrie
Kraepelinstrasse 2
8000 München 40, West Germany*

D. Le Bars
INSERM
Unité 161, Groupe de Recherche
de Neurophysiologie
Pharmacologique
2 rue d'Alésia,
75014 Paris, France

L. Lichtblau
Departments of Pharmacology and
Psychiatry
University of Minnesota
Minneapolis, Minnesota 55455

H.H. Loh
Department of Pharmacology
School of Medicine
University of California
at San Francisco
San Francisco, California 94143

A. Luini
Istituto di Ricerche Farmacologiche
"Mario Negri"
Via Eritrea, 62
20157 Milan, Italy

L.D. Lytle
Department of Psychology
University of California
Santa Barbara, California 93106

L. Manara
Istituto di Ricerche Farmacologiche
"Mario Negri"
Via Eritrea, 62
20157 Milan, Italy

T. Mennini
Istituto di Ricerche Farmacologiche
"Mario Negri"
Via Eritrea, 62
20157 Milan, Italy

R.B. Messing
Department of Psychology
University of California
Santa Barbara, California 93106

G. Meyer
Max-Planck-Institut für Psychiatrie
Department of Neuropharmacology
Kraepelinstrasse 2
8000 München 40, West Germany

S. Miksic
Department of Pharmacology
and Toxicology
University of Rhode Island
Kingston, Rhode Island 02881

J. Miller
Department of Pharmacology
Boston University
School of Medicine
80 East Concord Street
Boston, Massachusetts 02118

F. Miranda
Istituto di Ricerche Farmacologiche
"Mario Negri"
Via Eritrea, 62
20157 Milan, Italy

A.L. Misra
New York State Office of Drug
Abuse Services
Research Laboratory
Brooklyn, New York 11217

S.H. Ngai
Roche Institute of Molecular Biology
Nutley, New Jersey 07110
and Department of Anesthesiology and
Pharmacology
Columbia University College of
Physicians and Surgeons
New York, New York 10032

W.H. Oldendorf
Department of Neurology
UCLA School of Medicine
Los Angeles, California 90024

A. Oliverio
Cattedra di Psicologia Fisiologica
della Facoltà di Magistero
dell 'Università di Roma e
Laboratorio di Psicobiologia e
Psicofarmacologia, C.N.R.
Via Reno, 1
Roma, Italy

L.M. Orensanz Munoz
Departmento de Investigacion
Centro Nacional "Ramòn y Cajal"
and Facultad de Medicina
Universidad Autonoma
Madrid, Spain

L. Paalzow
Department of Pharmacology
Pharmaceutical Faculty
Biomedical Center
University of Uppsala
Uppsala, Sweden

L. Phebus
Department of Psychology
University of California
Santa Barbara, California 93106

J. Poulson
Department of Pharmacology
Faculty of Medicine
Queen's University
Kingston, Ontario, Canada

M.P. Pugnaire
Departamento de Investigacion
Centro Nacional "Ramòn y Cajal"
and Facultad de Medicina
Universidad Autonoma
Madrid, Spain

F. Racagni
Istituto di Farmacologia e
Farmacognosia
Università di Milano
Via A. Del Sarto, 21
Milan, Italy

M.J. Rance
Drug Metabolism Department
Reckitt and Colman Pharmaceutical
Division
Dansom Lane
Hull, HU8 7DS, United Kingdom

R. Rosenthal
Queens College of the City University
of New York
Flushing, New York 11367

C. Rosow
Department of Pharmacology
Boston University School of Medicine
80 East Concord Street
Boston, Massachusetts 02118

R. Samanin
Istituto di Ricerche Farmacologiche
"Mario Negri"
Via Eritrea, 62
20157 Milan, Italy

M. Satoh
Department of Pharmacology
Faculty of Pharmaceutical Sciences
Kyoto University
Kyoto 606, Japan

G. Serra
Istituto di Ricerche Farmacologiche
"Mario Negri"
Via Eritrea, 62
20157 Milan, Italy

J.S. Shillingford
Drug Metabolism Department
Allen and Hanbury Research Ltd.
Priory Road
Ware, Herts., United Kingdom

E.J. Simon
New York University Medical Center
550 First Avenue
New York, New York 10016

E. Somoza
Departamento de Investigacion
Centro Nacional "Ramòn y Cajal"
and Facultad de Medicina
Universidad Autonoma
Madrid, Spain

P.F. Spano
Istituto di Farmacologia e
Farmacognosia
Università di Milano
Via A. Del Sarto, 21
Milan, Italy

S.B. Sparber
Departments of Pharmacology and
Psychiatry
University of Minnesota
Minneapolis, Minnesota 55455

S. Spector
Roche Institute of Molecular Biology
Nutley, New Jersey 07110

M. Städele
Max-Planck-Institut für Psychiatrie
Department of Neuropharmacology
Kraepelinstrasse 2
8000 Munich 40, West Germany

H. Steinberg
Department of Pharmacology
University College London
Gower Street
London, WC1, England

H. Takagi
Department of Pharmacology
Faculty of Pharmaceutical Sciences
Kyoto University
Kyoto 606, Japan

A.E. Takemori
Department of Pharmacology
University of Minnesota
Health Sciences Center Medical
School
Minneapolis, Minnesota 55455

R.J. Tallarida
Department of Pharmacology
Temple University School of
Medicine
Philadelphia, Pennsylvania 19129

Hj. Teschemacher
Department of Neuropharmacology
Max-Planck-Institut für Psychiatrie
Kraepelinstrasse 2
8000 München 40, West Germany

M. Trabucchi
Istituto di Farmacologia e
Farmacognosia
Università di Milano
Via A. Del Sarto, 21
Milan, Italy

L.F. Tseng
Department of Pharmacology
University of California
San Francisco, California 94143

L. Valzelli
Istituto di Ricerche Farmacologiche
"Mario Negri"
Via Eritrea, 62
20157 Milan, Italy

S.J. Watson
Department of Psychiatry and
Behavioral Sciences
Stanford University
School of Medicine
Stanford, California 94305

E.L. Way
Department of Pharmacology
University of California
San Francisco, California 94143

E. Wei
Department of Environmental Health
  Sciences
School of Public Health
University of California
Berkeley, California 94705

I. Yano
Visiting Research Fellow
Department of Pharmacology
Wakayama Medical College
Wakayama, Japan

G. Zsilla
Semmelweis University of Medicine
Department of Pharmacology
Budapest, Hungary

1. CHOICE OF TEST SUBJECTS

AND METHODS

Factors Affecting the Action of Narcotics, edited by
M.L. Adler, L. Manara, and R. Samanin.
Raven Press, New York©1978.

General Characteristics of the Test Subject:

Introduction to the Topic

J.J.C. Jacob

Laboratory of Pharmacology - Pasteur Institute
F 75724 PARIS Cedex 15, France

Narcotic analgesics are studies with many test
subjects, i.e., a) a man or a whole animal; b) an
organ within an organism or an isolated organ in vitro
or slices of tissues; c) a cell in its normal
environment or cultured cells; d) more or less
purified extracts of brain, parts of brain, tissues,
or cultured cells, obtained from normal or narcotized
animals which are or are not tolerant and dependent.
The responses of these subjects to narcotics (or their
binding of narcotics) are specific or not specific, a
distinction which is not always easy, as responses
(or bindings) are often mixed ones. Among the
responses obtained in man and in whole animals, the
principal ones are inhibition of nociceptive reactions,
particular syndromes (bradycardia, bradypnea,sedation
or excitation according to species and dose, locomotor
disturbances, intestinal and pupillary reactions,etc.)
and induction of dependence and tolerance. Biochemical
and neurological correlates or mechanisms of these
effects are searched for at different levels of
organization.

A general characteristic of narcotics in man and
in the whole animal is that they are able to depress
almost all nociceptive reactions whatever the nature
of the applied stimulus (physical, chemical) and its
site of application (superficial, deep or mixed)(4);
similarly, they depress - with appropriate dosages -
all signs of abstinence in withdrawn dependent
subjects. Other drugs, on the contrary, depress only
a given nociceptive response (or set of responses) or
a given abstinence sign (or set of signs). In my

3

opinion, this indicates that all these nociceptive
reactions have in common a particular set of neurons
or neuronal components and similarily, that all
abstinence signs proceed from common primitive biochemical modifications; in other words, opioid
receptors are involved as the basic unit, receptors
being considered here as the macromolecules and not
only as their binding sites. Drugs other than narcotics are characterized by components (sets of neurons)
which vary from one response to another. This is
generally the case for acetylcholine, catecholamines,
and serotonin, and their depletors and antagonists;
these mediators (and others) would then appear to be
involved mainly in secondary mechanisms of particular
responses.

   However, the reactions of the test subject,although
all are depressed by narcotics, are not equally
sensitive to these drugs. The sensitivity of
nociceptive reactions has been related to the site of
application of the stimulus and to its strength; e.g.,
the peritoneal writhing test allows one to assess the
antinociceptive effect of weak analgesics and of mixed
agonist-antagonists which are ineffective with tests
using superficial stimuli; some of these latter tests
(tail-flick, hot-plate), however, are convenient when
the intensity of the stimulus is lowered (i.e., the
temperature of the water bath or of the hot plate).

   The sensitivity of a reaction has also been related
to the complexity of the underlying neuronal network
and/or its spinal or supraspinal localization. In the
method of Carroll and Lim (1), vocalization afterdischarge is more sensitive to narcotics than
vocalization per se, which is more so than responses
of the tail; we showed that in the hot-plate method,
jumping was more sensitive than licking, and licking
more so than withdrawal of the paws (6). However,in
usual experimental conditions, even simple responses
like tail-flick and withdrawal of the paws involve a
spinal component and a supraspinal control.

   Similarly, reactions produced by nociceptive"psychic"
stimuli appear to be particularly sensitive,
nociceptive being accepted here in its true etymological
sense (i.e., damaging or potentially damaging or
warning of a danger). These reactions reflect in some

manner the psychic processing of human pain; an
example is the greater sensitivity of the jump response
with repeated trials of the hot-plate test, because,
as we demonstrated, this response involves conditioning. Another example is the quieting we observed
with Michaud in dogs having received a low dose of
morphine (0.1 mg kg^{-1} I.V.) (7). This dose did not
affect "physical" nociception evoked by toe-pinching.
It is of the same order of magnitude as the dose used
in man.

Sensitivity to narcotics depends also on species,
strain, sex and age. Man was considered as being
especially susceptible to narcotics; however, the
differences with other species used in the laboratory
do not appear to be as great as was once thought when
one takes into account the preceding comments on the
nature of the reaction and also relates the dose, not
with the weight, but with the surface of the body.
Nevertheless, interspecies variations of pharmacokinetic and pharmacodynamic origin are sufficiently
great to render the extrapolation as difficult as and
sometimes more difficult than for other drugs. It is
especially difficult for a) psychological dependence,
since the dependence liability will depend on many
factors other than those which are determined by self-
administration experiments (2), b) mixed agonist-
antagonist compounds; for some of these drugs, the
proportion between the two properties and hence, the
analgesic effects and also the dependence potential
have been found to be different in man and in monkey
(3). Some authors have suggested that this resulted
from a difference in "receptors"; metabolic differences
in N-dealkylation must also be considered. It is
worth mentioning that the major properties of narcotics
i.e., antinociception, tolerance, and dependence
induction can be studied and compared in the same
animal species, thanks especially to the development
of acute techniques of tolerance and dependence; mice,
rats, dogs, and monkeys can be used, each species
having its advantages and its drawbacks (5).

Influence of sex is as important, and I will only
recall here that it was critical for rejecting the
hypothesis that tolerance was related to an inhibition
of the demethylation of narcotics as reflected by

hepatic enzyme activity; hepatic demethylase occurs only in males,tolerance in both sexes. Age is also known to be important (e.g., with regard to the toxicity of narcotics and to the development of tolerance).

Tissue extracts and isolated organs such as the guinea pig ileum and the mouse vas deferens have proved valuable models for characterizing the agonist and antagonist properties of series of compounds and for giving theoretical insight into the mechanism and mode of actions of narcotics. They are also almost indispensable tools for isolating and characterizing the natural ligands,and indeed, were used to isolate the first known active peptide: enkephalin.

REFERENCES

1. Carroll, M.N. and Lim, R.K.S. (1960): Arch.Int. Pharmacodyn.,125: 383-403.
2. Evaluation of dependence liability and dependence potential of drugs. (1975): Report of a Scientific Group OMS. Technical Report Series n.577,pp.3-55.
3. Fraser, H.F. (1974): In: Narcotic Antagonists, edited by M.C. Braude, pp.439-453. Raven Press, New York.
4. Jacob, J. (1973): In: Utilisation des Morphinomimé-tiques en Anesthesie et Réanimation, edited by J. Montagne, C.G.Nahas, J.C.Salamagne, P.Viars, and G. Vourc'h, pp. 63-70. Librairie Arnette, Paris.
5. Jacob, J. (1975): In: Neuropsychopharmacology, edited by H.Hippius, J.R.Boissier and R.Pichot, pp.279-286. Excerpta Medica, Amsterdam.
6. Jacob, J. and Blozovski, M.(1961): Arch.Int. Pharmacodyn., 133: 296-309.
7. Jacob, J.J. and Michaud, G.M. (1974): Psychol.Med., 4: 270-273.

Factors Affecting the Action of Narcotics, edited by
M.L. Adler, L. Manara, and R. Samanin.
Raven Press, New York © 1978.

Genetic Aspects in Narcotic Action

A. Oliverio[+] C. Castellano[+] F. Racagni[o] P.F. Spano[o]
M. Trabucchi[o] and F. Cattabeni[o]

[+]Cattedra di Psicologia Fisiologica della Facoltà di
Magistero dell'Università di Roma e Laboratorio di
Psicobiologia e Psicofarmacologia, C.N.R. Via Reno 1
Roma, Italy
[o]Istituto di Farmacologia e Farmacognosia, Università
di Milano, Via A. Del Sarto 21, Milano, Italy

In a number of studies of narcotics on animal
behavior, evidence has been obtained indicating that
cholinergic mechanisms at the CNS level, may explain in
part the effects of most narcotic agents in relation
to tolerance and abstinence in rats and mice (7, 14).
Serotoninergic mechanisms also seem to play a role in
morphine analgesia and opiate tolerance or physical
dependence (5, 30, 36, 38).

By using different measures of locomotor activity,
it has been shown that morphine exerts a stimulating
effect in mice (12, 32).   The effects of morphine
on locomotor activity, and its analgesic effects, were
related by some authors to a reduction of the release
of acetylcholine at the central cholinergic synapses
(11, 15, 25, 31), or to alterations in brain catecholamine content and turnover (1, 28, 35).

A number of studies show the role played by genetic
make-up in modulating the effects of morphine on the
behavior of rats and mice (10, 12, 20).   It has been
shown, in particular (10), that different strains of
inbred mice are characterized by different patterns of
morphine addiction. In recent experiments (22), the
effects of morphine on locomotor activity and analgesia
have been investigated in three inbred strains of mice:
C57BL/6J (C57), DBA/2J (DBA), and BALB/cJ (BALB).
This genetic approach seems a useful method to assess
what biochemical systems are involved in the various
behavioral effects which follow the administration of
morphine.

C57 mice exhibit high levels of exploratory activity and low levels of avoidance and maze learning,
while higher levels of avoidance but lower patterns of

7

locomotor activity are attained by DBA and BALB mice
(23).   In addition, a number of recent experiments
indicate that differences in brain chemicals also
characterize these strains of mice.   For example, C57
show lower acetylcholinesterase and choline-acetyl-
transferase activities in the temporal lobe, than the
other strains (8, 19).   In contrast, higher levels of
noradrenaline are present in the pons and medulla of
C57 mice (18), while the lower locomotor activity of
the other two strains seems to be positively correlated with lower levels and turnover of noradrenaline
(16, 19).
    On the basis of these behavioral and biochemical
differences, the sensitivity of these strains to
morphine-induced analgesia and motor activity was
determined.   Locomotor activity was measured in toggle-floor boxes, and it was shown that the strains
tested clearly differed as regards the morphine-induced
"running fit".   Following morphine administration, a
three-fold average increase was evident in the C57
strain, while a two-fold increment appeared in the
BALB mice compared with saline-injected controls.
No effect was evident when the opiate was injected
into DBA mice (Fig. 1).

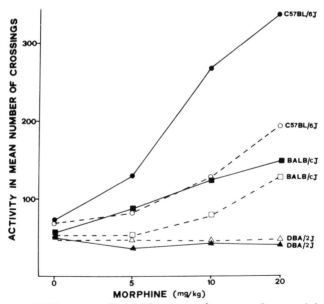

FIG. 1.   Effects of different doses of morphine on
the running activity of normal (solid lines) and tolerant (broken lines) mice.   Each group consisted of
10 mice tested 30 min after injection of morphine (22).

Analgesic effects of morphine were measured with
the hot-plate method (9, 12); the patterns of reactivity to the opiate by these three strains of mice
were the opposite of the activity patterns.   The C57
strain, in which morphine exerted a clear stimulating
effect on locomotor activity, appeared to be less
sensitive to the analgesic effect; DBA mice were very
sensitive to the analgesic effects of morphine, while
the same dose did not affect their locomotor behavior
(Fig. 2).

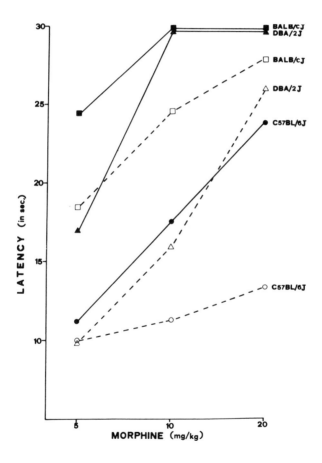

FIG. 2.   Morphine-induced analgesia in normal (solid
lines) and tolerant (broken lines) mice.   The
animals were tested 30 min after injection with different doses of morphine   (22).

In a further study (4), genetic analyses of the
effects of morphine on running activity and analgesia
were extended to the F_1 hybrids of the three strains
considered (C57, DBA and BALB).   From these experiments a clear dominance of the C57 strain over the
other two strains was evident.   Incomplete dominance
seemed to regulate the inheritance of morphine analgesia, in that the performance of C57 x BALB hybrid mice
was very similar to that of the C57 strain.   Because
of large estimates of environmental variance, it was
impossible to show that the backcross population
(C57 x BALB) x C57 and (C57 x BALB) x BALB, or (C57
x BALB) x C57 and (C57 x DBA) x DBA contained a
significant genetic component.   When the genetic
correlations between analgesia and locomotor activity
were calculated, the results were negative and large
enough to suggest that both behaviors were influenced
by many of the same genes.

Since negative correlations between analgesia and
running activity were evident, it was suggested that
the effects of the opiates on activity and analgesia
were likely to imply two different sites of action or
neurophysiologic systems, and that the biochemical
differences observed among the strains tested might
account for the dissociation between the two measures
and the strain-dependent effects of opiates.   An
initial response to this point has been given by
analysis of the interaction between septal lesions
and morphine-induced "running fit" and analgesia in
DBA and C57 mice (2).   Numerous data have shown that
there is a clear relationship between the distribution
of opiate receptors in the brain and the distribution
of neurotransmitters, and that among the areas rich
in opiate receptors are sites closely associated with
the limbic system, a critical area for eliciting
analgesia [13, 17, 37).   From our experiments it was
evident that morphine-induced "running fit" did not
change following septal lesions, while analgesia was
antagonized in both strains.   In the same study,
inhibition of the synthesis of noradrenaline by
pretreating mice with α-methyl-p-tyrosine (αMT)
resulted in a marked reduction of locomotor activity
both in C57 and in DBA mice.

Since it is well known that a decreased cholinergic
impact on the other regions of the limbic system
follows septal lesions (17, 25, 33), one of the more
likely explanations for the data obtained, may be that
reduction of cholinergic activity in the limbic system,
due to septal lesions, interferes with morphine analgesia.   The fact that only the analgesic behavior and

: antagonized by septal lesions,
;ite effect, has led to the
irophysiological and biochemical
morphine-induced running and
t, and that the limbic system
: behavior, but not the effects

also seems important when the
s of opiates with other drugs
ior of mice are assessed.
emonstrated (3) that the motor
BA mice may be affected by the
inations of heroin with ethanol,
ine, and that the type of
lepending on the strain conside-
articular, the combinations
r heroin + ethanol, clearly
ctivity of DBA mice, while the
f the C57 strain caused by
only by strychnine.
icity of the heroin + strychnine
of particular interest. This
sed higher toxicity than heroin
eroin, which was 200 mg/kg in
D mg/kg in DBA mice, was enhanced
l with a combination of heroin
D mg/kg and 100 mg/kg, respecti-
bination of the two drugs
r potentiated effect, proving
t which strychnine or heroin
t.   These results may have clear
ical implications, since many
n overdose of heroin, ought
ascribed to the use of adulte-
e effects of the opiate.
tion of the difference between
DBA) as regards their reactivi-
ided by recent studies of EEG
Oliverio (21) recorded the
oG) of saline-and morphine-
ice (Fig. 3).   No difference
rdings of ECoG activity in
these strains, while the normal
g sleeping showed generally
than C57 mice.   Morphine did
ttern of the DBA strain, while
and the appearance of slow
e evident in the ECoG of the
single acute opiate injection.
to 10 minutes after the injec-

8 mice, from one side to the other of the toggle-floor box. mean number of crossings (session 1 to V) of a group of Each session was 30 min long (31).

TABLE 1. Effects of heroin alone, or in combination with other drugs, on the locomotor activity of C57BL/6J and DBA/2J mice

	C57	DBA
Saline	37.0 ± 3.6	35.8 ± 1.1
Heroin 5 mg/kg	263.7 ± 7.6	28.5 ± 5.2
Amphetamine 2mg/kg	139.6 ± 5.1	48.7 ± 7.2
Strychnine 0.3 mg/kg	42.1 ± 2.4	29.7 ± 2.4
Ethanol 1 g/kg	38.0 ± 4.3	37.5 ± 3.5
Amphetamine 2 + Heroin 5	249.3 ± 2.7	98.2 ± 8.6
Strychnine 0.3 + Heroin 5	410.1 ± 6.3	33.4 ± 5.1
Ethanol 1 + Heroin 5	186.2 ± 3.7	79.5 ± 9.3

tion, lasted as long as 45-60 minutes, and was accompanied by behavioral activation.

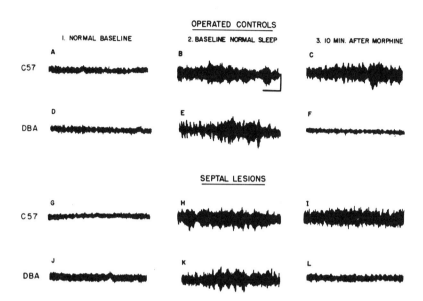

FIG. 3. Effects of a single injection of morphine on the EEG tracing recorded from the cortex in normal mice (operated controls) and in mice with lesions of the septum. Samples of polygraphic recordings during waking (1. normal baseline), slow wave sleep (2. baseline normal sleep) and 3. after the injection of morphine (20 mg/kg) in C57BL/6J and DBA/2J mice. Normal sleep EEG(B) and that after morphine injection (C) are similar in the C57BL/6J strain, while the waking EEG (D) and that after morphine injection (F) are similar in DBA mice. Septal lesions do not produce any major modification of the effects of morphine on the EEG patterns (21).

Septal lesions did not modify the morphine-induced ECoG patterns, nor the running response, but the analgesic effect was reduced. These results suggest that morphine-induced behavioral activation is correlated to a sleep-like ECoG pattern, and that a dissociation between ECoG and behavior, similar to that described for some anticholinergic drugs, occurs in C57 mice following administration of this opiate.

The fact that septal lesions antagonize morphine-induced analgesia, but not the "running fit" or the sleep-like ECoG activity, seems to support the hypothesis that locomotor or other excitatory patterns, rather than the analgesic effect of morphine, may be correlated to the ECoG responses.

As has been previously reported, a number of findings indicate that different biochemical mechanisms may account for the behavioral differences among inbred strains of mice and for their sensitivity to the effects of drugs.   Evidence exists, for example that strains of mice which have high alcohol preference, such as C57 mice, also have a different rate of ethanol clearance from the blood and different tissue sensitivity to alcohol, resulting in a faster metabolism of ethanol (6, 29).   Recent findings also indicate higher liver dehydrogenase activity in C57 than in BALB mice, and the latter strain has significantly less preference for alcohol than the former (6, 29).   It has also been shown (24) that different behavioral characteristics correspond to these biochemical differences, and that the same doses of ethanol decrease activity more markedly in C57 than in BALB mice.   It has also been demonstrated that the differences, in the effects of morphine on the locomotor and analgesic response of different strains of mice, may be related to biochemical differences in the brain. These findings indicate that the effects of morphine on locomotor activity and analgesia are related to two separate neurochemical patterns.

Trabucchi et al. (34) have shown that in C57 mice, which show more locomotor activity than DBA mice, in the absence of morphine, striatal adenylate cyclase is more stimulated by dopamine (Table 2).   Moreover, striatal dopaminergic neurons are activated mainly in C57 mice.   It has been demonstrated that 3-methoxy-tyramine and cAMP are increased by morphine administration only in the C57 strain (Table 3).

The same authors have shown that cholinergic pathways may be implicated in morphine-induced analgesia in the DBA strain.

Only in this strain was a decrement seen in acetylcholine turnover rate in limbic structures following morphine administration.

In the same study, a decrease in acetylcholine turnover rate was observed in the striatum of C57 mice, as a consequence of the activation of the dopamine turnover rate following morphine administration (Table 4).   This confirms the relationship existing between cholinergic and dopaminergic neurons in this nucleus.

TABLE 2.   Adenylate cyclase activity (pmoles cAMP/mg protein/min) in striatal homogenates of two different strains of mice

Condition	C57	DBA
Basal	232 ± 12	213 ± 3
DA 5 x 10^{-6}	371 ± 8 ⊞	337 ± 14 ⊞
DA 5 x 10^{-5}	434 ± 13 ⊞	408 ± 4 ⊞
M 5 x 10^{-5}	217 ± 5	209 ± 5
DA 5 x 10^{-6} + M 5 x 10^{-5}	348 ± 10 ⊞	325 ± 7 ⊞
DA 5 x 10^{-5} + M 5 x 10^{-5}	422 ± 7 ⊞	399 ± 8 ⊞

Effect of various concentrations of dopamine (DA) and morphine (M) on the accumulation of cAMP.   All values are expressed as the mean $\pm$ SEM of 4 determinations (27).

⊞ $p < 0.05$

TABLE 3. Effect of morphine on 3-methoxy-tyramine content (nmoles/g) in striatum and limbic system of different strains of mice injected with morphine (10 mg/kg i.p.)

Strain	Striatum		Limbic System	
	Saline	Morphine	Saline	Morphine
C57	0.53 ± 0.043	1.28 ± 0.20[+]	0.50 ± 0.033	0.48 ± 0.029
DBA	0.48 ± 0.049	0.28 ± 0.023[+]	0.46 ± 0.040	0.44 ± 0.039

The animals were killed $\frac{1}{2}$ h after morphine injection.
Values are Mean ± SEM of 5 determinations (27)

[+]$p < 0.05$

TABLE 4. Turnover rate of acetylcholine (μmoles/g/h) in striatum and limbic system of different strains of mice injected with morphine (10 mg/kg i.p.)

Strain	Striatum		Limbic System	
	Saline	Morphine	Saline	Morphine
C57	0.75 ± 0.033	0.40 ± 0.024[+]	0.36 ± 0.019	0.29 ± 0.030
DBA	1.0 ± 0.050	1.2 ± 0.048	0.40 ± 0.020	0.28 ± 0.018[+]

The animals were killed $\frac{1}{2}$ h after morphine injection.
Deuterated phosphorylcholine (20 μmoles/kg/min) was infused for 6 min immediately before killing by microwaves (26).
Data are Mean ± SEM of at least six determinations (26)

[+]$p < 0.05$

It was suggested that striatal dopaminergic systems
may be involved in the running fit which follows
morphine administration, since striatal dopaminergic
neurons are activated and the increased motor activity
is antagonized by antidopaminergic drugs in C57 mice.
Future biochemical and behavioral research will
assess whether other neuronal systems are involved
in modulation of the effects of narcotic drugs.
In this regard, a genetic approach in the mouse seems
to be very fruitful.

REFERENCES

1. Buxbaum, D.M., Yarbrough, G.G., and Carter, M.E.
    (1973): J. Pharmacol. Exp. Ther., 185: 317.
2. Castellano, C., Espinet-Llovera, B., and Oliverio,
    A. (1975): Naunyn-Schmiedeberg's Arch. Pharmacol.
    288: 355.
3. Castellano, C., Filibeck, U., and Oliverio, A.
    (1977): Psychopharmacology (in press)
4. Castellano, C., and Oliverio, A. (1976):
    Psychopharmacologia, 41: 197.
5. Cheney, D.L., and Goldstein, A. (1971):
    J. Pharmacol. Exp. Ther., 177: 309.
6. Damjanovich, R.P., and MacInnes, J.W. (1973):
    Life Sci., 13: 55.
7. Domino, E.F., and Wilson, A. (1973): J. Pharmacol.
    Exp. Ther., 184: 18.
8. Ebel, A., Hermetet, J.C., and Mandel, P. (1973):
    Nature N. Biol., 242: 46.
9. Eddy, N.B., and Leimback, D. (1953): J. Pharmacol.
    Exp. Ther., 107: 385.
10. Eriksson, K., and Kiianmaa, K. (1971): Ann. Med.
    Exp. Fen., 49: 73.
11. Giarman, N.J., and Pepeu, G. (1962): Br. J.
    Pharmacol., 19: 226.
12. Goldstein, A., and Sheehan, P. (1969): J. Pharmacol.
    Exp. Ther., , 169: 175.
13. Herz, A., Albus, K., Metys, J., Schubert, P., and
    Teschemaker, H. (1970): Neuropharmacology, 9:
    539.
14. Jhamandas, K., and Dickinson, G. (1973): Nature
    N. Biol., 245: 219.
15. Jhamandas, K., Pinsky, C., and Phillis, J.W. (1970):
    Nature, 238: 176.
16. Kempf, E., Greilsamer, J., Mack, G., and Mandel,
    P. (1974): Nature N. Biol., 247: 483.
17. Kuhar, M.J., Pert, B.C., and Snyder, S.H. (1973):
    Nature, 245: 447.

18. Mack, G., Greilsamer, J., Kempf, L., and Mandel,
    P. (1973): In: Abstr. IV Int. Meeting of the
    International Society of Neurochemistry, Tokyo.
19. Mandel, P., Ebel, A., Hermetet, J.C., Bovet, D.,
    and Oliverio, A. (1973): C.R. Acad. Sci.(Paris):
    276: 395.
20. Nichols, J.R., and Hsiao, S. (1967): Science, 157:
    561.
21. Oliverio, A. (1974): Brain Res., 82: 101.
22. Oliverio, A., and Castellano, C. (1974):
    Psychopharmacologia, 39: 13.
23. Oliverio, A., Castellano, C., and Messeri, P.
    (1972): J. Comp. Physiol. Psychol., 79: 459.
24. Oliverio, A., and Eleftheriou, E., (1977):
    Pharmacol. Behav., in press .
25. Pepeu, G., Mulas, A., Ruffi, A., and Sotgiu, P.
    (1971): Life Sci., 10: 181.
26. Racagni, G., Cheney, D.L., Zsilla, G., and Costa,
    E. (1977): Neuropharmacology, in press .
27. Racagni, G., Oliverio, A., Bruno, F., Maggi, A.,
    and Cattabeni, F. (1977): Brain Res., in press .
28. Rethy, C.R., Smith, C.B., and Villarreal, J.E.
    (1971): J. Pharmacol. Exp. Ther., 176: 472.
29. Rodgers, D.A., and McClearn, G.E. (1962):
    Q. J. Alcohol Stud., 23: 26.
30. Samanin, R., and Valzelli, L. (1972): Arch.
    Int. Pharmacodyn. Ther., 196: 138.
31. Sharkawi, M. (1970): Br. J. Pharmacol., 40: 86.
32. Shuster, L., Hannum, R.V., and Boyle, W.E.
    (1963): J. Pharmacol. Exp. Ther., 140: 149.
33. Srebro, B., Oderfeld-Nowak, B., Klodos, I.,
    Dabrowska, J., and Narkiewicz, O. (1973):
    Life Sci., 12: 261.
34. Trabucchi, M., Spano, P.F., Racagni, G., and
    Oliverio, A. (1977): Brain Res in press .
35. Villarreal, J.E., Guzman, M., and Smith, C.B.
    (1973): J. Pharmacol. Exp. Ther., 187: 1.
36. Way, E.L., Ho, I.K., and Loh, H.H. (1973):
    J. Pharmacol. Exp. Ther., 185: 108.
37. Wei, E., Loh,H.H., and Way, E.L. (1973):
    J. Pharmacol. Exp. Ther., 185: 108.
38. Yarbrough, G.G., Buxbaum, D.M. and Sanders-Bush,
    E. (1973): J. Pharmacol. Exp. Ther., 185: 328.

Factors Affecting the Action of Narcotics, edited by
M.L. Adler, L. Manara, and R. Samanin.
Raven Press, New York©1978.

Isolated Organs and Cultured Cells as Models for the
Study of Narcotic Action

H.W. Kosterlitz and J. Hughes

Unit for Research on Addictive Drugs,
University of Aberdeen
Aberdeen, AB9 1AS, Scotland

INTRODUCTION

The effects of opiates on the central nervous system
are so complex that many attempts have been made to
develop models in which the pharmacological actions of
these drugs can be measured with a sufficient degree of
confidence. Two types of models have been used; the
one depends on the displacement of a labelled ligand,
e.g. $\{^3H\}$-naloxone or$\{^3H\}$-dihydromorphine from the
opiate receptor by unlabelled opiates (see articles by
E.J. Simon and by V. Höllt in this volume). This
review will consider the use of representatives of other
types of models, namely the guinea-pig ileum and the
mouse vas deferens. Finally, the effects of narcotic
analgesics on cultures of neuroblastoma cells will be
discussed.

An examination of the action of opiates on neuronal
junctions outside the central nervous system has shown
that they depress impulse transmission at certain junctions of the autonomic nervous system by reduction in
transmitter release; the localization of these sites
is not specific for either species or organ. The
characteristics of this effect have been discussed by
Lees, Kosterlitz and Waterfield (30).

The earliest observation on the guinea-pig ileum was
made by Trendelenburg (42), who showed that distension
of the lumen of the isolated ileum of the guinea-pig
causes a peristaltic reflex which is inhibited by low
concentration of morphine; this effect of morphine is
absent in the ileum of the rabbit (36).

In the electrically stimulated ileum the depression
of the contraction of the longitudinal muscle is due to
a reduction in acetylcholine release (34); in the rabbit
morphine does not cause such reduction (30). Other
morphine-sensitive cholinergic junctions are those which
mediate slowing of the heart after stimulation of the

vagus nerve in the rat and rabbit but not in the guinea-pig (24).

So far, two morphine-sensitive noradrenergic junctions have been found, namely in the cat nictitating membrane (4,43) and in the vas deferens of the mouse but not the rat, guinea-pig, rabbit or gerbil (12,16). On the other hand, adrenergic junctions in the sino-auricular node of the cat (24) and the myenteric plexus of the guinea-pig ileum are not sensitive to morphine (13).

Finally, a model of quite a different nature will be considered in which cultures of neuroblastoma x glioma hybrid cell lines are used (20,41).

The value of an in vitro model for research into the action of morphine-like compounds depends on its ability to predict the agonist and antagonist potencies of such compounds. In the whole animal or in man the agonist activities are evident as analgesia, depression of respiration, euphoria and other clinical manifestations; analgesia would appear to be the best parameter for comparison with the agonist activities observed in in vitro preparations. Antagonist activities of a drug are measured in the whole animal by the reversal of the acute action of morphine-like compounds or by the induction of withdrawal after chronic administration; both parameters are suitable for comparison with in vitro preparations.

Myenteric Plexus of Guinea-Pig Ileum

This preparation has been used for a number of years for the assay of the agonist and antagonist actions of opiates (25,26,27). Agonist potencies of drugs with mainly agonist or with dual agonist and antagonist action are measured by the depression of the contraction of the longitudinal muscle induced by coaxial electrical stimulation of a segment of ileum or by field stimulation of a preparation of the myenteric plexus with attached longitudinal muscle. The antagonist potencies of drugs with mainly antagonist or with dual actions are estimated by the ability of an antagonist drug to reverse the depression caused by standard concentrations of morphine or normorphine.

Agonist Activities

When the logarithms of the relative potencies for human analgesia are plotted against those of the relative agonist potencies in the guinea-pig ileum, a linear relationship is obtained (Fig. 1). The value for codeine has been omitted for the calculation of the correlation coefficient (r = 0.926) and the regression

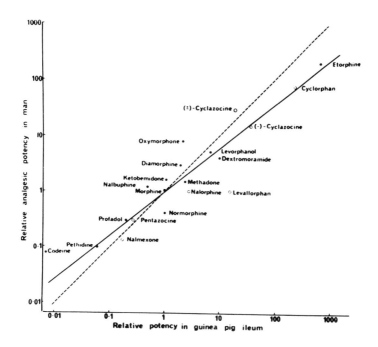

FIG. 1. Correlation between the relative agonist potencies of narcotic analgesics in guinea-pig ileum and
analgesia in man (morphine = 1). The effects in segments of guinea-pig ileum are measured by the depression
of the isometric contraction of the longitudinal muscle
evoked by coaxial stimulation (0.1 Hz, 0.5 msec, supramaximal voltage). The values are plotted on a logarithmic scale. Correlation coefficient without codeine,
r = 0.926 (n = 19). The solid line has been drawn from
log y = 0.79 log x -0.03, the slope being different
from unity (p < 0.02); the interrupted line has a slope
of 1. The slopes for the compounds with (o) and without (•) antagonist activity do not differ, and the
apparent shift of the values of the drugs with antagonist activity is not statistically significant.
Nalmexone is N-dimethylallyl-7,8-dihydro-14-hydroxy-
morphinone and nalbuphine is N-cyclobutylmethyl-7,8-
dihydro-14-hydroxymorphine. Reproduced with permission,
from Kosterlitz and Waterfield (25).

equation, because most of its action in man is probably
due to biotransformation to morphine (1). The slope
of the regression line is significantly smaller than
unity, indicating that without logarithmic transformation,

the relationship between the values for human analgesia and the guinea-pig values is not linear. Nevertheless, the predictive value of the guinea-pig ileum is obviously very high over the whole potency spectrum covering five orders of magnitude. This finding is remarkable because there are many uncertainties in the assessment of analgesia in human patients in whom variations in distribution, metabolism and excretion affect the results.

It is noteworthy that the relative agonist potencies of compounds with dual agonist and antagonist actions correlate well with the analgesic potencies in man although it would appear that the guinea-pig ileum may be particularly sensitive to the agonist activity of this type of drug.

Antagonist Activities

The antagonist potencies of compounds with only negligible agonist component (naloxone, naltrexone, Mr 1256 and GPA 2163) and of compounds with dual agonist and antagonist activities have been compared with their potencies to cause withdrawal symptoms in the morphine-dependent monkey as reported by the Department of Pharmacology of the University of Michigan (Fig. 2). The correlation between the two sets of logarithmic values is very close and the slope of the regression does not differ from unity.

Correlation with Inhibition of {^{3}H}-Naloxone Binding

It has been pointed out (25) that there is good correlation between the potencies of antagonists to reduce stereospecific naloxone binding in rat brain homogenates obtained in the presence of 100 mM Na^{+} (35) and the dissociation equilibrium constants (K_e) which are the reciprocals of the affinity constants and measure the antagonist potencies in the myenteric plexus of the guinea-pig ileum (27) (Fig. 3). A close correlation has also been shown by direct comparison in the guinea-pig ileum of pharmacological action and inhibition of {^{3}H}-naloxone binding (Fig. 4); moreover, there is good agreement between the inhibition of {^{3}H}-naloxone binding in the guinea-pig ileum and in the brain of rat (6) or guinea-pig (Kosterlitz and Leslie, unpublished observations).

Mouse vas Deferens

Agonist activities

This preparation has been developed only recently (16). As far as agonist compounds without significant

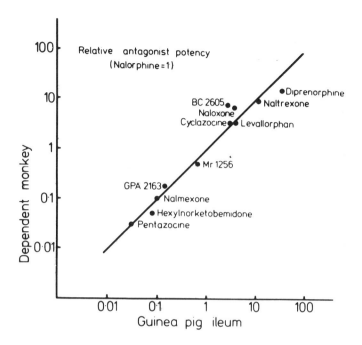

FIG. 2. <u>Correlation between the relative antagonist</u>
<u>potencies of narcotic analgesics in guinea-pig ileum</u>
<u>and morphine-dependent monkey (nalorphine = 1)</u>. The
effects in guinea-pig ileum are measured by their
antagonism of the depressant action of morphine or
normorphine on the contraction of the longitudinal
muscle evoked by coaxial stimulation as in Figure 1.
The values in the monkey are the amounts causing withdrawal (Department of Pharmacology, University of
Michigan). The values are plotted on a logarithmic
scale. Correlation coefficient, r = 0.974 (n = 11).
The line has been drawn from log y = 0.96 log x +0.03.
GPA 2163 is (-)-β-2-propargyl-5-phenyl-9-methyl-2'-
hydroxy-6,7-benzomorphan, Mr 1256 (+)-α-2-(3-furylmethyl)
-5,9-dimethyl-2'-hydroxy-6,7-benzomorphan and BC 2605,
or oxilorphan, (+)-N-cyclopropylmethyl-3,14-dihydroxy-
morphinan. Reproduced, with permission, from Kosterlitz
and Waterfield (25).

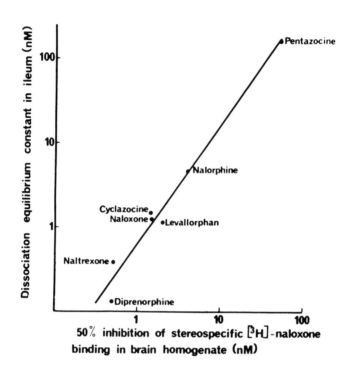

FIG. 3. Correlation between the potencies to reduce
stereospecific naloxone binding in brain homogenates
(35) and the dissociation equilibrium constants measuring antagonist potency in guinea-pig ileum (23,27).
Abscissa, concentration (ED_{50}) required to cause 50%
inhibition in stereospecific binding (x); ordinate,
dissociation equilibrium constant (K_e), i.e. concentration producing a dose-ratio of 2 (y). The values
(nM) are plotted on a logarithmic scale. Correlation
coefficient, r = 0.986 (n = 7). The line has been
drawn from log y = 1.41 log x -0.21. Reproduced, with
permission, from Kosterlitz and Waterfield (25).

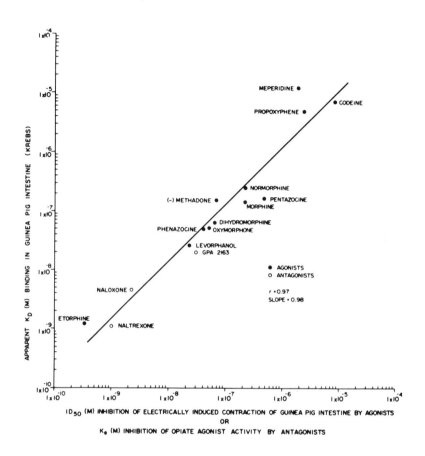

FIG. 4. Correlation between receptor binding and pharmacological activities of opiates in the guinea-pig intestine. The K_D values (determined by the inhibition of stereospecific ^{3}H-naloxone binding in homogenates of the guinea-pig intestine longitudinal muscle and myenteric plexus preparation) for a series of opiate agonists and antagonists are plotted against the ID_{50} concentration, for agonists, required to inhibit the electrically induced contractions of the guinea-pig intestine longitudinal muscle and myenteric plexus preparation by 50%, or the K_e value for antagonist inhibition of agonist activity in the same preparation. Reproduced, with permission, from Creese and Snyder (6).

antagonist properties are concerned, the relative
agonist potencies show a good correlation with the
values obtained in the guinea-pig ileum.

It has already been pointed out that in the guinea-
pig ileum, compounds with dual agonist and antagonist
actions such as, for instance, nalorphine and levallorphan, can be readily assayed for their agonist actions.
Provided the interval between the exposures to the
different concentrations is long enough, possibly 1 hr
or more, dose-response curves having slopes similar to
that of morphine are obtained (11). In the mouse vas
deferens, however, the dose-response curves for nalorphine and levallorphan are parallel to the abscissa
even when the interval between exposures to the drug is
lengthened (Fig. 5). For this reason, agonist potencies
obtained from the lowest concentration to give a depression of the response to electrical stimulation are
related to the normorphine concentration which produces
an identical depression. When this is done, there is a
close correlation between the relative agonist potencies
in the mouse vas deferens and those in the guinea-pig
ileum (Fig. 6).

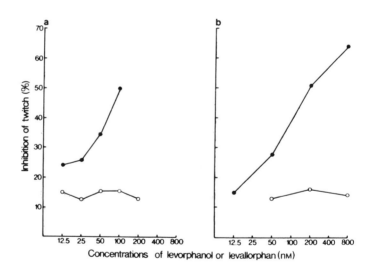

FIG. 5. Dose-response curves for the inhibition of the
evoked longitudinal contraction of the mouse vas
deferens. Abscissae, concentration of levorphanol (●)
or levallorphan (o); ordinates, inhibition of contraction (%). Dose-cycle 7 min in (a) and 40 min in (b).
Reproduced, with permission, from Hughes et al. (16).

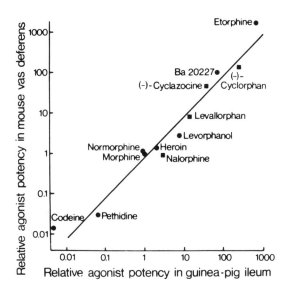

FIG. 6. Correlation between the relative potencies of
narcotic analgesics in the guinea-pig ileum and the
mouse vas deferens. Abscissae, relative agonist potency
in guinea-pig ileum (morphine = 1); ordinates, relative
agonist potency in mouse vas deferens (morphine = 1).
(●), Drugs with no significant antagonist action, (■)
drugs with dual agonist and antagonist actions. The
values are plotted on a logarithmic scale. Correlation
coefficient r = 0.979 (n = 12). The line has been
drawn from y = 1.02 x -0.07. Reproduced, with permission, from Hughes et al. (16).

Antagonist Activities.

The lack of an increase in the depressant response
to increasing concentrations of drugs with dual agonist
and antagonist actions makes the mouse vas deferens
particularly suitable for the estimation of the antagonist potency of such compounds. For instance, in the
guinea-pig ileum, cyclorphan is an agonist of such high
potency that the contraction is completely suppressed
before its antagonist activity becomes apparent. In
the mouse vas deferens, on the other hand, the antagonist activity of cyclorphan can be readily demonstrated
to give a K_e of 1.6 nM compared with a K_e of 3.7 nM for
naloxone (16). Closely related to this phenomenon is
the observation that with a mixture of normorphine and
nalorphine the agonist activities of the two drugs are

additive in the guinea-pig ileum while in the mouse vas
deferens the antagonist action of nalorphine reduces
the agonist activity of normorphine (Fig. 7). In order
to show the antagonist activity of nalorphine in the
guinea-pig ileum, the preparation has to be exposed to
nalorphine for several minutes before the addition of
morphine to the bath (11).

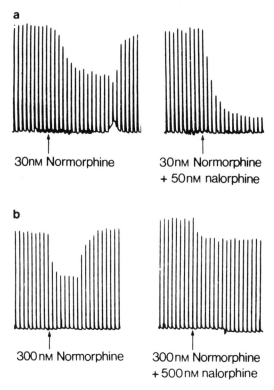

a

30nM Normorphine   30nM Normorphine
                            + 50nM nalorphine

b

300nM Normorphine   300nM Normorphine
                            +500nM nalorphine

FIG. 7. Comparison of the effects of mixtures of normorphine and nalorphine in (a) a segment of guinea-pig
ileum and (b) in the mouse vas deferens. Stimulation
was supramaximal at 0.1 Hz. The contractions of the
ileum were recorded isometrically and those of the vas
deferens isotonically. Reproduced, with permission,
from Hughes et al. (16).

Differences in Responses of Guinea-Pig Ileum and
Mouse vas Deferens

The findings obtained on the two in vitro models
suggest that their receptor populations are not identical. This view is supported by observations on a number

of benzomorphans which have been shown to be potent
analgesics without suppressing the abstinence syndrome
of morphine-dependent monkeys (2,32). It was of great
interest to find (18) that the agonist potencies of
these compounds are four times higher in the guinea-
pig ileum than in the mouse vas deferens (Table 1).
Moreover, in both in vitro models the benzomorphans,
which do not suppress the withdrawal syndrome in the
morphine-dependent monkey, require 3 to 7 times more
naloxone for antagonism of their agonist activity than
normorphine or the benzomorphans which substitute for
morphine in the dependent monkey (18).

The agonist potencies of the endogenous opioid pentapeptides, methionine-enkephalin and leucine-enkephalin,
differ greatly in the two preparations (17). In the
mouse vas deferens, methionine-enkephalin is 20 to 30
times more potent than normorphine while in the guinea-
pig ileum these two compounds are about equiactive.
This discrepancy is shown even more clearly when the
potency to inhibit $\{^3H\}$-leucine-enkephalin binding in
the guinea-pig brain is also measured (Table 2) (31).
While in the guinea-pig ileum, β-endorphin (β-lipotropin
61-91 or C fragment), methionine-enkephalin and morphine
have similar potencies, in the mouse vas deferens the
order of their potencies is methionine-enkephalin, β-
endorphin and, much weaker, morphine. For the inhibition of $\{^3H\}$-leucine-enkephalin binding the order is
β-endorphin, methionine-enkephalin and, again much
weaker, morphine. Of the compounds in Table 2 leucine-
enkephalin is the most potent agonist in the mouse vas
deferens but the weakest in the guinea-pig ileum; it
is a powerful inhibitor of $\{^3H\}$-leucine enkephalin
binding. Naloxone is very potent in both guinea-pig
ileum and mouse vas deferens when its antagonist action
is measured against morphine or normorphine but it is a
relatively weak inhibitor of $\{^3H\}$- leucine-enkephalin
binding.

Thus the evidence available at present would appear
to indicate that the receptor populations in the guinea
pig ileum, mouse vas deferens and brain homogenates are
similar but not identical. In this connection it is
important to recall that, as far as morphine, its
derivatives and its synthetic surrogates are concerned,
there is good correlation between the values found for
human analgesia and those obtained in the guinea-pig
ileum, the mouse vas deferens and the binding tests.
The discrepancies found recently indicate that the new
classes of compounds, namely, first, the benzomorphans
which do not substitute for morphine in the dependent
monkey and, secondly, the endogenous opioid peptides,
differ from the classical opiates in that they interact

TABLE 1. Relative agonist potencies of benzomorphans[a]

Compound	Suppression of withdrawal syndrome of morphine-dependent monkey[b]	Relative mean agonist potency (±S.E.) (normorphine = 1)			Mouse vas deferens/ Guinea-pig ileum
		Guinea-pig ileum	Mouse vas deferens		
Normorphine	yes	1	1		1
Phenazocine[c]	yes	13.3 ± 1.1 (4)	19.0 ± 3.6 (3)		1.4
NIH 8152[d]	yes	2.60± 0.29(4)	4.17± 0.52(4)		1.6
Ethylketocyclazocine[e]	no	397 ±43 (7)	99 ±11 (7)		0.25
Mr 1268[f]	no	1.49±0.15 (6)	0.34± 0.03(6)		0.23
Mr 1353[g]	no	5.55±0.50 (6)	1.54± 0.10(6)		0.28

[a]Modified from Hutchinson, et al. (18)

[b]Data obtained from Eddy and May (8); Deneau et al. (7) and Villarreal and Seevers (44)

[c](-)-α-5,9-dimethyl-2-phenethyl-2'-hydroxy-6,7-benzomorphan

[d](±)-β-2,9-dimethyl-5-n-propyl-2'-hydroxy-6,7-benzomorphan

[e](-)-α-5-ethyl-9-methyl-8-oxo-2-cyclopropylmethyl-2'-hydroxy-6,7-benzomorphan

[f](±)-α-5,9-dimethyl-2-(2-methyl-3-methylfuryl)-2'-hydroxy-6,7-benzomorphan

[g](±)-α-5,9-dimethyl-2-(3-methylfurfuryl)-2'-hydroxy-6,7-benzomorphan

TABLE 2. Potencies in three assays[a]

Compound	Agonist (mean ID$_{50}$±S.E.) or antagonist (mean Ke±S.E.) action (nM)		Inhibition (mean ID$_{50}$±S.E.) of {[^{3}H]-leucine-enkephalin binding in homogenate of guinea-pig brain
	Guinea-pig ileum	Mouse vas deferens	
β-Endorphin[b]	75 ± 6 (4)	53 ± 4 (4)	1.51 ± 0.19 (3)
Methionine^5-enkephalin[c]	96 ± 9 (31)	12.8± 1.2 (6)	2.07 ± 0.31 (10)
Leucine^5-enkephalin	463 ±59 (10)	7.8± 0.8 (9)	3.78 ± 0.72 (10)
Morphine	68 ±15 (6)	492 ±53 (7)	705 ± 239 (4)
Naloxone	1.89± 0.15 (12)	3.10±0.25 (6)	51 ± 11 (5)

[a]Modified from Lord et al. (31)

[b]β-lipotropin$_{61-91}$; results in the guinea-pig ileum and mouse vas deferens were obtained on the natural compound (Dr. D.G. Smyth) and the inhibition of binding on the synthetic compound (Dr. C.H. Li). The synthetic peptide gave 88 and 57 nM in the guinea-pig ileum and 67 and 69 nM in the mouse vas deferens.

[c]β-lipotropin$_{61-65}$

with groups of receptors which, while belonging to the
general class of opiate receptors, exhibit differences
in detail.

Some Applications of the in vitro Models

Use has been made of the two in vitro preparations
in a study of structure-activity relationships (25),
where problems of absorption, biotransformation and
excretion have been reduced, if not eliminated. Another
example is the effect which the degree of lipid solubility has on the potency and onset and duration of
action of a narcotic analgesic. If a drug is administered intravenously, potency, rate of onset and rate of
offset of action are facilitated by high lipid solubility (14). This relationship is very different in
isolated preparations (22). Lipid solubility has no
or only little effect on the potency and, in contrast
to the findings in the whole animal, a hydrophilic
compound, such as normorphine, has a much faster rate
of onset and offset of action than a more lipophilic
compound, such as etorphine or methadone. Since the
resultant effects of lipid solubility in vitro and
in vivo are in an opposite direction, an optimum may be
expected if a drug has a degree of lipid solubility
which ensures rapid penetration into the central nervous
system without seriously slowing down the rate of
receptor association and dissociation.
When guinea-pigs are made tolerant to morphine by
implantation of morphine pellets, the myenteric plexus-
longitudinal muscle preparation is also tolerant (9,37).
In preparations of the guinea-pig ileum and mouse vas
deferens obtained from animals made tolerant by pellet
implantation it can be shown that the two in vitro
models have become tolerant not only to morphine but
also to methionine-enkephalin; in other words, cross
tolerance has developed between morphine and enkephalin
(45).
Both the mouse vas deferens (15) and the guinea-pig
ileum (5,10,29) have been used as monitoring assays
during the isolation and purification of the endogenous
opioid peptides.

Neuroblastoma x Glioma Hybrid Cells

It has been shown that some cultured neuroblastoma
cell lines or neuroblastoma x glioma hybrid cell lines
possess opiate receptors as evidenced by inhibition of
PGE_1-stimulated cyclic AMP formation (41) or by stereospecific $\{^3H\}$-dihydro-morphine binding (20). The
inhibition of $\{^3H\}$-naloxone binding and the inhibition

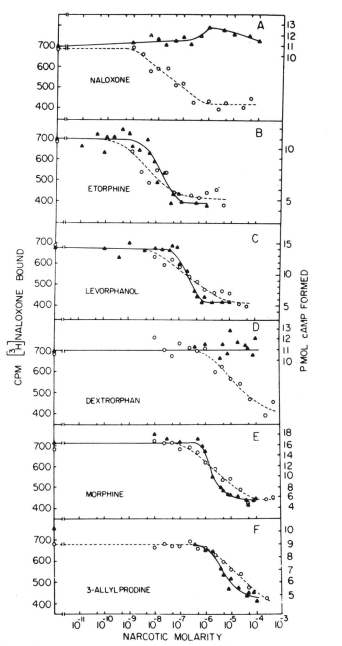

FIG. 8. The effectiveness of various narcotics as inhibitors of adenylate cyclase activity of NG108-15 homogenates is compared with their ability to displace {³H}-naloxone from the opiate receptor. Symbols represent the following: O, {³H}-naloxone bound to receptor; ▲, {³²p}-cAMP formed per 5 min per tube (250 µg of protein per tube). Reproduced, with permission, from Sharma et al. (39).

of adenyl cyclase activity have been used for the
assessment of the activity of opiates (39). While the
antagonist naloxone has a high affinity to the opiate
receptors of the neuroblastoma x glioma hybrid NG108-
15 (Fig. 8) it does not inhibit adenyl cyclase activity.
The values for half-maximal inhibition of {^{3}H}-naloxone
binding and enzyme activity agree well for the agonists
etorphine, morphine, 3-allylprodine and levorphanol
although the curves are not superimposable because the
effects of the drugs on adenyl cyclase activity, but
not on receptor binding, are cooperative processes.
The (+)-isomer dextrorphan is a much weaker inhibitor
of {^{3}H}-naloxone binding than the (-)-isomer levorphanol and has no effect on adenyl cyclase activity.
    An investigation of the phenomena of tolerance and
dependence on these hybrid cells has led to the hypothesis that a secondary and delayed increase in enzyme
activity during prolonged exposure to morphine counter-
acts the primary inhibition by morphine of enzyme
activity and is responsible for tolerance and dependence
(38).
    These morphine-sensitive cell lines have been used
for an analysis of the mode of action of the endogenous
opioid peptides. Methionine-enkephalin and leucine-
enkephalin show a primary inhibition and a delayed
secondary increase in adenyl cyclase activity after
prolonged exposure to the peptides, a sequence of events
similar to that found for morphine (3,19,21,28). These
findings strongly indicate that after prolonged exposure
of methionine-enkephalin and leucine-enkephalin tolerance and dependence is observed in neuroblastoma x
glioma hybrid cells as has been shown to occur in the
guinea-pig ileum and mouse vas deferens obtained from
morphine-dependent animals (45).

Brain Slices as in vitro Models

    It has recently been shown in slices of rat neo-
striatum that opiates, methionine-enkephalin and leucine-
enkephalin increase the concentration of cyclic GMP
(33). In slices of rat occipital cortex, preincubated
with {^{3}H}-noradrenaline, methionine-enkephalin decreases
the outflow of radioactive material evoked by electrical
field stimulation or by 20 mM K^+ (40).

ACKNOWLEDGEMENTS

    The Unit for Research on Addictive Drugs is support-
ed by grants from the U.S. National Institute on Drug
Abuse (DA-00662), the U.K. Medical Research Council and
the U.S. Committee on Problems of Drug Dependence.

REFERENCES

1. Adler, T.K. (1963): J. Pharmacol. Exp. Ther., 140: 155
2. Albertson, N.F. (1974): In: Narcotic Antagonists. Advances in Biochemical Psychopharmacology, vol.8, edited by M.C. Braude, L.S. Harris, E.L. May, J.P. Smith and J.E. Villarreal, p. 63. Raven Press, New York.
3. Brandt, M., Fischer, K., Moroder, L., Wünsch, E., and Hamprecht, B. (1976): FEBS Lett., 68: 38
4. Cairnie, A.B., Kosterlitz, H.W., and Taylor, D.W. (1961): Br.J.Pharmacol.Chemother., 17: 539
5. Cox, B.M., Goldstein, A., and Li, C.H. (1976): Proc. Natl.Acad.Sci., U.S.A., 73: 1821
6. Creese, I., and Snyder, S.H. (1975): J. Pharmacol. Exp.Ther., 194: 205
7. Deneau, G.A., Villarreal, J.E., and Seevers, M.H. (1966): Bulletin of the Committee on Problems of Drug Dependence, 28: Addendum 2, p.1.
8. Eddy, N.B., and May, E.L. (1966): In: Synthetic Analgesics. International Series of Monographs in Organic Chemistry, Vol. 8, edited by D.H.R. Barton, and W. von Doering, p. 113, Pergamon Press, Oxford.
9. Goldstein, A., and Schulz, R. (1973): Br. J. Pharmacol., 48: 655
10. Graf, L., Ronai, A.Z., Bajusz, S., Cseh, G., and Szekely, J.I. (1976): FEBS Lett., 64: 181
11. Gyang, E.A., and Kosterlitz, H.W. (1966): Br. J. Pharmacol. Chemother., 27: 514
12. Henderson, G., Hughes, J., and Kosterlitz, H.W. (1972): Br.J.Pharmacol., 46: 764
13. Henderson, G., Hughes, J., and Kosterlitz, H.W. (1975): Br.J.Pharmacol., 53: 505
14. Herz, A., and Teschemacher, H.-J. (1971): Adv. Drug Res., 6: 79
15. Hughes, J. (1975): Brain Res., 88: 295
16. Hughes, J., Kosterlitz, H.W., and Leslie, F.M. (1975): Br. J. Pharmacol., 53: 371
17. Hughes, J., Smith, T.W., Kosterlitz, H.W., Fothergill L.A., Morgan, B.A., and Morris, H.R. (1975): Nature, 258: 577
18. Hutchinson, M., Kosterlitz, H.W., Leslie, F.M., Waterfield, A.A. and Terenius, L. (1975): Br. J. Pharmacol., 55: 541
19. Klee, W.A., Lampert, A., and Nirenberg, M. (1976): In: Opiates and Endogenous Opioid Peptides, edited by H.W. Kosterlitz, p. 153. North-Holland Publishing Co., Amsterdam.
20. Klee, W.A., and Nirenberg, M. (1974): Proc. Nat. Acad. Sci., U.S.A., 71: 3474

21. Klee, W.A., and Nirenberg, M. (1976): Nature, 263: 609
22. Kosterlitz, H.W., Leslie, F.M. and Waterfield, A.A. (1975): Eur. J. Pharmacol., 32: 10
23. Kosterlitz, H.W., Lord, J.A.H., and Watt, A.J.(1972): In: Agonist and Antagonist Actions of Narcotic Analgesic Drugs, edited by H.W. Kosterlitz, H.O.J. Collier, and J.E. Villarreal, p. 45. Macmillan Press, London.
24. Kosterlitz, H.W., and Taylor, D.W. (1959): Br. J. Pharmacol. Chemother., 14: 209
25. Kosterlitz, H.W., and Waterfield, A.A. (1975): Ann. Rev. Pharmacol., 15: 29
26. Kosterlitz, H.W., Waterfield, A.A., and Berthoud, V. (1974): In: Narcotic Antagonists. Advances in Biochemical Psychopharmacology, vol. 8, edited by M.C. Braude, L.S. Harris, E.L. May, J.P. Smith and E.J. Villarreal, p. 319. Raven Press, New York.
27. Kosterlitz, H.W., and Watt, A.J. (1968): Br. J. Pharmacol. Chemother., 33: 266
28. Lampert, A., Nirenberg, M., and Klee, W.A. (1976): Proc. Natl. Acad. Sci., U.S.A., 73: 3165
29. Lazarus, L.H., Ling, N. and Guillemin, R. (1976): Proc. Natl. Acad. Sci., U.S.A., 73: 2156
30. Lees, G.M., Kosterlitz, H.W., and Waterfield, A.A. (1972): In: Agonist and Antagonist Actions of Narcotic Analgesic Drugs, edited by H.W. Kosterlitz, H.O.J. Collier and J.E. Villarreal, p. 142. Macmillan Press, London.
31. Lord, J.A.H., Waterfield, A.A., Hughes, J., and Kosterlitz, H.W. (1976): In: Opiates and Endogenous Opioid Peptides, edited by H.W. Kosterlitz, p.275. North-Holland Publishing Co., Amsterdam
32. Merz, H., Langbein, A., Stockhaus, K., Walther, G., and Wick, H. (1974): In: Narcotic Antagonists. Advanced in Biochemical Psychopharmacology, vol.8, edited by M.C. Braude, L.S. Harris, E.L. May, J. P. Smith, and J.E. Villarreal, p. 91. Raven Press, New York
33. Minneman, K.P., and Iversen, L.L. (1976): In: Opiates and Endogenous Opioid Peptides, edited by H.W. Kosterlitz, p. 137. North-Holland Publishing Co., Amsterdam.
34. Paton, W.D.M. (1957): Br. J. Pharmacol. Chemother., 12: 119
35. Pert, C.B., Pasternak, G., and Snyder, S.H. (1973): Science, 182: 1359
36. Schaumann, W. (1955): Br. J. Pharmacol. Chemother., 10: 456
37. Schulz, R., Cartwright, C., and Goldstein, A. (1974): Nature, 251: 329

38. Sharma, S.K., Klee, W.A., and Nirenberg, M. (1975):
    Proc.Natl.Acad.Sci., U.S.A., 72: 3092
39. Sharma, S.K., Nirenberg, M., and Klee, W.A. (1975):
    Proc. Natl.Acad.Sci., U.S.A., 72: 590
40. Taube, H.D., Borowski, E., Endo, T., and Starke,
    K. (1976): Eur. J. Pharmacol., 38: 377
41. Traber, J., Fischer, K., Latzin, S., and Hamprecht,
    B. (1974): FEBS Lett., 49: 260
42. Trendelenburg, P. (1917): Naunyn-Schmiedebergs
    Arch. Exp. Pathol. Pharmakol., 81: 55
43. Trendelenburg, U. (1957): Br. J. Pharmacol.
    Chemother., 12: 79
44. Villarreal, J.E., and Seevers, M.H. (1972): Bulletin
    of the Committee on Problems of Drug Dependence,
    34: Addendum 7, p. 1040.
45. Waterfield, A.A., Hughes, J., and Kosterlitz, H.W.
    (1975): Nature, 260: 624

Factors Affecting the Action of Narcotics, edited by
M.L. Adler, L. Manara, and R. Samanin.
Raven Press, New York © 1978.

Neurological Models for the Study of Narcotics :
Bradykinin-Induced Nociceptive Responses and Site
of Anti-Nociceptive Action of Morphine

H. Takagi and M. Satoh

Department of Pharmacology, Faculty of Pharmaceutical
Sciences, Kyoto University, Kyoto 606, Japan.

INTRODUCTION

The site and the mode of action of narcotics in
animals have been studied using various neurological
models as follows :
1) the spinal nociceptive reflex of the hind-limb,
   induced by mechanical somatic stimulation (52);
2) the ventral root reflex discharge, evoked by
   electrical stimulation of the peripheral nerves
   (26,46),
3) the licking reaction, elicited by electrical stimulation of the tooth pulp (20),
4) EEG-arousal responses induced by peripheral
   noxious stimulation (14,27),
5) the evoked potentials recorded from the pain afferent pathways following peripheral nerve stimulation (14,17,40),
6) the spontaneous and evoked unit activities recorded
   from the spinal dorsal horn following peripheral
   noxious stimulation (24,28,39,45,47).
In some of these studies it is not certain that the
stimulation applied, a single peripheral nerve stimulation, causes a painful sensation. However, bradykinin
is considered to be a potent pain producing substance,
since it induces pain in man (2,6,30), and nociceptive
response in animals (19).   Thus, it appears reasonable
to adopt bradykinin as an adequate stimulus of sensory
nerve endings when attempting to measure anti-nociceptive action of analgesics in animals. The usefulness of
bradykinin-induced nociceptive   reaction for measuring

of anti-nociceptive action of analgesics has already
been demonstrated by some researchers. Routes of
injection of bradykinin into animals include :
   1) intradermally into guinea pigs (10); 2) intraperitoneally into mice(15); 3) intra-arterially into
dogs(29)rats(1,5,11),rabbits(39,45,47) and cats(3).
   These studies are summarized in Table 1. The .intra-
arterial route of administration of bradykinin appears
to be most suitable for the study of narcotics, since
the bradykinin-induced response following intra-arterial injection is clearly evident in the majority of
individual animals used and the nociceptive response is
easily reproduced even after repeated application.
   Three neurological models for the study of narcotics
are presented in the following sections I, II and III.

I. BRADYKININ-INDUCED FLEXOR REFLEX OF THE RAT FORE-LIMB

   The application in rats of bradykinin-induced
nociception was first described by Deffenu et al.(11).
Small doses of bradykinin injected in a retrograde
manner into the right carotid artery of conscious rats
by way of a previously implanted catheter resulted in
a syndrome consisting of dextrorotation of the head,
flexion of the right fore-limb and occasionally
squeaking. These workers reported that subcutaneous
ED$_{50}$ of methadone bitartrate and codeine phosphate was
1.45 mg/kg and 32.0 mg/kg, respectively. Their
techniques were confirmed by Blane (5) and Abe et al.
(1) and were extended for application in evaluation of
the analgesic potency of morphine antagonists, such as
nalorphine and pentazocine.

Methods

   The technique we used (1) differed in minor detail
only from that described by Deffenu et al. (11) and
Blane (5). Male Wistar rats (230-300 g) were lightly
anesthetized with ether and a poly-ethylene cannula
(internal diameter of 0.5 mm) was inserted in a
retrograde manner into the right carotid artery and
secured there. A trochar was used to deliver the free
end through the skin of the dorsal surface in the

TABLE 1. Bradykinin-induced nociceptive responses

References	Route of Administration	Dose µg	Animal	Response
(10)	Intradermal	0.5	Guinea-Pig	Biting,scratching the injection site,"wet dog" response
(15)	Intraperitoneal	20	Mouse	Writhing
(29)	Intra-arterial: splenic artery	crude	Dog	Vocalization
(5,11)	Intra-arterial: carotid artery	0.125- 0.5	Rat	Flexion of fore-limb dextro-rotation of head
(1)	Intra-arterial: carotid artery	0.4 - 0.6	Rat	Flexion of fore-limb dextro-rotation of head movement of whole body
(13)	Intra-arterial: femoral artery	5.0 - 10	Rabbit	Flexor reflex of hind-limb
(39,45,47) 45,47	Intra-arterial: femoral artery	1.0 - 2.0	Rabbit	Increased activities of lamina V cells of spinal dorsal horn
(3)	Intra-arterial: popliteal artery	5.0	Cat	Increased activities of lamina V cells of spinal dorsal horn

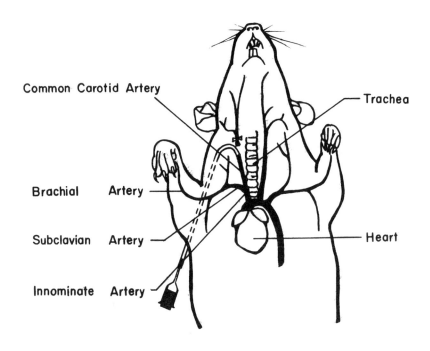

FIG. 1. Schematic illustration of the method

scapular region (Fig. 1). The skin wound in the neck
was closed by ligation. Experiments were begun 3 hr
after termination of the ether anesthesia. Synthetic
bradykinin (Protein Research Foundation, Mino, Osaka)
was dissolved in 0.9% saline and injected in a volume
of 0.2 ml through the cannula, and this cannula was
flushed with 0.2 ml of the vehicle immediately after
each bradykinin injection.

The minimum dose of bradykinin required to consistently produce three types of responses, flexion of the
right fore-limb, dextrorotation of the head and
movement of whole body (rotation, rearing, walking
etc.) was determined for each rat (Fig. 2). This dose
was commonly 0.4-0.6 µg/rat and animals not responding
to a dose of 0.6 µg were discarded. The responses
appeared within 5 sec and persisted for about 10 sec.

CONTROL

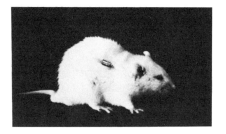

BRADYKININ—INDUCED RESPONSE

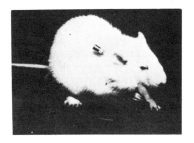
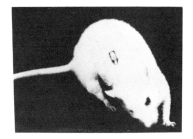

FLEXION OF THE
RIGHT FORELIMB

DEXTRO ROTATION
OF THE HEAD

FIG. 2. Behavioral changes after retrograde injection
of bradykinin into the right carotid artery.

Tachyphylaxis was not observed after repeated injection
of bradykinin at intervals of 15 min.

Disappearance of at least two out of the three types
of responses induced by bradykinin was taken as a
criterion for scoring an analgesic effect. With all
drugs, the ED_{50} values at the time of peak effect and
their 95% confidence limits were estimated using the
method of Litchfield and Wilcoxon (31).

Results and Discussion

ED_{50} values of some analgesics determined by the
bradykinin-test in rats are shown in Table 2. The
subcutaneous ED_{50} value for morphine was 2.5 (1.5-3.9)

TABLE 2. Analgesic Effect of Various Drugs Using
Bradykinin Test in the Rat

DRUGS	ED_{50} mg/kg (95% C.L.)	
Morphine	2.5 (1.5 - 3.9)	s.c.
Codeine	18.8 (12.8-27.6)	s.c.
Nalorphine	3.9 (1.6 - 9.4)	s.c.
Levallorphan	>100	s.c.
Pentazocine	7.6 (3.0 -19.0)	s.c.
RAM-301	no effect [a]	i.p.
RAM-302	no effect [a]	i.p.
Aminopyrine	58.0 (43.6-77.1)	i.p.
Aspirin	180.0 (62.1-522)	i.p.
Indomethacin	34.0 (14.7-78.2)	oral
Chlorpromazine	no effect [b]	i.p.
Levomepromazine	no effect [b]	i.p.

C.L. Confidence Limits
RAM-301 : N-allyl-14-hydroxydihydro-normorphine HCl
RAM-302 : N-propargyl-14-hydroxydihydro-normorphine
          HCl
[a]: up to 200 mg/kg   [b] : up to 10 mg/kg

mg/kg, this value being larger than that (1.1 mg/kg)
obtained by Blane (5). The discrepancy in these
results is attributed to different sensitivities to
morphine between the strains of animals used: Blane
used Sprague-Dawley rats while our experiments were
done on Wistar rats.

The bradykinin-induced response is not depressed
by larger doses of chlorpromazine or levomepromazine
(1,5).

The pharmacological characteristics of this
experimental system are as follows :

1) sensitivity to narcotic analgesics is high,
2) sensitivity to agonist-antagonist analgesics is good,
3) evaluation of non-narcotic analgesics is feasible,
4) the reflex is not influenced by subcutaneous administration of reserpine (2.5-5 mg/kg), atropine (4-30 mg/kg), hexamethonium (50 mg/kg), pronethalol (2.5-5 mg/kg),phenoxybenzamine (20-40 mg/kg),procaine (10-20 mg/kg), mephenesin (100 mg/kg) and diphenylhydantoin (200 mg/kg), none of which is analgesic (1),
5) pentobarbital depresses this reflex in an anesthetic dose, but not in a sedative dose(1).

The following points, however, appear to be drawbacks of this system :

1) assessment of the suppressive effect of drugs on bradykinin-induced response tends to be rather subjective, particularly in case of partial suppression,
2) damage of right side of the brain due to ligation of the right carotid artery may induce changes in sensitivity to analgesics,
3) analgesic effects are assessed on the basis of changes in motor "response" and the effects on motor "performance" are apt to be considered in some cases.

II. BRADYKININ-INDUCED FLEXOR REFLEX OF RABBIT HIND-LIMB

In an attempt to eliminate the disadvantages of the bradykinin-induced flexor reflex of rat fore-limb, we recorded on smoked paper the bradykinin-induced flexor reflex of the hind-limb and the recorded reflexes were used as a measure of the nociceptive reaction (13).

Methods

Albino rabbits of both sexes weighing 2.7-3.5 kg were anesthetized with ether and a polyethylene cannula cannula (0.9 mm in diameter) was inserted in a retrograde manner into the deep femoral artery on either side for the purposes of injecting bradykinin. In

some experiments, the spinal cord section was performed at the L_2 level. The experiments were started at
least 2 hr after the termination of the ether
anesthesia. Five or ten micrograms of bradykinin dissolved in 0.1 ml saline was injected through the cannula within 1 sec at intervals of 15 min. All drugs
were administered intravenously.

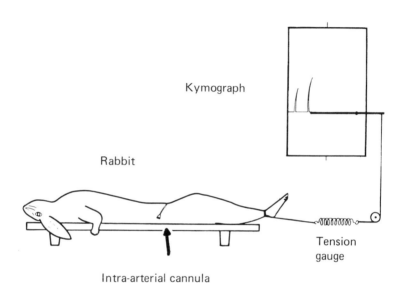

FIG. 3. Schematic illustration of the method

As illustrated in Fig.3, the rabbit was fixed in a
supine position and the hind-limb ipsilateral to the
cannulated side was linked to a kymographion through
a tension gauge (available range of 2-4 kg) buffing
slight movements of the hind-limb. In such a position
the rabbit was usually at rest and the hind-limbs were
maintained in a spontaneously extending but not flex-
ing position. When 5-10 µg of bradykinin was repeatedly injected into the femoral artery at intervals of
15 min, a flexor reflex of the ipsilateral hind-limb
was invariably elicited in each trial and recorded on

a smoked paper of the kymographion (Fig.4), whereas
other pseudo-affective reactions such as vocalization,
hyperpnea and a struggle of the upper body were not
consistently exhibited. The latencies of the ipsilateral hind-limb flexor reflex were 4-15 sec, corresponding to a fair degree with those of bradykinin
induced excitation of the lumbar dorsal horn lamina V
cells (see later section).

    Since the magnitudes of the flexor reflexes after
each bradykinin injection varied in the same rabbit,at
least four control trials were performed before the
administration of drugs. The effect of test drugs on
the flexor reflex was regarded as being inhibitory
when the magnitudes of the flexor reflexes following
at least two successive bradykinin injections were
less than 50% of the smallest control magnitude and
recovered to the control level.

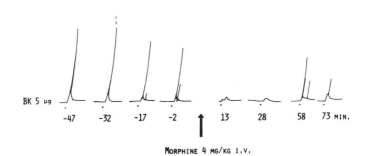

FIG. 4. Bradykinin-induced flexor reflex of the hind-
limb and inhibitory effect of morphine (4 mg/kg i.v.).

Results and Discussion

Morphine depressed the bradykinin-induced flexor
reflex in intact rabbits, in a dose-dependent manner.
A typical effect of morphine (4 mg/kg) is illustrated
in Fig.4. A depression of the bradykinin-induced
reflex was observed in 7 out of 9 rabbits within 13
min after morphine (4 mg/kg) and lasted for about 50
min. This depression was antagonized by a single
administration of nalorphine (0.5 mg/kg i.v.). Estimated intravenous ED50 value of morphine was 2.75 mg/kg.

Pentazocine (5 mg/kg) depressed the bradykinin-
induced response in 4 out of 6 cases. Indomethacin
(0.5 and 1.0 mg/kg), aspirin (10 and 20 mg/kg) and
aminopyrine (10 and 30 mg/kg) depressed in intact rabbits the bradykinin-induced response in a dose-dependent manner. The inhibitory effect of these drugs occurred within 30 min after administration and lasted
for 90-120 min.

The bradykinin-induced response was not depressed by
administration of diazepam or chlorpromazine in a dose
of 2 mg/kg, which caused a marked muscle relaxation
such as head drop.

In spinal rabbits, the magnitude of the bradykinin-
induced reflex was considerably smaller than that in
intact rabbits, indicating involvement of supraspinal
structures in the bradykinin-induced flexor reflex.In
all 4 animals, morphine in a dose of 6 mg/kg failed to
depress the bradykinin-induced reflex, suggesting that
morphine, in small doses, inhibits the bradykinin-
induced flexor reflex through its action on the supraspinal structure.

Pharmacological characteristics of this system are
as follows :
1) effect of drugs on bradykinin-induced response can
   be determined objectively,
2) function of the brain and spinal cord is not
   altered,
3) sensitivity to narcotic analgesics is high,
4) sensitivity to agonist-antagonist analgesics is
   also high,
5) evaluation of analgesic effect of non-narcotic
   analgesics is feasible,
6) the bradykinin-induced reflex is not modified by

either diazepam or chlorpromazine given in a muscle
relaxant dose .
The following points, however, appear to be drawbacks
of this system :
1) analgesic effects are assessed on the basis of
   changes in motor "response" and the effects on motor
   "performance" are apt to be considered in some
   cases,
2) the rather unnatural posture of the rabbit may have
   an influence on the response.

III. BRADYKININ-INDUCED ACTIVATION OF LAMINA V CELLS
        OF THE RABBIT SPINAL DORSAL HORN

   Satoh et al. (39) demonstrated that an intravenous
injection of bradykinin (1 or 2 μg) induced a marked
increase in the firing rates of the rabbit spinal
dorsal horn neurons which responded to noxious stimulation such as a squeeze of the skin. Similar results
concerning the bradykinin-induced responses of lamina V
cells of the spinal dorsal horn were also demonstrated
in cats (3).
   Rexed (37) divided the dorsal horn of the spinal
cord into 6 layers according to neuronal size, distribution and orientation. Among these 6 layers, it is
considered that lamina V cells play an important role
in transmission and integration of pain at the spinal
cord, since these cells respond to small myelinated
afferents activated by electrical stimulation of the
peripheral nerves or by mechanical stimulation of their
receptive fields (41,42,50,51) or by intra-arterial
injection of bradykinin (3,39,45,47).
   Satoh et al. (39) and Takagi et al.(47) found that
morphine, in small doses, inhibits the bradykinin-
induced activation of lamina V type cells of the spinal
dorsal horn. Moreover, Takagi et al.(47) reported that
a more marked inhibition of the bradykinin-induced
activities of lamina V type cells than of the spontaneous activity was seen after morphine administration.

Methods

   Male albino rabbits, weighing 2.5-3.0 kg, were
anaesthetized with ether, immobilized with gallamine

triethiodide (Flaxedil®), artificially ventilated and placed on a stereotaxic apparatus. The vertebral column was immobilized with metal clamps. Following laminectomy, the dura mater was opened and the cord exposed from L_5 to S_1 then covered with warm paraffin oil (37-38°C). In 10 experiments, the spinal cord section was performed at L_2 level. Recordings were started 3 hr after termination of the ether anaesthesia. Lidocaine was repeatedly applied to wound edges throughout the entire experiments. Extracellular unit activity was recorded from the left lamina V cells of L_6-L_7 segments using a tungsten microelectrode the tip of which was about 1-3 μ in diameter. The lamina V cells were selected according to the electrophysiological properties described by Wall (51) and Kitahata, Taub and Sato (25). Spike potentials were amplified and displayed on an oscilloscope and photographed. A schema of the method is illustrated in Fig. 5.

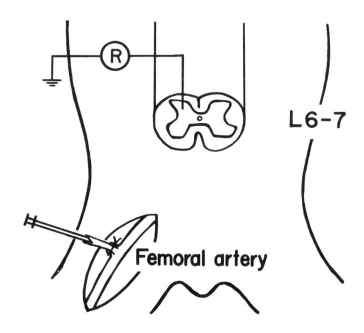

FIG. 5. Schematic illustration of the method

A polyethylene cannula of 0.9 mm in diameter was introduced in a retrograde manner into the left deep femoral artery and tied into place in such a way that the tip was just distal to the bifurcation. Bradykinin, synthesized by Protein Research Foundation (Mino, Osaka, Japan), was dissolved in saline (10 or 20 µg/ml) and 0.1 ml of the solution was rapidly (1 sec or less) injected into the femoral artery through the cannula at intervals of 10 min. The cannula was flushed with the vehicle (0.1-0.2 ml) 1-2 min after each bradykinin injection.

The number of unit discharges of each neuron for 60 sec before and after each bradykinin injection was counted using a small computer (Nihon Kohden ATAC 501-10S) and the former number was considered as spontaneous. The number of unit discharges of each neuron after bradykinin minus the number before bradykinin was considered as bradykinin-induced. The 95% confidence limits were calculated from 5 values of the bradykinin-induced discharges before administration of morphine. If the values following at least 2 successive bradykinin injections after morphine administration were either below or above the calculated 95% confidence limits, the effect of morphine was regarded as being inhibitory or facilitatory, respectively, and expressed as a percent change from control. A similar analysis of data was made to assess the effect of morphine on spontaneous activity, however, in this assessment, neurons without spontaneous activity were disregarded.

After termination of experiments in which a typical response to bradykinin injection was observed, the location of the recording electrode in the spinal cord was histologically confirmed. Tips of the electrodes were located in the area corresponding to the lamina V of cat's dorsal horn (37).

Morphine hydrochloride was injected i.v. and the doses are given in terms of the salt. Each animal was dispensed only one dose of morphine and the effect of morphine was observed at only one lamina V cell in each experiment.

Results and Discussion

   The rates of spontaneous unit activity of lamina V
cells of the spinal L_6-L_7 segments in intact rabbits
were less than 5 spikes/sec in 65% of cells tested
(n=52), 5-20 spikes/sec in 25% and more than 20 spikes
/sec in the other 10%. The rates in spinal rabbits,
however, were more than 5 spikes/sec in 75% of neurons
examined (n=32), in particular, more than 20 spikes/
sec in 40%. In a preliminary report where 65 dorsal
horn neurons were examined, 36 (55%) showed a marked
increase in rates of firing following the intra-arterial injection of 1-2 µg of bradykinin (39). Fig 6
demonstrates a typical increase in firing after a 2 µg

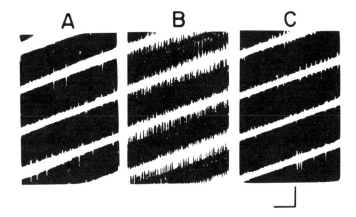

FIG. 6 Spontaneous activity and bradykinin-induced
response of a lamina V cell of the spinal dorsal horn
of the rabbit. Time scale : 0.1 sec. Calibration 200µV
A : Before bradykinin injection (spontaneous activity)
B : 20-25 sec after an arterial injection of 2 µg
    bradykinin into the femoral artery
C : 50-55 sec after the injection

bradykinin injection. Increase in the number of spikes
appeared with a latent period of 5-10 sec, reached a
maximum 15-30 sec after intra-arterial application of
bradykinin and then declined in 60-90 sec (Fig.6).
Maximum increase in the firing rate was 900%. In 13
(20%) of 65 neurons examined, activities were reduced
following bradykinin injection, with a time course
similar to that of the excitation, and 16 (25%) showed
no appreciable change. These modifications of the
activity of lamina V dorsal horn cells by intra-
arterial injection of bradykinin were due to the
peripheral action, as such could no longer be induced
after cutting L_6-L_7 dorsal roots. Although bradykinin
(1 or 2 μg) was repeatedly injected into the femoral
artery more than 20 times at intervals of 10 min in
each experiment, signs of tachyphylaxis or hypersensitivity to bradykinin were not observed.

A similar tendency was observed in cats using the
intra-arterial injection of bradykinin (3). These
authors reported that the injection of bradykinin
preferentially activated the lamina V cells (52%) and
produced few excitations in the lamina IV cells(13.7%).

In our studies of the effects of morphine, we used
only those neurons in which unitary activity increased
and was stable for more than 60 min following injection
of bradykinin.

Intravenous administration of 0.3 mg/kg of morphine
to intact rabbits decreased the number of bradykinin-
induced discharges of the lamina V cells to 10-50% of
the pre-morphine level in 10 out of 21 experiments and
this inhibition lasted for 35-60 min (Fig.7). An
increase of 150-180%, however, was observed in 5 cases.
In the other 6 experiments, it could not be ascertained
that morphine actually had an effect on the bradykinin
response. When 2.0 mg/kg of morphine was injected,
the inhibitory effect was observed in 6 out of 10
experiments, the facilitatory effect in 1 and no clear
effect in the other 3 cases (Table 3). The inhibitory
effect of morphine was antagonized by nalorphine (0.2
mg/kg) injected 20-30 min after morphine, while the
facilitatory effect of the drug was not always
antagonized by nalorphine. In spinal rabbits, morphine
in a dose of 2.0 mg/kg did not significantly decrease
the number of bradykinin-induced unit discharges, but

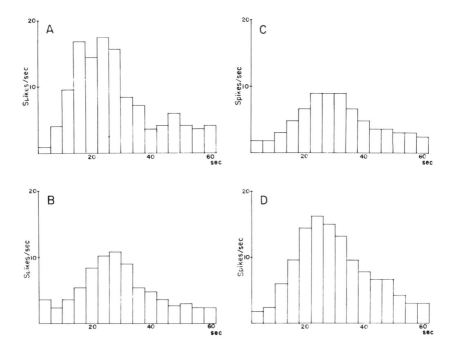

FIG. 7. Effect of morphine on the activity of a lamina V cell responding to intra-arterial injection of bradykinin into the femoral artery. Abscissa: Time after bradykinin injection (2 μg). Ordinate: Mean firing rate in periods of 4 sec duration.
A : control response
B, C, and D : 5,15 and 35 min after an administration
     of morphine (0.3 mg/kg i.v.), respectively.

the response was inhibited with a dose of 5.0 mg/kg (Table 3). This inhibition was   antagonized by nalorphine (0.5 mg/kg). These results suggest that morphine, in small doses, inhibits the sensory transmission of bradykinin-induced pain at the dorsal horn of the spinal cord, through its facilitatory action on the descending inhibitory mechanism; in larger doses the sensory transmission is directly inhibited at the level of the dorsal horn.
     Intravenous administration of 0.3 mg/kg of morphine

TABLE 3. Effects of various doses of morphine on the bradykinin-induced activities of lamina V cells in intact and spinal rabbits.

Doses mg/kg (i.v.)	Preparation	Inhibition	Facilitation	No Clear Effect
0.3	Intact	10	5	6
2.0	"	6	1	3
2.0	Spinal	0	2	4
5.0	"	3	0	1

to intact rabbits significantly inhibited the bradykinin-induced activities of lamina V cells in 45% of all the experiments, while inhibition of spontaneous activities was evident in 24% of all experiments. When 2.0 mg/kg of morphine was given, both bradykinin-induced response and spontaneous activity were suppressed in 60% and 56% of experiments, respectively.These results strongly indicate that it is the bradykinin-induced activity in lamina V cells which is more susceptible to morphine (47). Such also applies to pentazocine, since 5 mg/kg of the drug inhibited the bradykinin-induced activities in 5 but the spontaneous activities in only 2 out of 8 intact rabbits. On the contrary, pentobarbital in doses of 10-20 mg/kg suppressed the former in only 3 but the latter in 7 out of 14 rabbits tested.

On the other hand, Kitahata et al.(24) and Le Bars et al. (28) pointed out that morphine inhibits both the electrically and mechanically induced activities as well as the spontaneous activities of the lamina V cells. Phenoperidine (2 mg/kg), a potent morphine-like narcotic, also reportedly inhibits electrically induced activities as well as the spontaneous activities (4).

In our studies, we found that morphine was much less effective in suppressing the bradykinin-induced response in spinal rabbits than in intact rabbits. Kitahata et al. (24) showed that small doses of morphine (0.5-2.0 mg/kg) suppressed spontaneous as well as nociceptively induced activities of lamina V

cells in decerebrate spinal cats. Jurna and Grossmann
(23) also found that in spinal cats, 0.5 mg/kg of
morphine depressed the activity evoked in axons of the
ventrolateral tract of the spinal cord by stimulation
of Aδ - and C-fibers in the sural nerve. Discrepancies among these results are attributed to differences in animal species, forms of stimuli and other
experimental conditions. A comparative study of the
action of morphine on the spinal mechanism in both
intact and spinal animals was proved necessary before
drawing conclusions as to the main site of morphine
action on the spinal cord. With regard to the suppressive effects of small doses of morphine on hind-
limb reflexes of chronic spinal dogs as reported by
Martin et al.(32), we consider that the mechanism may
to some extent be attributed to the denervation supersensitivity to morphine with chronic spinal transection.

Pharmacological characteristics of this system are
as follows:
1) assessment of analgesic effect of narcotics can be
   based directly on changes in unit activities of
   the afferent system involved in the sensation of
   pain, and effects of the drugs on the motor system
   will not be an obstacle preventing an objective
   judgement,
2) effects of various drugs on the bradykinin-induced
   unit activity can be quantitatively measured,
3) sensitivity to narcotic analgesics is high,
4) sensitivity to agonist-antagonist analgesic
   (pentazocine) is good,
5) evaluation of the analgesic effect of non-narcotic
   analgesics (indomethacin, aminopyrine, aspirin
   etc.) is feasible; these drugs inhibit the
   bradykinin-induced activities when minute doses
   are administered into the same cannulated femoral
   artery (38),
6) the bradykinin-induced activities are not so easily
   depressed by pentobarbital (10-20 mg/kg).
Thus the bradykinin-induced unit activity of lamina
V cell of the spinal dorsal horn is indeed an excellent
model for determining the site and the mode of action
of analgesic drugs. The facilitatory action of
narcotics on the bradykinin-induced response was,

however, occasionally observed in this system, and the role this action plays in analgesia is now being investigated.

There is now considerable evidence that sites for anti-nociceptive action of morphine are located in some regions of the brain stem : the thalamus (7),the hypothalamus (16,21,48,49), the periaqueductal gray matter (20,22,35,43,48,49), the floor of the fourth ventricle (20) or the ventral surface of the brain stem (12). Moreover, Satoh and Takagi (40) found that analgesic doses of morphine enhanced the descending inhibitory control on the spinal sensory transmission originating from the lower brain stem, in particular, painful sensation induced by the intra-arterial injection of bradykinin (39,47).

Recently, we observed that : 1) a single micro-injection of morphine hydrochloride in a dose of 0.5 µg into the nucleus reticularis giganto-cellularis (NRGC) produced a marked analgesia in rats and this effect was reversed by subcutaneous administration of naloxone (44); 2) a single micro-injection of morphine hydrochloride in a dose of 40 µg into the rabbit NRGC inhibited the bradykinin-induced activities of the spinal dorsal horn lamina V cells (44); 3) an electrical stimulation of the rabbit NRGC inhibited the bradykinin-induced response of the spinal dorsal horn lamina V cells and this descending inhibitory system is, in part, catecholaminergic(45), and 4) an electrical stimulation of the rat NRGC produced behavioral analgesia (Takagi et al., unpublished data).

Some investigators have emphasized the peri-aqueductal gray matter (PGM) as a site for analgesic action of morphine (22,35,43,48,49). Takagi et al. (44), however, showed that the NRGC was more sensitive to morphine than the PGM in the rat in terms of the analgesic dose. Oliveras et al.(33) reported that electrical stimulation of the raphe obscurus and the raphe magnus nuclei of cats produced behavioral analgesia. This result was confirmed by ·Proudfit and Anderson (36) using rats. A single micro-injection of morphine hydrochloride (0.5 µg) into the nucleus raphe magnus, however, did not produce analgesia in the rat (44). This result suggests that an enhancement by

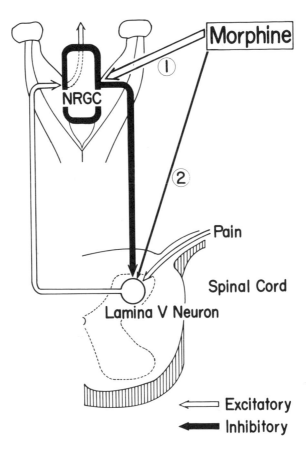

FIG. 8 Schema illustrating two types of mechanisms
of inhibitory action of morphine on the sensory
transmission of pain at the lamina V of spinal dorsal
horn. ① An enhancement of descending inhibitory
control on the lamina V neuron originating from the
nucleus reticularis gigantocellularis (NRGC).
② A direct inhibition of the lamina V neuron.

morphine of the descending inhibitory control from the
NRGC is not mediated via the nucleus raphe magnus.
In this connection, it is of interest that the descending inhibitory system from the NRGC is, in part,
catecholaminergic (45).

A role of the NRGC in nociception has been suggested; some neurons of the NRGC were found to be activated
by electrical stimulation of Aδ and C cutaneous afferents or noxious stimuli applied to their receptive
fields (9,53) or intra-arterial injection of bradykinin
(18). Peacock and Wolstencroft (34) showed a projection from the NRGC to the dorsal horn of the spinal
cord in the cat. These studies together with our
results suggest that there is a feed-back loop by which
the NRGC can control its own input and that this
control is enhanced by an analgesic dose of morphine
(Fig. 8). On the other hand, a direct action of
morphine at the level of the dorsal horn cannot be
excluded, as a direct application of morphine to the
extracellular space of the spinal dorsal horn neurons
of cats or the spinal (lumbar) subarachnoid space of
rats produced an inhibition of the neuronal response
to noxious stimuli or a potent analgesia, respectively
(8,54). Comparative studies of the action of morphine
on spinal structures involved in pain processes, such
as lamina V, in intact and spinal animals are necessary to determine   the relative pharmacological
importance of these two mechanisms. We found that
in spinal rather than intact rabbits, larger doses of
morphine were required for the inhibition of bradykinin
induced activities of the lamina V cells (47). Thus
the direct action of morphine on the dorsal horn probably plays only a minor role in analgesic action of
morphine applied systematically.

SUMMARY

Three neurological models using the bradykinin-
induced nociceptive responses were described and
pharmacological characteristics and feasible application to the study of narcotics were discussed. Data on
recent studies of the site of the anti-nociceptive
action of morphine were also discussed.

ACKNOWLEDGEMENTS

This study was supported by Scientific Research Funds
from the Ministry of Education, Japan.   Thanks are due
to M. Ohara for assistance with the manuscript.

REFERENCES

1.   Abe, T., Kaneko, T., and Takagi, H. (1971): Folia
     pharmacol. Jpn., 67: 9.
2.   Armstrong, D., Jepson, J.B., Keele, C.A., and
     Stewart, J.W. (1957): J. Physiol. (Lond.) 135: 350.
3.   Besson, J.M., Conseiller, C., Hamann, K.-F., and
     Maillard, M.C. (1972): J. Physiol. (Lond.) 221:
     189.
4.   Besson, J.M., Wyon-Maillard, M.C., Benoist, J.M.,
     Conseiller, C., and Hamann, K.-F. (1973):
     J. Pharmacol. Exp. Ther., 187: 239.
5.   Blane, G.F. (1967): J. Pharm. Pharmacol., 19: 367.
6.   Burch, G.E., and De Pasquale, N.P. (1962): Circ.
     Res., 10: 105.
7.   Buxbaum, D.M., Yarbrough, G.G., and Carter, M.E.
     (1970): Pharmacologist, 12: 211.
8.   Calvillo, O., Henry, J.L., and Neuman, R.S. (1974):
     Can. J. Physiol. Pharmacol., 52: 1207.
9.   Casey, K.L. (1969): Exp. Neurol., 25: 35.
10. Collier, H.O.J., and Lee, I.R. (1963): Br. J.
     Pharmacology Chemother., 21: 155.
11. Deffenu, G., Pegrassi, L., and Lumachi, B. (1966):
     J. Pharm. Pharmacol., 18: 135.
12. Dey, P.K., and Feldberg, W. (1975): J. Physiol.
     (Lond.), 248:40P.
13. Doi, T., Kawasaki, K., Akaike, A., Ohashi, M.,
     Satoh, M., and Takagi, H. (1976): Jpn. J. Pharmacol
     26: 634.
14. Domino, E.F. (1968): In: The Addictive States,
     edited by A. Wikler, p.117. William & Wilkins,
     Baltimore.
15. Emele, J.F., and Shanaman, J. (1963): Proc. Soc.
     Exp. Biol. Med., 114: 680.
16. Foster, R.S., Jenden, D.J., and Lomax, P. (1967):
     J. Pharmacol. Exp. Ther., 157: 185.
17. Fujita, S., Yasuhara, M., Yamamoto, S., and Ogiu,K.

(1954): Jpn. J. Pharmacol., 4: 41.

18. Guilbaud, G., Besson, J.M., Oliveras, J.L., and Wyon-Maillard, M.C. (1973): Brain Res., 63: 131.
19. Guzman, F., Braun, C., and Lim, R.K.S. (1962): Arch. Int. Pharmacodyn. Thér., 136: 353.
20. Herz, A., Albus, K., Metyš, J., Schubert, P., and Teschemacher, H.J. (1970): Neuropharmacology, 9: 539.
21. Jacquet, Y.F., and Lajtha, A. (1973): Science, 182: 490.
22. Jacquet, Y.F., and Lajtha, A. (1974): Science, 185: 1055.
23. Jurna, I., and Grossmann, W. (1976): Exp. Brain Res., 24: 473.
24. Kitahata, L.M., Kosaka, Y., Taub, A., Bonikos, K., and Hoffert, M. (1974): Anesthesiology, 41: 39.
25. Kitahata, L.M., Taub, A., and Sato, I. (1971): J. Pharmacol. Exp. Ther., 176: 101.
26. Koll, W., Haase, J., Block, G., and Mühlberg, B. (1963): Int. J. Neuropharmacol., 2: 57.
27. Kuromi, H., Satoh, M., and Takagi, H. (1972): Jpn. J. Pharmacol., 22: 264.
28. Le Bars, D., Menétrey, D., Conseiller, C., and Besson, J.M. (1975): Brain Res., 98: 261.
29. Lim, R.K.S., Guzman, F., Rodgers, D.W., Goto, K., Braun, C., Dickerson, G.D., and Engle, R. (1964): Arch. Int. Pharmacodyn. Thér., 152: 25.
30. Lim, R.K.S., Miller, D.G., Guzman, F., Rodgers, D.W., Rogers, R.W., Wang, S.K., Chao, P.Y., and Shih, T.Y. (1967): Clin. Pharmacol. Ther., 8: 521.
31. Litchfield, J.T. Jr., and Wilcoxon, F. (1949): J. Pharmacol. Exp. Ther., 96: 99.
32. Martin, W.R., Eades, C.G., Fraser, H.F., and Wikler, A. (1964): J. Pharmacol. Exp. Ther., 144:8.
33. Oliveras, J.L., Redjemi, F., Guilbaud, G., and Besson, J.M. (1975): Pain, 1: 139.
34. Peacock, M.J., and Wolstencroft, J.H. (1976): Neuroscience Letters, 2: 7.
35. Pert, A., and Yaksh, T. (1974): Brain Res., 80:135.
36. Proudfit, H.K., and Anderson, E.G. (1975): Brain Res., 98: 612.
37. Rexed, B. (1954): J. Comp. Neurol., 100: 297.
38. Satoh, M., Doi, T., Kawasaki, K., Akaike, A., and Takagi, H. (1976): Jpn. J. Pharmacol., 26: 309.

39. Satoh, M., Nakamura, N., and Takagi, H. (1971):
    Eur. J. Pharmacol., 16: 245.
40. Satoh, M., and Takagi, H. (1971): Eur. J. Pharmacol
    14: 60.
41. Selzer, M., and Spencer, W.A. (1969): Brain Res.,
    14: 331.
42. Selzer, M., and Spencer, W.A. (1969): Brain Res.,
    14: 349.
43. Sharpe, L.G., Garnett, J.E., and Cicero, T.J.,
    (1974):   Behav.Biol., 11: 303.
44. Takagi, H., Doi, T., and Akaike, A. (1976): In:
    Mode of Action of Opioids, edited by S. Archer,
    H.O.J. Collier, A. Goldstein, H.W. Kosterlitz,
    E.J. Simon, H. Takagi, and L. Terenius,p.191. North
    Holland Publ., Amsterdam
45. Takagi, H., Doi, T., and Kawasaki, K. (1975):
    Life Sci., 17: 67.
46. Takagi, H., Matsumura, M., Yanai, A., and Ogiu, K.
    (1955): Jpn. J. Pharmacol., 4: 176.
47. Takagi, H., Satoh, M., Doi, T., Kawasaki, K., and
    Akaike, A. (1976): Arch. Int. Pharmacodyn. Thér.,
    221: 96.
48. Tsou, K., and Jang, C.S. (1962): Acta Physiol.
    Sinica, 25: 119.
49. Tsou, K., and Jang, C.S. (1964): Scientia Sinica,
    8: 1099.
50. Wagman, I.H., and Price, D.D. (1969):
    J.Neurophysiol., 32: 803.
51. Wall, P.D. (1967): J. Physiol.(Lond.), 188: 403.
52. Wikler, A. (1950): Pharmacol. Rev., 2: 435.
53. Wolstencroft, J.H. (1964): J. Physiol.(Lond.),174:91.
54. Yaksh, T.L., and Rudy, T.A. (1976): Science, 192:
    1357.

Factors Affecting the Action of Narcotics, edited by
M.L. Adler, L. Manara, and R. Samanin.
Raven Press, New York © 1978.

The Use of Operant Behavior Methods to Study Aggression and
Effects of Acute and Chronic Morphine Administration in Rats

S.B. Sparber, V.F. Gellert[1], L. Lichtblau and R. Eisenberg+

Departments of Pharmacology and Psychiatry, University of
Minnesota, Minneapolis, Minnesota 55455 U.S.A.
+ Department of Pharmacology, University of Minnesota,
Duluth, Minnesota 55812 U.S.A.

INTRODUCTION

We have recently become interested in the behavioral and
biochemical consequences of opiate tolerance, dependence, and
withdrawal and have been exploring the feasibility of utilizing
operant behavioral methodologies to assess the degree of
tolerance and dependence, instead of the traditional subjective
methods of behavioral analyses in which semi-quantitative
estimates of running, jumping, teeth chattering, ptosis, restlessness, irritability, and a host of other measures have been used.
One major advantage realized with the use of an ongoing behavior
is that agents or manipulations which specifically block or
reverse the withdrawal syndrome will maintain or reinstate the
behavior, while manipulations which render the subject physically
or otherwise incapable of responding would further suppress
behavior previously suppressed by the withdrawal state. This is
important since many substances (e.g., high doses of atropine)
which are reported to suppress withdrawal signs have the capacity
to suppress many types of unconditioned and conditioned behavior
at the doses used and therefore, may be acting nonselectively.

Of additional importance is the fact that operant behavior
maintained by the same schedule of reinforcement can be used to
study the acute behavioral action of morphine and tolerance to
this pharmacological effect. In this manner the same behavior can
be used to study tolerance as well as dependence (via withdrawal),
instead of having to study two or more different types of
behaviors, such as tail-flick or paw-lifting in response to
noxious stimuli and jumping or wet-shakes, etc. as a behavioral
measure of withdrawal. One of the basic laws of behavior, when
viewed within an operant framework, is that patterns and types of
behavior are important determinants of the effects of drugs upon
behavior (see an excellent review of these factors by Kelleher
and Morse) (28). Within this context, it is not suprising to
encounter studies in which various treatment schedules block or
enhance one measure of analgesia or withdrawal and not other
measures, since different types of behavior are being utilized.
Studies of this type have led to tentative conclusions that

1. Present address: Dept. Pharmacol., Emory Univ., Atlanta, Georgia 30322

tolerance and dependence differ temporally (appearance and disappearance) and therefore are separable phenomena, while in fact no clear-cut separation of these phenomena has been demonstrated. Utilizing operant behavior may allow us to study tolerance and dependence with a single or identical variables so that questions relating to the separability of or mechanisms by which these phenomena develop may be more succinctly answered. This summary of some of the research we have been engaged in during the last couple of years will be presented in a somewhat chronological order.

Our interest in this area first evolved around the folklore descriptions of heroin addicts engaged in acts of aggression and violence in conjunction with a hypothesis that behavioral effects of drugs or withdrawal from them depended in great part upon the interaction of subjects within a social hierarchy. However, when reading the recent experimental literature dealing with morphine-withdrawal-induced aggression (6,17,30,39) it became immediately apparent that crowding or shock-induced episodes of squealing and attacking in rats were unsuitable for several reasons. Firstly, hyperirritability or hyperalgesia to noxious stimuli during withdrawal (52) may be responsible for apparent increases in aggression, instead of specific increases in aggressive behavior. This would be akin to increasing the shock intensity for non-withdrawn subjects, which in turn would lead to increased "aggression". Secondly, laboratory rats rarely engage in overt attack and the many ethological studies of social hierarchies in rodents indicate that dominance and submissive postures are more likely to maintain order within groups of rats. Instead of attempting to devise and/or learn a complex, subjective scoring method for quantifying agonistic or aggressive behavior, we decided to allow the rats to evaluate each other's postures, and we determined the hierarchal position of each subject of a pair by observing the distribution of lever-pressing behavior between the pair when placed together within an operant chamber before, during, and after acute and chronic morphine injections. It soon became apparent that rats maintained on a twice daily morphine injection schedule were experiencing withdrawal of varying intensities (depending upon the dose level) twice a day. Because the withdrawal was evident within 24 hr of initiating the injection schedule, a series of studies was undertaken in which shorter time intervals were utilized to study acute dependence and then acute tolerance.

Since the nature of the withdrawal state implies a generalized stressful condition, we attempted to verify this assumption by measuring plasma corticosterone levels of rats subjected to treatment schedules which produced significant behavioral changes that we were interpreting as withdrawal-induced.

I. MORPHINE WITHDRAWAL-INDUCED AGGRESSION AND DISRUPTION OF
    FIXED-RATIO OPERANT BEHAVIOR IN CHRONICALLY INJECTED RATS

Although they used groups of 6 male rats in their studies,

Boshka et al.(6) noted that the fighting they observed during
withdrawal occurred only between pairs of rats. In addition,
Crabtree and Moyer (12) reported that increased shock-elicited aggression during withdrawal was limited to paired male rats,little
being observed in female-female or male-female pairs.

This study was undertaken to determine if a combination of
techniques could be used to objectively quantify the aggressive or
agonistic behavior, as well as conditioned operant behavior depression, engendered by withdrawal from morphine. The design was
one in which social structures were restricted to pairs, rather
than groups, of rats. However, spontaneous fighting between pairs
of laboratory rats is essentially nonexistent (5). In addition,
withdrawal alone induces only sporadic overt aggression in isolated pairs of rats (14).

In view of these previous reports it was decided to combine
operant and ethological techniques using food as the reinforcing
stimulus and competition for it to study aggressive behavior. This
first section deals with the methods and results of acute and
chronic morphine administration and withdrawal in pairs of rats
where one or both members were subjected to drug treatment.

We have observed alterations in operant responding by individual rats as early as 24 hr after initiating a morphine SO_4 injection schedule in which 25 mg/kg was administered twice a day for 2
days and increased, in 25 mg/kg increments, to 100 mg/kg twice a
day, over an 8 day period. It appears that injection schedules of
this type (twice a day) cause cyclic episodes of withdrawal which
are responsible for the behavioral alterations and can compromise
studies on tolerance and dependence by virtue of the chronic
stress of twice daily episodes of withdrawal. To partially verify
this interpretation, a second experiment was undertaken in which
another group of rats was administered morphine on the same injection schedule and their plasma corticosterone levels were analyzed
every 2 hours starting 10 hours after their last injection of
morphine.

Subjects. Male,Long-Evans hooded rats obtained from Blue-Spruce
Farms(Altamont, N.Y.,USA) at 2-2 1/2 months of age served as subjects for these behavioral experiments. Upon arrival, they were
housed in community cages, 6 to a cage, in a constant environment
room with 12 hour light-dark cycles for several weeks. After being
placed in individual cages until their body weights reached 350-
400 g, they were partially food-deprived until they reached 80% of
their free-feeding weight. Water was available in their home cage
ad libitum throughout all experiments.

Apparatus. All paired and unpaired behavioral experiments were
conducted in standard operant chambers Model 143-22, BRS/LVE,
Beltsville, Md.) equipped with sound-attentuating and ventilating
devices. On one wall of the chamber were 2 operant levers,which
required a force of approximately 25 g to depress. Stimulus
lights and a food pellet delivery trough were likewise on the
front panel. Intermittent schedules of reinforcement were program-

med and data recorded by standard electro-mechanical equipment and cumulative recorders located in an adjacent room.

Procedure for evaluating aggressive behavior. Rats stabilized at 80% of their free-feeding weights were magazine-trained to eat 45 mg food pellets (P.J.Noyes, Lancaster,N.H.) automatically delivered to the food trough and were then shaped to press one lever for food pellets on a continuous reinforcement (crf) schedule. After responding had stabilized, a number of preliminary experiments were conducted to determine those conditions which would allow stable lever-pressing behavior with a moderate level of overt fighting when two rats were placed in the chamber at the same time. A moderate level of fighting was defined as consisting of one to several overt fights per 15 min paired session, the total duration of which would not exceed 60-120 sec, thus allowing either increases or decreases in fighting to be detected.

It was found that pairs consisting of rats whose operant behavior had been stable on an FR20 schedule on the same lever before pairing came closest to matching the criteria set. Under these conditions, initial pairings led to much struggling between the rats to get at the lever, which often resulted in overt fighting. However, within a few 15 min sessions most of the fighting had dissipated and a hierarchy emerged where one member of the pair emitted most or all of the responding (80-100%) and ate virtually all of the food pellets it had earned. The other member would sit quietly or autogroom at the other end of the chamber. Occasionally it would attempt to get at the bar or food trough , which would lead to struggling resulting in threat postures by the responding rat or overt fighting, ranging up to 20 sec per 15 min session.

The procedure for forming stable pairs for experimental use was first to shape individual FR20 responding and then to pair the rats by matching response rates and body weights, both within 10% of each other. They were then simultaneously placed in the chamber for 15 min sessions. Behavior was monitored by closed-circuit television (CCTV) and tape-recorded to allow subsequent analysis. The amount of time each member engaged in lever-pressing or both engaged in overt fighting behavior was recorded on a 3-channel print-out recorder by pressing one of 3 switches while viewing the behavior through the CCTV. The switch would close the appropriate relay between a pulse generator, set to send out 60 msec pulses every half-second, and the recorder, which printed out the number of 1/2 seconds of each behavior emitted by each rat per minute. Overt fighting behavior was recorded whenever both members of a pair assumed one of 3 postures: upright defensive (boxing) postures; actual wrestling, squealing, and biting; and dominant-submissive postures, which usually terminated a fight. These postures have been well defined and illustrated by Grant and Mackintosh (20) and usually occur in the above sequence. Daily, unpaired 15 min sessions (subject in operant chamber alone) were conducted in addition to (on the same day),or

instead of paired sessions to maintain stable FR20 responding by
both members of a pair. This also allowed a determination of the
effects of the various behavioral and drug manipulations upon unpaired response rates and how these rates compared with changes
in paired responding. In the latter instance, the unpaired
sessions acted as a control to determine if the subjects were
capable of the operant while in the paired condition. The members
of each stable pair were labelled dominant (Dom) or submissive
(Sub), determined by virtue of whether or not they had control of
the operant manipulandum. Paired behavior was considered stable
if the Dom rat controlled the lever for 80% or more of the 15 min
session, over 4 consecutive sessions.

Procedures for assessing the effects of morphine sulfate on unpaired and paired operant behavior. The effect of acute morphine
on unpaired and paired behavior was determined first. Five
pairs of drug-naive rats whose paired and unpaired operant
behavior had stabilized were used. 5 or 10 mg morphine SO_4 (MS)/
kg were administered, i.p., one half-hour before unpaired FR20
responding per 15 min session was evaluated. Following this, the
effect of 5 or 10 mg MS/kg on paired behavior was studied when
administered to the Sub or Dom member only, or when given to both
rats one half-hour prior to testing.

Chronic morphine administration to both members of each pair. The
control (saline) paired sessions of the above experiment revealed
that paired behavior remained unchanged in the absence of MS,
despite the intervening drug treatments. Subsequently, these
pairs were exposed to a chronic regimen of morphine treatment.
The sequence of drug administration and behavioral testing generally was on a 12 hr schedule. Briefly, both members of each pair
were administered 4 doses each of 25 mg, 50 mg and 75 mg MS/kg and
5 doses of 100 mg MS/kg with one injection given between 10 a.m.
and 12 noon and one between 10 p.m. and 12 midnight each day over
an 8 1/2 day period. Unpaired and paired operant behavior was
monitored 12 hr after the second and fourth injection,respective-
ly, of each dose level except after 75 mg MS/kg. An additional
paired session was run 6 hr after the fifth injection of 100 mg
MS/kg. The morning morphine injections were administered immediately after the operant behavior was monitored. After the fifth
dose of 100 mg MS/kg the drug was withheld and behavior monitored
for the next 6 consecutive days and also 9, 14, and 28 days after
morphine withdrawal.

Plasma corticosterone levels after chronic morphine. All of the
corticosterone experiments were performed on male rats (ARS
Sprague-Dawley, Madison, Wisc.) weighing approximately 250 g.They
were housed at a constant temperature(21°C) and in a light cycle
of 14 hr light/10 hr dark. Laboratory food and water were available ad libitum. Each animal was allowed to acclimate to the sur-
roundings and routine for at least 5 days before experimentation
was begun. Catheterization of the superior vena cavae and prepara-

tion of the dental acrylic fixture was done under pentobarbital anesthesia according to a modification of a procedure used by Brown and Hedge (7) and Martin (personal communication). To maintain patency, catheters were flushed daily with heparinized saline, 500 U/ml. The animals were divided into two groups : saline-treated and morphine-treated. On day 1, the day following surgery, drug treatment was begun. Morphine SO_4 was injected (i.p.) at 8 a.m. and 8 p.m. Dosage was increased every 2 days on the following schedule : 25, 50, 75, and 100 mg/kg per injection. Equivalent volumes of saline were injected into control animals. On the morning of day 8, each animal was placed in the experimental cage within a sound-attentuating chamber in order to become accustomed to being connected to the exteriorized blood sampling tube. Following the last injection at 8 p.m. on this day, each animal stayed in the experimental cage. Blood sampling commenced at 6 a.m. and continued every 2 hr until 4 p.m. of day 9. Each 0.6 ml blood sample was collected in a heparinized syringe. Following centrifugation the plasma was separated, quickly frozen, and stored at -10°C. The red blood cells were resuspended in saline and injected back into the animal from which they were collected; plasma corticosterone was determined by a modification of the fluorescence method of Glick et al. (19).

Unpaired and paired behavior after acute morphine administration. This procedure was conducted so the effects of acutely administered morphine on these behaviors could be compared and contrasted with the effects of withdrawal. The effect of 5 mg and 10 mg MS/kg on unpaired FR20 responding is shown in Table 1. These doses of morphine significantly decreased the number of responses emitted per 15 minute session by 22% and 36%, respectively. The distribution of responding by paired rats was unaffected after 5 mg or 10 mg MS/kg were administered to the Sub members (Fig. 1). However, two of the 5 pairs exhibited either reversal (pair 9-16) or disruption (pair 4-10) of their hierarchies after administration of morphine to the dominant members only. Interestingly, the hierarchies of these 2 pairs remained intact after morphine was administered to both members, while a third pair (14-17) exhibited paired-behavioral disruption as a shift in the distribution of responding between the Dom and Sub members of the pair (i.e., Dom < < 80%). The average amount of time spent fighting by the 5 pairs over the 4 saline control sessions was 7.5 seconds. This residual fighting was virtually eliminated after the Sub rats were administered 5 mg or 10 mg MS/kg (1.0 and 1.3 sec of fighting, respectively) and after both members were administered 10 mg MS/kg (0.3 sec of fighting).

Effect of chronic morphine administration and withdrawal on behavior: both members treated and withdrawn. Unpaired FR20 responding by all rats and control of the manipulandum by the Dom rat was compromised in a dose-related manner during chronic

TABLE 1. Effect of acute morphine administration on unpaired FR20 responding

Treatment[a]	Saline	5 mg MS/kg	10 mg MS/kg
Responses Emitted per 15 min Session	1965+66[b]	1534+132[c]	1260+324[c]
% of saline control	100+3.4	78.4+6.7	64.4+16.6

[a] Morphine sulfate (MS) or saline was administered i.p. $\frac{1}{2}$ hr before behavioral testing

[b] mean $\pm$ S.E. (N=10)

[c] $p < .01$ when compared to saline values (Student's two tailed t-test for paired observations)

morphine administration. Unpaired and paired behavioral sessions were conducted 12 hr after the second and fourth injection, respectively, at each dose level (i.e., 25 mg, and 100 mg MS/kg). During these periods responding on the part of the Sub rats, which was virtually nonexistent during control sessions, was greatly increased, while that of the Dom rats decreased in a reciprocal fashion. These behavioral changes appeared qualitatively similar to those seen after acute morphine administration to the Dom rat (Fig. 1). It was therefore possible that the depressant effects of these relatively high doses of morphine on behavior were still detectable 12 hr after administration. On the other hand, these behavioral changes may have been induced by the early stages of spontaneous withdrawal. Consequently, a fifth dose of 100 mg MS/kg was administered and paired behavior monitored 6 hr later. The hierarchies at this time were not different from control, indicating the behavioral disruption observed 12 hr after morphine was probably withdrawal-induced (Fig.2, Session 4; Table 2A).

No further morphine was given and the behavior of 3 remaining pairs was monitored through the 28th day of abstinence. All 3 pairs exhibited severe disruption of the hierarchies in that the Sub rats were in control of the manipulandum well above their individual ranges during the 4 saline sessions, while the Dom members relinquished control. Two of the pairs (4-10 and 9-16) exhibited this phenomenon through the ninth day of abstinence, which was accompanied by prolonged fighting episodes at various times during this period (Fig.2, sessions 5-11). The third pair (1-11) recovered by the fifth day of abstinence and did not

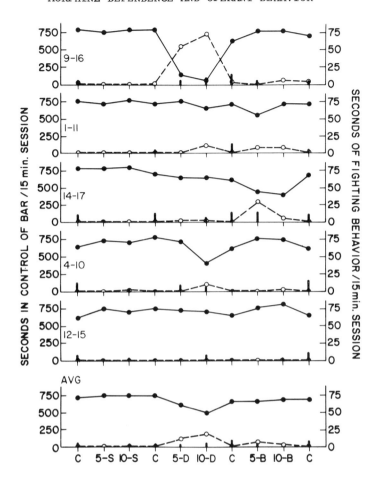

FIG. 1.   Action of acute morphine on paired responding and
          fighting behavior. S, D, or B after numerical values on
          the abscissa indicate 5 or 10 mg MS/kg administered to
          the submissive, dominant, or both members, respectively,
          of each pair 1/2 hr prior to behavioral sessions.
          C indicates control sessions in which both members
          received saline injections. When only one member was
          injected with MS the other member was injected with
          saline.
          Solid lines connecting points indicate lever-pressing
          behavior emitted by the Dom animal and dotted lines, the
          Sub animal, while the heavy vertical lines denote the
          amount of fighting behavior during the individual
          sessions. Note the scale for fighting behavior is 1/10
          that for lever-pressing behavior. Numbers in graphs to
          the right of the ordinates represent the pair members.
          AVG represents the averaged data for 5 pairs used in this
          study.

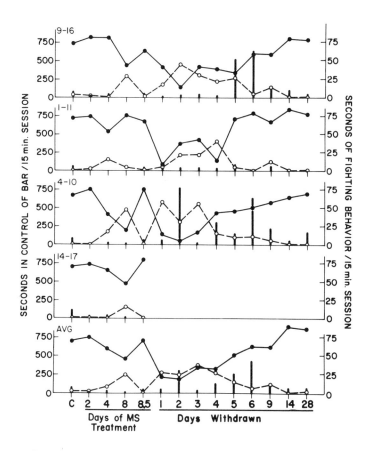

FIG. 2. <u>Distribution of paired responding and fighting behavior</u>
<u>during chronic morphine administration and withdrawal in both</u>
<u>members.</u> Numbers on the abscissa represent the behavioral ses-
sions as follows: C,the average of 4 control sessions; sessions 1-
3, behavior monitored 12 h after the fourth dose of 25 mg, 50
mg, and 100 mg MS/kg, respectively; session 4, behavior monitored
6 h after the fifth dose of 100 mg MS/kg; sessions 5-13, behavior
monitored 1-6,9,14, and 28 days, respectively, after the last dose
of morphine. Solid lines connecting points indicate lever-pressing
behavior emitted by the Dom member and dotted lines, the Sub animal, while the heavy vertical lines denote the amount of fighting
behavior during the sessions. Note the scale for fighting behavior is 1/10 that for lever-pressing behavior. Numbers in graphs to
the right of the ordinates represent the pair members. The bottom
panel labelled AVG illustrates the averaged data. The data obtained from pair 14-17 is not shown past the fourth session, because
the drinking tube in the home cage of rat 17 became clogged some-
time after the last dose of morphine. As a result,this member
ceased responding in the unpaired condition until several days
later when the problem was oorrected.In addition,one member of
pair 12-15(not shown) died during the period of morphine
administration.

TABLE 2. Effect of chronic morphine administration and withdrawal submissive rats

A. Behavior during morphine administration

		Control	25 mg MS/kg	50 mg MS/kg
Seconds in Control of the Bar	Dom	704 ± 22[b]	750 ± 25	605 ± 86
	Sub	10 ± 1.0	12 ± 6.8	86 ± 47
Seconds of fighting		7.5 ± 1.3	0.5 ± 0.5	2.2 ± 1.1
Unpaired FR-20 responses		1861 ± 48	1502 ± 84[e]	1504 ± 104[e]

B. Behavior during morphine withdrawal

Days of Abstinence		1	2	3	4
Seconds in Control of the Bar	Dom	209[d]± 104	184[d]± 95	337[d]± 84	317[d]± 89
	Sub	268 ± 160	238[d]± 114	354[d]± 102	258[d]± 78
Seconds of Fighting		4.5 ± 1.8	28 ± 25	3.0 ± 1.0	12 ± 9.3
Unpaired Responses		979[e]± 146	1443[e]± 82	1898 ± 81	2000 ± 101

[a] Unpaired and paired behavior was monitored 12 hr after the second
[b] Mean $\pm$ S.E. (paired N=4, unpaired N=8; during abstinence, paired
[c] Paired behavior at this time was monitored 6hr after morphine
[d] $p < .05$ when compared with control values (Student's 2-tailed t-
[e] $p < .01$ when compared with control values (Student's 2-tailed t-

on unpaired and paired responding and fighting by dominant and

100 mg MS/kg	100 mg MS/kg[c]	ANOVA
465 ± 117[d]	713 ± 36	F= 3.270, p < .02
241 ± 90[d]	3.3 ± 3.3	F=4.248, p < .005
0.8 ± 0.4	3.8 ± 1.2	F=2.174, p < .1
1458 ± 114[e]	---	F=5.918, p < .005

5	6	9	14	28	
496 ± 116	625 ± 83	600[d]± 31	755 ± 61	741 ± 29	F=5.595, p < .001
134 ± 61	54 ± 28	108[e]± 26	1.0 ± 0.3	3.5 ± 1.8	F=7.510, p < .001
25 ± 19	43 ± 21	14 ± 4.8	5.9 ± 2.9	6.5 ± 5.3	F= .908 p < .6
1971 ± 156	1994 ± 94	--	---	--	F=20.015 p < .001

and fourth dose of morphine sulfate (MS) respectively
N=3, unpaired N=6)
administration, unpaired responding was not evaluated
test for paired observations).

test for paired observations).

at any time display an increase in overt fighting. Paired
behaviors of all pairs were no different from control by the 14th
day of abstinence. Unpaired response rates were significantly
depressed during chronic morphine administration beginning with
the session 12 hr after the second dose of 25 mg/kg and 1 and 2
days after morphine was withheld (Table 2B).

Plasma corticosterone levels. As seen in Table 3, within 10-12 hr
after their last dose of MS, the animals in this experiment showed
a great increase in plasma corticosterone levels. This glucocorticoid remained significantly elevated for the duration of
plasma sampling, which lasted until 4 p.m. or at least 8 hr into
spontaneous withdrawal.

TABLE 3. Plasma corticosterone levels, measured every two hours
starting ten hours after the fourth and final 100 mg morphine
sulfate/kg dose

Time	Controls	Morphine
	μg/100 ml plasma	
6 a.m.	$(6.4, 3.7)^a$	7.7 ± 0.5
8 a.m.	6.8 ± 2.1	9.7 ± 2.1
10 a.m.	6.7 ± 1.5	17.6 ± 0.2^e
12 noon	7.4 ± 0.6	17.4 ± 3.5^b
2 p.m.	7.6 ± 1.1	18.6 ± 2.1^c
4 p.m.	6.1 ± 1.3	18.7 ± 2.0^d

[a] only 2 samples collected at this time, all other values represent
the mean $\pm$ S.E. of 4-5 rats

[b] p <.05 2 tailed Student's t-test for independent samples

c p <.01

[d] p <.005

[e] p <.001

The paired operant paradigm utilized in these experiments was
designed to incorporate a number of factors thought to contribute
to spontaneous aggression so that a continuous moderate level of
fighting between pairs of rats might be attained. These variables
include food competition (42), aversiveness of intermittent
schedules of reinforcement (25), and close subject proximity and

orientation (21, 54) made possible by competition for a single
response lever and food delivery trough. However, the results
are similar to those of Thompson and Bloom (50) in that the
initial fighting observed in the first pairings dissipated with
additional pairings. It is possible that responsing for food,
which has been shown to be incompatible with fighting behavior
(1), was responsible for the observed decrease in fighting.
Alternatively, novelty of an inanimate target or strangeness of
a second animal may elicit attack(36, 44). The paired rats may
have habituated to each other, thus decreasing overt aggressive
behavior (31).

While these variables undoubtedly contribute to the absence
of fighting observed in established pairs, the most important
factor appears to be the development of stable dominant-submissive hierarchies. Scott(43) has pointed out that the lack of
social organization is the major cause of fighting and mortality
in mice and rats.

The acute effects of 5 mg and 10 mg MS/kg on unpaired and
paired responding reflect the behavioral depressant effects of
the drug on individual FR responding (34,47,51). The anti-
aggressive, anti-psychotic drug profile of morphine (11) may
have additionally contributed to the disruption of 2 of the 5
hierarchies after acute administration to the Dom members (Fig.
1). The disappearance of this effect when both members were
administered the drug may have been due to aggressiveness being
reduced in both members, allowing the hierarchy to remain intact.

The increased fighting observed during withdrawal may be
related to irritable aggression (36), in that contact between
competing, hyperalgesic, and hyper-irritable rats (33,52) may
have initiated the aggression. Alternatively, the withdrawal
state may lead to disinhibition and/or loss of previous control
by the cue complex of the partner and social position, leading
to a breakdown of the established hierarchy which results in
increased fighting. Holtzman and Villarreal (23) have reported
that monkeys subjected to morphine withdrawal show great increases
in punished (by shock) responding for food pellets in those
animals which had low baseline rates of responding prior to
withdrawal. They concluded the effect of withdrawal on punished
behavior may be specific for behavior under aversive control, or
it may generally increase low rates of responding. Similarly,the
low or nonexistent rates of paired responding by Sub rats are also
presumably under aversive control. The cue complex of the Dom
rat, which normally maintains the Sub rat's low responding rates,
may no longer be attended to when the Sub rat is withdrawn. On
the other hand, the behavior of the withdrawn Dom rats may be
altered such that the stimuli which help maintain the hierarchy
are no longer emitted by this member.

Decreased paired responding by the Dom rats (Fig.2) during
withdrawal may be related to the decreased unpaired responding
early into withdrawal. This probably reflects a general
incapacity to respond because of the debilitating nature of the

syndrome. However, the paired responding by these members remained depressed even after unpaired response rates had recovered.
Additionally, withdrawal differentially increased paired responding by Sub members, even though unpaired responding was depressed
up to 50% 1-3 days after morphine was withheld.   Related to
these behavioral phenomena during withdrawal is the observation
that acute morphine administration to the Sub members eliminated
any residual aggression within the pairs but not when the Dom
members were given the same treatment. These results indicate
that the Sub member plays an integral role in both maintaining the
hierarchy and initiating aggressive episodes. This conclusion is
supported by a number of reports on the structure and maintenance
of dominant-submissive hierarchies (40,44).
     Uniquely interesting in the withdrawal experiments is that
identical treatments of the rats led to opposite results in paired
responding behavior,**depending**   on the hierarchal position occupied by the subjects.Paired responding by the Dom rats was decreased during withdrawal while this behavior was increased in
the Sub members. It is well known that the behavioral effects of
drugs are markedly influenced by the rate and temporal patterning
of on-going behavior(15,28). It is possible that withdrawal from
physical dependence-producing drugs may have similar rate-and
temporal-dependent effects on behavior. Moreover,it has been shown
that central biochemical changes induced by drugs or stressful
conditions are greatly influenced by the types of behavior the
animals are engaged in at the time treatment is administered(41,48).
There may have been interaction between hierarchal position and
morphine withdrawal which led to the behavioral differences
observed.
     It has been known for many years that acute morphine administra-
tion produces large increases in circulating glucocorticoids(45).
From the data presented in Table 3, it is apparent that the elevation is short-lived or that tolerance had depevolped to any such
effect because animals injected with saline showed similar corticosterone levels as the rats injected with morphine but sampled 8-
10 hr after 100 mg MS/kg. The only reasonable interpretation of
the tripling of this hormone in plasma is that it is a reflection
of a stress reaction to a chronic injection schedule in which 12
hr or longer may separate successive doses of morphine. Subjective
symptoms of withdrawal, including wet-dog shakes,ejaculation,and
irritability,were among those observed in this group of animals
upon handling at the time of their next injection,within days of
initiating the experiment.The question of whether or not morphine
withdrawal-induced aggression is a primary consequence unique to
this class of drugs or secondary to sub-acute stress in general,
remains to be elucidated.

II.PLASMA CORTICOSTERONE LEVELS IN RATS IMPLANTED WITH 75 mg
                     MORPHINE PELLETS

     Having observed the probability that animals on intermittent
injection schedules of morphine undergo cyclic episodes of with-

drawal,we undertook a series of experiments to determine is subcutaneous implantation of morphine pellets could eliminate what
appeared to be secondary effects of morphine administration(i.e.,
subacute stress). While implanting morphine pellets,as originally
suggested by Huidobro and Maggiolo(24)and formulated by Gibson and
Tingstad(18),resulted in an initial 25% suppression(P <.05, 2-
tailed paired t-test) of FR20 operant behavior the following day,
within 2 days behavior was back to control rates.Subsequent challenge by injections of naloxone over the succeeding 35 days indicated that equivalent(constant)degrees of disruption of the operant and associated body weight loss could be obtained for at least
11 days after a single pellet implantation(Gellert and Sparber,
submitted for publication).However,more recent studies with other
batches of morphine pellets indicated that significant differences
in degree of dependence(measured as body weight loss or as a withdrawal symptom profile)upon injection of naloxone,may be obtained
with morphine pellets from different sources(35).With this in mind
we analyzed plasma corticosterone levels of rats implanted with
75mg morphine pellets which gave a "stable"degree of dependence
for at least 6 days after subcutaneous implantation.
Subjects.Subjects were adult Sprague-Dawley males implanted with
intravenous catheters as described previously.Additionally,they
were implanted subcutaneously with either 75mg morphine pellets or
lactose placebo pellets and administered a dose of 0.4 mg of
naloxone HCl/kg(i.v.) three days later.

The results of this experiment are depicted in Fig.3.Two important factors should be considered.Firstly,the maximal increase in
plasma corticosterone occurred one hr after naloxone,decreasing
from a threefold elevation at this time to about two times the basal level 3hr after injection of the antagonist.This time course
of effect is almost identical to the operant behavioral disruption
observed after administration of various doses of naloxone to
morphine-pelleted rats in the study mentioned above(Gellert and
Sparber,submitted for publication).Secondly,basal levels of plasma
corticosterone were significantly elevated to twice that of placebo-implanted controls,prior to injection with naloxone.Naloxone,at
the dose employed,had no effect upon plasma corticosterone levels
in the control subjects.The elevated basal corticosterone levels
in morphine-pelleted rats raised the question of whether or not
pellet implantation techniques,while giving a reasonably constant
plasma or brain level of morphine for several days(3 4,38)might no
also be responsible for secondary and tertiary physiological or
biochemical changes which would mask or otherwise interfere with
studies in which primary mechanisms of opiate tolerance and /or
dependence are being sought.

III. ACUTE DEPENDENCE AND TOLERANCE

The only obvious alternative remaining was to resurrect and re-
examine the observation reported by Wikler and Carter(55)which
suggested that a single dose of morphine was adequate to produce
some form of physical dependence in the dog.Relatively large doses

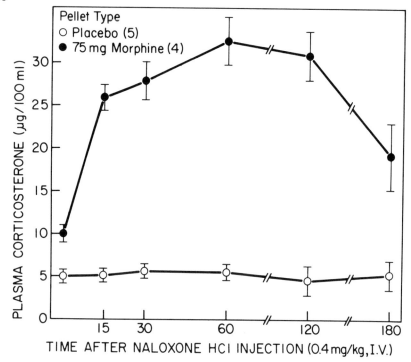

FIG. 3. <u>Plasma corticosterone levels in male rats implanted subcutaneously with 75 mg morphine or lactose placebo pellets.</u>
Numbers in parentheses next to appropriate legends denote the number of subjects in each group. Differences between morphine-implanted rats and placebo-implanted rats,both before and after
naloxone injection, are significant.
($p < .01$, 2-tailed test).

of morphine or slow release suspensions or infusions of morphine
have been used in several species but by and large,it has been
necessary to utilize antagonists to precipitate the various
symptoms used to assess physical dependence(8,9,29,32).As a consequence,interpretations of the results have tended to support
the idea that antagonists administered within minutes or hours of
a single dose of an opiate induce symptoms which, although
similar to those that have been used to measure dependence-with-
drawal, in fact may be masking the depressant properties of the
opiates, allowing stimulant properties to emerge and induce the
symptoms. Alternatively, the presence of the opiate might unmask
a stimulatory or other action of naloxone, which in turn could
cause jumping or other symptoms in mice (2,29). This latter
possibility is an attractive alternative in light of reports
that naloxone can itself induce behavioral effects at high
doses (e.g. >10 mg/kg) which may be augmented by pretreatment
with non-opiate agents such as theophylline and/or 5HTP (10).

Recently, however, Smits (46) reported significant increases in jumping by mice given subcutaneous injections of morphine in doses as low as 2 mg/kg, followed 1 hour later by doses of 2 mg and 16 mg/kg naloxone (i.p.), although 2 mg naloxone/kg produced the same number of jumps, regardless of whether the mice were pretreated with 2, 8, or 32 mg morphine/kg (s.c.) one hour previously. However, as suggested by Smits' data (46) and reviewed by Jacob (26), the acute pharmacological depressant effects of morphine have to be overcome if the antagonist is administered too soon after morphine, instead of at a time when the concentration of morphine in the CNS (or wherever else it might be acting) is low enough so as not to mask the withdrawal signs being observed and/or quantified. One advantage of conditioned behavior is that termination of the initial suppression of the operant by the acute depressant properties of morphine can be determined precisely because of continuous monitoring of the behavior. When the subject's behavior has returned towards baseline rates, the antagonist can be administered to determine if an otherwise behaviorally inactive dose of the antagonist will disrupt behavior. An example of how this procedure might be used to study individual differences in responsivity to opiates or antagonists among rats of the same strain or groups of rats from different sources (or of different strains) is depicted in Fig. 4. This subject was one of a group of male Long-Evans rats(Simonsen, Gilroy, Calif.) we received during the winter of 1975. They turned out to be much more sensitive to the effects of morphine than subsequent shipments of the "same" strain we received from the same source. A single dose of 15 mg MS/kg (11.3 mg morphine/kg, i.p.) completely suppressed FR responding for up to 7 hours. The subject depicted in the figure started to respond in a fairly regular manner about 4 hr and 15 min after this dose of morphine. After receiving 55 reinforcers (an arbitrary criterion) it was injected with saline and allowed to respond for another 15 min. Naloxone HCl, in a dose of 1 mg/kg (i.p.), completely and immediately suppressed responding during the succeeding 1 hr period the rat was left in the operant chamber. We have, on several occasions, allowed animals to remain in the operant chamber for several hours after challenge with 1-5 mg/kg naloxone following a single dose of 15 mg morphine/kg 3-5 hr earlier, without observing resumption of responding prior to removal from the chamber. Observations of this type support the idea that strain differences can profoundly influence studies of acute or single dose dependence or tolerance (37).

Additionally, because of the problems relating to interpretation of data acquired with the use of another agent(naloxone), we have used the same protocol and time course to determine whether single dose tolerance develops to the acute behavioral depressant properties of morphine. As in the previous experiments, plasma corticosterone was monitored as an additional measure of withdrawal, the implication again being made that stress of withdrawal will increase plasma glucocorticoids.

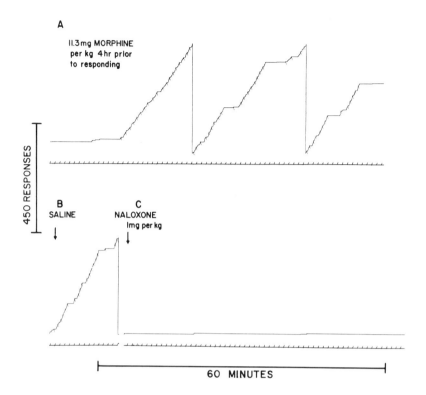

FIG. 4. Cumulative record of a male Long-Evans hooded rat given
a single dose of 15 mg MS/kg (11.3 mg morphine/kg) and placed in
the operant chamber immediately (A). Fixed-ratio 20 (for food
pellets) was completely suppressed for more than 4 hr, after which
time responding resumed at a reduced rate. When 55 reinforcers
were earned, the rat was injected with saline (B), which did not
affect responding. Fifteen min later an injection of 1 mg
naloxone HCl/kg (C) completely suppressed behavior for the next
hour. Rats given saline instead of naloxone at this time continue
to respond for the entire hour. Naloxone, at this dose, does not
suppress responding in morphine-naive subjects.

Naloxone-Precipitated Disruption of Operant Behavior in Rats
Given a Single Dose of Morphine Three Hours Earlier

Subjects. Adult male Long-Evans hooded rats (Simonson, Gilroy,
Calif. U.S.A.), approximately 3 months old at the start of the
experiment and weighing about 425 g, served as subjects.
They were housed in individual cages, deprived to 80% of their
free-feeding weights, and maintained as described previously for
the subjects used in the aggression study.
As in that study, 45 mg food pellets (P.J. Noyes Co.,Lancaster,

N.H.) were used as reinforcers with which to shape and maintain lever-pressing responses on fixed-ratio (FR) schedules of various amplitudes.   Different ratio requirements were utilized so that effects observed could not be assumed to be associated with a specific rate of behavior but could generalize across this parameter.   Behavioral sessions were conducted in standard operant boxes (Model 143-22, BRS/LVE, Beltsville, Md. U.S.A.) enclosed in sound-attenuating chambers equipped with closed-circuit video cameras.   Schedule and other environmental parameters were controlled and responses recorded by a computer-based interact system (BRS/LVE, Beltsville, Md. U.S.A.) in another room.   After responding had stabilized on a FR15 schedule of reinforcement, subjects were assigned to experimental or control groups in a semi-random manner such that animals were equally distributed between groups, based upon their individual response rates.   It had been previously established that 2.5 mg naloxone/kg was without significant effects upon FR behavior during various session lengths ranging from 15 min to 1 hr.   We replicated these experiments and were satisfied that this dose was without behavioral effects in these animals.

On the day of the morphine injection, the subjects were placed in the operant chambers for 5 min to collect baseline data for each rat.   They were then injected with 15 mg morphine/kg i.p. and returned to their home cages.   Three hours later they were placed within the operant chamber for a second 5 minute session to confirm that their behavior was not significantly different from baseline.   They were then injected with either 2.5 mg naloxone/kg or an equal volume of saline and returned to the operant chamber for analysis of their behavior over the succeeding 15 minutes.
Another group of rats, shaped to lever press on a FR5 schedule of reinforcement, was handled in an identical fashion except they were administered 30 mg morphine/kg three hours prior to challange with 2.5 mg naloxone/kg.

The results of this experiment indicate that administration of naloxone to rats which have been treated 3 hr previously with a single injection of morphine suppresses operant behavior immediately, and the degree of suppression is related to the dose of morphine given earlier.   Additionally, the effect is not restricted to a specific ratio requirement and hence, response rate.   Responses emitted by rats maintained on the FR15 schedule averaged about 100/min, while rats maintained on the FR5 schedule were emitting about 50 responses/min (post-reinforcement pauses are included in the estimates of responding/unit of time).   When 2.5 mg naloxone/kg was given to four rats pretreated 3 hr earlier with 15 mg morphine/kg, their response rate during the subsequent 15 minute period was suppressed significantly to

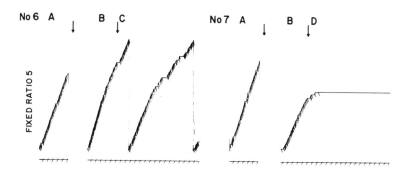

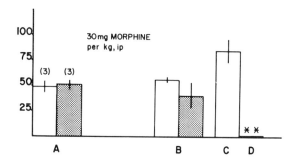

FIG. 5. <u>Suppression of FR5 responding for food pellet reinforcers</u>
<u>by 2.5 mg naloxone/kg injected into rats treated 3 hr previously</u>
<u>with 30 mg morphine/kg.</u> The upper portion of the figure shows
sample cumulative records of one subject in each group responding during a 5 min session immediately prior to morphine administration (A), during a 5 min session 3 hr later and immediately
prior to saline or naloxone administration(B), and during the
ensuing 15 min session after saline (C) or naloxone (D). The
event pen beneath the cumulative recorder pen denotes a 1 min time
base. Arrows indicate the points of injection. The bottom
portion of the figure represents the means (± S.E.) for each
group. The histograms above A show responses/min for the group
to be given saline (open) and the group to be given naloxone
(stippled)3 hr later. The histograms above B show responses/min
of each group 5 min immediately before saline or naloxone while
the histograms above C and D show the mean percent of baseline
(A). Notice the group given saline is responding at 75% of baseline while the group injected with naloxone is responding at
about 0% of baseline.   Numbers in parentheses denote the number
of subjects in each group.
** p < .01, Student's 2 tailed t-test.

about 35% of control (4 subjects injected with 2.5 mg naloxone/
kg 3 hr after saline). Fig. 5 shows the complete, immediate suppression of FR responding by 2.5 mg naloxone/kg 3 hr after 30 mg
morphine/kg.The complete suppression of responding after naloxone
was given to the latter group clearly shows the dose-related
nature of the phenomenon. Because behavior maintained by lower
ratio schedules is generally more resistant to disruption than
that maintained by schedules requiring greater response output
on the part of the subject, it is a more conservative estimate
of the effects of naloxone than that which would have been
observed had the group maintained on the FR15 schedule been
given the higher dose of morphine.

Plasma Corticosterone Levels in Rats Injected with a Single
Dose of Morphine and Challenged Two Hours Later with Naloxone

Because it appeared that a single dose of morphine can
produce dependence of a type which is manifest by suppression
of operant behavior when challenged with naloxone within a few
hours, it seemed appropriate to determine if a similar response
to naloxone would be manifest as an increase in plasma corticosterone levels. While a demonstration of a "stress reaction"
of this type would not in itself prove a state of physical
dependence (in contrast to a form of behavioral dependence unrelated to physical dependence) it would strengthen that notion.

Subjects. The source of subjects and methods used for this
experiment were as those described previously for corticosterone
determinations. After having recovered from the intravenous
catheter implantations, the animals were sampled for basal
plasma corticosterone levels. Immediately afterward they were
injected through the catheters with 10 mg MS/kg or saline.
(Because this strain seemed to be more sensitive to morphine
and the route of administration was i.v., lower doses of
morphine and naloxone were used). Subsequent samples were taken
at 15, 120, 135, and 180 minutes after injection of morphine.
Naloxone HCl (0.4 mg/kg) was injected through the catheters of
both groups immediately after the 120 minutes blood sample
was taken.

Within 15 minutes of the intravenous administration of
10 mg MS/kg plasma corticosterone levels went from about
4 µg/100 ml to about 17 µg/100 ml. The group administered
saline was not affected by the injection procedure. Two hr
after the first injection, while still elevated significantly
above the control group, the morphine group's plasma corticosterone levels had fallen back to about 10 µg/100 ml.
Administration of naloxone to half of each group resulted in
an immediate (15 minutes later) significant increase in plasma
corticosterone levels in the   morphine-treated group so that
it was twice that of its counterpart given saline instead of
naloxone.   The plasma corticosterone levels of the group

given naloxone 2 hr after saline, were not different from its
counterpart given saline 2 hr after saline (Fig. 6).
Interestingly, by 180 minutes after i.v. morphine administration,
the plasma corticosterone levels of the group given saline

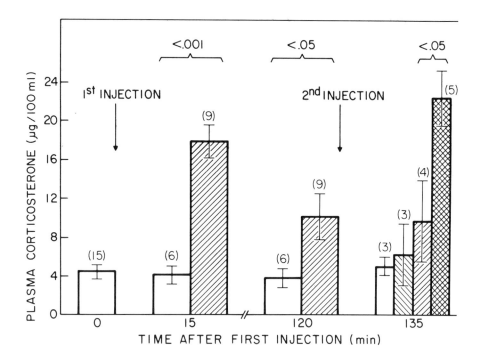

FIG. 6. Plasma corticosterone levels in response to intravenous
injections of MS (10 mg/kg) or naloxone HCl (0.4 mg/kg).
Catheterized rats had their blood sampled immediately before
saline or morphine. Additional samples were drawn at 15, 120,
135 and 180 min (data not shown) to determine the effects of
morphine and/or naloxone on plasma corticosterone levels. The
group injected with morphine is depicted by the histogram with
right to left descending diagonal lines while subgroups given
naloxone are depicted by histograms with left to right descending
diagonal lines. Values represent the means + S.E. and numbers
in parentheses denote the number of subjects in each group (wide
histograms) and subgroup (narrow histograms).
Statistical comparisons are between bracketed groups and the
level of significance was derived using Student's 2-tailed t-test
for independent samples.

instead of naloxone   had reversed their downward trend
and climbed to a mean of 17.3 (+ 2.2) μg/100 ml from 9.8
(+ 4.2) μg/100 ml 45 minutes before (p < .05, 1-tailed paired
t-test), indicating that spontaneous withdrawal might be
occurring.

We have previously observed operant behavior return between
2-5 hr after single doses of 10-30 mg of morphine/
kg but have not carried out the behavior observation periods
long enough to determine if another dip in behavior (suppression) could be seen during this period of "spontaneous withdrawal".   We did, however, originally observe what appeared
to be spontaneous withdrawal-induced suppression of operant
behavior 10-12 hr after the second dose of 25 mg MS/kg (unpaired
behavior monitored during the aggression study).

Tolerance to the Behavioral Suppressant Effects of Morphine by a Single Dose of Morphine Three Hours Earlier.

Naloxone has a pharmacology of its own, being capable of
suppressing FR operant behavior about 25% in rats at a dose of
10 mg/kg (Gellert and Sparber, submitted for publication).
It will also suppress eating behavior of 48 hr starved rats
given food noncontingently (22) and lower threshold to noxious
stimuli as well (27).   Whether this activity is related to
its interaction with endogenous morphine-like substances at the
receptor level remains to be elucidated.   As mentioned
previously, utilization of antagonists to demonstrate dependence
via the precipitation of withdrawal-like behaviors carries
with it the obvious drawbacks of interpretation.

Tolerance to opiates has never been clearly separated from
dependence, although many investigators claim to have separated
them temporally (perhaps owing mainly to the fact that different
"behaviors" were used to study tolerance and dependence, each
behavior being differentially sensitive to morphine's action).
One advantage which a study of tolerance affords is that a
second drug (naloxone) is not necessary to demonstrate
clearly the phenomenon.   Additionally, since morphine itself
suppresses operant (and obviously other) behavior, we could
use the same protocol as that used in the acute dependence
study to determine if tolerance develops over a different time
course than does dependence.

Subjects.   Methods and subjects were identical to those described for the acute dependence study. One slight modification
was used. Instead of allowing the subjects to remain in the
operant chamber for 5 min to collect daily baseline data and 5
min beginning 3 hr after morphine injection and prior to challenge with a dose of morphine,etc.,the animals were allowed 10
min in the chamber, injected immediately afterwards with saline,
3.75 mg or 7.5 mg morphine/kg, and placed back in their home
cages.   The 10 min session starting 3 hr after the first

injection was used to verify that behavior was at least back
to baseline rates. The second or challenge injection of
morphine (the first dose of morphine given to the group administered saline 3 hr previously) at a dose of 3.75 mg/kg was
administered and the rats placed immediately back in the operant
chamber for an additional 30 min, so that the suppressant
effects of morphine on behavior could be evaluated. Initially
it was thought that residual morphine from the first injection
might mask any tolerance to the second dose of morphine. The
demonstration by Dahlstrom et al. (13) that within 3 hr of an
intravenous injection of 2.5 mg morphine/kg, the concentration of
morphine in rat brain was less than the estimate of variability
(S.E.) of the peak brain concentration at 15 min prompted us to
disregard this potential problem and assume that an observation
indicating significant tolerance would be an understimate, if
anything, for the reason given above.

The results of this experiment (Table 4) clearly show tolerance to the behavioral suppressant effects of morphine given 3 hr
after an initial dose of morphine. The data for the last 30 min
of responding suggest, at first glance, that all groups were
suppressed by 3.75 mg morphine/kg. In fact, this was not the
case. FR responding subsides during a long session (40 min session in this case) because of satiation effects, so that the
73.3% and 78.3% of initial baseline rates in the morphine-pretreated groups is an underestimate of percent of control response
rates which would have been engendered during an equivalent session length. During the 5 days prior to injection with saline
or morphine, the rats were run for 30 min sessions as the terminal part of the shaping and stabilizing procedure. If responding
during the 30 min period after 3.75 mg morphine/kg is compared
with responding during the 30 min sessions run prior to the day
of injection, one sees a more clear-cut, almost complete tolerance. The rats given saline prior to morphine are responding at
41.8% (+14.7%,M + S.E.) of the baseline. Those pretreated with
3.75 mg or 7.5 mg morphine/kg are responding at 82.6% (+ 9.6%) or
85.6% (+8.3%)of 30 min "control" session baselines,respectively,
both of the latter groups (pretreated) rates being not
significantly different from their 30 min "controls".
It is therefore apparent that during the 3 hr interval, tolerance developed to at least one of the pharmacological actions of
morphine, after doses which are generally used for analgesia
studies. These data tend to extend or strengthen our acute
dependence data, as well as those of Smits (46), which indicate
that biochemical and physiological changes responsible for the
phenomena of tolerance and/or dependence,may start within a short
time (minutes to hours) after single doses of morphine which are
within the range of those used for studies of analgesia.
Such data raise questions about interpretation of experiments
in which pretreatment of animals with single, large analgesic
doses of morphine produced an increase in the capacity of naloxone

TABLE 4. Single Dose Morphine Tolerance

Initial Injection	10 min session prior to initial injection	10 min session prior to 3.75 mg/kg Morphine challenge	30 min session following 3.75 mg/kg Morphine challenge
Saline	102.6 ± 12.4[a]	116.4 ± 11.8[a] (115.4 ± 8.3)[b]	39.8 ± 13.8[c] $(\mathbf{38.0} \pm 13.2)$[b,d]
Morphine 3.75 mg/kg	106.2 ± 12.5	135.3 ± 19.6 (125.3 ± 5.8)	79.0 ± 12.2 (73.3 ± 5.6)
Morphine 7.5 mg/kg	103.9 ± 12.3	$120.6' \pm 16.6$ (116.2 ± 6.1)	80.9 ± 10.8 (78.3 ± 6.0)

[a] Mean $\pm$ S.E. responses/min for 5 rats/group on a FR15 schedule of reinforcement
[b] Mean % $\pm$ S.E. responses/min of initial 10 min session
[c] Mean $\pm$ S.E. responses/min for 30 minutes following morphine challenge
[d] $p < .02$ (ANOVA)

to antagonize analgesia caused by a second dose of morphine (2-24 hr later), compared with saline-pretreated animals (49,53). Since hyperalgesia-hyperirritability is a hallmark of withdrawal and corticosterone levels in plasma are elevated, it may be that animals exposed to identical intensities of noxious stimuli, determined by setting a dial, are in fact being subjected to more intense stimuli, as they perceive it, during withdrawal. Or, pituitary-adrenal activation resulting from withdrawal may antagonize the analgesic effect of morphine or allow greater accessibility of the antagonist to its receptor(s). The suggestion of spontaneous withdrawal 2-3 hr after about 7.5 mg morphine (10 mg MS)/kg i.v., coupled with the demonstrated tolerance to 3.75 mg or 7.5 mg morphine/kg, i.p., in both instances without the presence of an exogenous antagonist, is pertinent in two respects. Firstly, it strengthens the idea that tolerance and/or dependence are responsible for symptoms observed after a single low dose of morphine, instead of the unmasking of a stimulatory action of either a high dose of morphine or naloxone. Secondly, it questions the necessity of having to invoke an idea of a conformational change in the opiate-antagonist-receptor complex to explain enhanced efficacy of antagonists after a single dose of morphine.

CONCLUSIONS

The results of the aggression experiments demonstrate the utility of the operant competitive paradigm in objectively assessing agonistic behavior in rats. With it, increases in aggressiveness within individual members of a pair of rats can be determined by increases in overt fighting and/or changes in the distribution of responding between dominant and submissive members of a pair. Additionally, we are able to detect increases in what appear to be 2 types of aggressive behavior within morphine-withdrawn pairs of rats. Specifically, the increase in successful attempts to get at the response manipulandum and food trough by the withdrawn Sub rats reflects an increase in what appears to be spontaneous, inter-male competitive aggression. The dramatic increases in overt fighting when the Dom rats were withdrawn we interpret as an exaggerated irritable aggressive response by this member to the normal or elevated number of contacts initiated by Sub rats. The paradigm has the advantages of (1) objectively quantifying changes in aggressive behavior within pairs of rats,(2) identifying the behavior of the individual members of a pair and evaluating the contribution of each to the change in paired behavior and (3) accomplishing these ends without the aid of sensitizing agents (amphetamine or noxious stimuli). Additionally, it is apparent that injection schedules in which rats are administered morphine twice a day induce in these animals states of withdrawal during the injection periods which can confound studies on the physiology and biochemistry of tolerance/dependence.

Presently, the most parsimonious interpretation of our (and

other) tolerance dependence data, in our eyes at least, must include the phenomena of tolerance and dependence within a mutually inclusive framework. This implies that tolerance is the flip-side of dependence and is another, more subtle measure of withdrawal. Since increased reactivity and heightened level of arousal of the CNS is experienced during withdrawal, greater amounts of morphine are required to bring the organism's reactivity to its internal and external environment to that originally attained after the initial dose(s) of morphine. Because tolerance/dependence to opiates may occur rapidly, could it be that the positive reinforcing properties of opiates with high abuse liability (i.e., short t 1/2's) are mechanistically indistinguishable from their negative reinforcing properties and are part of the same process along an intensity continuum?. It may be that the moderate increased level of arousal of the CNS early into severe withdrawal, or during the course of mild withdrawal, is reinforcing and is partially responsible for drug-seeking and drug-taking behavior. This hypothesis, of course, would strain the dualistic nature of the medical model of addiction which implies that opiates produce euphoria via a direct depressant effect. If this were true, one would predict that animals dependent upon opiates would self administer very low doses of an antagonist. Such an effect has recently been reported by Downs and Woods (16), who showed that two morphine-dependent monkeys would self-administer 2 μg of naloxone/kg/infusion contingent upon responding on a second-order fixed – ratio schedule. In one monkey the naloxone infusion maintained behavior (which is disrupted by higher doses of naloxone) for only 8 sessions while in the second monkey, behavior (self-infusion of naloxone) was maintained for only 15 sessions. Since maximal morphine dosages were held constant at 10 mg/kg/day, a reasonable question to ask is whether or not dependence was maintained or whether the animals kept self-administering 10 mg/kg/day, the maximum allowed. Because of the varied behavioral and drug history of the subjects used in this study, it is difficult to completely interpret the data. However, the suggestion,that, under certain circumstances, narcotic antagonists can act as positive reinforcers needs further investigation.

ACKNOWLEDGEMENTS

Naloxone HCl was generously donated by Endo Laboratories, Garden City, N.Y.
Technical assistance of Ms. L.H. Fossom is gratefully acknowledged
Supported in part by grants from the U.S.P.H.S., GM01117,MH08565 and DA00532.

REFERENCES

1. Baisinger, J., and Roberts, C.L.(1972): J.Exp.Anal.Behav., 18: 535-540.

2. Barthelemy, C., and Jacob, J. (1972). J.Pharmacol.(Paris), 3: 530.
3. Berkowitz, B.A., Cerrets, K.V., and Spector, S. (1974): J.Pharmacol.Exp.Ther., 191: 527-534.
4. Blüsig, J., Herz, A., Reinhold, K., and Zieglgansberger, S. (1973): Psychopharmacologia, 33: 19-38.
5. Boreman, J., and Price, E. (1972): Anim.Behav., 20:534-542.
6. Boshka, S.C., Weisman, H.M., and Thor, D.H. (1966): Psychol. Res., 16: 541-543.
7. Brown, M.R., and Hedge, G.A. (1972): Neuroendocrinology, 9: 158-174.
8. Cheney, D.L., and Goldstein, A. (1971): Nature, 232: 477-478.
9. Collier, H.O.J., Francis, D.L., and Schneider, C. (1972): Nature, 237: 220-223.
10.Collier, H.O.J., Francis, D.L., Henderson, G., and Schneider, C. (1974): Nature, 249: 471-473.
11.Cook, L., and Weidley, E. (1957): Ann.N.Y.Acad.Sci., 66: 740-752.
12.Crabtree, J.M., and Moyer, K.E.(1973): Physiol.Behav., 11: 337-343.
13.Dahlstrom, B., Paalzow, G., and Paalzow, L. (1975): Life Sci., 17: 11-16.
14.Davis, M.H., and Khalsa, J.H. (1971): Life Sci., 10: 1321-1327.
15.Dews, P.B. (1958): J.Pharmacol.Exp.Ther., 122: 137-147.
16.Downs, D.A., and Woods, J.H. (1975): Pharmacol.Rev., 27: 397-406.
17.Gianutsos, G., Hynes, M.D., Puri, S.K., Drawbough, R.B., and Lal, H. (1974): Psychopharmacologia, 34: 37-44.
18.Gibson, R.D., and Tingstad, J.E. (1970): J.Pharm.Sci., 59: 426-427.
19.Glick, D., von Redlich, D., and Levine, S. (1964): Endocrinology, 74: 653-655.
20.Grant, E.C., and Mackintosh, J.H. (1963): Behaviour, 21:246-259.
21.Hinde, R.A.(1969): J.Psychosom.Res., 13: 213-219.
22.Holtzman, S.G. (1974): J.Pharmacol.Exp.Ther., 189: 51-60.
23.Holtzman, S.G., and Villarreal, J.E. (1973): J.Pharmacol.Exp. Ther., 184: 528-541.
24.Huidobro,F., and Maggiolo, C. (1961): Acta Physiol.Latinamer., 11: 201-209.
25.Hutchinson, R.R., Azrin, H.H., and Hunt, G.M. (1968):J.Exp. Anal.Behav., 11: 489-495.
26.Jacob, J.J.C. (1975): In: Proc.IX Congress of the Collegium Internat.Neuropsychopharmacology, Paris 7-12 July, 1974. Excerpta Medica, Amsterdam.
27. Jacob, J.J., and Michaud, G.M. (1974): Psychol.Med., 4: 270-273.
28. Kelleher, R.T., and Morse, W.H. (1968): Ergeb.Physiol.Biol. Chem.Exp.Pharmakol., 60: 1-56.
29.Kosersky, D.S., Harris, R.A., and Harris, L.S. (1974): Eur.J.

Pharmacol., 26: 122-124.
30. Lal, H., O'Brien, J., and Puri, S.K. (1971): Psychopharmacolo-gia, 22: 217-223.
31. Lorenz, K.(1966):On Aggression, Harcourt, Brace and World; New York.
32. Martin, W.R., and Eades, C.G. (1961): J.Pharmacol.Exp.Ther., 133: 262-270.
33. Martin, W.R., Wikler, A., Eades, C.G., and Pescor, F.T. (1963): Psychopharmacologia, 4: 247-260.
34. McMillan, D.E., and Morse, W.H. (1967): J.Pharmacol.Exp.Ther., 157: 175-184.
35. Meyer, D.R., and Sparber, S.B.(1976): Pharmacol. Biochem. Behav., 5: 603-607.
36. Moyer, K.E. (1968): Comm.Behav.Biol.(part A): 2: 65-87.
37. Mushlin, B.E., Grell, R., and Cochin, J. (1976): J.Pharmacol. Exp.Ther., 196: 280-287.
38. Patrick, G.A., Dewey, W.L., Spaulding, T.C., and Harris, L.S. (1975): J.Pharmacol.Exp.Ther., 193: 876-883.
39. Puri, S.K., and Lal, H. (1974): Psychopharmacologia, 35: 237-241.
40. Rowell, T.E. (1974): Behav.Biol., 11: 131-154.
41. Schoenfeld, R.I., and Seiden, L.S. (1969):J.Pharmacol.Exp. Ther., 167: 319-327.
42. Scott, J.P., and Frederickson, E. (1951): Physiol.Zool., 24: 273-309.
43. Scott, J.P. (1958): Aggression, University of Chicago Press, Chicago.
44. Seward, J.P (1945,1946): J.Comp.Psychol., 38: 175-197; 213-224; 225-238; V.39: 51-76.
45. Sloan, J.W. (1971): In: Narcotic Drugs, Biochemical Pharmacology, edited by D.H. Clouet, pp.262-282. Plenum Press, New York.
46. Smits, S.E.(1975): Res.Commun.Chem.Pathol.Pharmacol., 10: 651-661.
47. Sparber, S.B., Tilson, H.A., and Peterson, D.W. (1973): Pharmacol.Biochem.Behav., 1: 133-136.
48. Stolk, J.M., Conner, R.L., Levine, S., and Barchas, J.D. (1974): J.Pharmacol.Exp.Ther., 190: 193-209.
49. Takemori, A.E., Oka, T., and Nishiyama, N. (1973): J.Pharmacol. Exp.Ther., 186: 261-265.
50. Thompson, T.I., and Bloom, W. (1966): Psychon.Sci., 5: 335-336.
51. Thompson, T., Trombley, J., Luke, D., and Lott, D. (1970): Psychopharmacologia, 17: 182-192.
52. Tilson, H.A., Rech, R.H., and Stolman, S. (1973): Psychopharmacologia, 28: 287-300.
53. Tulunay, F.C.,and Takemori,A.E. (1974): J.Pharmacol.Exp.Ther., 190: 401-407.
54. Ulrich,R.,and Azrin,N.H. (1962):J.Exp.Anal.Behav.,5:511-520.
55. Wikler,A.,and Carter, R.L. (1953): J.Pharmacol.Exp.Ther., 109: 92-101.

Factors Affecting the Action of Narcotics, edited by
M.L. Adler, L. Manara, and R. Samanin.
Raven Press, New York©1978.

Factors to be Considered in Using Brain Lesions to
Study the Central Sites of Action of Narcotics

Martin W. Adler and Ellen B. Geller

Temple University School of Medicine
Department of Pharmacology
Philadelphia, Penna 19140 U.S.A.

INTRODUCTION

Destruction of discrete areas of the brain is a
technique that has been used for many decades not
only to study the normal physiological function of a
particular brain region but also to determine the site
of action of a variety of centrally acting drugs. One
need only scan the papers of the Symposium to see the
large percentage of investigators who either use
lesions in their own research or refer to the lesion
work of others in formulating and testing various
hypotheses relating to the actions of the opiates. It
is worthwhile, therefore, to examine the utility of
brain damage as a technique for studying narcotic
actions and to analyze the role that the specific
lesion plays in determining the effects of these drugs.
This discussion will be divided into 3 sections:
1) type of lesion;
2) chronicity of lesion;
3) locus of lesion.

Type of Lesion

Of the variety of means by which lesions can be
produced, only a few are employed for laboratory
studies of drug actions. These methods fall into five
broad (although not mutually exclusive) classes:
electrolytic, radiofrequency, ablation, cryogenic, and
chemical. Techniques such as knife cuts which entirely sever the neuronal connections to an area are really

93

modifications of the basic methods. Brain damage, by
whatever method, may be unilateral or bilateral. As
this factor is an important consideration in evaluating the results of lesion studies, one must be cogni-
zant of crossed and uncrossed afferent and efferent
anatomical pathways when unilateral lesions are used.

Electrolytic lesions may be further characterized
as anodal or cathodal, and a variety of metals can
serve as electrodes.   The size of the electrode,
characteristics of the metal, properties of the insu-
lating material, and current intensity and duration,
may be crucial factors. For example, if the current
used to create a lesion results in the deposition of
the electrode metal, a chronic irritative focus can
result (24). Both the duration and the intensity of
the current contribute to the size of the lesion (11).
The size of the electrode is also of critical importance, especially in small animals, since brain damage
is caused by the lowering of the electrode even in the
absence of an electrical current. Similar in some
respects to the electrolytic lesion, the radiofrequency lesion produces essentially no metallic deposition
and somewhat less damage to surrounding blood vessels
(23). For small, discrete areas of damage, however,
it may be advantageous to use electrolytic lesions
since one can achieve greater control of the lesion
size with a thin electrode and anodal current (15).
In the ablation technique, the entire tissue is
removed either by suction or by surgical resection (1,
18). Cryogenic lesions are like electrolytic, radiofrequency, and ablation techniques, in that all cells
in the area of the lesion are destroyed, or at least,
injured; the lesion is non-specific with respect to
the type of cell or tissue. An interesting application of the cooling technique is in making reversible
lesions in the brain, a task that cannot be accomplished with the other methods. A paper by Byck and
Dirlik (9) discusses the technique in detail. Which
of these four methods yields the sharpest delineation
of the damaged area and the most precise localization
of the lesion, is probably more a function of the
surgeon than of the method itself. All are useful
in investigating the influence of a particular anatomical locus.

The fifth type of lesion is the chemical lesion, as exemplified by 6-hydroxydopamine (6-OHDA) or 5,6 and 5,7-dihydroxytryptamine (DHT). Injected into various areas of the brain in low doses, these chemicals are relatively specific in that they will cause a selective destruction of certain nerve terminals (7,8,21). Little unspecific damage occurs with 6-OHDA as compared to other lesion techniques, and the extent of the lesion can be controlled by selection of an appropriate concentration of the drug (17). 5,6-DHT, on the other hand, is selective for indoleamine neurons only within a limited dose range and, in sufficiently high doses, can produce degenerative changes in peripheral noradrenergic and central catecholaminergic neurons (7) as well as unspecific damage to cells surrounding the injection cannula(8). Although even less specific than 5,6-DHT, 5,7-DHT is not as toxic and can be used effectively in conjunction with 6-OHDA pretreatment (8). When upsetting the natural balance of neurotransmitters in the brain, however, it should be remembered that these systems are not isolated entities and that a disturbance in one may exert some effect on another (20). Nevertheless, chemical lesions are a valuable method for investigating the influence of a particular neurotransmitter.

Chronicity of Lesion

A lesion may be produced at varying periods of time before drugs are tested. Although we have known for many years that the chronicity of a lesion is an important determinant of the response to drugs, this factor is all too often ignored. The classic work of Cannon and Rosenblueth (10) demonstrated the significance of the time course of a lesion on drug responses. If an acute lesion alters the response to a drug, one does not know if the change is due to damage to the lesioned area itself with its specific neurons (or to areas connecting with the lesion locus) or, alternatively, if the altered response is a reflection of edema, increased cerebrospinal fluid (CSF) pressure, or breakdown of the blood-brain barrier (BBB). With a drug such as morphine, the integrity of the BBB assumes critical importance since morphine penetrates poorly into the central nervous system(CNS) under normal BBB conditions. As an example of the difficulties in interpreting results with acute lesions, we might cite the work of Kerr and Pozuelo(19) and that of Teitelbaum et al. (29). Both of these laboratories have demonstrated a loss of tolerance to morphine in the rat after certain lesions (thalamus for Teitelbaum, ventromedial hypothalamus for Kerr). Yet both agree that they may be dealing, at least in part, with an altered BBB rather than simply an altered neuronal sensitivity to morphine (19,28).

The chronic lesion (i.e., one that has been placed months or years prior to testing) can also modify drug effects. Again, a variety of factors may affect the interpretation of the results. We observed, for instance, that the response to amphetamine and that to the convulsant drug, flurothyl, after acute bilateral cortical ablations in rats differed from the effect seen with chronic lesions (1,2). A diminished response resulted from acute lesions (one week), but an increased sensitivity to the drugs appeared after chronic lesions (3 months). The reversal occurred 2 to 8 weeks after the lesion, depending on the particular cortical locus. Just as one has to consider edema, altered CSF pressure, and BBB changes with acute lesions, chronic lesions may be associated with neuronal sprouting (22), loss of dendritic spines (30), and denervation supersensitivity (10,26). All of these factors must be taken into account in evaluating changes in drug responsivity following chronic lesions.

Locus of Lesion

Lesion experiments provide an invaluable tool for determining the sites of action of drugs. Used in conjunction with electrical stimulation experiments and electrophysiological recordings, they can precisely define the anatomical locus. It should be obvious that without histological verification of all lesion sites, one cannot be certain as to the exact extent of the lesion. Biochemical measurements cannot substitute for histological verification.

If it is observed that a lesion in a certain region modifies the action of a particular drug, what conclusions can be drawn from this finding? There are four basic ways in which such a result may be interpreted: 1) the anatomical site itself is a principal locus of action of the drug; 2) the anatomical site normally functions in maintaining levels throughout the brain of a particular chemical necessary for the action of the drug; 3) the anatomical site is important only in that crucial fiber pathways carrying impulses affected by the drug pass through the area; 4) the anatomical site alters the general level of cerebral excitability. Let us examine each of these possibilities in regard to the actions of narcotics.

The simplest interpretation one may give to the finding that a specific lesion modifies an action of a narcotic is that the anatomical site of the lesion is the critical area for that particular narcotic effect. If one is testing narcotics, for example, the lesioned area might contain the opiate receptors or specific neurons responsible for the particular action of the narcotic. As a case in point, we can look at the effects of thalamic lesions on the physical signs of narcotic withdrawal. On several occasions, it was observed that patients subjected to basal thalamotomies for the relief of intractable pain did not manifest physical signs of abstinence even though they had been previously dependent on narcotics (16,27). In attempting to duplicate this result in the morphine-dependent rat in collaboration with Dr. Gildenberg, we found that we could alter only certain specific signs of abstinence with acute lesions. Lesions of the centre median and parafascicularis (PF) nuclei lowered the incidence of wet-dog shakes and writhing, while jumping appeared to decrease only with lesions of the PF (3). Our interpretation of these results is that specific areas of the brain are involved with specific signs of narcotic abstinence. The possible relationship between the specificity of lesion locus with respect to signs of abstinence and the location of opiate receptors presents an intriguing avenue for future research.

A second interpretation to be considered if a lesion alters a drug effect is that the anatomical site of the lesion is essential for the maintenance of a particular chemical in the brain. Evidence that a lesion changes brain levels of that chemical in addition to some drug action may imply a causal relationship between the two. To illustrate, we can point to the effect that lesions of the locus coeruleus have on catecholamines and that which raphe lesions have on serotonin. The reports from Dr. Samanin and his co-workers that midbrain raphe lesions not only decrease forebrain levels of 5-HT but diminish the antinociceptive activity of morphine are representative of how one can interpret lesion effects on the basis of a specific neurochemical system (4, 25).

A third possible explanation for an altered effect of a drug after a brain lesion presumes that the lesion is located in an area containing anatomical pathways critical to the drug action (rather than the specific target neurons). In order to evaluate this possibility, one must place lesions in areas where the fiber pathways arise and note whether effects are similar to those observed following the original lesion. The multitude of interconnections between the various nuclei that comprise the limbic system, for instance, necessitates placement of lesions in several parts of the system before assigning a particular action to one site. Any conclusion as to the site of critical importance would result from an analysis of the afferent connections to and from the lesion locus. Studies by Wikler and his colleagues (31), Costall and Naylor (13), Foltz and White (14) and Charpentier (12) point to the limbic system as being involved in at least some actions of morphine. We have looked at the effect of acute and chronic lesions of this system on morphine abstinence and, in many cases, it appears that the effects we have noted are found with lesions throughout the system, rather than specific to one nucleus (3).

The fourth interpretation maintains that the particular lesion affects the general level of cerebral excitability. This view is particularly important when considering some of the actions of narcotics. We know that morphine is a drug which possesses both excitatory and inhibitory properties and that the relative balance between the two is, to some degree, species - dependent. If a certain lesion alters general cerebral excitability, it may influence a particular narcotic action merely by virtue of its changing the responsiveness of neurons to the drug. For example, it was demonstrated several years ago that a characteristic of the morphine abstinence syndrome in the rat was a decrease in seizure threshold (6). Recently, we also reported that acute morphine produces a dose-related anticonvulsant effect in the rat (5). One must allow for possible changes in CNS excitability in assessing the role of a specific lesion on other actions of morphine.

In summary, lesion experiments provide an excellent and indispensable means of investigating the sites and mechanisms of narcotic action, as long as care is exercised in interpreting the results of these experiments. When combined with neurochemical and neurophysiological studies, lesioning is an important means of studying narcotic action. With the spectacu-lar advances being made in the field of opiate receptors, one can envision an even greater importance of lesion studies in the future.

ACKNOWLEDGEMENTS

The authors would like to express their thanks to Lorraine Costella for typing the manuscript. This work was supported in part by U.S.P.H.S. grant DA 00049 and DA 00376 from the National Institute on Drug Abuse and research grant 719 from the North Atlantic Treaty Organization.

REFERENCES

1. Adler, M.W. (1961): J.Pharmacol.Exp.Ther., 134: 214-221.
2. Adler, M.W. (1966): J.Pharmacol.Exp.Ther., 153: 396-400.
3. Adler, M.W., Geller, E.B., Beeton, P.B., Klemfuss, H., and Gildenberg, P.L. manuscript in preparation.
4. Adler, M.W., Kostowski, W., Recchia, M., and Samanin, R. (1975): Eur.J.Pharmacol., 32: 39-44.

5. Adler, M.W., Lin, C.H., Keinath, S.H., Braverman, S.,and Geller, E.B. (1976): J.Pharmacol. Exp.Ther., 198: 655-660.

6. Adler, M.W., Lin, C.H., Smith, K.P., Tresky, R., and Gildenberg, P.L. (1974): Psychopharmacologia, 35: 243-247.

7. Baumgarten, H.G., Bjorklund, A., Lachenmayer, L., Nobin, A., and Stenevi, V. (1971): Acta physiol. Scand., suppl. 373: 1-15.

8. Baumgarten, H.G., and Lachenmayer, L. (1972): Z. Zellforsch.Mikroskop.Anat., 135: 399-414.

9. Byck, R., and Dirlik, P. (1963): Science, 139: 1216-1218.

10.Cannon, W.B., and Rosenblueth, A. (1949): The Supersensitivity of Denervated Structures, MacMillan Co., New York.

11.Carpenter, M.B., and Whittier, J.R. (1952): J.Comp. Neurol., 97: 73-117.

12.Charpentier,J.(1967):Psychopharmacologia,11:95-121.

13.Costall, B., and Naylor, R.J. (1974): Psychopharmacologia, 35: 203-213.

14.Foltz, E.L., and White, L.E. Jr. (1957): J.Neurosurg., 14: 655-673.

15.Gildenberg, P.L. (1957): Conf.Neurol.,17:299-309.

16.Gildenberg, P.L., personal communication.

17.Hokfelt, T., and Ungerstedt, U. (1973): Brain Res., 60: 269-297.

18.Kennard, M.W., Spencer, S., and Fountain, G. (1941): J. Neurophysiol., 4: 512-524.

19.Kerr, F.W.L., and Pozuelo, J. (1971): Mayo Clin. Proc., 46: 653-665.

20.Kostowski, W., Samanin, R., Bareggi, S.R., Marc, V., Garattini, S., and Valzelli, L. (1974): Brain Res., 82: 178-182.

21.Kostrzewa, R.M., and Jacobowitz, D.M. (1974): Pharmacol.Rev., 26: 199-288.

22.McCouch, G.P., Austin, G.M., Liu, C.N., and Liu, C. Y. (1958): J.Neurophysiol., 21: 205-216.

23.Reynolds, R.W.(1963): Science, 141: 930-932.

24.Reynolds, R.W.(1963): Am.J.Physiol., 204: 60-62.

25.Samanin, R., Gumulka, W., and Valzelli, L. (1970): Eur.J.Pharmacol., 10: 339-343.

26.Sharpless, S.K. (1964): Ann.Rev.Physiol., 26: 357-388.

27.Spiegel, E.A., Wycis, H.T., Szekely, E.G.,
    Gildenberg, P.L., and Zanes, C.(1964): J.Internat.
    Coll.Surg., 42: 160-168.
28.Teitelbaum, H., personal communication.
29.Teitelbaum, H., Catravas, G.N., and McFarland, W.L.
    (1974): Science, 185: 449-451.
30.Ward, A.A.Jr. (1966): In: Nerve as a Tissue, edited
    by K. Rodahl and B. Issekutz,Jr . Harper & Row,
    New York.
31.Wikler, A., Norrell, H., and Miller, D. (1972):
    Exp.Neurol., 34: 543-557.

Factors Affecting the Action of Narcotics, edited by
M.L. Adler, L. Manara, and R. Samanin.
Raven Press, New York ©1978.

Effect of Morphine on the Transmission of Painful
Messages at the Spinal Level

Jean Marie Besson and Daniel Le Bars

INSERM, Unité 161, Groupe de Recherche de Neurophysiol.
Pharmacologique, 2 rue d'Alésia, 75014 Paris, France.

INTRODUCTION

Since evidence has been advanced showing a central
site for the analgesic action of narcotics (77) many
electrophysiological investigators have tried to
localize central nervous structures involved in pain
mechanisms and also sensitive to these drugs. Nevertheless, the interpretation of works related to supraspinal structures is not easy for the following
reasons:
   - A large number of these studies concerned macro-
physiological phenomena (evoked potentials, EEG, etc.)
which are difficult to interpret per se.
   - From a methodological point of view, the macro-
physiological phenomena such as the data obtained by
recording supraspinal evoked potentials are not always
relevant to pain. In most cases, the supraspinal
evoked potentials have a short latency (at the utmost
a few tens of milliseconds); but it is well known
that the latency of spinal cell responses induced by
the activation of unmyelinated C fibres* is at least

----

* The leading role of the thin fibres ($A\delta$ and C) in the
transmission of painful messages is well known; initial
evidence obtained in animals by Adrian (3) and
Zotterman (137) has been confirmed in man by stimulating cutaneous nerves (27,70) or recording single fibres
with transcutaneous microelectrodes (50,121,124).
The recent review by Burgess and Perl (24) provides
information related to nociceptive fibres.

200-300 milliseconds. Thus, the painful messages have not
yet reached the first spinal relays when the supraspinal evoked potentials occur. Consequently, in most
cases, any pharmacological manipulation of such evoked
potentials cannot be related to analgesia.

- In spite of recent progress, our physiological
knowledge of pain mechanisms at the higher central
nervous structures is still insufficient and, thus,
the electrophysiological approach to narcotic action
at these levels is incomplete.

The present review will not go into all the entire
data related to the modalities of the antinociceptive
action of morphine. An attempt at drawing attention
to recent data and hypotheses will be made with special
references to spinal mechanisms. The gate control
theory of pain proposed by Melzack and Wall (89) led
during the last decade to many investigations and to
the concept of the management of both transmission and
integration of painful messages at the spinal level
(see ref. 14). For instance, the cells receiving
nociceptive afferences, and the cells at the origin of
ascending pathways (spinothalamic, spinoreticulo-
thalamic and spino-cervico-thalamic tracts) were
localized and characterized. Nowadays, the spinal cord
cannot be considered as a "cable" connecting peripheral
receptors to the brain: At the spinal level various
control systems have an effect on the transmission of
cutaneous messages. These controls are both of local
(segmental) and supraspinal origin (mainly from the
brainstem). They lead to a modulation of afferent
messages activating dorsal horn interneurons which
project directly or indirectly onto the higher central
structures.

On the basis of these integrative properties of the
spinal cord, two hypotheses (Fig.1), which are not
mutually exclusive, have been advanced to explain the
depressive effect of morphine on the transmission of
painful messages at this level.
1) A direct depressive action
2) An indirect effect by strengthening descending inhibitory controls of brainstem origin.

As schematically indicated on Fig.1, these two major
hypotheses have to be completed: for instance effects
of narcotics on higher supraspinal structures (Fig.1:3)

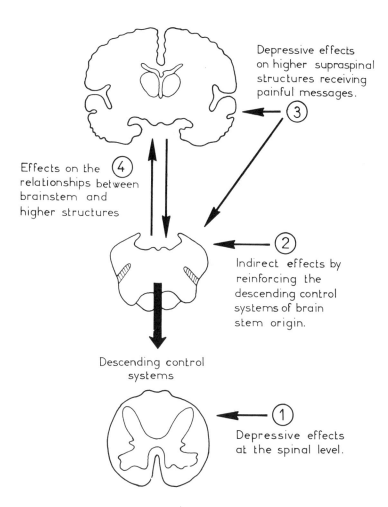

Depressive effects
on higher supraspinal
structures receiving
painful messages.

③

Effects on the ④
relationships between
brainstem and
higher structures

②

Indirect effects by
reinforcing the
descending control
systems of brain
stem origin.

Descending control
systems

①

Depressive effects
at the spinal level.

Fig. 1. Schematic representation of some hypotheses on
the sites of the antinociceptive action of morphine.

are well known and their effects on the relationships
between brainstem and higher structures (Fig.1:4) cannot be excluded.

I. Direct Depressive Effect of Morphine at the Spinal
Cord Level

This data was obtained on animals whose spinal cord

was acutely or chronically cut (spinal preparations).
Initial investigations concerned spinal reflexes and
more recent approaches considered the effects of
morphine on the activities of dorsal horn interneurons
involved in the transmission of painful messages.

a) Effects of Morphine on Spinal Reflexes

Wikler (131) and Wikler and Frank (132) clearly
showed in the spinal dog that morphine (5 mg/kg) or
methadone (2 mg/kg) greatly depressed polysynaptic
nociceptive reflexes. These results were confirmed by
many authors (18,58,66,68,87). It is worthwhile pointing out that larger doses of morphine (15 mg/kg) are
needed to depress monosynaptic reflexes.
The depressive effects of morphine are specific since
they are immediately reversed by nalorphine or naloxone.
These results, obtained in the three last decades,
are homogenous and give clear evidence of a direct
depressive effect of narcotics at the spinal cord level.
Nevertheless they are mainly concerned with motor
reflexes and were not necessarily related to analgesia.
We have tried to approach the problem of the effects
of morphine (28,71,72,73,74) and synthetic narcotics
(16,31) on various activities of dorsal horn cells
involved in pain processes.

b) Effect of Morphine on Dorsal Horn Cell Activities

Available data provide strong evidence that lamina V
dorsal horn cells (according to Rexed,104) play a major
role in the integration and transmission of painful
messages. As initially described by Wall (129) and
Hillman and Wall (54) these units are activated by
cutaneous stimulations applied to their large peripheral receptive fields. A threshold gradient between
the field center and its periphery is often observed:
low intensity stimuli are effective in the center
while more intense ones (pinch, pressure, pin-prick)are
required to obtain a response at the periphery. Their
firing rate is generally directly related to the
peripheral stimulus strength including those at the
most noxious levels. They are preferentially activated
by small cutaneous afferent fibres A$\gamma$and C (46,90,100,

101, 128), by intra-arterial injections of bradykinin
into the limbs (13,15) and by visceral stimulation (99,
112).   Lamina V type cell activities are modulated both
by segmental and supraspinal controls (see references
in 14).   Recent anatomical and electrophysiological
studies showed that some of them are at the origin of
spino-cervico-thalamic and spinothalamic ascending
pathways in several species (9,20,21,22,23,43,122,133).

These data, showing the role of lamina V type
cells in pain processes, underline their importance in
the study of analgesics at the spinal level.   For this
purpose, long duration extracellular recordings were
made in the spinal cat, using glass micropipettes fil-
led with KCl 3M.   Recorded cells were characterized
according to their electrophysiological properties and
localized by extracellular injections of pontamine sky
blue (28,71,72,73,74).

The effects of morphine (2 mg/kg i.v.) were studied
on various types of cellular activities: spontaneous
activity, responses to natural cutaneous stimulation
of strong intensity, responses to supramaximal transcutaneous electrical stimulation applied in the center
of the peripheral receptive field.   In addition,
responses to threshold electrical stimulation were
also studied.

The results of these studies indicate that morphine
and morphine-like agents substantially depress both
spontaneous and evoked activities.   Spontaneous firing
rate was reduced to 49% of its mean initial value;
responses to intense natural stimulation (strong
pinches) were decreased by 50%; responses to supramaximal electrical stimulation were reduced to 67% of
their mean initial level.   In this case, morphine preferentially depresses responses of long latency and
duration which are due to the activation of small afferent fibres.   On the other hand the first short lasting component of the responses to supramaximal electrical stimulation and the responses to threshold electrical stimulation, which are both due to the activation
of large myelinated fibres, were unaffected by the
drug.   The depressive effects of morphine are specific
since they were immediately reversed by the administration of an opiate antagonist (nalorphine or naloxone).

These data clearly show a direct depressive effect

of morphine at the spinal level since a supraspinal
site of action of the drug (by strengthening descending inhibitory controls) was excluded in these experiments, because of the spinal cervical transection.
They are in good agreement with previous reports on
spinal reflexes (see above) and with more recent electrophysiological studies.   For instance Kitahata et
al. (65) also observed a depression of spontaneous
activity of Lamina I and V interneurons after intravenous morphine administration.   Nevertheless this effect was, in their study, of very short duration (10
minutes) contrasting with our time course curves
(lasting at least 40 minutes) which were much more
consistent with analgesia obtained in clinical practice.   A direct depressive effect on dorsal horn interneurons   was likewise obtained during iontophoretic
application of morphine (25, 32, 136).   With few
exceptions (32) these works showed that morphine depresses responses induced by peripheral nociceptive
stimulation (pinch, radiant heat).   Furthermore, the
specificity of these effects is established since they
are reversed by both iontophoretic and intravenous
administration of naloxone.   Additional experiments by
the above authors using intravenous injections of
morphine gave results similar to ours.
   The same conclusions can be put forward when studying the effects of morphine-like agents on dorsal horn
interneurons : phenoperidine (16), fentanyl (26,59),
meperidine (26) and levorphanol (136).   In the same way
lamina V interneurons   are depressed by Viminol (31),
a synthetic derivative of pyrrylethanolamines.   In
this case, using several stereoisomers of Viminol, a
significative correlation has been shown between the
analgesic properties of the isomers (appraised by classical pharmacological tests) and their depressive effects upon lamina V interneurons..
   These data indicate that dorsal horn unit responses
to nociceptive stimulations are preferentially depressed by morphine and morphine-like agents while responses
induced by weak stimuli are unaffected.   In other
words, a dissociative effect of these drugs is observed
on responses of individual convergent dorsal horn units
to both nocuous and innocuous stimuli.
   We have attempted to pinpoint the effects of

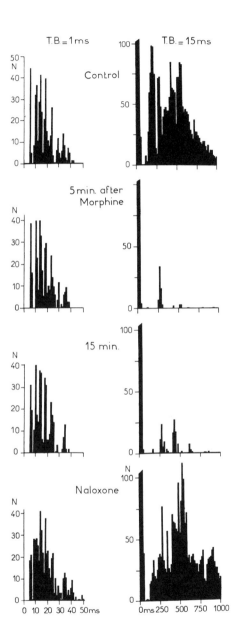

FIG. 2. Effects of morphine on responses of a dorsal
horn Lamina V type cell to stimulation of the sural
nerve (see text).

morphine on responses elicited by the stimulation of
large and thin afferent fibres (71). The responses of
lamina V type cells were induced by electrical stimulation of the sural nerve; they were generally polymodal
and their different components were classified in
responses due to Aα , Aγ and C fibres input according
to their latency related to the conduction velocity of
each group of fibres (23,39,40). Figure 2 shows post-
stimuli histograms obtained by the accumulation of 50
responses of a lamina V cell induced by the sural nerve
stimulation. On the left, only the first component
(brief latency, short duration) of the responses
related to myelinated large fibres input is shown;
morphine (2 mg/kg,i.v.) has very little effect, if any,
on this component. On the right,with a 15 times longer
time base, the entire response is shown; the first
short-lasting component is truncated, but the late
long-lasting (about 800 milliseconds) one related to
unmyelinated C fibres input can be observed. There is
dramatic reduction of this last activity after morphine
administration and total recovery following naloxone
injection. The upper part of Fig.3 shows the mean
results obtained in this study. Responses elicited by
Aα fibre input were unaffected; responses elicited by
A γ fibre input were decreased by 40%, and responses
elicited by C fibre input were decreased by 70%.

Knowing the role of small diameter afferent fibres
in pain processes (17,73,124,137), the preferential
depressive effects of morphine on the responses of
lamina V type cells to activities in this kind of fibre
could, to some extent, explain the analgesic properties
of this drug especially as the opiate antagonist
naloxone specifically reversed this action.

Although the effects of morphine were studied on
various preparations including squid giant axons (38),
Renshaw cells (29,33,35), mammal peripheral fibres (67,
127) etc., the detailed mechanisms of the depressive
effects described above are still unknown. A peripheral site of action seems to be excluded (67,77); as
shown in the lower part of Fig. 3 the neurogram of C
fibres recorded on the sural nerve is not affected by
morphine or naloxone. Thus, the depressive effect is
relevant to a central site of action. The differential
effects on responses evoked in the same cell by differ-

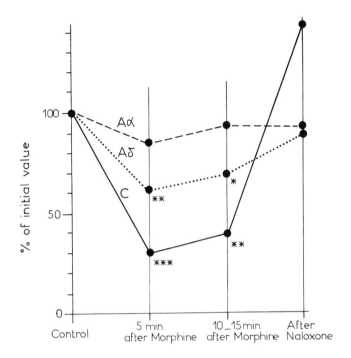

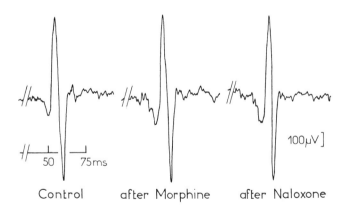

FIG.3. <u>Top</u>: mean curves showing the differential effects
of morphine and naloxone on responses of lamina V cells
to A and C fibre stimulation.
<u>Bottom</u>: In contrast, on the sural nerve the peripheral
action potential (average of 50 responses)due to C fibre
activation is not affected by administration of the two
drugs.

ent groups of fibres might suggest a presynaptic site
of action, already proposed by different authors (25,
64). But a direct post-synaptic site of action has
now been demonstrated (136). Nevertheless, action on
synaptic transmission of small diameter afferent fibres
or on the interneuronal network cannot be excluded.

The studies described, on spinal preparations,
clearly show a depressive effect of morphine as early
as the first spinal relays of pain pathways. The
recent finding (97,115) of specific opiate receptors
at the level of the substantia gelatinosa of Rolando
(Laminae II and III of the dorsal horn) supports this
conclusion, because of the proposed inhibitory role of
this structure on other dorsal horn cell activities(89)

II. Indirect Effect by Strengthening Descending
Inhibitory Controls

This hypothesis is supported by three kinds of data
using various methodologies: electrophysiological
investigations using intravenous injections of morphine,
studies using intraventricular and intracerebral
injections of morphine, and experiments showing an
analogy between morphine analgesia and analgesia induced by electrical stimulation of some brain stem
structures.

a) Electrophysiological Studies Using Intravenous Injections of Morphine

As early as 1955, Takagi's group (117) postulated
that the depressive effect of morphine on spinal re -
flexes could mainly be explained by the strengthening
of descending inhibitory controls of brainstem origin.
Comparing this depressive effect in intact, thalamic,
decerebrated and spinal preparations, they show in all
except the spinal preparation, a depressive effect of
morphine on polysynaptic discharges induced by sciatic
nerve stimulations. Complementary experiments (110,
111) confirmed their hypothesis. Nevertheless, as
mentioned above, it is difficult to reject that
morphine may have a direct spinal depressive effect;
furthermore these results were much debated (63,72,73,
114). For instance, in the decerebrate cat, we were

unable to demonstrate exacerbation of inhibitory controls of brainstem origin on lamina V type cell
activities; the effect of morphine was surprisingly
small on this type of preparation (72,73).
This lack of effect could be interpreted on the basis
of recent physiological data which show that the brainstem powerfully and tonically inhibited the dorsal
horn cell activities, especially those induced by
noxious stimuli (15,20,51). Thus the dorsal horn
interneurons are already strongly inhibited prior to
any pharmacological manipulation. Direct electrophysiological evidence of an increase in the descending
inhibitory controls after morphine administration must
therefore be sought for in intact preparations.
Nevertheless the following alternative methodological
approaches strongly support the initial hypothesis.

b) <u>Pharmacological Studies Using Intraventricular and
    Intracerebral Injection of Morphine</u>

Applying micro amounts of morphine to ventricular
(2,55,78), hypothalamic (37,79,80) and gray matter
surrounding the third ventricle (123) or the aqueduct
(61,62,74,113,130,135) induced strong analgesia. This
suggests that opiate receptors related to analgesia
are located in the vicinity of the ventricular system.
With the object of localizing the sites involved, Herz
and coworkers (10,52,53,120,125) perfected a method
for injection of morphine in restricted areas of the
ventricular system in the chronic rabbit; autoradiographic controls indicated that morphine was only dif-
fusing within the bordering inner surface of this
system. Analgesic tests were the threshold variation
of responses to tooth pulp electrical stimulation on
one hand, and thermal or electrical stimulation of the
hindlimb on the other (52,125). Morphine administered
in the rostral part of the fourth ventricle induced an
almost complete blockade of the segmental nociceptive
reactions whereas more rostral administration was ineffective. In these experiments, the intraventricular
route was 500 to 1000 times more potent than the
intravenous one. In complementary studies, these
authors showed that the administration of opiate
antagonists (nalorphine, levallorphan) in the fourth

ventricle almost abolished the analgesic properties of
systemic injections of morphine (10,52,125). They
suggested that the main active site was located in
the rostral part of the fossa rhomboides. In addition,
binding autoradiographic localization of morphine diffusion with its analgesic effect enabled them to prove
that this site was 1 mm from the inner surface of the
ventricle (120). By this route, the latency of the
analgesic properties of opiates is in function of their
liposolubility; for instance morphine acted slowly
whereas fentanyl shows a quicker onset.

These results are in good agreement with Takagi's
hypothesis and emphasize the brainstem periventricular
structures as a main morphological substrate for
narcotic analgesia. For Herz et al. the effects
observed are not related to a direct spinal mechanism
since the C^{14} morphine concentration was insufficient
at this level when administered intraventricularly.
It seems harder to pinpoint morphine's modality of
action when administered by the intravenous route;
experiments in which systemic injection of morphine
was associated with central administration of an
antagonist do not exclude a direct spinal site of
action for the opiates because of the fast vascular
resorption of the antagonist;very shortly after
ventricular injection, levallorphan was present in
detectable amounts at the spinal lumbar level (53).
Thus the antagonistic effect of levallorphan might be
at the segmental level and may, to some extent, play
a part in the discontinuance of analgesia. Nevertheless, Herz and coworkers suggested that the analgesic effect of opiates is mainly related to a brainstem mechanism.

To explain this mechanism, one might postulate that
morphine strengthens the descending inhibitory controls of brainstem origin. However, the inhibitory
bulbar reticular formation is located in the ventral
part of the brainstem (34,81,82) and microinjection of
morphine at this level does not inhibit nociceptive
spinal reflexes (125). Therefore, these authors suggested that this inhibitory system might be activated
indirectly, when morphine acts on the floor of the
rostral part of the fossa rhomboides, but still do not
exclude the possibility of a blockade of descending

facilitatory mechanisms.

c) Analogy Between Morphine Analgesia and Analgesia Induced by Stimulation of Some Brainstem Structures.

   The first observation was reported by Reynolds(105);
electrical stimulation of the periaqueductal gray
matter in the rat induced strong enough analgesia to
perform a laparotomy. This initial observation was
investigated in detail by Liebeskind and coworkers(42,
85,86) in the same species and confirmed in the cat
(47,76,88,92,96), monkey (44) and man (1,106,107).
Some characteristics of this analgesia obtained in the
rat are described by Akil et al. in this volume. We
will underline that in the cat, at the mesencephalic
level, the analgesic effects are obtained by stimulating the ventral part of the periaqueductal gray matter
(92, 96), near the dorsal raphe nucleus, rich in
serotoninergic cell bodies. We recently confirmed (94,
95,103) the role of serotoninergic structures in this
phenomenon by observing particularly strong analgesic
effects induced by the stimulation of posterior nuclei
of the raphe (mainly Magnus nucleus). These results
have been confirmed in the rat (91,102).
   All these data suggest that this kind of analgesia
is a result of active processes inducing a blockade of
the pain pathway in the central nervous system. One
of these processes might be activation of descending
inhibitory systems which control the transmission of
nociceptive messages at the spinal level. Thus,
central stimulation resulted in suppression of polysynaptic reflexes (85,86) in the rat and of the jaw
opening reflex obtained by tooth pulp stimulation in
the cat (96). Microphysiological data gave convincing
evidence of such an activation. In the cat,we demonstrated powerful inhibitory effects on dorsal horn
lamina V type cell activities during stimulation of
both the ventral part of the periaqueductal gray matter
in the vicinity of the dorsal raphe nucleus (76,92)
and the raphe magnus (49). These inhibitory effects
were preferentially on responses induced by nociceptive
stimuli while those induced by light cutaneous stimuli
were unaffected. The morphological substrate of this
inhibitory pathway is described since the posterior

raphe nuclei have dense tryptaminergic spinal
projections (19,30, 116).

Although close functional similarity between
morphine analgesia and analgesia induced by central
stimulation has still to be demonstrated, evidence of
striking analogies between them is already to hand.

1) Strong analgesia has been obtained by microinjections of morphine at periaqueductal and periventricular sites (52,61,62,79,98,113,123,135). Morphine
analgesia induced by systemic injection is reduced
by microinjection of opiate antagonists in these areas.

2) Both the periaqueductal gray matter and the
periventricular structures are rich in opiate binding
sites (69).
Other binding sites have been described (Amygdala,
Corpus striatum...), but neither electrical stimulation
nor morphine microinjection induced analgesia at these
levels.

3) Repeated microinjections of morphine in the
periaqueductal gray matter induced a tolerance
phenomenon; cross tolerance between systemic and intracerebral injections has also been described (62).
Similar tolerance phenomena are obtained with repeated
central stimulation (84). Cross tolerance between
morphine analgesia and analgesia induced by central
stimulation was observed, the latter being less effective in a morphine tolerant animal (83).

4) Various neurochemical and neuropharmacological
arguments reinforce the analogy between the two kinds
of analgesia. Findings on catecholamines show many
contradictions, while those related to serotonin are
more easily interpretable.

Akil and Liebeskind (5) showed that dopamine and
norepinephrine had opposite effects on the analgesia
induced by central stimulation, the former facilitatory,
the latter inhibitory. However it is hard to compare
these findings with those related to morphine analgesia
since there are numerous contradictions in these studies.

On the other hand, the part played by serotoninergic
mechanisms seems well established in both kinds of
analgesia. In the cat, analgesia is mainly obtained
by stimulating raphe nuclei (92,95). In the rat, this
analgesia is reduced after pretreatment with para-
chlorophenylalanine (pCPA), a serotonin synthesis

inhibitor; administration of 5-hydroxytryptophan
restores it to its initial level (5,6). In the same
way, morphine analgesia is reduced after pCPA administration (36,45,75,118,126).

Analgesia induced by microinjection of morphine
into the periaqueductal gray matter is reduced after
administration of cinanserin, a serotoninergic receptor blocker (134). Lastly, stimulating the dorsal
raphe nucleus potentiates morphine analgesic effects
(109) while destroying it reduces them (108).

5) As mentioned above, the analgesic effects of
central stimulation might be explained by activation
of descending pathways which inhibit the activities
of dorsal horn interneurons involved in the transmission of pain messages. Inhibition of these interneurons is suppressed after administration of LSD
(47) which blocks the serotoninergic neuron activities (4). Recently Basbaum et al. (11) described
a suppression of the analgesia induced by central
stimulation by cutting bulbo-spinal serotoninergic
fibres.

Some experiments suggest that descending serotoninergic pathways contribute to morphine analgesia.
This analgesia is greatly reduced after electrolytic
lesion of the raphe magnus nucleus (102) which presents
dense spinal projections. Evidence is obtained by
5-6 dihydroxytryptamine (5-6 DHT) injection within the
lateral ventricles; this treatment reduces the lumbar
serotonin content without affecting the amount of
serotonin in the brainstem (12). This selective
reduction of spinal serotonin content is associated
with a large decrease of morphine analgesia (41,126).

6) A direct argument underlines the analogy between
both types of analgesia: the analgesia induced by
central stimulation is greatly reduced after the
administration of the specific opiate antagonist,
naloxone. This observation was reported in the rat
(7,8), cat (93,94) and in man (1,107). The recent
finding of morphine-like substances in the brain (56,
57,119) could offer an explanation for the analgesic
properties of central stimulation : this manipulation
presumably induces the release of morphine-like
substances. This hypothesis is supported by the finding of Jacob et al. (60) that naloxone, given alone,

decreases the response threshold to nociceptive
stimuli in both the rat and the mouse.

SUMMARY

Recent neuropharmacological studies have brought to
light various mechanisms related to morphine analgesia.
However, these studies mainly concern the spinal
level as current knowledge of the physiology of pain
at supraspinal levels is noticeably scant. At the
spinal level, morphine acts upon painful messages by
two processes :
- A direct depressive action
- An indirect effect by strengthening the descending
  inhibitory controls of brainstem origin
The relative importance of these two mechanisms
has still to be investigated. However, it is evident
that the spinal target is certainly not involved alone
in morphine analgesia; for instance in man, owing to
the doses used in clinical practice, it seems likely
that morphine's action on the **awareness** of painful
sensations plays a prominent part.

REFERENCES

1. Adams, J.E. (1976): Pain, 2: 161-166.
2. Adler, T.K. (1964): Fed.Proc., 23: 283.
3. Adrian, E.D. (1931): Proc.R.Soc.B., 109: 1-18.
4. Aghajanian, G.K., Foote, W.E., and Sheard, M.H.
   (1968): Science, 161: 706-708.
5. Akil, H., and Liebeskind, J.C. (1975): Brain Res.,
   94: 279-296.
6. Akil, H., and Mayer, D.J. (1972): Brain Res., 44:
   692-697.
7. Akil, H., Mayer, D.J., and Liebeskind, J.C. (1972):
   C.R.Acad.Sci.(Paris), 274: 3603-3605.
8. Akil, H., Mayer, D.J., and Liebeskind, J.C. (1976):
   Science, 191: 961-962.
9. Albe-Fessard, D., Levante, A., and Lamour, Y. (1974):
   Brain Res., 65: 503-509.
10. Albus, K., Schott, M.,and Herz, A. (1970): Eur.J.
    Pharmacol., 12: 53-64.
11. Basbaum, A.I., Marley,N., and O'Keefe, J.(1975): In:
    Proc.1st.World Congress on Pain, Florence. p.268.

12. Baumgarten, H.G., Evetts, K.D., Holman, R.B.,
    Iversen, L.L., Vogt, M., and Wilson, G. (1972):
    J.Neurochem., 19: 1587-1597.
13. Besson, J.M., Conseiller, C., Hamann, K.F., and
    Maillard, M.C. (1972): J.Physiol.(Lond.),221:189-
    205.
14. Besson, J.M., and Guilbaud, G. (1976): In:
    Mechanisms in Transmission of Signals for Conscious
    Behavior, edited by T. Desiraju, pp.138-162.
    Elsevier, Amsterdam.
15. Besson, J.M., Guilbaud, G., and Le Bars, D. (1975):
    J.Physiol.(Lond.),248: 725-739.
16. Besson, J.M., Wyon-Maillard, M.C., Benoist, J.M.,
    Conseiller, C., and Hamann, K.F. (1973):
    J.Pharmacol.Exp.Ther., 187: 239-245.
17. Bessou, P., and Perl, E.R. (1969): J.Neurophysiol.,
    32: 1025-1043.
18. Bodo, R.C., and Brooks, C.Mc.C. (1937): J.Pharmacol.
    Exp.Ther., 61: 82-88.
19. Brodal, A., Taber, E., and Walberg, F. (1960):
    J.Comp.Neurol., 144: 239-259.
20. Brown, A.G. (1971): J.Physiol.(Lond.), 219:103-125.
21. Brown, A.G., and Franz, D.N. (1969): Exp.Brain Res.,
    7: 231-249.
22. Bryan, R.N., Coulter, J.D., and Willis, W.D.(1974):
    Exp.Neurol., 42: 574-586.
23. Bryan, R.N., Trevino, D.L., Coulter, J.D., and
    Willis, W.D. (1973): Exp.Brain Res., 17: 177-189.
24. Burgess, P.R., and Perl, E.R. (1973): In:Handbook
    of Sensory Physiology, Vol.2: Somatosensory System,
    edited by A.Iggo, pp.29-78. Springer, Heidelberg.
25. Calvillo, O., Henry, J.L., and Neuman, R.S. (1974):
    Can.J.Physiol.Pharmacol., 52: 1207-1211.
26. Calvillo, O., Henry, J.L., and Neuman, R.S. (1975):
    In: Proceedings First World Congress on Pain,
    Florence, Italy, p. 259.
27. Collins, W.F., Nulsen, F.E., and Randt, C.T. (1960):
    Arch.Neurol., 3: 381-385.
28. Conseiller, C., Menetrey D., Le Bars, D. and Besson,
    J.M. (1972): J.Physiol.(Paris), 65: suppl.220-221.
29. Curtis, D.R., and Duggan, A.W. (1969): Agents and
    Actions, 1: 14-19.
30. Dahlstrom, A., and Fuxe, K. (1965): Acta Physiol.
    Scand., 64: suppl.247, 5-36.

31.Della Bella, D., Benelli, G. and Besson, J.M. (1975) Life Sci., 17: 73-74.

32.Dostrovsky, J., and Pomeranz, B. (1973): Nature(New Biol.) 246: 222-224.

33.Duggan, A.W., and Curtis, D.R. (1972): Neuropharmacology, 11: 189-196.

34.Engberg, I., Lundberg, A., and Ryall, R.W. (1968): J.Physiol.(Lond.), 194: 201-224.

35.Felper, L.P., Sinclair, J.G., and Yim, G.K.W.(1970): Neuropharmacology, 9: 203-210.

36.Fenessy, M.R. and Lee, J.R. (1970): J.Pharm. Pharmacol., 22: 930-935.

37.Foster, R.S., Jenden, D.J., and Lomax, P. (1967): J.Pharmacol.Exp.Ther., 157: 185-195.

38.Frazier, D.T., Murayama, K., Abbott, N.J., and Naramashi, T. (1972): Proc.Soc.Exp.Biol., 139: 434-438.

39.Gasser, H.S. (1960): J.Gen.Physiol., 43: 937-940.

40.Gasser, H.S., and Erlanger, J. (1927): Am.J.Physiol. 80: 522-547.

41.Genovese, E., Zonta, N. and Mantegazza, P. (1973): Psychopharmacology, 32: 359-364.

42.Giesler, G.J., and Liebeskind, J.C. (1976): Pain, 2: 43-48.

43.Giesler, G.J., Menetrey,D., Guilbaud, G., and Besson, J.M. (1976): Brain Res., 118: 320-324.

44.Goodman, S.J., and Holcombe, V. (1975): Proc.First World Congress on Pain, Florence, Italy, p.264.

45.Gorlitz, B.D., and Frey, H.H. (1972): Eur.J. Pharmacol., 20: 171-180.

46.Gregor, M., and Zimmermann, M. (1972): J.Physiol. (Lond.), 221: 255-276.

47.Guilbaud, G., Besson, J.M., Liebeskind, J.C., and Oliveras, J.L. (1972): C.R.Acad.Sci.(Paris), 275: 1055-1057.

48.Guilbaud, G., Besson, J.M., Oliveras, J.L., and Liebeskind, J.C. (1973): Brain Res., 61: 417-422.

49.Guilbaud, G., Oliveras, J.L., Giesler, G.J., and Besson, J.M. (1977): Brain Res., 126: 355-360.

50.Hallin, R.G., and Torebjork, H.E. (1973): Exp.Brain Res., 16: 309-320.

51.Handwerker, H.O., Iggo, A., and Zimmermann, M. (1975): Pain, 1: 147-165.

52. Herz, A., Albus, K., Metys, J., Schubert, P., and Teschemacher, Hj. (1970): Neuropharmacology, 9: 539-551.

53. Herz, A., and Teschemacher, Hj. (1971): Adv. Drug. Res., 6: 79-119.

54. Hillman, P., and Wall, P.D. (1969): Exp.Brain Res., 9: 284-306.

55. Horlington, M., and Lockett, M.T. (1959): J.Pharm. Pharmacol., 11: 415-420.

56. Hughes, J. (1975): Brain Res., 88: 295-308.

57. Hughes, J., Smith, T.W., Kosterlitz, H.W., Fothergill, L.A., Morgan, B.A., and Morris, H.R. (1975): Nature(Lond), 258: 577-579.

58. Irwin, S., Houde, R.W., Bennett, D.R., Hendershot, L.C., and Seevers, M.H. (1951): J.Pharmacol. Exp. Ther., 101: 132-143.

59. Iwata, N., and Sakai, Y. (1971): Jpn.J.Pharmacol., 9: 284-306.

60. Jacob, J.J., Tremblay, E.C., and Colomber, M.C. (1974): Psychopharmacologia, 37: 217-223.

61. Jacquet, Y.F., and Lajtha, A. (1974): Science, 185: 1055-1057.

62. Jacquet, Y.F., and Lajtha, A. (1976): Brain Res., 103: 501-513.

63. Jurna, I., and Grossmann, W. (1976): Exp.Brain Res., 24: 473-484.

64. Jurna, I., Grossmann, W., and Theres, C. (1973): Neuropharmacology, 12: 983-993.

65. Kitahata, L.M., Kosaka, Y., Taub, A., Bonikos, K., and Hoffert, M. (1974): Anesthesiol., 41: 39-48.

66. Koll, W., Haase, J., Block, G., and Muhlberg, B. (1963): Int.J.Neuropharmacol., 2: 57-65.

67. Kosterlitz, H.W., and Wallis, D.I. (1964): Br.J. Pharmacol.Chemother., 22: 499-510.

68. Krivoy, W., Kroeger, D., and Zimmermann, E. (1973): Br.J.Pharmacol., 47: 457-464.

69. Kuhar, M.J., Pert, C.B., and Snyder, S.H. (1973): Nature(Lond), 245: 447-450.

70. Landau, W.M., and Bishop, G.H. (1958): Science, 128: 712-714.

71. Le Bars, D., Guilbaud, G., Jurna, I., and Besson, J.M. (1976): Brain Res., 115: 518-524.

72. Le Bars, D., Menetrey, D., and Besson, J.M. (1976): Brain Res., 113: 293-310.

73.Le Bars, D., Menetrey, D., Conseiller, C.,and
    Besson, J.M.(1974) : C.R.Acad.Sci.(Paris), 273:
    1369-1371.
74.Le Bars, D., Menetrey, D., Conseiller, C., and
    Besson, J.M. (1975): Brain Res., 98: 261-277.
75.Lee, J.R., and Fenessy, M.R. (1970): Eur.J.
    Pharmacol., 12: 65-70.
76.Liebeskind, J.C., Guilbaud, G., Besson, J.M., and
    Oliveras, J.L. (1973): Brain Res., 50: 441-446.
77.Lim, R.K.S., Guzman, F., Rodgers, D.W., Goto, K.,
    Braun, C., Dickerson, G.D., and Enge, R.J. (1964):
    Arch.Int.Pharmacodyn.Ther., 152: 25-58.
78.Lockett, M.F., and Davis, M.M. (1958): J.Pharm.
    Pharmacol., 10: 80-85.
79.Lotti, V.J., Lomax, P.,and George,R. (1965):
    J.Pharmacol.Exp.Ther., 150 : 135-139.
80.Lotti, V.J., Lomax, P., and George, R. (1966):
    Int.J.Neuropharmacol., 5: 35-42.
81.Lundberg, A. (1966): In: Muscular Afferents and
    Motor Control, edited by R.Granit, pp.275-304.
    Wiley, New York.
82.Magoun, H.W., and Rhines, R.L. (1946): J.Neuro-
    physiol., 9: 165-171.
83.Mayer, D.J. (1975): Neurosci.Res.Prog.Bull., 13:
    94-99.
84.Mayer, D.J., and Hayes, R. (1975): Science, 188:
    941-943.
85.Mayer, D.J., and Liebeskind, J.C. (1974): Brain Res.
    68: 73-93.
86.Mayer, D.J., Wolfle, T.L., Akil, H., Carder, B.,and
    Liebeskind, J.C. (1971): Science, 174: 1351-1354.
87.Mc Clane, T.K., and Martin, W.R. (1967): Int.J.
    Neuropharmacol., 6: 89-98.
88.Melzack, R., and Melinkoff, D.F. (1974): Exp.Neurol.
    43: 369-374.
89.Melzack, R., and Wall, P.D. (1965): Science, 150:
    971-979.
90.Mendell, L.M. (1966): Exp.Neurol., 16: 316-332.
91.Oleson, T.D., and Liebeskind, J.C. (1975):
    Physiologist, 18: 338.
92.Oliveras, J.L., Besson, J.M., Guilbaud, G., and
    Liebeskind, J.C. (1974): Exp.Brain Res., 20:32-44.
93.Oliveras, J.L., Guilbaud, G., and Besson, J.M.
    (1975): J.Physiol.(Paris), 164A.

94.Oliveras, J.L., Hosobuchi, Y., Redjemi, F.,
   Guilbaud, G., and Besson, J.M. (1977): Brain Res.
   120: 221-229.
95.Oliveras, J.L., Redjemi, F., Guilbaud, G., and
   Besson, J.M. (1975): Pain, 1: 139-145.
96.Oliveras, J.L., Woda, A., Guilbaud, G., and Besson,
   J.M. (1974): Brain Res., 72: 328-331.
97.Pert, C.B., Kuhar, M.J., and Snyder, S.M. (1975):
   Life Sci., 16: 1849-1854.
98.Pert, A., and Yaksh, T. (1974): Brain Res., 80:
   135-140.
99.Pomeranz, B., Wall, P.D., and Weber, W.V. (1968):
   J.Physiol.(Lond.), 199: 511-532.
100.Price, D.D., and Browe, A.C. (1973): Brain Res.,
   64: 425-429.
101.Price, D.D., and Wagman, I.H. (1970): Exp.Neurol.,
   29: 383-399.
102.Proudfit, H.K., and Anderson, E.G.(1975): Brain
   Res., 48: 612-618.
103.Redjemi, F., Oliveras, J.L., Guilbaud, G., and
   Besson, J.M. (1974): C.R.Acad.Sci.(Paris), 279:
   1105-1107.
104.Rexed, B. (1952): J.Comp.Neurol., 16: 415-495.
105.Reynolds, D.V. (1969): Science, 164: 444-445.
106.Richardson, D.E., and Akil, H. (1973): Ann.
   Meeting Amer.Ass.Neurol.Surg.
107.Richardson, D.E., and Akil, H. (1976): J.Neurosurg.
   (in press)
108.Samanin, R., Gumulka, W.,and Valzelli, L. (1970):
   Eur.J.Pharmacol., 10: 339-343.
109.Samanin, R., and Valzelli, L.(1971): Eur.J.
   Pharmacol., 16: 298-302.
110.Satoh, M., Nakamura, N., and Takagi, H. (1971):
   Eur.J.Pharmacol., 16: 245-247.
111.Satoh, M., and Takagi, H. (1971): Eur.J.Pharmacol.,
   14: 60-65.
112.Selzer, M., and Spencer, W.A. (1969): Brain Res.,
   14: 331-348.
113.Sharpe, L.G., Garnett, J.E., and Cicero, T.J.
   (1974): Behav.Biol., 11: 303-313.
114.Sinclair, J.G. (1973): Eur.J.Pharmacol., 21:111-114.
115.Snyder, S.H. (1975): Nature(Lond), 257: 185-189.
116.Taber, E., Brodal, A., and Walberg, F. (1960):
   J.Comp.Neurol., 114: 161-187.

117.Takagi, H., Matsunara, M., Yanai, A., and Ogiu, K. (1955): Jpn.J.Pharmacol., 4: 176-187.
118.Tenen, S.S. (1968): Psychopharmacologia, 12:278-285.
119.Terenius, L., and Wahlstrom, A. (1975): Life Sci., 16: 1759-1769.
120.Teschemacher, Hj., Schubert, P., and Herz,A.(1973): Neuropharmacology, 12: 123-131.
121.Torebjork, H.E., and Hallin, R.G. (1972): Exp. Brain Res., 137: 347-360.
122.Trevino, D.L., Coulter, J.D., and Willis, W.D. (1973): J.Neurophysiol., 36: 750-761.
123.Tsou, K., and Jang, C.S. (1964): Scientia Sinica, 13: 1099-1109.
124.Van Hess, J., and Gybels, J. (1972): Brain Res., 48: 397-400.
125.Vigouret, J.M., Teschemacher, Hj., Albus, K., and Herz, A. (1973): Neuropharmacology, 12: 111-121.
126.Vogt, M. (1974): J.Physiol.(Lond.), 236: 483-498.
127.Wagers, P.K., and Smith, C.M. (1960): J.Pharmacol. Exp.Ther., 130: 89-105.
128.Wagman, I.H., and Price, D.D. (1969):J.Neurophysiol. 32: 803-816.
129.Wall, P.D. (1967):J.Physiol.(Lond.), 188: 403-423.
130.Wei, E., Sigel, S., and Way, E.L. (1975): J.Pharmacol.Exp.Ther., 193: 56-63.
131.Wikler, A. (1944): J.Pharmacol.Exp.Ther., 80: 176-187.
132.Wikler, A., and Frank, K. (1948): J.Pharmacol.Exp. Ther., 94: 382-400.
133.Willis, W.D., Trevino, D.L., Coulter, J.D., and Maunz, R.A. (1974): J.Neurophysiol.,37: 358-372.
134.Yaksh, T.L., Du Chateau, J.C., and Rudy, T.A. (1976): Brain Res.,104: 367-372.
135.Yaksh, T.L., Rudy, T.A., and Yeung, J.C. (1975): Proc.Soc.Neurosci., 1: 283.
136.Zieglgansberger, W., and Bayerl, H. (1976): Brain Res.,115: 111-128.
137.Zotterman, Y. (1933): Acta Med.Scand., 80: 185-242.

Factors Affecting the Action of Narcotics, edited by
M.L. Adler, L. Manara, and R. Samanin.
Raven Press, New York ©1978.

Importance of In Vitro Measurements of Adrenocortical
Steroid Synthesis in Assessing Locus of Morphine
Effects

Walter B. Essman and Richard Rosenthal

Queens College, of the
City University of New York
Flushing, N.Y., U.S.A.

INTRODUCTION

Although there has been some interest in the relationship between adrenal steroid synthesis and the effects of morphine, there has been little detailed
investigation of the issue. It has been known for some
time that chronic treatment with morphine causes alterations in adrenal function, and much has been made of
the central effect of morphine on the hypothalamic-
pituitary regulation of the adrenal cortex. Male rats
acutely treated with morphine showed more than a tenfold increase in adrenal corticosterone concentration
and more than a twenty-fold increase in serum corticosterone by one hour after treatment (2). The acute
treatment of male rats and mice with morphine produced
marked increases in plasma corticosterone within one
hour, and male rabbits given morphine acutely showed
increased plasma corticosterone in July and a decreased
level after morphine in January. Rats and mice did
not show such seasonal variations (4). Repeated
morphine treatment to male rats increased adrenal
weight but decreased adrenal corticosterone production
in vitro (3).
In adult male rats, serum testosterone levels were
reduced by 70% within six hours after implantation of
morphine pellets. Serum testosterone was decreased to
about 20% of control levels in male rats after five
days of morphine treatment. Such reductions in serum
testosterone levels by morphine were shown to subse-

quently affect the weight, secretory activity, and
cytoarchitectural features of the secondary sex organs
(1).

Although limited observations for adrenal steroid
concentration or synthesis are interesting, little
attempt has been made to separate the central from the
peripheral effects of morphine and also to delineate
the extent to which sex differences might contribute
to adrenocortical steroid synthesis. In order to deal
with these issues directly, the in vitro synthesis of
four adrenocortical steroids was measured in tissue
from adult male and female mice, and the direct effects
of morphine upon the synthesis of these steroids was
assessed.

METHODS AND RESULTS

Adrenocortical tissue removed from 65 day old male
and female mice at approximately 2 P.M. was prepared
as a 10% (W/V) homogenate in 0.32M sucrose, using
pooled sets of tissue samples. An aliquot of 0.1 ml of
homogenate was incubated in 1.7 ml of Krebs-Henseleit
solution with 0.1 ml of C^{14}-Na Acetate (1.25 µCi/ml);
to each of the incubation mixtures, 0.1 ml of morphine
sulfate in a concentration of 10^{-7}M, 10^{-6}M, 10^{-5}M,
10^{-4}M, or 10^{-3}M was added, and a control addition of
0.9% NaCl was also made. The incubation was carried
out for 45 minutes in a shaker bath at 37°C, under a
gas mixture of 95% O_2 and 5% CO_2. The reaction was
stopped by the addition of 2 ml of ice cold distilled
water, and the mixture was combined with 2 ml of acetone, shaken, and centrifuged for 10 minutes at 3000
r.p.m.. The organic layer was removed and 0.1 ml aliquots
were applied by micropipette to appropriate chromatography papers. Silica gel (SG) paper was used with a
benzene:acetone (1:1) solvent system to separate
cholesterol and corticosterone (Rf value = 0.888, 14.3
cm from origin, and 0.472, 7.6 cm from origin, respectively); alumina paper with a benzene:ethanol (19:1)
solvent system was used to separate testosterone and
17-β estradiol (Rf = 0.869, 14.0 cm from origin, and
0.441, 7.1 cm from origin, respectively). The samples
were chromatographed, along with appropriate standards,
for 10 minutes; the chromatograms were dried for 30

minutes, and using a standardized template, 1.0^2 inch
of chromatographed sample at each standardized point
was removed, eluted, and solubilized in scintillation
fluid (toluene with omnifluor); all samples were thus
run in triplicate and counted in a liquid scintillation counter. For separate 0.1 ml aliquots of the
original homogenate, protein determinations were carried out.

Baseline rates of cholesterol synthesis did not
differ between adrenal tissue from male and female mice
(120.9 ± 4.3 nM/mg protein and 123.9 ± 7.1 nM/mg
protein, respectively). Morphine did not affect
cholesterol synthesis appreciably, except at 10^{-3}M,
where male adrenals showed a 14% increase in synthesis
(p < .05) and female adrenals showed a 22% increase
(p < .02).

Corticosterone synthesis did not differ between
male and female adrenal tissue (218.0 ± 0.2 nM/mg
protein and 225.2 ± 9.6 nM/mg protein, respectively)
and morphine over a range of 10^{-7} to 10^{-3} M failed to
alter corticosterone synthesis in either male or female
adrenal tissue.

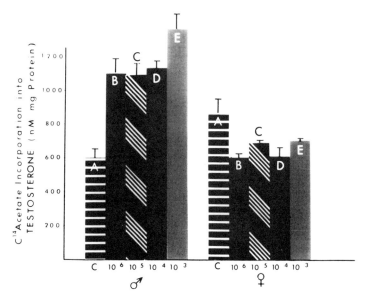

FIG. 1. Testosterone synthesis (n Moles/mg protein)
by adrenal tissue, in vitro, from male and female mice:
effects of morphine.

Differences in basal rates of testosterone synthesis *in vitro* between male and female adrenal tissue and the effects of morphine over a concentration range of 10^{-6}M to 10^{-3}M have been summarized in Figure 1. An interesting paradoxical effect was observed for the sex differences in morphine action upon *in vitro* testosterone synthesis, such that in tissue from male mice there was almost a doubling of the rate of synthesis. There was a relationship between morphine concentration and altered synthesis rate (S = 0.40, p < .06; 82.50 nM/mg protein/10^1 M morphine) to suggest an incremental relationship with a high degree of statistical significance (p < .001).

For adrenal tissue derived from female mice, it is apparent that testosterone synthesis was decreased by morphine (S = 0.40, p < .06; 67.0 nM/mg protein/10^1M morphine) and that the decreased synthesis at all concentrations was significantly lower than controls (p < .01).

The synthesis of 17-β estradiol in male adrenal tissue did not differ from the rate observed for female adrenals, except that for the latter, morphine caused a significant inhibition of synthesis at all concentrations (Figure 2). In male adrenal tissue no statistically significant alteration in 17-β estradiol occurred from any of the concentrations of morphine utilized *in vitro.* For the female adrenal tissue significant decreases in 17-β estradiol occurred over the entire range of morphine concentration (p < .01). It is therefore apparent that differences in 17-β estradiol synthesis, although not manifest under baseline conditions for adrenal cortex from male and female mice, are apparent in the differential response of such synthesis to morphine.

DISCUSSION AND CONCLUSIONS

It is apparent from the foregoing *in vitro* studies, in contrast to experiments in which animals were treated with morphine *in vivo*, that corticosterone synthesis was not affected by morphine over a wide range of concentration. The absence of a morphine effect *in vitro* suggests that the basis for increased corticosterone observed in *in vivo* studies (2,4) or decreased

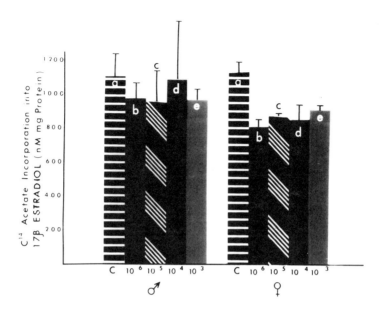

FIG. 2.   17-β Estradiol synthesis (n Moles/mg protein) by adrenal tissue, in vitro, from male and female mice: effects of morphine.

---

production measured in vitro after in vivo treatment (3) may be the stimulation of the hypothalamic-pituitary axis, rather than any direct effect on the adrenal.

Cholesterol synthesis, similarly, not only did not differ between male and female adrenal, but like corticosterone synthesis was unaffected by morphine. It is of some interest to observe that the two major components of the pathways for adrenal steroid synthesis were not affected by morphine and did not show any sex differences.   The major indices of male and female sex hormones, testosterone and 17-β estradiol, were affected by morphine, and did differ with respect to how synthesis was affected by morphine. It seems apparent, therefore, that the reduced testosterone levels resulting from morphine in vivo in male rats (1) probably again represent a central rather than a peripheral

effect, particularly in view of the findings that
luteinizing hormone levels were markedly reduced by
morphine. The increased in vitro synthesis of testosterone by male adrenal and decreased synthesis by
female adrenal as a result of morphine, suggests that
the narcotic is capable of exerting a direct peripheral
effect that is sex-dependent. The nature of this dependency may depend on differences in enzyme activity,
or possibly seasonal variables which were not examined
in this study.

Differences in the effects of morphine on adrenal
17-β estradiol synthesis, again appear sex related.
This most potent estrogen is clearly synthesized at
equal rates in male and female mouse adrenal, but
morphine has a significant inhibitory effect, as with
testosterone, only in female adrenal. Although the
secretory rates of testosterone as well as 17-β estradiol may be differentiated between male and female
adrenal tissue, there is no real evidence for differen-
tiating basal control synthesis rates of these molecules on the basis of sex differences. The only
consistent finding is that the direct effect of morphine on the female adrenal, acts to reduce the in
vitro synthesis of both molecules. The lack of effect
of morphine on 17-β estradiol synthesis by the male
adrenal cortex, may be contrasted with its stimulatory
effect on testosterone synthesis by the same tissue.

The present studies have indicated a need to examine
the direct effects of morphine on the adrenal cortex,
indipendent of the central effects of this narcotic;
moreover, little data are available in a comparison
of male and female differences in adrenocortical synthesis, or the plasma concentrations of derived
hormones.

Although the present findings cannot exclude the
influence of the hypothalamic-pituitary axis on sex-
related differentiation of the adrenal cortex, the
differences in the action of morphine on steroid synthesis appear to reside in the unique endogenous
characteristics of the adrenal tissue.*

---

* Recent data from our laboratory have shown that the
synthesis of testosterone and 17-β estradiol by the
adrenal cortex from fetal female sheep (113-115 days
of gestation), was significantly inhibited by 10^{-6}M

ACKNOWLEDGEMENTS

The results reported in these studies were derived from research supported, in part, by a grant from the Council for Tobacco Research - U.S.A.

REFERENCES

1. Cicero, T.J., Meyer, E.R., Bell, R.D.,and Koch, G. A. (1976): Endocrinology, 98: 367-372.
2. Kuwamura, T., Nagao, S., Nakaura, S., Kawashima, K., Tanaka, S., Omori, Y.,and Nakoa, T. (1973): Endocrinol.Jpn., 20: 359-364.
3. Kuwamura, T., Nakaura, S., Nagao, S., Kawashima, K., Tanaka, S., Omori, Y., and Nakato, T. (1974): Jpn. J. Pharmacol., 24: 89-95.
4. Sable-Amplis, R., Agid, R.,and Abadie, D. (1974): Biochem.Pharmacol., 23: 2111-2118.

morphine (magnitude of inhibition 75 and 56%, respectively). Corticosterone synthesis in the fetal sheep adrenal, however, was significantly increased (36%) at the same concentration of morphine.

Factors Affecting the Action of Narcotics, edited by
M.L. Adler, L. Manara, and R. Samanin.
Raven Press, New York©1978.

Factors Influencing the Manifestation of
Dependence in Rats

J. Bläsig, G. Meyer and M. Städele

Max-Planck-Institut für Psychiatrie
Department of Neuropharmacology
Kraepelinstrasse 2, 8000 Munich 40, W-Germany

INTRODUCTION

With chronic exposure to opiates, adaptive processes
are initiated which compensate for the drug effects and
give rise to tolerance and dependence. The degree of
tolerance can easily be quantified with the determination of the loss of efficacy of the drug, whereas the
intensity of physical dependence can only indirectly be
implied by the character of the withdrawal syndrome
that appears when the drug supply is interrupted or
morphine antagonists are applied. A variety of problems
arise when this complex abstinence behavior is to be
taken as a measure for the underlying opiate dependence.

A. Changes in Withdrawal Symptomatology in Correlation
with Different Degrees of Dependence

Withdrawal behavior is a function of counterregula-
tory mechanisms against morphine action and, thus, is
the negative of the acute effects of the drug. These
acute effects are known to change not only quantitatively but also qualitatively with the dose of morphine
applied. It is therefore not surprising that the
qualitative pattern of withdrawal signs also depends
upon the dose of morphine maintaining a given degree
of dependence. This was shown in a study in which the
precipitated withdrawal symptomatology of increasingly
dependent rats (maintained on increasing amounts of
morphine) was evaluated (see 2). From these experiments,
it became obvious that only a few withdrawal signs
were correlated in a positive way with the degree of
underlying dependence. Signs such as writhing, wet
dog shaking, ptosis, and diarrhea were strongly expressed in weakly dependent rats but were less evident in
higher dependence groups, whereas other signs such as
jumping, teeth-chattering, and chromodacryorrhea showed

the opposite relationship to the degree of dependence.
A similar change in the pattern of signs was observed
upon the recovery from a high degree of dependence
after the cessation of morphine-pellet implantation
(see Fig. 1). Since absorption of morphine from a

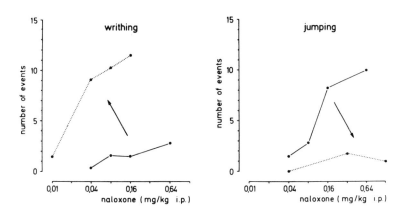

FIG. 1. Changes in the dose-response curves of two
different withdrawal signs upon increase in the length
of time between last implantation of pellets and
precipitation of withdrawal
Rats had received 1 pellet on the 1st, two pellets on
the 4th, and 3 pellets on the 7th day, each pellet
containing 75 mg morphine base and bulk constituents.
Withdrawal was precipitated 3 days ●——● or 8 days
●---● later without previous removal of the pellets.
The ordinate gives the number of events observed over
a time of 30 min after administration of the antagonist,
the abscissae give the doses of naloxone.
Each point represents the mean value of at least 10
rats. For details of experimental approach, definition
of signs, and preparation of pellets, see Bläsig et al.
(2).

pellet slowly decreases after about 3 days because of
encapsulation of the pellet by fibrous tissue (2,16,
21), the degree of dependence gradually declines after
the 4th day, unless further pellets are implanted.
As evident from the figure, with increasing length of
time between last pellet implantation and the precipitation of withdrawal, the course of changes that took

place in the shape of dose-response curves for jumping
and writhing were opposite to each other. The jumping
curve flattened, that is, the sign no longer occurred
with the same frequency seen 3 days after the last
implantation. On the other hand, the writhing curve
steepened, indicating an increase in the manifestation
of this sign. Comparable observations regarding the
qualitative changes in withdrawal symptomatology were
made in rats by Hoffmeister and Schlichting (13) and in
dogs by Martin et al. (15).
    These findings point out that some caution must be
used when the withdrawal syndrome is quantified by
scoring withdrawal signs according to point ranking
systems (see 11,12,21,22). Moreover, the observations
explain discrepancies in the literature regarding the
relative appropriateness of the different signs for
withdrawal assessment. While writhing, for example,
was considered by some authors to be important (5,13,
14), others have more or less neglected it (7,8,11,17).
Probably these groups were dealing with different
degrees of dependence and had therefore observed different patterns of signs.

    B. Some Aspects Concerning the Quantification of
                Withdrawal Jumping

1. Comparison of Jumping Thresholds in Rats and Mice

    As a rule, practical considerations will dictate
that only one or a few withdrawal signs be used for the
assessment of underlying dependence. Of all behavioral
or vegetative signs observed, jumping is usually the
best-suited since its frequency is positively related
to the degree of underlying dependence (2), and since
it can be easily evaluated in an objective way.   In
principle, both species, rats and mice, show this sign
from a certain minimum degree of dependence onwards.
However, in mice this sign reaches a high intensity
more rapidly because of two facts. First, in mice high
degrees of dependence can be induced within a much
shorter time in comparison to rats because the former
species tolerates higher initial doses of morphine.
Moreover, in mice lower degrees of dependence are needed for the manifestation of jumping as compared to
rats, meaning that the latter species apparently pos-
esses higher thresholds for this sign. This is demonstrated in figure 2 in which the morphine brain concentrations maintaining different degrees of dependence
in mice and rats were related to the highest numbers of
jumps that could be obtained by administration of a
supramaximum dose of an antagonist, naloxone, in these

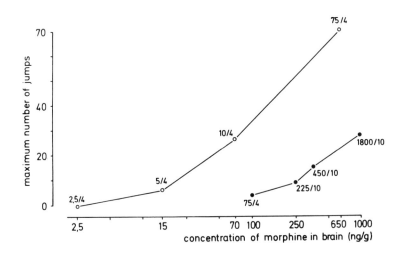

FIG. 2. Maximum frequencies of jumps obtained in
differently dependent rats (●——●) and mice (o——o)
in correlation to the brain concentration of morphine
measured at the time of withdrawal precipitation
The numbers for maximum jumps were obtained by taking
the mean values from the plateau region of the dose-
response curves (for mice see fig. 3). Codes give the
total amount of morphine (mg) implanted (first number)
and time of morphine exposure in days (second number).
Mice always received 1 pellet containing different
amounts of morphine base, while rats received different
amounts of pellets, each pellet containing 75 mg
morphine base. All pellets had a total weight of 150
mg, containing morphine and bulk constituents (2).
Brain concentrations of morphine were measured with
gas-liquid chromatography according to Dahlström et al.
(10). Each value represents a mean of at least 5
brains.

animals. Obviously rats, in comparison to mice, had to
adapt to approximately a tenfold higher brain concentration of morphine before naloxone was able to precipitate
this sign. Probably, in the experiments in rats reported in recent literature such high degrees of dependence
were not reached, which may explain why jumping has
been rarely used as a parameter for assessing dependence in this species.

2. Comparison of dose-response curves for jumping in mice with different degrees of dependence

When selecting the withdrawal sign, jumping, as a parameter for the assessment of dependence, the question arises how this sign can be best evaluated. In 1969 Way's group (21) presented evidence for an inverse relationship between the degree of dependence and the dose of antagonist necessary for the precipitation of this sign. This finding, implying a parallel shift to the left of the dose-response curves for jumping with an increase in dependence, has given rise to the assumption that during dependence development the affinity of morphine antagonists for the opiate receptors increases. Especially because of interest in this latter question, we looked at the shapes of dose-response curves for jumping in mice with increasing degrees of dependence. Jumping was evaluated according to two different methods. In one case, the percentage of animals showing this sign was taken as the response to naloxone (quantal method); in the other case, the frequencies of jumps obtained were correlated with the different doses of naloxone (variable method). Two striking facts (see fig. 3a and b) became evident with these methods: a) With increasing degrees of dependence, the dose-response curves steepened while at the same time the maximum effects increased. b) The curves always reached their individual maxima within the same dose range of naloxone, approximately 1 mg/kg i.p.

Apparently with an increase in dependence, the jumping curves do not shift to the left in a parallel way. Instead, the amount of effect induced by naloxone continually increases. Such an increase in the maximum effect is, however, observable with the use of the quantal method only as long as no 100% effects are obtained.

From these types of curves no support is thus given to the assumption that dependence development is associated with an increase in the affinity of naloxone for its specific binding sites, as has been suggested from other kinds of experiments (18,19,20). On the other hand, the findings show the maximum number of jumps obtained to be a good index for the degree of dependence, whereas the use of the quantal method has the disadvantage of being restricted to those degrees of dependence at which jumping is inducible in high percentages of animals. The second finding, that the plateau of the jumping curves is always reached at about the same dose of naloxone, is probably a reflection of the saturation of specific receptors occupied by naloxone. This suggestion is also supported by

evidence obtained by in vivo receptor binding studies
(Bläsig et al., unpublished results).

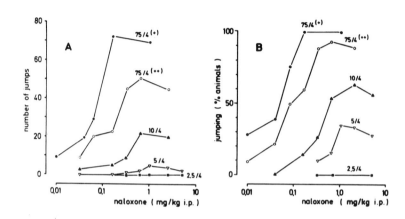

FIG. 3. Dose-response curves for jumping in mice having different degrees of dependence. Codes give the
total amount of morphine (mg) implanted per pellet
(first number), and time of morphine exposure in days
(second number). The same data was used for each
method of evaluation. In A) the different doses of
naloxone are correlated with the number of jumps, in
B) with % of animals showing at least 2 jumps.
Points represent the mean of at least 10 animals. Mice
had a body weight of 20 g (+) or 30 g (++) at time of
first pellet implantation.
For further details see fig. 2

---

3. Jumping induced by various antagonists and partial
   agonists and its suppression by morphine

    When dependence is assessed by the maximum number of
jumps that can be precipitated, the same antagonist
must always be used. This became evident from a study
in which the jumping-precipitating properties of various
antagonists and partial agonists were compared (3).
Such experiments showed that the dose-response curves
of the individual substances for jumping were not
parallel but varied in steepness. Whereas the position
of the individual curves on the abscissa paralleled the

affinities of the compounds for specific receptor sites
in brain homogenates, the steepness of the curves was
related to the agonistic properties of the substances
as judged from the ratio of their binding in sodium-
free and sodium-containing medium. Thus, the "purest"
antagonist, naloxone, induced the lowest maximum level
of jumping, while cyclazocine and some newly synthesized benzomorphane derivatives, although far less
potent when judged according to the ED_{50}, induced
several-fold higher numbers of jumps. Apparently other
effects of the partial agonists than those shared with
naloxone are responsible for their higher "intrinsic
activity" to induce jumping, whatever the cause of it
may be.

In order to further characterize the nature of these
effects, the ability of morphine to suppress the jumping induced by the various partial agonists was investigated. Results of such experiments are presented in
Fig. 4. This figure compares the doses of morphine
that were needed to suppress jumping induced in equally
dependent rats by the same doses (2 mg/kg i.p.) of the
different substances. As evident from the figure, the
least amount of morphine is necessary for the suppression of SH 254-induced jumping, although this substance caused the highest number of jumps. On the
other hand, the effects of the same dose of naloxone
precipitating the lowest level of jumping could not be
antagonized by the highest amount of morphine applied
in these experiments. These findings show that the
jumping-inducing effects of the partial agonists are
completely reversible by morphine. The doses needed
are not correlated with the maximum effectiveness of
the substances but with their potency, which in turn
parallels their affinities towards specific receptor
sites in vitro (see 3). The findings, moreover,
suggest that the observations made by Cheney et al. (6)
in rats cannot be taken as evidence that during toler-
ance/dependence development the opiate receptors change
in such a way as to make competition between opiate
agonists and antagonists no longer possible. Instead,
the results show that, like suppression of abrupt withdrawal, the suppression of precipitated withdrawal can
also be used for checking unknown substances for dependence liability.

C. Abrupt Withdrawal in Correlation to the Disappearance
        of Morphine from the Brain

When morphine supply in rats is interrupted by
removal of morphine pellets, roughly the same withdrawal signs appear as those observed during precipitated withdrawal. As seen from Fig. 5, the individual

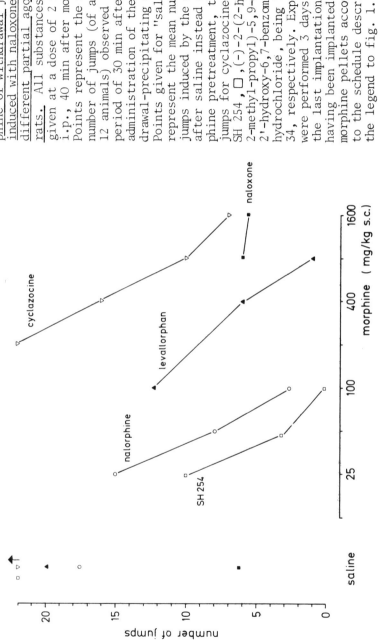

FIG. 4. Suppression by morphine of withdrawal jumping induced with naloxone or with different partial agonists in rats. All substances were given at a dose of 2 mg/kg i.p., 40 min after morphine. Points represent the mean number of jumps (of at least 12 animals) observed over a period of 30 min after the administration of the withdrawal-precipitating drugs. Points given for "saline" represent the mean number of jumps induced by the drugs after saline instead of morphine pretreatment, the mean jumps for cyclazocine, ▽, and SH 254, □, (-)-2-(2-hydroxy-2-methyl-propyl)-5,9-dimethyl-2'-hydroxy-6,7-benzomorphane hydrochloride, being 25 and 34, respectively. Experiments were performed 3 days after the last implantation in rats having been implanted with morphine pellets according to the schedule described in the legend to fig. 1.

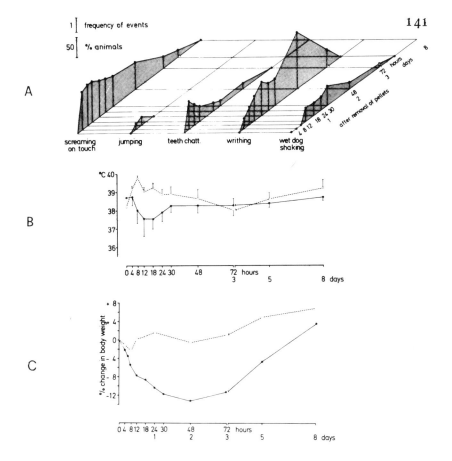

FIG. 5. The time course of the appearance of various
withdrawal signs after the removal of morphine pellets
in rats. Pellets were implanted according to the
schedule described in the legend of Fig. 1. Three days
after the last implantation all the pellets were removed.
A) Except for screaming on touch, the frequency (ordinates) of each sign was counted over a period of 30 min
at increasing times (oblique abscissae) after pellet
removal. In the case of screaming on touch the percentage of animals showing the sign was evaluated. All
points represent the mean of at least 8 observations.
B) Body temperature was measured by the insertion of a
thermistor-probe into the esophagus of rats from which
morphine pellets were removed (●——●), and of control
rats (o---o) from which placebo pellets were removed.
Points represent the mean ± SD of at least 8 rats.
C) % body weight change of rats after removal of
morphine pellets (●——●) and after removal of placebo
pellets (o---o). Each point gives the mean of at least
8 rats. Body weight at the time of pellet removal
varied between 200 and 250 g.

signs varied considerably according to onset, peak, and duration. While jumping was only observable during the first 8 hours after pellet removal, writhing and wet dog shaking were maximally expressed after about 48 hours. On the other hand, body temperature tended to normalize after 12 hours, whereas maximum body weight loss was not reached until 48 hours. Apparently those signs that can be precipitated during the earlier stages of the development of dependence, such as screaming on touch, wet dog shaking, and writhing (see 2), disappear latest upon recovery from dependence after the interruption of morphine supply. On the other hand, jumping, which affords a rather high degree of dependence before it can be induced by naloxone, is only expressed during the very first period after pellet removal. The phenomenon of threshold differences between the individual signs is thus apparent from both types of withdrawal induction.

For the characterization of the mechanisms behind the development of dependence it is important to know if the prolonged physiological disturbances seen in abstinent subjects are linked to the disappearance of morphine from the brain. Fig. 6 shows that morphine leaves the brain in two phases after pellet removal. While during the first 12 hours there is a rapid decline in concentration, further decrease is rather protracted. Thus, on the 4th day after pellet removal the concentration of morphine in the brain is still about 10 ng/g, a level which roughly equals that reached by 1 mg/kg of morphine given subcutaneously to naive rats (4). In line with this finding of a very slow disappearance of morphine from the brain is the observation of a long-lasting sensitivity to naloxone in abruptly withdrawn rats. Even 8 days after pellet removal (Bläsig et al., unpublished results), signs such as screaming on touch can still be precipitated, suggesting that some morphine is still present at its specific receptor sites. A similar biphasic disappearance of morphine was observed by Berkowitz et al. (1) in the plasma of rats after pellet removal. In these experiments morphine was detectable in the plasma for about 20 days. Moreover, our findings seem to be related to the observation made by Cox et al. (9) that the recovery of tolerance towards analgesia after the interruption of morphine exposure also occurs in two steps, that is to say, first, in a short phase during which the level of tolerance rapidly decreases and second in a longer phase, during which time, tolerance slowly fades over several days. Our finding is, however, not in line with the observation made in mice (16) showing that morphine very rapidly disappears from the brain within 6-8 hours after removal of a 75-mg morphine pellet.

It has to be concluded from our data showing a slow decay of the morphine concentration in the brain, that the long duration of physiological disturbances seen after abrupt withdrawal of morphine, is dependent, at least to a certain extent, on the long persistence of small amounts of morphine in the brain.

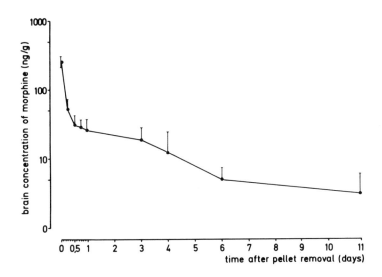

FIG. 6. The time course of the decay of the concentration of morphine in the brain after the removal of pellets from rats 3 days after the last implantation. Rats had received 1 pellet on the 1st, 2 pellets on the 4th, and 3 pellets on the 7th day. Brain concentrations of morphine were determined by gas-liquid chromatography according to Dahlström et al. (10). Points give the mean ± SD of at least 6 brains.

SUMMARY

Precipitated morphine withdrawal in rats changes qualitatively with the degree of underlying dependence. This is due to the fact that a) the adaptation to morphine must advance to a distinct threshold level for each individual sign, and that b) some signs seem to be suppressed by the occurrence of other signs. From this it follows that a sign, for instance, jumping, which is positively correlated to the degree of dependence, is an appropriate gauge for the assessment of dependence.

In mice the minimum degree of dependence required for jumping to appear is lower than in rats.

There are different ways to quantify the occurrence of jumping - either by counting its frequency (variable method) or by determing the dose of naloxone which induces this sign in 50% of animals (quantal method). The methods give very similar results and show that the dose-response curves for jumping steepen with an increase in underlying dependence instead of shifting to the left in a parallel way. These findings do not support the hypothesis that, with an increase in dependence, the affinity of opiate antagonists towards the specific receptor sites increases.

When quantifying dependence by counting the maximum number of jumps, it is necessary to always use the same antagonist, since the frequency of jumps obtained in equally dependent rats is different when different antagonists or partial agonists are used. Apparently the ability of the individual substances to induce jumping is related to their affinities to the specific receptor sites, while their maximal efficiency seems to be linked to their agonistic properties.

The minimum dose needed to induce jumping, and not the maximal efficiency of the substances, determines the amount of morphine necessary to antagonize their effects in dependent rats.

As a whole, precipitated withdrawal is strikingly similar to abrupt withdrawal. Those withdrawal signs that can be precipitated at the least advanced level of dependence are the latest to disappear after the interruption of morphine supply; while jumping is only manifested when dependence is highly developed (in rats), it appears only during a short, initial phase of abrupt withdrawal. The prolonged duration of abrupt withdrawal is probably not only a function of the recovery rate of the dependence mechanisms involved but is, moreover, dependent on the slow decay of the morphine concentration in the brain.

ACKNOWLEDGEMENT

The authors wish to thank Jane Dum for stylistic revision of the English text. The study was supported by the Bundesministerium für Jugend, Familie und Gesundheit, Bonn, W-Germany.

REFERENCES

1. Berkowitz, B.A., Cerreta, K.V., and Spector, S. (1974): J. Pharmacol. Exp. Ther., 191: 527
2. Bläsig, J., Herz, A., Reinhold, K., and Zieglgänsberger, S. (1973): Psychopharmacologia, 33: 19
3. Bläsig, J., Höllt, V., Herz, A., and Paschelke, G. (1976): Psychopharmacologia, 46: 41
4. Bläsig, J., Höllt, V., Meyer, G., and Herz, A.(1976): In: Opiates and Endogenous Opioid Peptides, edited by H.W. Kosterlitz, pp. 391-394. Elsevier,Amsterdam.
5. Buckett, W.R. (1964): Psychopharmacologia, 6: 410
6. Cheney, D.L., Judson, B.A., and Goldstein, A. (1972): J. Pharmacol. Exp. Ther., 184: 404
7. Cicero, T.J., and Meyer, E.R. (1973): J. Pharmacol. Exp. Ther., 184: 404
8. Collier, H.O.J., Francis, D.L., and Schneider, C. (1972): Nature, 237: 220
9. Cox, B.M., Ginsburg, M., and Willis, J. (1975): Br. J. Pharmacol., 53: 383
10. Dahlström, B., and Paalzow, L. (1975): J. Pharm. Pharmacol., 27: 172
11. Frederickson, R.C.A., and Smits, S.E. (1973): Res. Commun.Chem.Pathol.Pharmacol., 5: 867
12. Halbach, H. and Eddy, N.B. (1963): Bull. WHO, 28: 139
13. Hoffmeister, F., and Schlichting, U. (1972): In: Schmerz, Grundlagen-Pharmakologie-Therapie, edited by R. Janzen, W. Keidel, A. Herz and C.Steichele, p. 290, Thieme, Stuttgart.
14. Lorenzetti, O.J., and Sancilio, L.F. (1970): Arch. Int. Pharmacodyn. Ther., 183: 391
15. Martin, W.R., Eades, C.G., Thompson, W.O., Thompson, J.A., and Flanary, H.G. (1974): J. Pharmacol. Exp. Ther., 189: 759
16. Patrick, G.A., Dewey, W.J., Spaulding, T.C. and Harris, L.S. (1975): J. Pharmacol.Exp.Ther., 193: 876
17. Schwartz, A.S., and Eidelberg, E. (1970): Life Sci., 9: 613.
18. Shen, W.J., and Way, L. (1975): In: The Opiate Narcotics, Neurochemical Mechanisms in Analgesia and Dependence. The International Narcotic

Research Club Conference, May 21-24, p. 77
19. Takemori, A.E., Oka, T., and Nishiyama, N. (1973): J. Pharmacol. Exp. Ther., 186: 261
20. Tulunay, F.C., and Takemori, A.E. (1974): J. Pharmacol. Exp. Ther., 190: 395
21. Way, E.L., Loh, H.H. and Shen, F. (1969): J. Pharmacol. Exp. Ther., 167: 1
22. Wei, E. (1973): Psychopharmacologia, 28: 35

Factors Affecting the Action of Narcotics, edited by
M.L. Adler, L. Manara, and R. Samanin.
Raven Press, New York©1978.

Interaction of Opiates with Agents which cause
Withdrawal-like Syndromes

Eddie Wei

Department of Environmental Health Sciences
School of Public Health
University of California
Berkeley, California, U.S.A.

INTRODUCTION

The hypothesis (22,23) that opiates act as inhibitory
modulators of neurotransmission raises questions
concerning the nature of excitatory substances which
may be normally present in the same neuronal pathways.
Microinjection studies have shown that the principal
supraspinal sites of morphine action are located in
the medial brainstem (27). It might be expected that
activation of excitatory mechanisms in the medial
brainstem would precipitate a withdrawal-like syndrome
in normal animals, and that these actions would be
blocked by opiates. To investigate the endogenous
mechanisms which may counterbalance opiate actions,
Collier (7) has proposed the study of drugs which
produce "quasi-abstinence" effects: a "quasi-abstinence"
effect being defined as "an effect resembling one
elicited by withdrawal of a drug on which an animal has
been made dependent, but produced by another treatment
in a naive animal never exposed to drug nor to a like-
acting congener that induces, such dependence".
Two behavioral manifestations are especially characteristic of morphine-withdrawal in rodents and may be
useful for study as examples of "quasi-abstinence"
effects. The first is escape behavior, which is
manifested either as repeated jumps of withdrawing
animals off an elevated platform or as attempts of the
animal to escape from its container (32,35,39). A
second sign characteristic of withdrawal is repetitive
shaking movements of the body (47). This behavior,
termed by Wilker et al. (47) as "wet dog shakes", is
evident in abrupt (26) as well as antagonist-precipitated
withdrawal (14). The agents which promote escape
behavior in normal animals have been described elsewhere (11,21,24,45,46). In this paper, the conditions

147

and agents for stimulating and inhibiting shaking in normal animals will be briefly reviewed. Preliminary data on the interaction of agents which cause shaking with the process of morphine physical dependence will also be presented.

Non-Pharmacological Stimuli which Provoke Shaking

Head-shaking, the rhythmic, alternating, left and right rotations of the head about the longest axis of the body, was first studied in decerebrate and normal cats by Sherrington in 1917 (31). He described head-shaking as a component of the pinna reflex and noted that 1) the receptive field for this reflex was principally in the concha and meatus of the ear, 2) tactile and thermal stimuli readily provoked head shaking, a drop of fluid in the ear or a puff of air being effective stimuli, 3) the reflex was relatively resistant to chloroform or ether anesthesia, 4) attention mechanisms could suppress this reflex, 5) the stimuli provoking head-shaking had affective qualities which were different from nociception, and 6) the biological function of head-shaking was to protect the animal against irritant materials being deposited within the ear. These astute observations define the essential characteristics of shaking and the non-pharmacological conditions which provoke this behavior.

In rodents and other fur-coated animals, shaking of the head and body is observed as part of normal behavior and is classified by ethologists as "maintenance" behavior, along with grooming, washing, digging, licking of the penis, eating and drinking (33). Examples of conditions which provoke shaking in mice and rats are listed in Table 1. Some of these conditions may be species-specific. For example, we find that hamsters and gerbils do not shake after immersion in water, but when sand is poured on these rodents (who normally live in a desert habitat) they will shake and dig. The experimental conditions listed in Table 1 show that shaking, as a behavioral element, can readily be obtained under defined conditions and subjected to pharmacological analysis.

Pharmacological Stimulants and Inhibitors of Shaking

Reports of drugs which induce shaking in normal animals have appeared periodically in the literature, and examples are listed in chronological order in Table 2. So far no systematic effort has been made to compare the activities of these agents or to study their mechanisms of action. The chemical structures of

some of the more novel compounds are shown in Figure 1.
    I have recently studied the pharmacology of AG-3-5
(38).   This compound when administered at doses of 1 to
8 mg/kg will provoke shaking in mice, rats, gerbils,
hamsters, guinea pigs, rabbits, cats and dogs.   The
dose-effect relationship of AG-3-5 to shaking in rats
is shown in Figure 2.   Interestingly, of 32 rats tested

TABLE 1.   Examples of non-pharmacological stimuli which
           provoke shaking in rodents.

	Reference
Tactile stimulation of the ear with a fine hair or a puff of air	(1,13)
Dusting mice with charcoal	(29)
Application of xylene, an irritating solvent, onto the pinna	(3)
Immersion in water	(40)
Experimentally-induced seizures	(6)

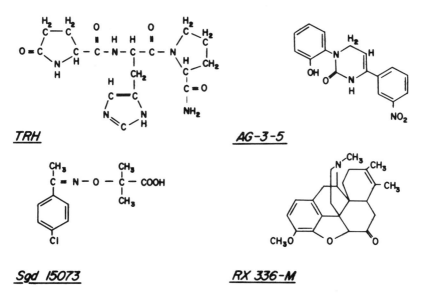

FIG. 1.   Chemical structures of compounds which provoke
          shaking

TABLE 2. Pharmacological stimulants of shaking

Condition or Agent	Reference
Abrupt withdrawal in morphine-dependent rats	(26,47)
Head shakes with prenderol	(2)
Head twitches with 5-hydroxytryptamine	(8)
Pentazocine	(30)
Levallorphan-precipitated withdrawal in morphine-dependent rats	(14)
AG-3-5	(4, 38)
Naloxone-precipitated withdrawal in morphine-dependent rats	(36)
TRH and analogs	(28,41,42)
Naloxone administration to rats treated chronically with delta[9]-tetra-hydrocannabinol	(18)
Benzylideneaminooxy-carbonic acid derivatives	(19)
RX-336M	(9)

with doses of 4,8 or 16 mg/kg of AG-3-5, 66 percent of the animals made on the average 21 escape attempts from their containers in the 5 to 10 minute interval after AG-3-5 injection. As mentioned previously, escape behavior is, like shaking, a characteristic sign of morphine abstinence. Other signs, such as teeth chattering and salivation, normally seen in morphine-abstinent rats, were not, however, observed in the AG-3-5 treated rats. The effects of AG-3-5 on shaking closely resembles that of Sgd 8473 and Sgd 15073, recently described by Jahn and Mixich (19).

A diverse number of agents can inhibit shaking (Table 3). These include: opiates (e.g. morphine and methadone), antischizophrenic drugs (e.g. chlorpromazine, perphenazine, haloperidol, reserpine), centrally-acting muscarinic agents (e.g. arecoline , physostigmine, diisopropylfluorophosphate: reversible with scopolamine) and agents which enhance adrenergic activity (e.g. imipramine, clonidine, d-amphetamine). Sedative-hypnotics (e.g. sodium pentobarbital) attenuate shaking

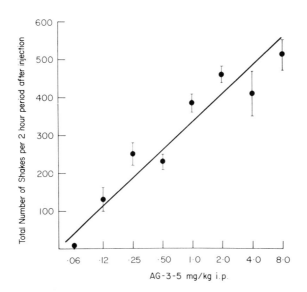

FIG. 2.   Dose-effect relationship of AG-3-5 on shaking
behavior in the rat.

produced by AG-3-5 and Sgd 15073 but do not abolish
this response even when the animal has reached the
plane of surgical anesthesia.   By contrast, sodium
pentobarbital anesthesia lowers the threshold dose for
thyrotropin-releasing hormone (TRH)-induced and naloxone-
precipitated shaking when the dose is compared to that
required to produce shaking in the conscious animal.
Possibly, the hypothermia associated with anesthesia
increases the effectiveness of stimuli which activate
thermogenetic shaking, whereas in the conscious animal,
at normal body temperature, the principal stimulus for
shaking may be sensory irritation.

Interactions of Compounds which Cause Shaking
with Morphine Physical Dependence

From the brief review of the literature, tabulated
in the previous sections, it is apparent that non-
pharmacological stimuli can activate shaking.   In addition, a unique reciprocal relationship appears to exist
between the acute inhibitory effect of morphine on

TABLE 3. Examples of conditions or agents which inhibit shaking

Stimuli for shaking	Inhibitory condition or agent	Reference
In the conscious animals:		
a) the pinna reflex stimulated by a fine hair	muscle relaxants, neuroleptics, opiates	(13,20,48)
b) antagonist-precipitated withdrawal in morphine-dependent rats	elevated body temperatures, d-amphetamine, clonidine diphenylhydantoin, delta9-tetrahydrocannabinol	(10,15,17,34, 44)
c) abrupt withdrawal in morphine-dependent rats	morphine, haloperidol, imipramine	(5,25)
d) benzylideneaminooxy-carbonic acid derivatives	opiates, clonidine	(19)
e) AG-3-5	opiates, clonidine	(38)
In barbiturate-anesthetized rats:		
a) immersion in ice water	for a), b) & c): morphine, clonidine and central injections of	(37,43)
b) application of xylene to the pinna	norepinephrine, epinephrine,	
c) central injections of TRH	carbachol, cholinesterase inhibitors	

shaking and the spontaneous shaking which occurs during withdrawal. Since physical dependence on opiates is generally considered to be a consequence of adaptive changes to the drug effect (16), the question may be asked: Can agents producing the "quasi-abstinence" effect of shaking mimic or activate endogenous mechanisms which will counteract the opiate actions leading to the development of physical dependence? Experiments were therefore carried out with AG-3-5 and TRH to see whether these drugs can affect the development of physical dependence on morphine.

AG-3-5 suspended in corn oil or corn oil alone was administered for three days to male rats implanted with a specially-formulated morphine pellet (12). Ten hours after the last dose of AG-3-5, animals were challenged with naloxone hydrochloride and the withdrawal syndrome observed under standardized conditions (39). The results in Table 4 show that although the incidence of shaking during withdrawal was decreased by AG-3-5, the other criteria of withdrawal, escape responses and weight loss, were unaffected by AG-3-5 pretreatment. Thus, AG-3-5, at doses which were pharmacologically active, does not counteract the development of physical dependence. An interesting incidental observation noted in these experiments was the finding that chronic oral administration of corn oil prevented the appearance of teeth chattering during withdrawal. The reason for this effect is not known.

To study the effects of TRH on the development of morphine physical dependence it was necessary to have a method for chronically delivering this peptide into the critical brain receptor areas. The recent development of the osmotic minipump (Alzet ^{TM} Osmotic Minipump System, Alza Corp., Palo Alto, California), an implantable device which permits the delivery of a small volume of drug solution at a constant rate, enabled us to overcome this methodological problem.

Animals were anesthetized with sodium pentobarbital and L-shaped cannulas were implanted into the periaqueductal gray region of the brain. The cannula was then connected to a minipump which was prefilled with either distilled water, naloxone hydrochloride or TRH. Six hours after being connected to the minipump, the animal was implanted subcutaneously with a morphine pellet. The abstinence syndrome was then precipitated with naloxone, 10 mg/kg i.p., 63 to 65 hours after morphine pellet implantation. As shown in Table 4, naloxone hydrochloride infused into the periaqueductal gray-fourth ventricular spaces at a total dose of 490 μg per animal per 70 hours, almost completely blocked the appearance of the withdrawal syndrome. Infusions of TRH into the periaqueductal gray was not, however,

TABLE 4. Effects of AG-3-5, naloxone, and TRH on the development of physical dependence on morphine[a]

Chemical	Unit dose	N	% Animals Showing Withdrawal Sign			% Weight Loss 3 hr after Naloxone
			Teeth Chattering	Escape Responses	Wet Shakes	
corn oil	1 ml/kg[b]	8	0	100	62	9.2 ± 0.6
AG-3-5	10 mg/kg[c]	7	43	100	14	8.8 ± 0.6
distilled H_2O	98 μl[d]	13	85	85	46	7.0 ± 0.3
naloxone HCl	98 μg[d]	8	0[e]	37	75	4.6 ± 0.6[e]
naloxone HCl	490 μg[d]	8	12[e]	12[e]	12[e]	3.7 ± 0.8[e]
TRH	980 μg[d]	8	75	75	50	6.3 ± 0.4

[a]Physical dependence was induced by subcutaneous implant of 1 pellet containing 75 mg of morphine base. Three days later withdrawal was precipitated by naloxone HCl 10 mg/kg i.p.: 15 min observation period of withdrawal signs.

[b]Administered twice daily for 3 days, oral route.

[c]Suspended in corn oil and administered twice daily for 3 days, oral route.

[d]Drugs dissolved in sterile distilled water, the estimated dose per animal per 70 hr infusion period calculated as concentration of drug in infusate x 1.4 μl/hr flow rate of minipump x 70 hr infusion period.

[e]$p < 0.05$ vs distilled water controls.

effective in attenuating the intensity of withdrawal (Table 4).

SUMMARY

The factors which antagonize narcotic actions can act by affecting the access or binding of the opiate to its receptor or by physiological antagonism of the drug effect. To characterize the neural substrates and modulators which exert physiological antagonism of opiate effects, Collier (7) proposed the study of agents or conditions which produce "quasi-abstinence" effects. The quasi-abstinence sign, shaking, can be elicited by non-pharmacological stimuli and by a number of chemicals. Two drugs which cause shaking, TRH and AG-3-5, were studied to see whether they can antagonize the development of morphine physical dependence. Chronic administration of these drugs failed to attenuate the development of dependence. However, under similar conditions, naloxone hydrochloride, a specific antagonist which prevents opiates binding to the receptor, inhibited the development of physical dependence.

ACKNOWLEDGEMENTS

The assitance of J.B. Cunningham is acknowledged. The osmotic minipumps used in this study were generously donated by Alza Corp., Palo Alto, California. AG-3-5 (1- [2-hydroxyphenyl]-4 [3-nitrophenyl]-1,2,3,6-tetra-hydropyrimidine-2-one) is a patented compund (U.S. Patent No. 3,821,221) of Delmar Chemical Co., Quebec, Canada. This study was supported by PHS Grant DA-00091.

REFERENCES

1. Askew, H.R., Leibrecht, B.C. and Ratner, S.C. (1969): J. Comp. Physiol. Psychol., 67: 497
2. Blum, B. (1962): Arch. Int. Pharmacodyn. Ther., 137: 128
3. Boulton, C.S. and Handley, S.L. (1973): Psychopharmacologia, 31: 205
4. Burford, R.G. and Chappel, C.I. (1972): In: Abstracts of the 5th International Congress on Pharmacology p. 33. San Francisco.
5. Colasanti, B. and Khazan, N. (1975): Neuropharmacology 14: 361
6. Colasanti, B.K., Kosa, J.E. and Craig, C.R. (1975): Psychopharmacologia, 44:33
7. Collier, H.O.J. (1974): Pharmacology, 11: 58
8. Corne, S.J., Pickering, R.W. and Warner, B.T. (1963): Br. J. Pharmacol., 20: 106
9. Cowan, A. and MacFarlane, I.R. (1976): Psychopharmacologia, 45: 277

10. Fertiziger, A.P., Lynch, J.J. and Stein, E. (1974): Brain Res., 78: 331
11. Francis, D.L., Roy, A.C. and Collier, H.O.J.(1975): Life Sci.,16: 1901
12. Gibson, R.D. and Tingstad, J.E. (1970): J. Pharm. Sci., 59: 426
13. Goodsell, J.S., Toman, J.E.P., Everett, G.M. and Richards, R.K. (1954): J. Pharmacol. Exp. Ther., 110: 251.
14. Grumbach, L. (1969): In: Proceedings of the 31st NAS-NRC Committee on Problems of Drug Dependence p. 5775.
15. Herz, A., Blasig, J. and Papeschi, R. (1974): Psychopharmacologia, 39: 121.
16. Himmelsbach, C.K. (1943): Fed. Proc., 2: 201
17. Hine, B., Friedman, E., Torrelio, M. and Gershon, S. (1975): Science, 187: 443.
18. Hirschhorn, I.D. and Rosecrans, J.A. (1974): Psychopharmacologia, 36: 243
19. Jahn, U. and Mixich, G. (1976): Psychopharmacologia, 46: 191
20. Janssen, P.A.J. (1961): J. Pharm. Pharmacol., 13: 513.
21. Koppanyi, T., Maling, H.M., Saul, W. and Brodie, B.B. (1970): J. Pharmacol. Exp. Ther., 172: 170.
22. Kosterlitz, H.W. and Hughes, J.W. (1975): Life Sci. 16: 91.
23. Krivoy, W. and Zimmerman, E. (1973): In: Chemical Modulation of Brain Function: A Tribute to J.E.P. Toman, edited by H.C. Sabelli, p. 111. Raven Press, New York.
24. Lal, H., Colpaert, F.C. and Laduron, P. (1975): Eur. J. Pharmacol., 30: 113
25. Lal, H. and Numan, R. (1976): Life Sci.,18: 163
26. Martin, W.R., Wikler, A., Eades, C.G. and Pescor, F.T. (1963): Psychopharmacologia, 4: 247.
27. Pert, A. and Yaksh, T. (1974): Brain Res., 80: 135.
28. Prange, A.J., Jr., Breese, G.R., Cott, J.M., Martin, B.R., Cooper, B.R., Wilson, I.C. and Plotnikoff, N.P. (1974): Life Sci., 14: 447.
29. Rohte, O. (1969): Psychopharmacologia, 14: 18.
30. Schneider, C. (1968): Nature (Lond.),220: 586.
31. Sherrington, C.S. (1917): J. Physiol. (Lond.), 51: 404.
32. Siegel, R.K., Gusewelle, B.E. and Jarvik, M.E. (1975): Int. Pharmacopsychiat., 10: 17.
33. Silverman, A. (1965): Br. J. Pharmacol., 24: 579.
34. Tseng, L.F., Loh, H.H. and Wei, E.T. (1975): Eur. J. Pharmacol., 30: 93
35. Way, E.L., Loh, H.H. and Shen, F.H. (1969): J. Pharmacol. Exp. Ther., 167: 1

36. Wei, E. (1973): Life Sci., 12: 385.
37. Wei, E. (1975): Life Sci., 17: 17
38. Wei, E. (1976): J. Pharm. Pharmacol. (in press)
39. Wei, E., Loh, H.H. and Way, E.L. (1973): J. Pharmacol. Exp. Ther., 184: 398.
40. Wei, E., Loh, H.H. and Way, E.L. (1973): Life Sci., 12: 489.
41. Wei, E., Loh, H. and Way, E.L. (1976): Eur. J. Pharmacol., 36: 227.
42. Wei, E., Sigel, S., Loh, H. and Way, E.L. (1975): Nature (Lond.), 253: 739
43. Wei, E., Sigel, S. and Way, E.L. (1975): J.Pharmacol. Exp. Ther., 193: 56
44. Wei, E., Tseng, L.F., Loh, H. and Way, E.L. (1974): Nature (Lond.), 247: 398.
45. Weissman, A. (1971): Psychopharmacologia, 21: 60.
46. Weissman, A. (1973): J. Pharmacol. Exp. Ther., 184: 11.
47. Wikler, A., Green, P.C., Smith, H.D. and Pescor, F.T. (1960): Fed. Proc., 19: 22
48. Witkin, L.B., Spitaletta, P. and Plummer, A.J. (1959): J. Pharmacol. Exp. Ther., 126: 330.

2. ROUTE OF ADMINISTRATION, DRUG BINDING, DISTRIBUTION AND METABOLISM

Factors Affecting the Action of Narcotics, edited by
M.L. Adler, L. Manara, and R. Samanin.
Raven Press, New York©1978.

Direct Application of Narcotics into the Brain

A. Herz and Hj. Teschemacher

Department of Neuropharmacology
Max-Planck-Institut für Psychiatrie
Kraepelinstrasse 2, 8000 München 40
Germany

INTRODUCTION

There are several general aspects which render the
direct application of drugs into the brain a promising
method of experimental pharmacology. This form of application circumvents the blood-brain-barrier (BBB),
which is difficult to overcome by compounds with low
lipid solubility, avoids catabolic breakdown in peripheral organs and conserves scarce substances. Another
feature of this approach is that it makes it possible
to study sites of action in the brain, and under certain
circumstances, the mechanism of action.

When drugs are injected into the lateral ventricle
the many structures lining the ventricular system (VS)
as well as parts of the external surface of the brain come
into contact with the drug. The spread of the drug
within the VS can be restricted by a plug, inserted
into different parts of the VS. Besides intraventricular application, the direct injection of small amounts
of drug into defined brain areas (microinjection) is
often used. Finally, a particular type of direct drug
application is represented by the microiontophoretic
method which permits recording of the electrical activity
of individual neurones to which the drug has been applied. All these methods have been widely used in
opiate research. In particular, they have proved very
valuable following the recent detection of endogenous
ligands for the opiate receptors (8, 19) in analysis
of the effects of these substances on the central nervous
system.

The purpose of this article is to outline aspects
and problems of general significance when applying
opiates and opioids directly into the brain. Particular

161

emphasis will be given to the pharmacokinetic aspects of such experiments from which the importance of the physico-chemical properties of the substance will become obvious.

Application into the Ventricular System (VS)

Since the intraventricular application of codeine in mice by Adler (1) this method has often been used for studying opiate effects in various species. Not only analgesia but also other specific opiate effects, such as sedation, catalepsia and respiratory depression are induced in various species by opiates with this form of application. After repeated intraventricular application tolerance and physical dependence also develop (4,20). A detailed study on the pharmacokinetic problems involved in this method showed that the physico-chemical properties of the applied opiates exert strong influence on the characteristics of action and must be considered in interpretation of the results (6).
Fig. 1 compares the antinociceptive effect of a representative hydrophilic (morphine), and lipophilic (fentanyl) narcotic after intravenous and intraventricular injection. Two essential points should be noted: The doses needed to induce similar effects after each mode of application and the time course of these effects. While in the case of morphine the ratio of equieffective dosage (i. ventr./i.v.) is about 1 : 500 (taking the body weight into account), this proportion is roughly 1:5 in the case of fentanyl. This is mainly due to the different abilities of the drugs to overcome the BBB after systemic administration, although differences in permeation into brain tissue are also of importance. Thus after intraventricular injection morphine for example, reaches its maximum effect much later than after intravenous injection; for details see (6).
To study such questions in more detail labelled narcotics with low and high lipophilicity were injected i. ventr. in rabbits. At increasing intervals after injection the concentration of the substances in the cerebro-spinal fluid (CSF), and in the brain tissue as well as the permeation into blood, were determined (Table 1). From the table it can be seen that the concentration of the hydrophilic compounds in the CSF remains high for a considerable time after injection, while the lipophilic compounds disappear rapidly from this compartment. In brain tissue the concentration of morphine and dihydromorphine remains constant for at least one hour, whereas in the case of the two lipophilic compounds, etorphine and fentanyl, it declines rapidly. This latter finding is explained by the large amount of

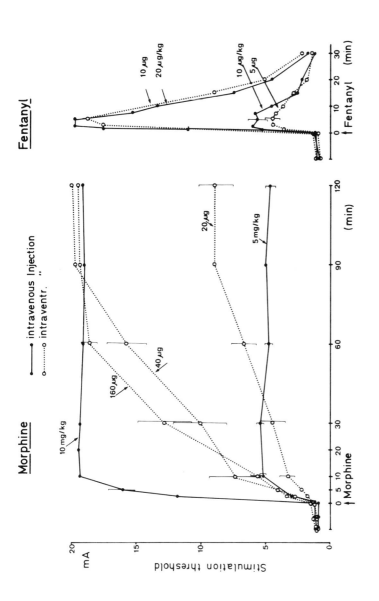

FIG. 1. Antinociceptive effect of morphine and fentanyl after intravenous and intra-ventricular application in rabbits. The licking reaction induced by electrical tooth pulp stimulation was used as test. For details see (6).

substance that passes into the blood stream within the
first 5 min after injection. Similar differences in
the persistence of the substances in brain tissue after
intraventricular injection are observed when the drugs
are injected directly into the tissue (see later) (for
details see 18).

Obviously there is a clear parallelism between the
persistence of the substances in brain tissue after intraventricular injection and the duration of the antinociceptive effect (see fig. 1). Moreover, the speed
of onset of this analgesic effect proved to be related
to the progressive permeation of the substance from the
ventricular space into the brain tissue (6, 18). From
this it can be concluded that the receptors involved in
the antinociceptive effect of the opiates are not
located immediately on the ventricular surface, but
somewhat distant. Though there is no real barrier, comparable to the BBB, between the ventricular space and
the brain tissue, the hydrophilic compounds obviously
need some time to reach these receptors. This is explained by the well known fact that hydrophilic compounds have difficulty crossing biological membranes.

TABLE 1. Distribution of opiates after intraventricular and
intracerebral injection in rabbits

	PK Heptane/ Water	Intraventricular injection							Intra-cerebral injection
		5 min			15 min		60 min		60 min
		CSF	Br	Bl	CSF	Br	CSF	Br	Br
Dihydro-morphine	<0.00001	48	15	3	56	20	12	15	43
Morphine	<0.00001	42	30	5	38	22	13	24	61
Etorphine	1.42	25	28	50	9	4	2	-	7
Fentanyl	19.35	20	33	38	6	7	2	-	7

Radioactivity found in the cerebro-spinal fluid (CSF), brain
tissue (Br) and blood (Bl) at various times after injection of
^{14}C-morphine, ^{3}H-dihydromorphine, ^{3}H-etorphine and ^{3}H-fentanyl
into the lateral ventricle of rabbits or into brain tissue in %
of quantity injected. The partition coefficients (PK) heptane/
water, pH 7.4 are also given. For details see(18).

A quite different time-course of effect is found in
isolated organs, as, for example, in the myenteric
plexus-longitudinal muscle of the guinea-pig ileum. In
this preparation hydrophilic narcotics show a much more
rapid onset of effect than lipophilic compounds (11).
This is an indication that in this preparation only a
few membranes have to be passed by the drug on the way
to the receptor.

In spite of the slow permeation of hydrophilic
compounds to the site of action in the brain after intraventricular application, these compounds are finally
very effective as they are held back in the brain.   The
lipophilic compounds, on the other hand, show a lower
efficiency as they leave the brain more rapidly. Nevertheless, the antinociceptive potency of a series of
narcotic analgesics, measured following intraventricular
injection into rabbits, is a much better reflection of
the receptor activity of these compounds than the
potency found after systemic application.   This also
agrees with a recent study in which the stereospecific
binding of a series of narcotic analgesics was compared
with their antinociceptive effects after intravenous
and intraventricular application (16).

Recently intraventricular drug application has become
essential for investigation of the action of endogenous
ligands of the opiate receptor on the central nervous
system.   Fig. 2 compares the antinociceptive effect of
enkephalin, endorphins and normorphine (3, 17).   Though
very effective in the isolated myenteric plexus-longitudinal muscle of the guinea-pig ileum and in the
mouse vas deferens (8), even high dosages of enkephalin
revealed only a very weak and short lasting   antinociceptive effect after intraventricular injection in
rats.   This contrasts greatly with the intense and long
lasting effect seen in response to a purified extract
of porcine pituitary gland containing longer chain
peptides (17).   Besides analgesia the endorphins also
induced strong catalepsia and respiratory depression.
Microelectrophoretic studies showed that enkephalin is
very effective when applied directly to cerebral neurones
(25) (see later).   This indicates that the weakness of
the effect produced by intraventricular application has
to be explained pharmacokinetically.   Because both
peptides are probably rather hydrophilic compounds the
pentapeptide is expected to have no greater difficulties
reaching the site of action than the endorphins which
have a much higher molecular weight.   It is suggested,
therefore, that the pentapeptide, in contrast to the
endorphins, is rapidly metabolized in the brain.   This
is supported by other evidence.   This is an interesting
example showing that even after intraventricular
injection interference from metabolism may become

critical when endogenous   constituents of the brain are
applied from outside.

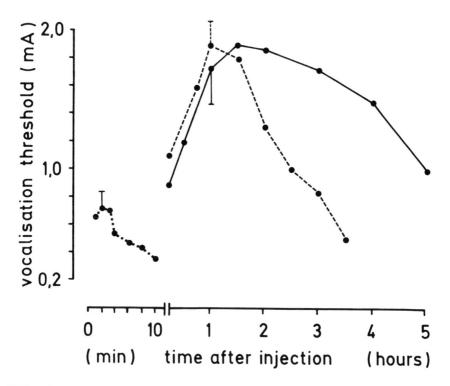

FIG. 2.   Antinociceptive effect of methionine-enkephalin,
endorphins and normorphine after intraventricular injection in rats.   Vocalization induced by electrical
stimulation of the tail was used as test.   For details
see (3).

●————● Endorphin ∿100 μg
●·······● Methionine-enkephalin 300 μg
●------● Normorphine 20 μg

Application into Restricted Parts of the
Ventricular System

As many periventricular structures and even sites on
the outer surface of the brain are reached by a drug
after intraventricular application, only limited information about drug sites of action can be obtained this
way. This disadvantage can, however, be partially
overcome if the spread of the drug within the VS is

restricted by a plug inserted into certain parts of the VS (2). Particularly in combination with a autoradiographic check of the spread of the injected labelled drug , this method proved useful when investigating the sites of the antinociceptive action of opiates in rabbits (5). The 'plug method' was developed in our laboratory because microinjection into restricted parts of the brain gave inconsistent results, probably due to spread of the drug beyond the target area (see next paragraph).

After the first study concerning the sites of action of morphine during the development of physical dependence in rabbits (7) we used this method in a similar study in rats (13). Naloxone injected into the lateral ventricle in rats with a plug inserted into the aqueductus mesencephali precipitated only weak withdrawal symptoms, while, when injected into the aqueduct or into the 4th ventricle, it precipitated a nearly complete spectrum of withdrawal symptoms as seen following systemic injection or injection into the ventricular system without restriction.

To get more detailed information, experiments with labelled naloxone were performed in which the spread of the drug in each individual experiment was evaluated autoradiographically. An example is given in fig. 3. Only weak withdrawal signs were observed in the experiment represented on the left in which the structure lining the lateral and 3rd ventricle as well as the anterior parts of the aqueduct were heavily labelled. Strong withdrawal, characterized by intense jumping, however, was present in the experiment represented on the right. The anterior parts of the VS were completely free of radioactivity while intense labelling was present in the fossa rhomboidea and, to some degree, also in the most posterior part of the periaqueductal grey matter. Injection of the antagonist onto the ventral surface of the brain stem (where intense radioactivity was also found in the experiments illustrated) was ineffective. The evaluation of a series of experiments, varying the location of the plug and using different injection sites, indicated that the most sensitive areas for precipitation of withdrawal were in the anterior parts of the fossa rhomboidea and possibly also in the most posterior part of the periaqueductal grey matter (Laschka et al., in preparation). As the sites of action of opiates and opiate antagonists are most probably identical, structures in this area are suggested to be of particular significance for the development of physical dependence on opiates.

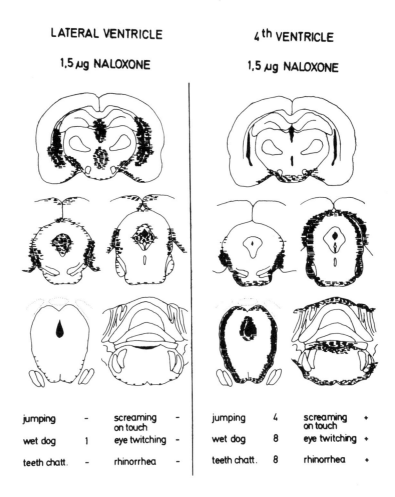

FIG. 3. <u>Distribution of radioactivity (as evaluated from autoradiographs) and precipitated withdrawal signs</u> after injection of 1.5 µg 3H-naloxone into different parts of the VS of tolerant/dependent rats. Rats were made tolerant/dependent by implantation of 6 morphine pellets (75 mg) within 7 days; withdrawal was precipitated at the 10th day. Animals were killed 10 min after naloxone injection. An eucerine plug was inserted in the aqueduct 5 min before naloxone was injected either into the lateral ventricle (left side) or the 4th ventricle (right side). The shaded area indicates distribution of radioactivity.
For details see (13) and Laschka, in preparation .

Microinjection into Brain Tissue

In a series of experiments the microinjection method was used to evaluate sites of acute and chronic action of opiates in the brain. Besides mesencephalic and rhombencephalic areas, thalamic and hypothalamic sites were found responsible for the analgesic action of morphine. Some of the discrepancies between the results of various laboratories may be explained by spread of the drug beyond the target area. In this context the physico-chemical properties of the substance used are also of considerable significance. Table 1 shows that lipophilic compounds leave the brain much more rapidly than hydrophilic ones; the same difference also holds true for diffusion within the brain, that is, lipophilic substances will tend to spread more rapidly.

From the fact that most narcotic effects were induced by intraventricular application of opiates in rabbits and rats (5, unpublished results), and that a strong withdrawal pattern could be precipitated by i. ventr. injection of opiate antagonists in dependent rabbits and rats (7,12), it can be concluded that most sites of action of morphine are located periventricularly. Therefore, one may expect that after microinjection into these areas the drug also reaches the ventricular space. The absolute size of the brain seems to be of importance in this context, rendering microinjection experiments in rats more critical than in monkeys (14). This does not mean that under well controlled conditions and using refined microinjection techniques reliable results cannot be obtained in rats too (9, 10,23). It may be helpful to check on the spread by means of labelled drugs (13). Valuable information can also be provided through comparison of the dosages effective on microinjection and i.ventr. injection. If they are in the same range, caution is indicated in interpretation of the findings.

In an effort to overcome such problems, crystal suspensions instead of solutions were applied under the assumption that the spread of the drug might thus be reduced (21). In practice, however, this technique leads to new problems in that the exact dosage is difficult to control and the amounts actually applied are considerably above those effective when administered in solution intraventricularly. Thus, the same authors used naloxone solutions in a recent study which indicated that, besides the periaqueductal 4th ventricle region, the medial hypothalamus was also sensitive to naloxone in morphine dependent rats (22).

Microiontophoretic Application

The microiontophoretic application of narcotics, widely used in the past few years (15), offers information about the action of these drugs at the single neurone level and, in particular, intracellular recording is a fruitful tool to investigate their mechanisms of action (24). It is essential, when using this method, to distinguish between specific effects (mediated by the opiate receptors) and non-specific (e.g. local anaesthetic) effects. Comparison of the effects of pharmacologically active and inactive opiate isomers (e.g. levorphanol vs dextrorphan) and the use of specific antagonists revealed that the inhibition of spontaneous and glutamate-induced discharge activity observed in various brain regions represents a specific opiate effect,while the excitation observed, especially after higher dosages,seemed to be non-specific (15). This view is supported by the recent finding that microiontophoretically applied methionine and leucine-enkephalin mimic the inhibitory effects of opiates,but not the excitatory ones (25). The demonstration of a specific effect of enkephalin at the neuronal level in the brain is also important in view of the very low efficacy of this endogenous ligand of the opiate receptor after i. ventr. injection (see paragraph on intraventricular injection). A task for further microiontophoretic work with opiates will be to relate their actions at the single neurone level with the opiate-induced changes in various functional systems of the brain.

SUMMARY

The various methods available for direct application of drugs into the brain have been widely used in opiate research. The pharmacological actions obtained by intraventricular application of opiates in rodents are very similar to those observed after systemic injection. The ratio of equieffective doses on each route of application and the onset and duration of effect largely depend, however, on the physico-chemical properties of the substances. Application of the drugs into restricted parts of the ventricular system showed that important sites for acute and chronic opiate actions are located in the periaqueductal/-4th ventricle area. Microinjection of opiates into defined brain structures may give more detailed information about these sites, provided that the spread of drug is kept under consideration and is well controlled. The microiontophoretic application of opiates to single neurones in various brain structures revealed their main effect to be inhibition of neuronal discharge activity. These methods for direct application of drugs into the brain have proved particularly valuable when investigating the actions of endogenous ligands of the opiate receptor.

ACKNOWLEDGMENT

The authors wish to thank Mrs. Dum for stylistic revision of the manuscript.

REFERENCES

1. Adler, T.K. (1963) : J. Pharmacol. Exp. Ther.,140: 155.
2. Albus, K. (1971) : Physiol. Behav.,8 : 569-571.
3. Bläsig, J., and Herz, A. (1976) : Naunyn Schmiedebergs Arch. Pharmacol., 294:297-300.
4. Eidelberg, E., and Barstrow, C.A. (1971) : Science, 174:74-76.
5. Herz, A., Albus, K., Metỹs, J., Schubert, P., and Teschemacher, H. (1970) : Neuropharmacology, 9 : 539-551.
6. Herz, A., and Teschemacher, H. (1971) : Adv. Drug Res., 6 : 79-119.
7. Herz, A., Teschemacher, H., Albus, K., and Zieglgänsberger, S. (1972) : Psychopharmacologia, 26 : 219-235.
8. Hughes, J., Smith, T.W., Kosterlitz, H.W.,Fothergill, L.A., Morgan B.A., and Morris, H.R. (1975) : Nature, 258 : 577-579.
9. Jacquet, Y. (1975) : In : Methods in Narcotics Research, edited by S. Ehrenpreis and A. Neidle, pp. 33-58, M. Dekker, New York.
10. Jacquet, Y., and Lajtha, A. (1973) : Science , 182: 490-492.
11. Kosterlitz,H.W., Leslie, F.M., and Waterfield, A.A. (1975) : Eur. J. Pharmacol, 32 : 10-16.
12. Laschka, E., Herz, A., and Bläsig, J. (1976) : Psychopharmacologia, 46 : 133-139.
13. Laschka, E., Teschemacher, H., Mehraein, P., and Herz, A. (1976) : Psychopharmacologia, 46 : 141-147.
14. Pert, A., and Yaksh, T. (1974):Brain Res., 80 : 135-140.
15. Satoh, M., Zieglgänsberger, W., and Herz, A. (1976) Brain Res.,115 : 95-110.
16. Terenius, L. (1974) : J. Pharm. Pharmacol., 26 : 146-148.
17. Teschemacher, H., Bläsig, J., and Kromer, W. (1976) Naunyn Schmiedebergs Arch.Pharmacol., (in press).

18. Teschemacher, H., Niedner, J., and Schubert, P. (1976) : Neuropharmacology, (in press).
19. Teschemacher, H., Opheim, K.E., Cox, B.M., and Goldstein, A. (1975) : Life Sci., 16 : 1771-1776.
20. Watanabe, K. (1971) : Jpn. J. Pharmacol., 21 :383-391.
21. Wei, E., Loh, H.H., and Way, E.L. (1973) : J. Pharmacol. Exp. Ther., 185 : 108-115.
22. Wei, E., Sigel, S.H., Loh, H.H., and Way, E.L. (1975) : J. Pharmacol. Exp. Ther., 195 : 480-487.
23. Yaksh, T.L., Yeung, J.C., and Rudy, T.A. (1976) : Brain Res. ,114 : 83-103.
24. Zieglgänsberger, W., and Bayerl, H. (1976) : Brain Res., 115 : 111-128.
25. Zieglgänsberger, W., Fry, J.P., Herz, A., Moroder, L., and Wünsch, E. (1976) : Brain Res., 115 : 160-164.

Factors Affecting the Action of Narcotics, edited by
M.L. Adler, L. Manara, and R. Samanin.
Raven Press, New York©1978.

The Use of Self-Administration for Assessing
the Action of the Opiates

Harold L. Altshuler

Neuropsychopharmacology Section
Texas Research Institute of Mental Sciences

and

Department of Pharmacology
Baylor College of Medicine
Texas Medical Center
Houston, Texas 77025
USA

INTRODUCTION

The use of mood-altering chemicals for their reinforcing properties has been associated with human
societies for all of recorded history. Although many
substances have been used by man for that purpose, none
have attained the prominence or social destructiveness
of the opiates and alcohol. Both drugs have been an
intimate part of the human experience and, while the
abuse of alcohol is the most prevalent and costly of
human drug abuse habits, opiate abuse presents a
striking and profoundly interesting syndrome. The opiate
narcotics such as morphine, heroin, codeine, and
methadone produce a syndrome of drug dependence characterized by compulsive drug-seeking, physical dependence
and tolerance, and a complex of self and socially
destructive behaviors.
Accompanying the changes in social awareness of the
problems of drug abuse has been a steady progression of
methodical and systematic research on opiate pharmacology.
Much of the research has, by necessity, been conducted
with laboratory animals, and the development of an
appropriate animal model was important. A number of
animal models have been studied but none have been as
useful as that of self-administration, which capitalizes
on the fact that the drugs of abuse serve as behavioral
reinforcers and maintain operant responding. The model
has provided a tool to evaluate many opiates, as well
as other classes of drug. This chapter will review
self-administration as a means of assessing the action
of the narcotics and present some data about a modification

173

of the intravenous self-administration model which
provides a new dimension in the evaluation of certain
opiates.

Self-Administration Research Methods

There are three main technical approaches to self-
administration studies: intravenous self-infusion of a
drug, self-administration by oral consumption of drugs
in drinking water or food, and self-infusion of the
drug directly into the gastrointestinal tract.

Intravenous Self-Administration

Intravenous self-administration has been the mainstay
of self-administration research for about 15 years. The
techniques for implantation of chronic indwelling
vascular catheters had been known for several years
when Weeks (34) developed a system that would allow an
animal to self-infuse drugs by depressing a response
lever in its cage. Weeks' original studies were conducted with rats and provided the germinal information
from which all other procedures evolved. Within a short
time other researchers (27,32) adapted Weeks' procedure
for studies in rhesus monkeys. Although there have
been several changes in the techniques of intravenous
self-administration, and several attempts to improve
the technical aspects of the procedure, it remains
essentially unchanged. Figure 1 presents an example
of the type of drug-intake data obtained in studies of
morphine self-administration by monkeys.

In intravenous self-administration, a silicone-rubber
catheter is implanted chronically in the animal's
jugular or femoral vein and tunneled subcutaneously
from the vein to the upper back, where it leaves the
body and connects to an infusion pump. The development
of restraint and protection devices for the animal and
the cannula was needed, and Weeks and Davis (35)devised
a saddle and backpack which met the need. Yanagita et
al. (42) and Deneau et al. (10) sucessfully modified
the design for studies with monkeys. In the early
systems, the drug injections and response contigencies
were controlled by electromechanical relay equipment
and the infusions were delivered by means of a syringe
infusion pump and solenoid valve (10,42). At the
present time, most laboratories control the self-administration chambers with minicomputers and deliver the
drug doses with peristaltic infusion pumps.

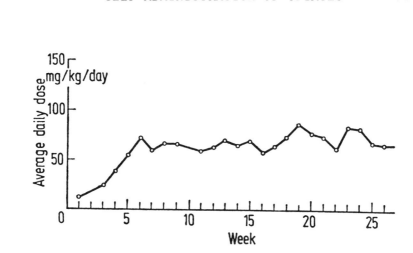

FIG. 1.   Intravenous self-administration of morphine
sulfate by a representative rhesus monkey allowed drug
access for 26 weeks

Note that animal increased its drug intake for first
5 weeks and then stabilized at an average daily intake
of about 70 mg/kg/day. This pattern is typical for
animals allowed access to drug 24 hrs/day on a continuous
reinforcement schedule.   From Deneau et al. (10), with
permission.

Oral Self Administration

The oral self-administration procedure is a simple
method of providing animals with drugs, and it has been
one of the most widely used methods for inducing volun-
tary drug consumption (5,21,22,23,26,31,36). Animals
are usually given a choice of several solutions, one
containing drug and the other containing water or a
liquid food source. The water or liquid food is usually
flavored with an aversive agent such as quinine.   The
usual way to establish oral self-administration of drugs
is to make the animal physically dependent on the drug
at the start of the study and to provide free access
afterward (36). Although parenteral pretreatment is
often used to produce physical dependence, the same
result can be accomplished by providing drug solutions
as the animal's only source of fluid.
Figure 2 presents an example of the type of result
obtained in oral self-administration studies. Fairly
precise estimates of solution intake may be obtained in
such studies (22,31). In addition, it is possible,

although difficult, to induce rats to drink morphine
solutions without first making them dependent upon
opiates (26,31). Oral self-administration procedures
may be subject to a great deal of variability. For
example, Schuster and Thompson (28) have suggested that
rats tend to persevere on a certain bottle position
and that their choices might be due more to the position
of the bottle than to the drug it contains. These
authors also have suggested that subtle differences in
the drinking tubes might provide sources of investigative
error which could be overlooked.

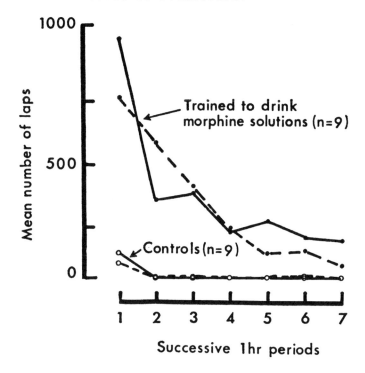

FIG. 2. Differences in water and morphine solution
intake for control and morphine-trained rats

Number of laps were recorded on a counter on the fluid
source. Solid lines represent rats deprived of fluids
overnight, dashed lines rats allowed to drink prior to
choice trial. Note that animals trained to drink
morphine solutions consumed much more morphine or water
than did control animals. From Stolerman and Kumar
(31), with permission.

The field of alcoholism research provides many studies of schedule-induced polydipsia to produce ethanol self-administration by rats and monkeys (24,25). It is surprising that relatively few researchers (23) have used that method to establish opiate self-administration by rats or monkeys. Polydipsia procedures raise many questions about the effects of excessive fluid intake on the pharmacological effects observed.

Intragastric Self-Administration

A few years after the establishment of intravenous self-administration in monkeys, Yanagita et al. (38,39, 41) recognized the need for an intragastric self-administration technique. Attempts to produce oral self-administration of drugs by subhuman primates had been generally unsuccessful, and the data contained many artifacts because of suspicious concern of the monkeys for their food or water and their tendency to reject drug-laced food or water unless it was the only source available or they were drug-dependent.
Yanagita's technique for intragastric self-administration used a nasogastric cannula and was moderately successful in studies with ethanol and certain insoluble barbiturates. He reported success with the technique, although he used it to only a limited extent to study the opiates. Little additional work was done with intragastric self-administration until the early 1970s, when four groups simultaneously developed intragastric self-administration procedures for laboratory animals. Three of the groups, those of Gotestam (17), Trojniar et al. (33), and Smith et al. (30), studied intragastric self-administration in rats: Smith's (30) and Trojniar's (33) groups examined the intragastric self-administration of the opiates. They demonstrated that rats would self-administer morphine by that route if first made physically dependent on the drug. Our laboratories developed a procedure (1,2,3,4) for intragastric self-administration of a number of drugs of abuse by the rhesus monkey. That technique uses a silastic cannula implanted directly into the monkey's stomach and will be described in detail below.

Factors in Opiate Self-Administration

Although many factors affect the patterns, rate, and magnitude of opiate self-administration, they fall into three major categories. Obviously, the pharmacological nature of the drug under examination is the primary determinant of its self-administration parameters (6.10,12). Other major determinants are the schedules of reinforcement

(12,15) and the magnitude of the reinforcement. Many investigators (28,29,37) have examined the relationship between reinforcement magnitude (dose) and response rates. There has also been a good deal of interest in examining several of the other major factors that determine the self-administration of opiates and their effects, such as manipulations in neurochemical state, environmental variables, and such antecedent variables as previous self-administration history (18).

Behavioral Variables that Control Self-Administration Rates

Schuster and Thompson (28) defined the factors that control the rate of self-administration behavior as (a) the reinforcement contigencies, (b) the reinforcing efficacy of the drug, and (c) the nonspecific rate-modifying effects of the drug. While the rate of self-administration of a drug may not be the best descriptor of its reinforcing efficacy, rate has been demonstrated to be an extremely useful means of determining the pharmacological effects and efficacy of drugs when they are serving as reinforcers. The typical response patterns for opiates, especially for morphine, when examined with fixed-ratio (FR) schedules, consist of binges of high response rates followed by brief periods of abstinence (39). With the intravenous self-administration model, periods of high responding and the inter-response periods are often minutes in duration, but they are hours or days long with the intragastric procedures (4).

The FR schedule is a relatively simple schedule and it has been used extensively to compare the reinforcement properties of a number of drugs, including morphine, codeine, and methadone. Woods and Schuster (37) reported that in time-limited sessions, morphine (100 mg/kg/infusion) maintained response rates of about 0.3 per second on a FR-20 schedule, while under the same conditions, methadone (100 mg/kg/infusion) maintained response rates of 0.9 responses per second. It is important to note that all of these experiments with FR schedules were conducted when the animals had only very limited periods of drug exposure and, consequently, were presumed to be nondependent. Although the FR schedules summarized above typify the way in which drugs can be compared for reinforcing properties, it is surprising that there have been so few studies of opiate self-administration maintained by fixed-interval (FI) schedules. In fact, FI schedules have been used primarily as parts of more complex sequences of chained schedules (15).

Effects of Reinforcement Magnitude

Several investigators (28,37) have examined the relationship between drug dose (per infusion) and total drug intake. Monkeys and rats tend to self-administer relatively constant session-to-session total drug doses by compensating for changes in dose/infusion with changes in response rates. Thus, when they are allowed to self-administer solutions that deliver low doses they tend to self-administer more infusions in a given period and consume about the same amount of drug each session. Such data are particularly applicable to paradigms in which the animals have limited periods of drug availability (i.e. , 2 to 4 hours). However, when drug availability is unlimited (24 hours/day), the animals tend to increase their drug dosage as they develop tolerance to the opiates; consequently, adjustments in the animal's responding tend to be obliterated by changes resulting from the development of opiate dependence (10, 39, 40, 42).

Effects of Neurochemical Manipulations

The ability of different neurochemical manipulations to alter opiate self-administration has been investigated in several laboratories. The assumption of such studies is that certain neurochemical systems are critically important determinants of the reinforcing properties of the opiates. Davis and Smith et al. (7, 9) have evaluated the ability of such drugs as alphamethylparatyrosine, which deplete central stores of catecholamines, to disrupt self-administration of several drugs, including morphine. These studies have produced provocative results, demonstrating an apparent decrease in response rates and total responding for morphine. Alphamethylparatyrosine and diethylthiocarbamate blocked morphine self-administration, but dopamine receptor blockers such as haloperidol did not. Davis and Smith (8) also explored the effects of drugs that affect cholinergic systems, finding that opiate self-administration could be blocked with atropine. These authors suggest that both cholinergic and catecholaminergic systems act together as substrate through which the reinforcing properties of morphine are manifest. Surprisingly, there have been no recent reports of attempts to replicate their work.

Agonist-Antagonist Interactions

Several groups (11,13,14,16,19,20,40) have examined the way in which the opiate antagonists change the

patterns, rates, and magnitude of self-administration
of opiate agonists. Leander et al. (23) have shown in
rats that opiate antagonists will increase response
rates for morphine at low doses and decrease responding
at higher doses. Similar results have been reported
by Goldberg et al. (13,14,15,16) and others (20) on the
effects of nalorphine and naloxone on morphine self-
administration by rhesus monkeys. They showed that low
doses of both drugs will produce higher rates of
responding for morphine, while high doses of the antagonists decrease responding. Presumably, those changes
result from the competitive antagonism of the agonist,
with partial blockade producing increased responding
and complete blockade preventing self-administration
by preventing reinforcement. Figures 3 and 4 summarize
representative results from experiments evaluating the
effects of antagonists on morphine self-administration.

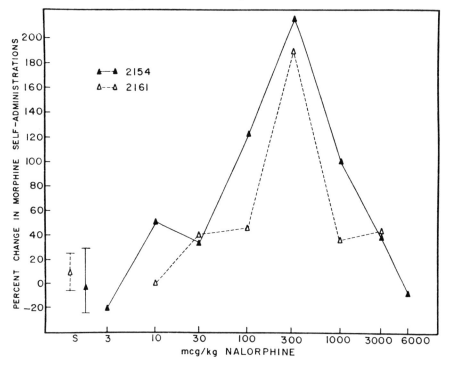

FIG. 3. Effects of nalorphine pretreatment on morphine
self-administration by two representative monkeys

Note that morphine self-administration increased by
almost 200% after pretreatment with 300 mcg/kg of nalorphine. After 6000 mcg/kg of nalorphine, morphine self-
administration was slightly lower than control levels.
From Goldberg et al. (16), with permission.

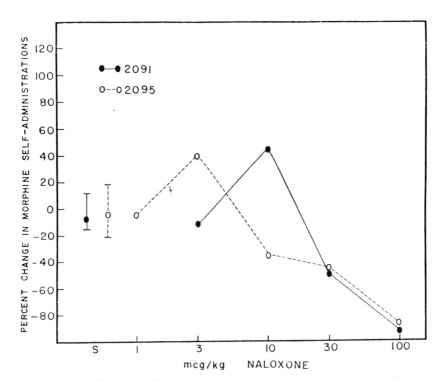

FIG. 4.   Effects of naloxone pretreatment on morphine
self-administration by two representative rhesus monkeys

At doses of 3 mcg/kg for monkey 2095 and 10 mcg/kg for
monkey 2091, morphine self-administration increased
about 50% and was extinguished after 100 mcg/kg of
naloxone.   In contrast to data shown on Figure 3, note
that a pure antagonist like naloxone is able to   ex-
tinguish self-administration, while a partial antagonist
like nalorphine does not.   From Goldberg et al. (16),
with permission.

The antagonist drugs alone seem to have negative
reinforcing properties in self-administration and other
operant paradigms. Hoffmeister and Wuttke (19, 20)have
shown that nalorphine, but not naloxone,   maintains
avoidance and escape behaviors in naive rhesus monkeys.
They interpret these differences as resulting from the
fact that nalorphine has partial agonist properties
which naloxone lacks.   Others (11, 14) have found that
naloxone can serve as a negative reinforcing agent,

especially in drug-dependent animals. In rhesus monkeys
which had a history of opiate dependence but were not
physically dependent at the time, weak partial antagonists such as propiranfumarate and pentazocine had
positive reinforcing properties (19,20) qualitatively
similar to those of heroin and codeine. On the other
hand, nalorphine and cyclazocine are apparently aversive
under those conditions. The developing data base raises
several provocative questions concerning the aversive
or negatively reinforcing properties of the opiate
antagonists.

One of the unique and attractive aspects of self-
administration methodology is that the animal model has
many similarities to human drug abuse patterns. Most
of the data available currently about drug self-administration by experimental animals have been obtained
by the intravenous method. Except for some studies of
oral self-administration, descriptions of self-administration parameters associated with drugs usually
consumed orally by human beings is scanty. The problems
associated with oral self-administration techniques
have been described, and it is generally agreed that
such techniques have serious limitations. Intragastric
self-administration techniques have been developed for
rats and monkeys in an attempt to circumvent the
problems of oral self-administration,while still providing
an animal model for consumption via the gastrointestinal
tract. I shall summarize some recent studies done in
our laboratory with an intragastric self-administration
technique in subhuman primates and describe its application to one of the opiates consumed orally by man,
methadone hydrochloride.

Intragastric Self-Administration of Methadone by Rhesus Monkeys

Although methadone hydrochloride is dispensed to a
large number of people in treatment programs for heroin
dependence, there are still major gaps in our knowledge
of the psychopharmacology of the drug. Most studies of
methadone self-administration have used the intravenous
route of administration, but the drug is consumed by
patients orally. Our studies were undertaken to develop
and evaluate an animal model in which the drug is self-
administered intragastrically so that the behavioral
consequences of methadone self-administration could be
examined in a way that has relevance to the clinical
situation.

METHODS

Animal Subjects. Twenty-one rhesus monkeys (Macaca mulatta) weighing 4 to 6 kg, were used in the experiments. All animals were drug-naive at the start of the study and were maintained in an accredited (American Association for Accreditation of Laboratory Animal Care) primate colony in accordance with the standards established by the U.S. Department of Agricultural and the National Institutes of Health. The animals had food (Purina 25 monkey chow) and water available ad lib throughout the study.

Intragastric Cannula. The cannula used in these studies was made of silicone-rubber tubing (0.040 in. i.d. x 0.085 in. o.d.). A 15-mm diameter disc was formed from silicone-rubber cement about 3 cm from one end of the cannula. After the disc was cured, a piece of Teflon intracardiac patch material, 25 mm in diameter, was sewn to it. The cannula was steam-sterilized before surgical implantation. Figure 5 is an artist's sketch of the cannula.

Surgical Procedure. The animals were fasted for about 16 hours before the operation. Thirty minutes before the operation, they were pretreated with atropine sulfate (0.1 mg/kg/s.c.) and anesthetized with sodium pentobarbital (30 mg/kg i.v.). An upper-left quadrant abdominal incision was made, the stomach exteriorized, and other abdominal viscera packed away from the surgical field. The end of the cannula was inserted through a small stab wound at the greater curvature of the stomach. After insertion, the stab wound was closed with a purse-string stitch of surgical silk (4-0) and the Teflon patch sutured to the serosal surface of the stomach. The implantation procedure is summarized in Figure 6. The long end of the cannula was guided out of the peritoneal cavity through a small puncture wound in the abdominal musculature, the abdomen closed in three layers, and the cannula tunneled subcutaneously to a point between the shoulder blades and connected to the infusion tubing at the fitting in the monkey harness. The monkey was maintained on a soft diet for 5 days following the procedure.

Control Studies. After the animal had recovered, saline was made available for intragastric self-administration on a 24 hour/day continuous-reinforcement (CFR) schedule. The animal was allowed to press a lever randomly to deliver intragastric infusions of saline (1.0 ml) until such random responding for saline had either extinguished completely or decreased to an extremely low rate(1 to 2 per day).

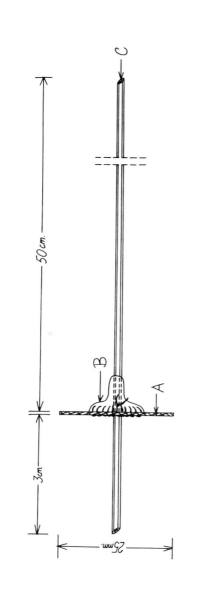

FIG. 5.   Schematic diagram of gastric cannula

A, 25 mm-diameter Teflon patch; B, molded and trimmed SILASTIC adhesive disc to which Teflon patch is sewn; C, silicone-rubber tubing, 0.04"i.d. x 0.085" o.d.   From Altshuler et al., (4), with permission.

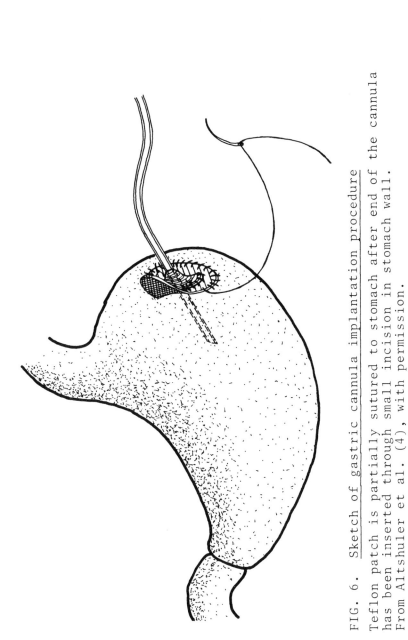

FIG. 6. Sketch of gastric cannula implantation procedure
Teflon patch is partially sutured to stomach after end of the cannula
has been inserted through small incision in stomach wall.
From Altshuler et al. (4), with permission.

Acquisition of Self-Administration.   After random
responding for saline had stopped, methadone was placed
in the drug reservoir bottle and the monkeys were
allowed to initiate self-administration of methadone on
a CRF-24 hour/day schedule. Each animal was allowed
30 days to initiate self-administration spontaneously.
The criteria for successful acquisition of methadone
self-administration were that the animal began responding
for the drug within 30 days of the first day of drug
availability and continued self-administration for at
least 30 days after the first response.
     The data presented in this chapter are of two types:
(a) 24-hour summaries of drug intake by individual
animals, and (b) the mean 24-hour intake obtained from
four animals studied simultaneously for 32 days.

RESULTS

Acquisition

     Ninety percent of the attempts (19/21) to establish
intragastric self-administration of methadone resulted
in acquisition of responding for methadone on a 24-
hour/day CRF schedule. Most animals initiated bar-
pressing within one or two days from the onset of drug
availability and maintained their self-administration
behavior for periods ranging from 35 days to six months.

Patterns of Intragastric Self-Administration

     In general, the patterns of methadone intragastric
self-administration tended to be cyclical, the animal
consuming high drug doses for several days and relatively
low doses on other days. The monkeys tended to self-
administer   relatively large doses initially, then
reduce and stabilize the daily doses in the early days
of the trial, and increase drug intake toward the later
stages. Figure 7 shows the daily self-administration
patterns for a representative animal which had methadone
available for self-administration on a 24-hour/day CRF
schedule.
     Figure 8 summarizes the mean intragastric self-
administration pattern for four of the seven animals
which were self-administering methadone at the same
time chronologically. Note that even when the animals'
mean drug intake is considered, there is still considerable day-to-day fluctuation in drug intake.

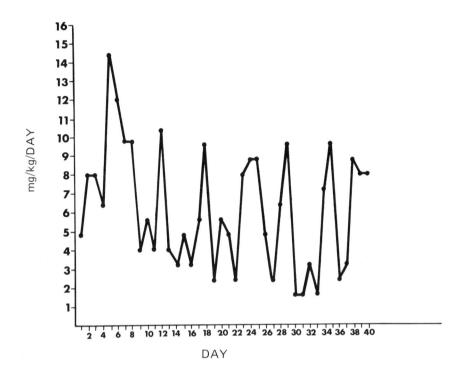

FIG. 7. Intragastric self-administration of methadone by representative animal

Graph summarizes intragastric self-administration history of representative rhesus monkey which had methadone hydrochloride available on 24 hr/day CRF schedule; ordinate: animal's drug intake. Animal consumed large dose for about the first 10 days of drug availability and stabilized drug intake thereafter. Cyclic nature of intragastric self-administration was characterized by several days of high drug intake alternating with several days of low drug intake.

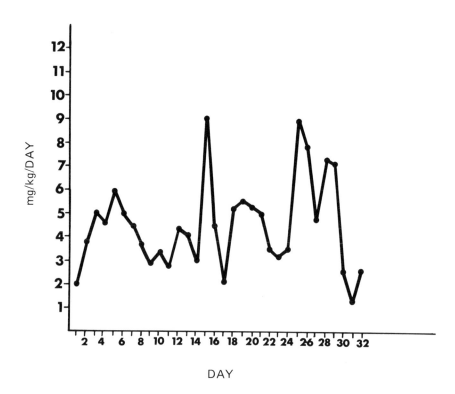

FIG. 8.   <u>Mean daily methadone intake of four animals</u>

Graph summarizes mean daily methadone intake of four
rhesus monkeys which had methadone available at the
same time on 24 hr/day, CRF schedule; ordinate : mean
drug intake for group. Note that mean daily methadone
dose was about 4 mg/kg/day and that methadone self-
administration is cyclical even when group means are
considered.

DISCUSSION

The self-administration paradigm is a powerful tool for laboratory studies of the drugs of abuse, their action, and the way in which they control behavior. Since Weeks (34) established self-administration as a useful model of drug abuse, scientists from many disciplines have become involved in the research, brought together by the common goal of understanding the mechanisms by which drugs serve as reinforcers. Their efforts produced much new information relevant to clinical medicine as well as basic research. The experiments with intragastric self-administration reported here demonstrated that the method is applicable to studies of such opiates as methadone and that it has potential application to long-term self-administration studies with direct clinical relevance.

Two major questions, however, needed to be answered before the usefulness of the procedure could be demonstrated. It was necessary to prove that the surgical technique for preparing subhuman primates for intragastric self-administration was well tolerated by the monkeys and that it was reasonably durable. The fact that we have maintained the animals in the self-administration system for periods of as long as two years is evidence that the technological aspects of the system meet those criteria.

The psychological principles that underly acquisition of intragastric self-administration are different from those of intravenous self-administration. In the latter case, reinforcement resulting from the behavioral response (lever press) occurs rapidly after the response, so that the animal is able to associate the sensation produced by the drug with the behavioral response. In the case of intragastric or oral self-administration, there is a fairly lengthy interval between the time the animal performs the behavioral task and the time it experiences the psychological and physiological effects of the drug. The drug must be absorbed into the blood-stream from the gastrointestinal tract before it becomes available to the central nervous system. The prediction was that such a delay would prevent animals from acquiring self-administration behavior without a great deal of shaping, since such shaping is often required in most other types of delayed-reinforcement paradigms. We have shown, however, that most monkeys are capable of acquiring self-administration behavior of most drugs of abuse with relative ease and without prior shaping.

Oral self-administration also involves a delayed-reinforcement paradigm and it is acquired by most animals, although much behavioral and pharmacological shaping is usually required. Oral self-administration experiments are difficult to do well, but they have been important in increasing understanding of some of the parameters of oral consumption of ethanol. Oral self-administration has the advantage of needing no surgical interventions nor extensive equipment. Intragastric self-administration, on the other hand,although it requires surgical procedures and expensive instrumentation, conforms to the principles of operant psychology and allows quantitative measures of drug-seeking behavior.

From the standpoint of sensitivity and ease of quantification, intravenous self-administration is nearly an ideal technique for evaluating drug-seeking behavior by laboratory animals. A great deal of information about the actions of the opiates and other drugs of abuse has been obtained through intravenous self-administration experiments. But with all its advantages, intravenous self-administration lacks some of the virtues of intragastric self-administration, especially the applicability to abuse syndromes associated with oral consumption of drugs by human beings. In addition, our recent experience shows that intragastric self-administration preparations are more durable and have a longer laboratory life than intravenous preparations.

In summary, self-administration preparations have been useful for evaluating the actions and relative reinforcing properties of drugs of abuse. In this paradigm, the drug serves as a primary reinforcer of drug-seeking behavior and as such maintains operant behavior in a way that models closely the syndrome associated with human drug abuse. At the present time, the self-administration model of drug abuse is the best animal model available for studies of abuse liability and physiological and psychological phenomena associated with drug dependence.

ACKNOWLEDGEMENTS

I would like to acknowledge the capable assistance of J. Boger, S. Marcks, and L. Gonzalez in the preparation of this manuscript, Mrs. Kendra Jackson for the typing of the manuscript and Ms. L. Feldman for her editing assistance.
This research was supported in part by PMAF Grant 5311.

REFERENCES

1. Altshuler, H.L., Deneau, G.A., Weaver, S.S., and Roach, M.K. (1974) :Pharmacologist,16:238.
2. Altshuler, H.L., and Phillips, P.E. (1976) : In: Drug Discrimination and State Dependent Learning, edited by B.T. Ho, Academic Press, New York (in press).
3. Altshuler, H.L., Weaver, S.S., and Phillips P.E. (1975) : Fed. Proc., 34:3211.
4. Altshuler, H.L., Weaver, S., and Phillips, P.E. (1975) : Life Sci., 17:883-890.
5. Beach, H.D. (1957): Can. J. Psychol., 11:104-112.
6. Collins, R.J., and Weeks, J.R. (1965) : Arch. Exp. Pathol., 249:509-514.
7. Davis, W.M., and Smith, S.G. (1972) : Curr. Ther. Res., 14:814-819.
8. Davis, W.M., and Smith, S.G. (1974) : Life Sci.,16: 237-246.
9. Davis, W.M., Smith, S.G., and Khalsa, J.A. (1975): Pharmacol. Biochem. Behav.,3:477-484.
10. Deneau, G., Yanagita, T., and Seevers, M.H. (1969): Psychopharmacologia,16:30-48.
11. Downs, D.A., and Woods, J.H. (1974) : Committee on Problems of Drug Dependence,36:826-833.
12. Ferster, C.B., and Skinner, B.F. (1957): Schedules of Reinforcement. Appleton-Century-Crofts,New York.
13. Goldberg, S.R., Hoffmeister, F., and Schlichting, U.U. (1972) : In : Drug Addiction, Vol. 1 : Experimental Pharmacology, edited by J.M. Singh, L. Miller, and H. Lal, pp. 31-48, Futura Publishing Co., Mount Kisco, New York.
14. Goldberg, S.R., Hoffmeister, F., Schlichting, U.U., and Wuttke, W. (1971): J. Pharmacol. Exp. Ther., 179:268-276.
15. Goldberg, S.R., Kelleher, R.T., and Morse, W.H. (1975) : Fed. Proc., 34:1771-1776.
16. Goldberg, S.R., Woods, J.H., and Schuster, C.R. (1971) : J. Pharmacol. Exp. Ther., 176:464-471.
17. Gotestam, K.G. (1973): Psychopharmacologia, 28:87-94.
18. Hoffmeister, F., and Schlichting, U.U. (1972) : Psychopharmacologia,23:55-74.
19. Hoffmeister, F., and Wuttke, W. (1973) : Psychopharmacologia,33:247-258.
20. Hoffmeister, F., and Wuttke, W. (1973) : Adv.Biochem. Psychopharmacol.,8:361-369.
21. Khavari, K.A., and Risner, M.E. (1973): Psychopharmacologia,30:45-60.

22. Khavari, K.A., and Risner, M.E. (1973) : Psycho-
    pharmacologia, 30:291-302.
23. Leander, J.D., McMillan, D.E., and Harris, L.S.
    (1973) : Committee on Problems of Drug Dependence,
    NRC-NAS.,35:411-422.
24. Mello, N..K. (1973) : Pharmacol. Biochem. Behav.,1:
    89-101.
25. Mello, N.K., and Mendelson, J.H. (1971) : Physiol.
    Behav., 7: 827-836.
26. Risner, M.E., and Khavari, K.A. (1973) : Psycho-
    pharmacologia,28:51-61.
27. Schuster, C.R., and Thompson, T. (1963): Committee
    on Drug Addiction and Narcotics, NRC-NAS, Vol. 25,
    Ann Arbor, Michigan.
28. Schuster, C.R., and Thompson, T. (1969): Annu. Rev.
    Pharmacol., 9:483-509.
29. Schuster, C.R., and Woods, J.H. (1968) : Int. J.
    Addict., 3:223-230.
30. Smith, S.G., Werner, T.E., and Davis, W.M. (1974):
    Proc. Soc. Neurosci., 4:645.
31. Stolerman, I.P., and Kumar, R. (1972): Psycho -
    pharmacologia, 26: 19-28.
32. Thompson, T., and Schuster, C.R. (1964) : Psycho-
    pharmacologia, 5: 87-94.
33. Trojniar, W., Cytawa, J., Frydrychowski, A., and
    Luszawska, D. (1974) : Psychopharmacologia, 37:
    359.
34. Weeks, J.R. (1962) : Science, 138: 143-144.
35. Weeks, J.R., Davis, J.D.(1964) : J. Appl. Physiol.,
    19:540-541.
36. Wikler, A., Martin, W.R., Prescor, F.T., and Eades,
    C.G. (1963) : Psychopharmacologia, 5:55-76.
37. Woods, J.H., Schuster, C.R. (1968) : Int. J.Addict.,
    3:231-237.
38. Yanagita, T. (1968) : Bulletin of the Committee
    on the Problems of Drug Dependence, NRC-NAS, 30:
    5631-5640.
39. Yanagita, T. (1973) : Bull. Narc., 25:7-17.
40. Yanagita, T. (1973) : Committee on Problems of
    Drug Dependence, NRC-NAS, 35:527-531.
41. Yanagita, T., Ando, K., Takahashi, S., and Ishida,
    K., (1969) : Proceedings of the Committee on the
    Problems of Drug Dependence, NRC-NAS, 31:6039-6051.
42. Yanagita, T., Deneau, G.A.,and Seevers, M.H. (1963) :
    Committee on Drug Addiction and Narcotics, NRC-
    NAS, vol. 25, Ann Arbor, Michigan.

Factors Affecting the Action of Narcotics, edited by
M.L. Adler, L. Manara, and R. Samanin.
Raven Press, New York©1978.

In Vitro Studies on Opiate Receptors
and Their Action

Eric J. Simon

New York University Medical Center
550 First Ave.
New York, N.Y. 10016,U.S.A.

It is my task to review in rather brief outline the
fastest moving field in opiate research and perhaps, in
all of pharmacology. I propose to do this by first
sketching in the background necessary for those not
working directly in this area.I shall then try to adhere
to the title of this symposium by concentrating primarily
on factors that affect interactions between opiates,
endogenous ligands and their receptors.

Discovery of Opiate Receptors

The presence of specific binding sites or receptors
for opiates in the brain has been suspected for decades.
The major reasons for the receptor hypothesis involved the great
structural and steric specificity exhibited by narcotic
analgesics in most of their pharmacological effects
and the finding that relatively small changes in molecular
structure could result in the formation of highly
specific and powerful opiate antagonists.

Earlier attempts to demonstrate specific receptors
by measuring that portion of the binding of opiates to
brain homogenate which is sensitive to displacement by
antagonists were unsuccessful (25). However, in 1973
stereospecific binding sites for opiates in rat brain
homogenate were discovered simultaneously in three laboratories (14,19,22).All utilized modifications of a method
for measuring stereospecific binding first proposed by
Goldstein et al. (2). Typical recent results in our
laboratory of stereospecific binding measurements are
presented in Table 1.

Since that time much evidence has been accumulated
suggesting that these stereospecific binding sites are
indeed the long sought pharmacological opiate receptors.
Binding is saturable and occurs at concentrations of
drugs in a range appropriate for pharmacological action.

TABLE 1. Stereospecific Bindings Assays by Filtration Procedure - Typical Results

Drug	Conc. (M)	D (CPM)	L (CPM)	D-L (CPM)	pmoles bound mg protein
Etorphine	2.5×10^{-10}	4100	540	3560	0.09
	1.0×10^{-9}	7800	2000	5800	0.15
Naltrexone	1.0×10^{-9}	3013	560	2453	0.08
	2.5×10^{-9}	5360	1340	4020	0.17

Membranes derived from rat brain P_2 fraction were preincubated with $10^{-6}M$ dextrorphan (D) or $10^{-6}M$ levorphanol (L) for 5 min. Samples were then incubated with ^3H-etorphine (20 Ci/mmole) or ^3H-naltrexone (15 Ci/mmole) for 15 min at 37°. Samples were filtered through Whatman GF/B filters. Filters were washed twice with 4 ml of cold Tris buffer, pH 7.4, dried and counted in a liquid scintillation spectrometer in a toluene based scintillation cocktail.

The sites have been found to be restricted to nervous
tissue. Distribution studies carried out in brains of
humans (4) and monkeys (9), demonstrated that   most
of the anatomical regions exhibiting high levels of
stereospecific opiate binding are in, or associated
with, the limbic system, a region of the brain long suspected as a site of certain of the actions of narcotic
analgesic drugs. Correlation between affinity for in
vitro binding and pharmacological potency has been
shown to be excellent for a large number of drugs (14,
19, 22, 26 and Stahl, Van Bever, Janssen and Simon, unpublished results). These experiments probably provide
the strongest support for the pharmacological relevance
of the binding sites.

Discovery of Endogenous Opiate-Like Peptides

The demonstration that specific opiate receptors
exist in many animals including man and the recognition
that they must convey some selective advantage on the
organism that carries them to have survived evolution,
led to a search for a physiological function for these
receptors.
Attempts to bind known neurotransmitters or hormones
were largely unsuccessful. This led a number of
laboratories to look in extracts of brain for the existence of novel materials with opiate-like activity.
Such a substance was first demonstrated in animal brain
by Hughes (5) and by Terenius and Wahlström (23) and more recently
by Pasternak et al. (10). Teschemacher et al. (24)
isolated a substance with opiate-like properties from
bovine pituitary glands. The substances were identified
by their ability to inhibit electrically stimulated
contractions of isolated guinea pig ileum or mouse vas
deferens and by their ability to compete with labeled
opiates for receptor binding . Hughes et al. (6) recently characterized the structure of the opiate-like
material isolated and purified from pig brain. The active
principle consists of the two pentapeptides H-Tyr-Gly-
Gly-Phe-Met-OH and H-Tyr-Gly-Gly-Phe-Leu-OH which they
named methionine (Met) enkephalin and leucine (Leu)
enkephalin. The same peptides have been identified in
extracts of bovine brain by Simantov and Snyder (17),
but here Leu-enkephalin predominates, unlike pig brain
where Met-enkephalin was found to be the major peptide.
Hughes et al. (6) made the interesting observation that
Met-enkephalin is present as amino acid residues 61-65
in the structure of the pituitary hormone β-lipotropin
(β-LPH). More recently a number of peptides with opiate-
like activity has been isolated from pig hypothalami
by Guillemin et al. (3). All represent portions of

β-LPH of varying lengths starting with the tyrosine in portion 61 at the N-terminal end. The generic term generally accepted for endogenous opiate-like peptides is endorphin (for endogenous and morphine), proposed by this author. Their physiological role is unknown,though evidence that they can produce at least short-lived analgesia, when injected intraventricularly, is beginning to appear. Such studies are rendered difficult by the rapid hydrolysis of endorphins by peptidases.

Effects of Enzymes on Opiate Receptor Binding

The stereospecific binding of opiates is highly sensitive to low concentrations of proteolytic enzymes such as pronase, trypsin and chymotrypsin (12,19). Binding is also inhibited by the presence of phospho-lipase A, though the source of this enzyme is critical. Phospholipase A from the venom of Crotalus adamanteus is without effect (19), while Pasternak and Snyder (12) found the enzyme from Russell's viper and bee venom to be highly effective. Interestingly, these authors ob-tained little inhibition with phospholipase A from the venom of Crotalus terrificus terrificus. Phospholipase C, ribonuclease, deoxyribonuclease and neuraminidase have little or no effect or opiate binding.

Effect of Ions on Receptor Binding

The addition of salt to the incubation mixture was found by us (19) to inhibit binding of etorphine, while no such inhibition was found for naloxone binding (14). Our suggestion that this discrepancy might represent a general difference in the way agonists and antagonists bind to the receptor was borne out. Pert and Snyder (15) found that salt decreased agonist binding while it enhanced antagonist binding. They discovered further that this discriminatory effect is exhibited specifically by sodium ions and to a lesser extent by lithium, while all other cations including the other alkali metals, inhibit the binding of both agonists and antagonists.Manganese and magnesium salts have been reported to enhance agonist binding while they depress antagonist binding (11). This effect is observed most clearly when sodium is also present and may represent a reversal of the sodium effect by the divalent ions.
The effect of sodium has been subjected to detailed scrutiny. We have provided evidence (21) that the addition of sodium during binding results in increased affinity of the receptors for antagonists and decreased affinity for agonists. Part of the evidence is presen-ted in Fig. 1 which shows a saturation curve and

Scatchard plot for /⁻³H_7 naltrexone binding in the presence and absence of 100mM NaCl. Similar but opposite data have been obtained for the binding of the agonist etorphine. No change in the number of binding sites was observed.

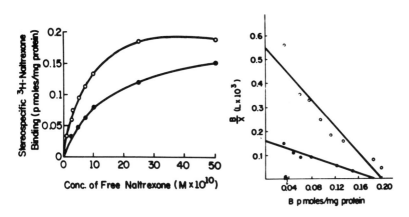

FIG. 1. <u>Saturation curves and Scatchard plots for stereospecific binding of ³H-naltrexone.</u> Rat brain P₂ fraction (1.2 mg of protein per ml) was preincubated for 5 minutes with levorphanol or dextrorphan (10⁻⁶M), followed by 15 minute incubation with various concentrations of ³H-naltrexone (specific activity 15.3 Ci/mmol). ●, 0.5 M Tris-HCl, pH 7.4; o, 0.10 M NaCl in 0.05 M Tris-HCl, pH 7.4. B, picomoles of drug bound per mg of protein, X, concentration of unbound drug (molar). From Simon et al. (21), with permission from Williams and Wilkins Co.

These results are most readily explained by an allosteric model in which the attachment of sodium to an allosteric site results in a conformational change in the receptor molecule. Pert and Snyder (15) reported results suggesting changes in the number of binding sites with no change in binding affinity. Despite the difference in experimental results the authors have postulated a similar allosteric model.

Effects of Protein Reagents

Stereospecific opiate binding has been shown to be sensitive to a variety of reagents known to react with functional groups of proteins (13, 19, 22). The best studied of these are the SH reagents (18), in particular the alkylating agent N-ethylmaleimide (NEM), which effectively destroys receptor binding. The rate of destruction follows pseudo-first order kinetics with a half-time (t $\frac{1}{2}$) of 8 minutes at 37° (Fig. 2). The presence of a drug capable of binding to the receptor protects against destruction by NEM. These data suggest the location of an essential SH group near the opiate binding site.

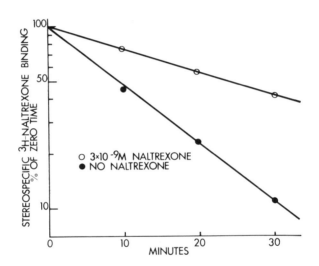

FIG. 2. <u>Kinetics of receptor inactivation by NEM and protection by unlabeled naltrexone.</u> A rat brain P_2 fraction was incubated with NEM (0.5 mM). Reaction was stopped by addition of tris-(2-carboxyethyl)-phosphine (2.5mM) which rapidly destroys NEM. Stereospecific binding of ^{3}H-naltrexone was assayed as previously described. Results are expressed as percent of sample incubated zero time with NEM. From Simon and Groth (18).

Of considerable interest was the unexpected finding
that the addition of NaCl protects against inactivation
by NEM ($t\frac{1}{2}$ increases from 8 minutes to 30 minutes).
This again is most readily explained by a conformational change
in the receptor. Evidence was obtained that this conformational change has the same ion specificity (Table
2) and sodium dose-response (Fig. 3) as the change in
antagonist and agonist affinities produced by sodium.
These results, therefore, constitute independent evidence for the allosteric model of the receptor.

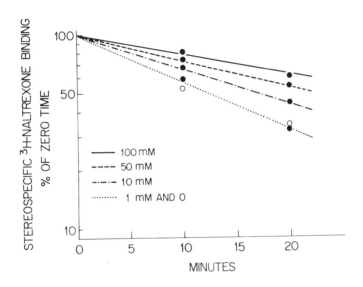

FIG. 3. <u>Kinetics of inactivation of stereospecific</u>
<u>binding of / ^{3}H / naltrexone by NEM in the presence of</u>
<u>various concentrations of NaCl.</u> Incubations with NEM
were carried out in the concentrations of NaCl shown.
From Simon and Groth (18).

Developmental Changes in Opiate Receptors

Studies carried out by Neil Clendeninn in our laboratory (Clendeninn and Simon, unpublished results) show
that stereospecific binding of opiates can be detected
in 14 day fetuses of rats, the earliest we were able to
examine, as depicted in Fig. 4. The level of binding
was 6-8 times lower than that observed in the brain of
adult rats. The period of most rapid increase ended at
3 weeks postnatally, a more gradual increase in binding

TABLE 2. Effect of Cations on Receptor Inactivation by NEM

Time of Preincubation	Tris Only	KCl	RbCl	CsCl	LiCl	NaCl
(Min)			^{3}H-naltrexone binding (% of zero time)			
5	73	72	75	-	81	85
10	45	51	51	50	65	78
20	22	24	27	24	42	65
30	12	11	17	12	32	48

All preincubations were carried out in the presence of 0.5 mM NEM in 50 mM Tris with appropriate salt to final concentrations of 100 mM. From Simon and Groth (18).

continued into adulthood (10 weeks). Similar studies
in guinea pigs indicated that late fetuses and neonatal
animals had the same level of receptor binding as adult
animals. Earlier fetuses had lower levels; development,
thus, took place entirely prior to birth. In both
species developmental changes were shown to be due to
an increase in the number of receptor sites but not in
affinity.

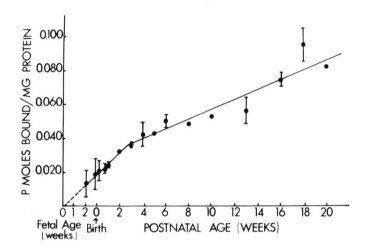

FIG. 4. <u>Ontogeny of opiate receptors in rat brain.</u>
Brain homogenate (1-2 mg of protein/ml) was assayed for
stereospecific binding of $\sqrt{^3H}$ naltrexone (spec. act.
15.3 Ci/mMole). Each point represents the average ±S.D.
of at least 3 experiments.

The development of opiate receptors parallels closely
major neurological development in the two species
studied, which in rats continues until 21 days postnatally, while the guinea pig is born with an essentially mature nervous system (7). This suggests that
opiate receptors are integral and important parts of the
central nervous system but permits no conclusions about
association of receptors with a given part of the nervous
system.

Effects of Chronic Morphine Treatment on Receptor
Binding and Levels of Enkephalins

The hypothesis that tolerance and dependence are due
to changes in the number of properties of opiate receptors
predates the discovery of the receptors by some years

(1). Recently, the idea that changes due to chronic opiate treatment may be reflected in changes in the level of endorphins has also become attractive.

Attempts to show changes in either the number or affinities of opiate receptors during chronic morphiniza-tion of rats have been unsuccessful (8). Increases in receptor binding after administration of opiates were found but were not correlated with the development of tolerance and dependence (16). In fact, this increase was produced most effectively by injecting antagonists, such as naloxone.

Most of the earlier studies were done with whole rat brain (minus cerebellum), which suggested to us that changes in small specific regions could be oscured by the presence of large parts of the brain in which no change occurs. In collaboration with Dr. K. Bonnet (Bonnet, Hiller and Simon, unpublished results) we therefore studied binding of $\sqrt{\ }^3$H $\overline{\ }$naltrexone in three specific regions of the brains of naive and addicted rats, the caudate nucleus, peri-aqueductal gray area and the medial thalamus. Fig. 5 shows saturation curves for $\sqrt{\ }^3$H $\overline{\ }$naltrexone binding (in 100mM NaCl) for homo-genates of medial thalamus from naive and addicted rats. No changes were observed in the medial thalamus, nor in the other areas examined, for either number or affinity of binding sites. The addicted animals were sacrificed after treatment with subcutaneous morphine pellets for 72 hours.

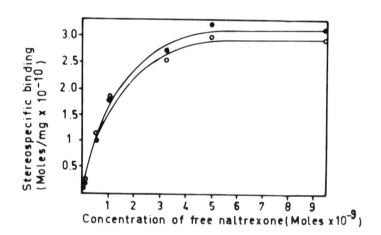

FIG. 5. Saturation curves for $\sqrt{\ }$3H $\overline{\ }$naltrexone binding to medial thalamus homogenate from brains of morphine dependent and control rats.

o Dependent   • Control

The possibility that longer periods of pelleting are
needed is currently under investigation. However,since
the differences in affinity one might expect are quite
large and should be observable at 72 hours, the results
appear to be negative, suggesting that the changes
leading to tolerance and dependence do not take place
at the level of opiate-receptor interaction.

Attempts to show differences in level of opiate-like
endogenous peptides are in progress in a number of laboratories, but no published results are known to the
author at the time of writing.

Terenius and Wahlström reported last July at the
International Congress of Pharmacology in Helsinki that they
have evidence for the production of yet a new opiate-
like substance during chronic morphine treatment. This
substance behaves like an antagonist in the presence of
sodium salts and has been named naloxone-like factor
(NLF). It is attractive to speculate that the production
of NLF and a reduction in the synthesis of endorphins
might explain the development of tolerance to and
dependence on opiates.

Effect of Conditions of Rearing on Opiate Receptors in Mouse Brain

Recent experiments (Bonnet, Hiller and Simon, unpublished results) in which C57Bl/6J mice reared in
total isolation were compared to mice reared under normal
aggregated conditions gave indication of a change in
opiate receptor binding. After 5 months of rearing in
isolation (beginning with weaning) homogenates of whole
brain showed a significant decrease in receptor binding
of $/^3$H_7etorphine when compared to control mice. The
mice reared in isolation also exhibit a decreased
sensitivity to morphine analgesia. This result appears
to be sensitive to the mouse strain used since DeFeudis
(private communication) found exactly opposite results
when he used Swiss albino mice.

Attempts at Solubilization of Opiate Receptors

I cannot conclude this review without mentioning our
recent attempts to solubilize and ultimately to purify
the opiate receptor. We recently reported (20) that we
were able to solubilize an $/^3$H_7etorphine macromolecular
complex from brain derived plasma membrane, using the
non-ionic detergent BRIJ36T, which no longer sediments
at 100,000xg and has an apparent molecular weight of
350,000. This complex exhibits properties which suggest
that it is an etorphine-receptor complex, including
stereospecificity of etorphine binding and sensitivity
to protein reagents, heat and proteolytic enzymes. How-

ever, dissociation of the solubilized complex did not
result in a free receptor moiety able to rebind drug in
solution.

More recently we have obtained deoxycholate extracts
of brain membranes which no longer sediment at 20,000xg
but still sediment at 100,000xg. These extracts are
able to bind $\underline{/}^{-3}H\underline{7}$ etorphine stereospecifically measured by chromatography on XAD-4 columns (20). Attempts
at further subdivision of this material have so far
resulted in complete loss of activity. Although the
deoxycholate-extracted material is still rather large,
it is considerably smaller than the original membrane
fragments. Efforts to purify this material are in progress.

FINAL CONCLUSIONS

The discovery of specific opiate receptors in animal
and human brain and, more recently, of endogenous
peptides with opiate-like activities, including binding
to opiate receptors, has clearly revolutionized research on the biochemistry of opiate action. Research
in this area is moving so rapidly that aspects of this
discussion may be obsolete by the time it is published.
There remain many important unanswered questions and it
is too early to predict where this research will lead
and what its practical clinical implications may be.
The recent abundance of coverage of research in this
field by the news media and the attraction to this area
of many excellent laboratories indicate that hope is
running high for further significant findings.

The present report has of necessity focused on aspects of the work of particular interest to the author
and has omitted other important facets. Among the most
important areas not covered here are the recent reports
suggesting that opiate binding to receptors may trigger
changes in the activity of the enzymes which synthesize
cyclic nucleotides and the use of neuroblastoma x glioma
hybrids in cell culture as models for the study of
opiate action (see the review by Kosterlitz, in this
volume). It is hoped that these important developments
will be covered by other participants in this conference.

ACKNOWLEDGEMENTS

The portion of the work performed in the author's
laboratory was supported by Grant DA-00017 from the
National Institute of Drug Abuse.

REFERENCES

1. Collier, H.O.J. (1965) : Nature, 205: 181.
2. Goldstein, A., Lowney, K.I., and Pal, B.K. (1971) :
   Proc.   Natl. Acad. Sci. (USA), 68 : 1742.
3. Guillemin, R., Ling, N.,and Burgus, R. (1976) :
   C.R. Acad. Sci. (Paris), 282 : 783.
4. Hiller, J.M., Pearson, J.,and Simon, E.J. (1973) :
   Res. Commun. Chem. Pathol. Pharmacol. 6 : 1052.
5. Hughes, J. (1975) : Brain Res. 88 : 295.
6. Hughes, J., Smith, T.W., Kosterlitz, H.W.,Fothergill,
   L.A., Morgan B.A.,and Morris, H.R. (1975) : Nature,
   258 : 577.
7. Jones, D.C., Dittmer, M.M., and Reading, L.C. (1974)
   Brain Res., 70: 245.
8. Klee, W.A., and Streaty, R.A. (1974) : Nature, 248:
   61.
9. Kuhar, M.J., Pert, C.B.,and Snyder, S.H. (1973) :
   Nature, 245: 447.
10. Pasternak, G.W., Goodman, R., and Snyder, S.H.
    (1975) : Life Sci., 16 : 1765.
11. Pasternak , G.W., Snowman, A.M., and Snyder, S.H.
    (1975) : Mol. Pharmacol. 11 : 735.
12. Pasternak, G.W., and Snyder, S.H. (1973) : Mol.
    Pharmacol. 10 : 183.
13. Pasternak, G.W., Wilson, H.A., and Snyder, S.H.
    (1975) : Mol. Pharmacol. 11 : 340.
14. Pert, C.B., and Snyder, S.H. (1973) : Science, 179:
    1011.
15. Pert, C.B., and Snyder, S.H. (1974) : Mol.Pharmacol.
    10 : 868.
16. Pert, C.B., and Snyder, S.H. (1976) : Biochem.
    Pharmacol. 25 : 847.
17. Simantov, R., and Snyder, S.H. (1976) : Life Sci.,
    18 : 781.
18. Simon, E.J., and Groth, J. (1975) : Proc. Natl.
    Acad. Sci. (USA), 72 : 2404.
19. Simon, E.J., Hiller, J.M.,and Edelman, I. (1973):
    Proc. Natl. Acad. Sci. (USA), 70 : 1947.
20. Simon, E.J., Hiller, J.M., and Edelman, I. (1975):
    Science, 190 : 389.
21. Simon, E.J., Hiller, J.M., Groth, J., and Edelman,I.
    (1975) : J. Pharmacol. Exp. Ther., 192 : 531.
22. Terenius, L. (1973) : Acta Pharmacol. Toxicol. 32:
    317.
23. Terenius, L., and Wahlström, A. (1974) : Acta
    Pharmacol. Toxicol. 35 : Suppl. 1. : 55.
24. Teschemacher, H., Opheim, K.E., Cox, B.M., and
    Goldstein, A. (1975) : Life Sci, 16 : 1771.
25. Van Praag, D., and Simon,E.J.(1966):Proc.Soc.Exper.
    Biol. Med., 122 : 6.

26. Wilson, R.S., Rogers, M.E., Pert, C.B.,and Snyder,
    S.H. (1975) : <u>J. Med. Chem.</u> , <u>18</u> : 240.

Factors Affecting the Action of Narcotics, edited by
M.L. Adler, L. Manara, and R. Samanin.
Raven Press, New York©1978.

The In Vivo Occupation of Opiate Receptors

Volker Höllt

Department of Neuropharmacology
Max-Planck-Institut für Psychiatrie
Kraepelinstrasse 2, 8000 München 40, Germany

INTRODUCTION

During the last few years considerable effort has
been directed towards the study of opiate receptor
binding in vitro (13,15,16). In contrast, few studies
have been made of receptor occupation by opiates in vivo.
In order to carry out such in vivo binding studies
radioactively labelled opiates are injected into animals
and measurements made of the concentration of radioactive
opiate present in the brain. It might be expected that
the simultaneous injection of high doses of non-labelled
opiate antagonists would decrease the concentration of
the radioactive opiate in the brain, since the 'displacement" of this radioactive opiate by antagonists
should reflect the removal of labelled drug from receptor sites. Early experiments, however, revealed
certain discrepancies. Mulé et al. (12), for example,
found that nalorphine, injected simultaneously with
[14]C-morphine, increased the concentration of this
radioactive opiate in dog brain, whereas Johannesson
and Milthers (8) observed no change in ^{14}C-morphine concentrations in the brains of rats treated with nalorphine; Wuepper et al. (17) found that nalorphine
decreased ^{14}C-levorphanol in dog brain. One reason
for the conflicting results may be that labelled
opiate were used which do not have a high affinity for
opiate receptors. A high affinity for these receptors
would appear to be important, since displacement of a
labelled opiate from brain by opiate antagonists can
only be expected when a major portion of the brain concentration of the tracer represents receptor bound drug.
In addition, the labelled opiate should ideally be administered in a small dose giving rise to a brain concentration below that necessary for complete saturation
of opiate receptors. At such low brain concentrations
the proportion of free and unspecifically bound drug
can be considered to be small in comparison with the
amount of opiate complexed with the receptors. The de-

207

tection of such small quantities of radioactive opiates or opiate antagonists in the brain requires that the labelled drug have a high specific activity.

When the above considerations are taken into account and low doses of highly labelled agonists or antagonists are injected into animals together with high doses of unlabelled antagonists, a consistent decrease is seen in the concentration of radioactive drugs in the brain. This was first reported by Dobbs (2) who observed a considerable decrease in the concentration of radioactivity in the rat brain when the agonist ^{3}H-etorphine was injected systemically together with the antagonist cyprenorphine. This finding was later confirmed by Cerletti et al. (1), who described a consistenly decreased accumulation of ^{3}H-etorphine in the brains of rats treated with any of various narcotic antagonists concurrently with the labelled opiate. Mulé et al. (11) after intracisternal administration of ^{3}H-etorphine reported a somewhat similar finding limited to a subcellular fraction containing less than one per cent of the total radioactivity in brain, while the latter was apparently unaffected. A considerable displacement from rat brain of labelled antagonists showing a high affinity to the opiate receptor (diprenorphine, naltrexone and naloxone) after treatment with high doses of unlabelled antagonists has been reported by Pert et al. (13) and by our group (5).

In the present paper we present further evidence that the decrease in concentration of high affinity tracers in the rat brain, seen after treatment of these animals with non-radioactive opiate antagonists, is due to removal of the opiate from specific receptor sites. Occupation of specific opiate receptors by these labeled opiates is suggested by the stereospecificity and saturability of this in vivo binding, its characteristic distribution in the brain and by the close correlation that exists between this in vivo binding and the pharmacological effects of the drugs.

Stereospecificity of Opiate Receptor Occupation In Vivo

It has been demonstrated that the D(-)-isomers of opiates, unlike the L (+)-isomers, are able to displace other opiates from their specific binding sites in vitro (within a reasonable concentration range, below 10^{-6}M) (14). Moreover, experiments performed in vivo have revealed that the D(-)-, but not the L(+)-isomers of opiate antagonists reduce the high affinity binding of opiate agonists in the brain. Mulé et al. (11) found that (-)-cyclorphan reduced ^{3}H-etorphine accumulation

in subfractions of osmotically shocked mitochondrial
fractions containing less than one per cent of total
radioactivity in the brain of rats, whereas (+)-
cyclorphan was inactive. In agreement with these results Pert et al. (13) observed a pronounced displacement
of ^{3}H-diprenorphine from rat brain by levallorphan,but
not by dextrallorphan. In a previous paper (5) we reported similar results in that levallorphan but not
dextrallorphan reduced the accumulation of ^{3}H-naltrexone
in mouse brain. Recently, we reported that the pharmacologically active opiate antagonist Mr 2266 (a N-methyl-
furyl benzomorphan derivative) reduced the brain levels
of ^{3}H-diprenorphine in mice whereas its isomer Mr 2267
was inactive in this respect (7). The clear stereospecific effects of opiate antagonists observed in the above
in vivo displacement experiments provide evidence that
specific receptor sites are involved. Steric factors,
however, may also influence the distribution, metabolism
and excretion of the tracer opiates. Further experiments
were therefore performed in order to obtain additional
evidence that the displacement of the tracer opiates
from brain reflects their removal from opiate receptor
sites.

Saturability of the Displacement from Binding Sites In Vivo

Fig. 1 illustrates the displacement of ^{3}H-diprenorphine
from mouse brain in vivo. Here, 0.2 µg/kg of this labelled opiate antagonist was injected i.v. into mice
either alone, or together with increasing doses of unlabelled diprenorphine. It can be seen that the concentration of radioactivity in the brain 15 minutes
after injection decreases up to about 85% in the dose
range of 3 to 300 µg/kg of simultaneously injected non-
labelled drug, whereas at higher doses of up to 10 mg/
kg no further reduction was observed. The shape of this
displacement curve was very similar to that observed
in vitro , when a tracer opiate is displaced from a
limited number of receptor sites by increasing doses of
the unlabelled drug. The constant concentration of the
labelled compound remaining after displacement of the
majority of the label was interpreted as being due to
unspecific and non-saturable binding of the compound.
Assuming that similar principles apply in vivo, the
saturable displacement of 3H-diprenorphine was analysed
according to Lineweaver and Burk (shown in the insert
of Fig. 1). It was found that about 30 pmoles of ^{3}H-
diprenorphine/g brain could be maximally displaced in
vivo, a value which is very similar to the number of
binding sites estimated from in vitro binding studies.
Similar results were obtained when the in vivo displacement

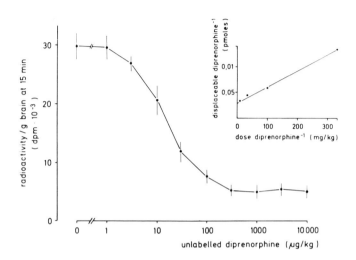

FIG. 1.   Displacement of ^{3}H-diprenorphine

0.2 μg/kg or 10 μCi/kg of ^{3}H-diprenorphine (spec.activity
22.3 Ci/mmole) was injected intravenously into mice
either alone or together with increasing doses of unlabelled diprenorphine.   15 min later brain samples were
taken and combusted, prior to liquid scintillation
counting. Each point is the mean of 8 observations.
Vertical bars represent standard deviation of the mean.

^{3}H-diprenorphine : A gift from NIDA, Rockville, U.S.A.;
unlabelled diprenorphine: A gift from Reckitt & Colman,
Kingston-upon-Hull, England.

of ^{3}H-naloxone and ^{3}H-naltrexone was analysed (5).   It
should be emphasized, however, that such a simple
estimate of the number of opiate receptor sites in vivo
can yield approximate values only, since the occupation
of receptor in vivo is complex and probably influenced
by several time dependent processes, which will be
discussed later.

Comparison of In Vivo Displacement
with In Vitro Binding

Recently, we showed that the extent to which labelled opiate antagonists can be maximally displaced from
brain by the simultaneous injection of very high doses

of unlabelled antagonists appears to be correlated with
the in vitro binding affinity of these tracers to the
receptors. The rank order of the displacement effect
was as follows; diprenorphine > naltrexone > naloxone.
The same rank order was found for the in vitro binding
affinity of these compounds to opiate receptors (6).
These results appear to be consistent since for a given
concentration of drug in the brain the fraction of labelled compound attached to receptors will depend on
their binding affinity for these receptors. On the
other hand, the proportion of tracer drug in the brain
that can be displaced by unlabelled antagonists will
also depend upon the extent of unspecific drug binding.
Furthermore, differences in apparent specific opiate
receptor occupation in vivo could arise through differences in the time courses of receptor occupation by
various agonists and antagonists. The low binding
affinities of ^{3}H-morphine, ^{3}H-dihydromorphine and ^{3}H-
fentanyl appear to be the reason why we were unable to
find any displacement with these drugs.

Further evidence for different in vivo affinities
of opiates is seen in experiments in which a labelled
opiate agonist is displaced from brain after the simultaneous injection of increasing amounts of various
opiate antagonists. The relative potencies of these
antagonists found for displacement of radioactive opiate
from the brain are closely correlated with their potencies for antagonism of opiate-induced analgesia (7).

Regional Displacement of Opiate Agonists and Antagonists In Vivo

Receptor binding studies carried out in vitro have
revealed a characteristic distribution of opiate receptors in the brain (4,9). Fig. 2 shows the in vivo
displacement of ^{3}H-diprenorphine from various areas of
rat brain by a high dose of unlabelled diprenorphine.
The low displacement of ^{3}H-diprenorphine from the cerebellum is in contrast to the high displacement from
other brain areas and correlates with the low receptor
density in this brain region, as evaluated by in vitro
binding studies (4,9). Recently, in vivo experiments
in which the agonist ^{3}H-etorphine was injected together
with saturation doses of the unlabelled antagonist
naltrexone revealed an even smaller displacement of the
labelled agonist from the cerebellum (7). This lower
displacement from the cerebellum of opiate agonists as
compared with opiate antagonists seems to indicate that
there are more "antagonist receptors" than "agonist receptors" in this brain area. A similar finding was
obtained from in vitro binding studies (10).

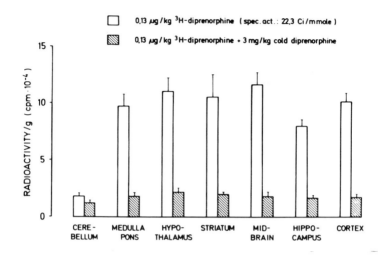

FIG. 2.   Displacement of ³H-diprenorphine in various brain areas.

0.13 µg/kg or 6 µCi/kg ³H-diprenorphine was injected i.v. into rats either alone (open bars) or together with 3000 µg/kg of unlabelled diprenorphine (hatched bars). 30 min after injection the animals were killed, their brains dissected out according to Glowinski and Iversen (3) and the radioactivity of the various brain areas determined. Each point is the mean of 8 observations. Vertical bars represent standard deviation of the mean.

The displacement of either opiate agonists or antagonists from the cerebellum seemed to be negligible when compared with that in other brain areas. This offers the possibility of using the concentration of tracer opiate in this brain area as "correction factor" or "internal standard" for opiate that is accumulating in brain but not bound to opiate receptors. Thus, the ratio of labelled opiate concentration in brain/cerebellum can be used as a measure of specific receptor occupation by opiates in vivo. This is shown in Fig.3, which illustrates results obtained with ³H-buprenorphine, a potent opiate antagonist with agonistic properties. Displacement of ³H-buprenorphine from brain by increasing doses of unlabelled buprenorphine (upper part of the figure) is compared with the decrease of the brain/cerebellum ratio (lower part of the figure) in the same animals. It can be seen that at doses of unlabelled buprenorphine of 1000 µg/kg and above a maximum displacement

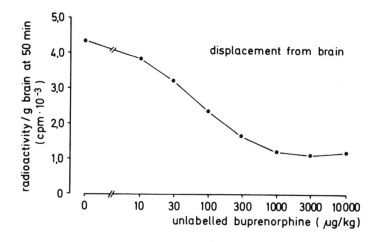

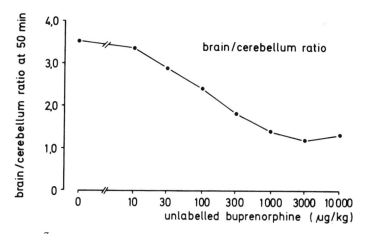

FIG. 3. ³H-buprenorphine : Comparison of displacement and the brain/cerebellum ratio

0.3 μg/kg or 15 μCi/kg ³H-buprenorphine (spec. activity 28 Ci/mmole) was injected i.v. into mice either alone or together with increasing doses of unlabelled buprenorphine. 50 min later radioactivity in the brain was determined. Upper part of the figure: Radioactivity in the whole brain; lower part of the figure : Ratio of radioactivity in the brain (minus cerebellum) to that in the cerebellum. Each point represents the mean of 6 determinations. Labelled and unlabelled buprenorphine were a gift from Reckitt & Colman, Kingston-upon Hull, England.

of the labelled drug is obtained. In the same dose
range the brain/cerebellum ratio of ^{3}H-buprenorphine
declines to a value of about 1, indicating that all
opiate receptors are occupied. The fact that, after
injection of large doses of unlabelled drug, the concentration of the tracer in the brain is markedly decreased whereas the concentration of the labelled
compound in the cerebellum is almost unaffected, is an
indication that the displacement is not caused by saturable mechanisms other than those at the receptor level,
such as transport processes through blood brain barrier,
metabolism, or excretion. Such processes would also be
expected to affect the concentration in the cerebellum
in the same way as in other brain regions.

The Effect of Opiate Agonists

As described above, a dose-dependent displacement of
radioactive opiates from brain could be observed when
the tracer opiate was injected together with high doses
of unlabelled antagonists or partial antagonists. In
marked contrast, however, the injection of tracer opiates
together with increasing doses of unlabelled opiate
agonists leads paradoxically to an increase in the
concentration of radioactive opiate in the brain. Fig.
4 illustrates the results obtained from an experiment
in which a small dose of the agonist ^{3}H-etorphine was
injected i.v. into mice together with increasing doses
of either non-radioactive etorphine or the antagonist
naltrexone. Whereas naltrexone was able to reduce
^{3}H-etorphine concentration in brain in a dose-dependent
manner the (non radioactive) etorphine caused an increase in ^{3}H-etorphine concentration until a maximum
occurred after injection of about 30 µg/kg of etorphine,
although a decline was observed after injection of
higher doses.
A similar increase in brain opiate concentration
could be observed if other agonists such as morphine or
fentanyl were injected together with the radioactive
opiate. This surprising result is in contrast to in
vitro binding studies in which a tracer opiate could be
displaced from the receptor sites either by agonists
or by antagonists. Moreover, it could be shown that
the increase in ^{3}H-etorphine concentration in brain was
also seen in the cerebellum, an area apparently almost
devoid of opiate receptor. The ratio of ^{3}H-etorphine
concentration in the brain to that in the cerebellum
decreased dose dependently with increasing doses of unlabelled agonists, reflecting saturation of specific
receptor sites by the drug. The cause of the increased
accumulation of the ^{3}H-etorphine in the brain after increasing doses of opiate agonists is unclear.

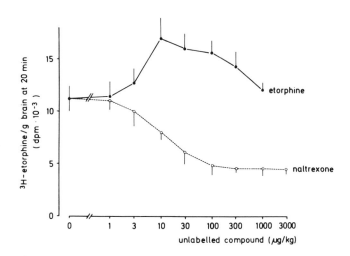

FIG. 4. Displacement of ^{3}H-etorphine

0.1 μg/kg or 10 μCi/kg ^{3}H-etorphine (spec. activity 41
Ci/mmole) was injected i.v. into mice either alone, or
together with increasing doses of unlabelled etorphine
or naltrexone. The radioactivity of the brains was
measured 20 min later. Each point is the mean of 8
observations. Vertical bars represents standard deviation of the mean.
^{3}H-etorphine : The Radiochemical Centre, Amersham,
England. Non-radioactive etorphine : A gift from Reckitt & Colman
Kingston-upon-Hull, England; unlabelled naltrexone: A
gift from Endo Laboratories, Brussels, Belgium.

The effect appears to be induced by pharmacological
effects of the opiate agonists which change the pharmacokinetics of the compound.
    Despite these additional effects of opiate agonists,
receptor occupation studies can still be performed by
measuring the ratio of radioactive opiate concentration
in brain and cerebellum.

    Comparison of the In Vivo Displacement of Opiates
            with their Pharmacological Actions

    The close correlation between the data obtained with
the in vivo displacement technique and that obtained by
in vitro binding studies provides strong evidence that
the decrease in the brain concentration of labelled

opiates after injection of high doses of unlabelled antagonists reflects their removal from specific receptor
sites. Further support for this assumption is given by
the close correlation between the ability of opiate
antagonists to antagonize opiate-induced analgesia and
their ability to displace radioactivity labelled opiates
from the brain. A comparison of the analgesic response
of mice to etorphine and the estimate of receptor occupation by the drug is depicted in figure 5.

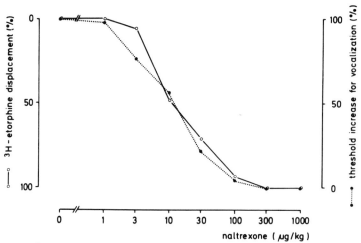

FIG. 5. ^{3}H-etorphine: Comparison of displacement and
the reversal of analgesia

30 μg/kg or 20 μCi/kg ^{3}H-etorphine was injected i.v.in-
to mice either alone, or together with increasing doses
of unlabelled naltrexone. 20 min after drug injection
measurements were made of either the radioactivity in
the brain or the analgesic response as judged by an increase in the threshold of electrical stimulation of the
feet inducing vocalization. (Electrical stimulation:
Constant current, frequency 1 Hz, duration 300 msec.).
Both data were normalized as the percentage of the
maximum effect. Each point represents the mean of 12
observations.

This figure shows reversal of the analgesic effect of a
30 μg/kg dose of ^{3}H-etorphine by the simultaneous application of naltrexone. The decrease of the analgesic
response is compared with displacement of the labelled
etorphine from brain by the same doses of the antagonist.
It can be seen that the reversal of analgesia occurs

within the same dose range as that necessary for the
displacement of ^{3}H-etorphine from brain. A similar
close correlation has been found between the displacement
of ^{3}H-naltrexone from brain by increasing doses of non-
radioactive naltrexone and manifestation of the withdrawal-induced jumping in tolerant/dependent mice (5).

Time Course of Opiate Receptor Occupation <u>In Vivo</u>

An important aspect of the <u>in vivo</u> receptor occupation
studies was to analyse the kinetics of the binding of
opiates in the brain. Fig. 6 shows the results of one
such study in which the concentration of ^{3}H-diprenorphine
in mouse brain was measured at different times after
the i.v. injection of two different doses of the drug.

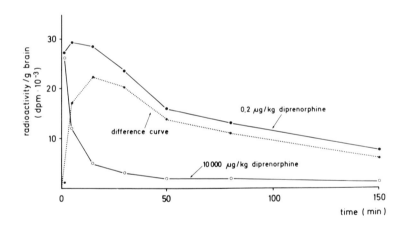

FIG. 6. <u>Time course of ^{3}H-diprenorphine</u>

0.2 µg/kg or 10 µCi/kg ^{3}H-diprenorphine was injected
i.v. into mice either alone (upper curve) or together
with 10,000 µg/kg unlabelled diprenorphine (lower curve).
The radioactivity was determined several time intervals
after the injection. The dotted curve gives the difference between the upper and the lower curves. Each
point represents the mean of 12 animals.

The lower curve shows the time-course of the radioactivity in brain following the injection of 0.2 µg/kg
^{3}H-diprenorphine together with a 50,000-fold
dose of unlabelled diprenorphine. This dose of the

unlabelled drug was high enough to displace ^{3}H-diprenorphine from
the receptors completely at each time interval studied
following the injection. It can be seen that in this
experiment the radioactivity in the brain was highest
at 1.5 minutes, the earliest time point taken, followed
by a rapid decline. The very fast penetration of ^{3}H-
diprenorphine into the brain and its subsequent rapid
elimination is characteristic of a lipophilic compound.
In contrast, when ^{3}H-diprenorphine was injected in the
tracer dose of 0.2 µg/kg alone, the radioactivity in
the brain at 1.5 minutes was about the same as that
seen after injection of tracer plus unlabelled drug.
Fig. 6 shows, however, that after injection of a tracer
dose alone ^{3}H-diprenorphine concentration in the brain
increased to a maximum at about 5-10 minutes followed
by a slow decline. The dotted curve of figure 6 gives
the difference between the upper and the lower curves.
It presumably describes the time course of ^{3}H-diprenorphine
binding to specific opiate receptors in the brain. This
time course is influenced by the rates of association
to and dissociation from the receptors, as well as by
the elimination of the drug from brain in vivo. Studies
are in progress to analyse these different kinetic
parameters (Höllt et al., in preparation). In preliminary
experiments a good correlation between the receptor
association times of various labelled opiate antagonists
(naloxone, naltrexone, buprenorphine and diprenorphine)
in vitro and the time course of receptor occupation
in vivo was found. For a more quantitative kinetic
analysis of the time courses in these studies, total
radioactivities (as shown in Fig. 6) as concentration
equivalent for the labelled compounds should not be
used. Solvent extraction of the labelled tracers from
brain followed by thin layer chromatography revealed
that at time intervals longer than 20 minutes a pronounced degradation of the highly labelled compounds
takes place. This degradation was primarily due to a
decomposition of these highly labelled drugs under in
vivo conditions and only to a minor extent due to
metabolism, since most of the changed labelled opiates
represent volatile radioactivity. Interestingly, a
much smaller proportion of degradation products was
found in the brain after injection of a small dose of
the labelled tracer than after higher doses. This
might indicate that receptor bound drug in brain is
protected from degradation in vivo.

SUMMARY

In experiments to identify opiate receptor binding in vivo, a labelled opiate was injected into animals together with high doses of non-radioactive opiates or opiate antagonists. A consistent displacement of the tracer opiate from brain by the unlabelled compounds could be observed only when labelled tracers were used which have a high specific activity and/or a high affinity for the receptors. In this in vivo displacement of opiate by various drugs correlated with the binding affinities of these drugs for opiate receptors in vitro and also fulfilled the criteria which are used for the identification of opiate receptor binding in vitro, namely stereospecificity and saturability. Moreover, the degree of opiate displacement in various brain areas correlated with the known distribution of opiate receptors and also with the pharmacological effects in the whole animal. The low receptor density in the cerebellum offers the possibility of using the brain/cerebellum ratio of opiates as an index of specific receptor occupation in vivo. The displacement technique therefore offers the possibility of analysing the kinetics and parameters of the receptor-occupation by opiates in living animals.

ACKNOWLEDGEMENT

The author wishes to thank Dr. J. Fry for stylistic revision of the manuscript.

REFERENCES

1. Cerletti, C., Manara, L., and Mennini, T. (1974) : Br. J. Pharmacol., 52: 440P.
2. Dobbs, H.E. (1968) : J. Pharmacol. Exp. Ther., 169: 406-414.
3. Glowinski, J. and Iversen, L.L. (1966) : J.Neurochem. 13 : 655-669.
4. Hiller, J.M.,Pearson , J., and Simon, E.J. (1973): Research Commun. Chem. Pathol. Pharmacol.,6 :1052-1062.
5. Höllt, V., Dum, J., Bläsig, J., Schubert, P., and Herz, A. (1975) : Life Sci. , 16 : 1823-1828.
6. Höllt, V., Haarmann, J., and Herz, A. (1976) : Arzneim. Forsch.,26 : 1102-1104.
7. Höllt, V., and Herz, A. (1976) : In : International Narcotic Research Conf. Aberdeen,(in press).
8. Johannesson, T., and Milthers, K. (1963) : Acta Pharmacol. Toxicol.,20 : 80-89.
9. Kuhar, M.J., Pert, C.B., and Snyder, S.H. (1973) : Nature ,245 : 447-450.

10. Lee, G.Y., Akera, T., Stolman, S., and Brody, T.M. (1975) : J. Pharmacol. Exp. Ther.,194 : 583-592.
11. Mulé, S.J., Casella, G., and Clouet, D.H. (1975) : Psychopharmacologia,44 : 125-129.
12. Mulé, S.J., Woods, L.A., and Mellett, L.B. (1962): J. Pharmacol. Exp. Ther.,136 : 242-249.
13. Pert, C.B., Kuhar, M.J., and Snyder, S.H. (1975) : Life Sci.,17 : 1849-1854.
14. Pert, C.B., and Snyder, S.H. (1973) : Science,179: 1011-1014.
15. Simon, E.J., Hiller, J.M., and Edelman, J. (1973): Proc.Natl. Acad. Sci. USA,70 : 1947-1949.
16. Terenius, L. (1973) : Acta Pharmacol. Toxicol.,32: 317-320.
17. Wuepper, K.D., Yeh, S.Y., and Woods, L.A. (1967): Proc. Soc. Exp. Biol. Med.,124 : 1146-1150.

Factors Affecting the Action of Narcotics, edited by
M.L. Adler, L. Manara, and R. Samanin.
Raven Press, New York©1978.

Factors Affecting Passage of Opiates through
the Blood-Brain Barrier

William H. Oldendorf
Dept. of Neurology, UCLA School of Medicine
Los Angeles, California 90024 and
VA Brentwood Hospital, Los Angeles
California 90073, USA

INTRODUCTION

To directly affect central nervous system (CNS)cells,
the pharmacokinetics of a drug must be such that appreciable quantities appear in the extracellular fluid
(ECF) environment of these cells. If one assumes a drug
has survived its exposure to intestinal lumen contents
(if orally administered), has penetrated the gut wall into
the portal venous circulation, has escaped liver en-
trapment, and is in the systemic blood plasma, the major
factor governing its distribution to brain ECF is the
blood-brain barrier (BBB).

"BBB" is a term which denotes the failure of many
blood-plasma solutes to achieve significant concentrations in brain. This concept has persisted since
Ehrlich's demonstration nearly a century ago that certain
optical dyes were uniquely excluded from brain after intravenous injection. Although BBB implies that there
is an impermeable obstacle between blood and brain, our
fund of common information would suggest this barrier
is selectively permeable rather than impermeable. We
know, for example, that certain drugs, such as thiopental,
result in an immediate CNS effect after intravenous injection. Additionally, the brain is metabolically active
and obviously is receiving its substrates from blood
plasma. So, even though some foreign substances such
as fluoroscein or trypan blue are excluded from brain
by the BBB, other solutes such as thiopental and glucose
are not.

METHODS AND RESULTS

The BBB is selectively permeable. Its degree of
permeability varies for different substances through a
very wide range from immeasurably low to immeasurably
high. During the past decade we have measured BBB
permeability to about 150 test solutes covering a wide

221

range of metabolic substrates, metabolic intermediates,
drugs and various substances of possible interest in
brain function. More than 10,000 individual rat studies
have been performed using a simple rat model, injecting
radiolabeled test substance into the carotid artery nd
and measuring its single-pass clearance by brain,
relative to simultaneously injected reference substance
(1,2,5,6,7,8,9,10,11,12,13,14). From these many studies
has emerged a reasonably coherent picture of the molecular factors governing BBB permeability. I will
discuss here only those factors which appear to me to
bear significantly on the distribution of narcotics to
brain.
     During the past decade it has become generally ac-
cepted that the BBB is a result of certain unique structural characteristics of CNS capillaries. The wall of
the brain capillary is the BBB (3).
     Whereas capillary walls in other tissues (general
capillaries) are freely permeable to all small molecules
less than 20,000-40,000 MW and slightly permeable to
molecules of any size (4), the permeability of the BBB
is not based upon size but rather upon other molecular
characteristics.
     The structural differences between general and brain
capillaries are diagrammatically summarized in Fig. 1.
Fig. 1A indicates the generalization that exchange
between the blood plasma and adjacent extracapillary
ECF is largely by extracellular routes, whereas in brain,
exchange must take place directly through the capillary wall and is thus transcellular (Fig. 2). Fig. 1B
shows these structural differences more explicity.
     We have studied morphine, codeine, and heroin as a
group (11) because they span a considerable range of
residual polarity of the free-base. Although many other
morphine derivatives might have been studied, one might
reasonably extrapolate results with these 3 derivatives
based upon the residual polarity of the free -base.
     When C^{14}-labeled morphine is injected into the
carotid artery simultaneously with the diffusible reference substance (in this case ^{3}H-tryptamine) (10), we
have established that approximately 1.37% remains in
the brain tissue, exclusive of any residual blood content, 5 seconds after carotid arterial injection into
the rat (see Table 1). When C^{14}-codeine is similarly
injected, 26% remains in the brain after 15 seconds
relative to a diffusible reference which, in this case,
is ^{3}H-water.   When heroin is studied similarly to
codeine, 68% remains in brain (Fig. 3).

TABLE 1.

Regional % extraction of ^{14}C-morphine
after carotid injection in rat

Anatomical Region	% extraction (mean ± S.D.)		
Olfactory Lobes (both)	0.55	+	0.05
Left-Cerebral Cortex	1.25	+	0.17
Right-Cerebral Cortex	1.96	+	0.25
Hypothalamus	1.58	+	0.41
Epithalamus (left)	1.18	+	0.83
Epithalamus (right)	1.51	+	0.25
Corpora Quadrigemina and Mesencaphalon	1.18	+	0.48
Cerebellum	1.46	+	0.53
Medulla	1.63	+	0.73
All regions combined	1.37		

Decapitation 5 seconds after injection of ^{14}C-morphine, ^{3}H-tryptamine (diffusible reference) and ^{113m}In-EDTA (non diffusible reference) (10).

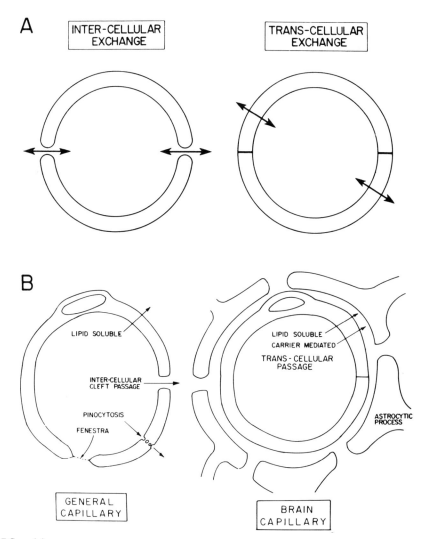

FIG. 1A.

The fundamental difference between the routes of
exchange of solutes between the blood plasma and the
adjacent more stationary extracellular fluid of general
capillaries vs. brain capillaries (BBB). In general
capillaries, the major route of exchange for small
molecules is between the cells via intercellular clefts.
In brain, the extracellular paths are sealed shut and
exchange must take place directly through the capillary
cell.

FIG. 1B.

The major differences between general capillaries and brain capillaries are shown more explicitly. Small molecules can equilibrate between the moving ECF(blood plasma) in the non-neural general capillary by diffusion through the intercellular cleft. A fenestra is shown at the bottom of the general capillary. This is a fusion of the inner and outer cell membranes but its role in trans-capillary exchange is unclear. These fenestrae are especially numerous in capillary walls passing considerable quantities of fluid such as in choroid plexus and renal glomerulus. Pinocytotic vesicles are quite common in general capillaries and may make up a substantial part of the capillary cytoplasmic volume. There are only 3-6% as many vesicles in brain capillaries. Exchange across the wall by pinocytosis is relatively inefficient but probably is independent of molecular size and even very large macromolecules can traverse the wall by this route.

In the brain capillary these non-specific routes of extracellular exchange are missing. In the general capillary intracellular cleft passage and pinocytosis do not require that the molecule actually enter the plasma membrane of the capillary cell, and these may properly be thought of as extracellular routes. There is no direct contact with the capillary cell cytoplasm. In the brain capillary the exchange between plasma and adjacent ECF must take place directly through the capillary cells and this requires that the molecules leave the blood plasma and enter the membrane. It must survive exposure to the capillary cell cytoplasm and repeat the membrane penetration at the other cell membrane. The major obvious structural differences between brain capillaries and general capillaries are 1. Fusion of membranes obliterating the intercellular cleft. 2. A paucity of pinocytotic vesicles. 3. An absence of fenestrae, and 4. Relatively large numbers of mitochondria in brain capillary cells. In the rat brain there are about five times as many mitochondria as in sekletal muscle capillary cells, suggesting that the blood-brain barrier has a capability of performing considerably more metabolic work than capillaries in other tissues. The BBB may be utilizing this energy largely in pumping ions into and out of the brain. The rectangle encompassing a segment of the wall of the brain capillary cell is shown diagrammatically in Fig. 2.

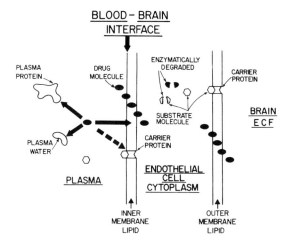

FIG. 2

A diagrammatic representation of the plasma-capillary
cell membrane interface corresponding to the rectangle
in Fig. 1. The black ovals represent drug molecules
and the hexagons represent metabolic substrates such
as glucose. The inner surface of the inner membrane
of the brain capillary cell, is the actual plasma-brain
interface. The molecular characteristics of the solute
in plasma governing BBB penetration largely represent
the ability of the solute to leave blood plasma and
enter the inner membrane of the brain capillary cell.
There are four relevant molecular species at this
plasma-brain interface. These are blood plasma water
and protein molecules and plasma membrane lipid and
protein molecules. The relative affinity of the plasma
solute for these four species governs the ability of
the molecules to make the transition from plasma into
capillary cell membrane. The affinity of such a solute
for the plasma water and membrane lipid are largely
predictable based upon knowledge of the polarity of the
molecule but the criteria governing affinity for the
plasma protein and for the membrane proteins are very
much less predictable. Even if a solute can successfully
penetrate the inner membrane, it is for a time exposed
to the full complement of enzymes contained in the
capillary cell cytoplasm and it may undergo enzymatic
degradation.
Some drugs are very strongly bound by blood protein
and are thus unavailable for BBB penetration. Affinity
for the membrane carrier protein is unpredictable. The
entry into brain of some drugs may be accelerated by
virtue of this route. The ability of drugs in free
solution in plasma to penetrate BBB, is largely determined
by the relative affinity for plasma water and membrane lipid.

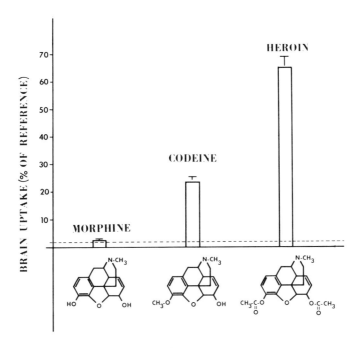

FIG. 3.

Morphine,codeine and heroin,make a useful group of
narcotics because they span a considerable range of
polarity. The olive oil/water partition coefficient of
morphine is about 0.016, codeine 0.15, and heroin 0.2,
presumably almost entirely owing to the different sub-
stitutions at the hydroxyl sites of morphine. When
the brain uptake of these three compounds is measured
during a single rat brain blood passage, approximately
1.5% of the morphine, 25% of the codeine, and 65% of
the heroin are cleared. Because most of the heroin
carried into the brain is deposited there, its regional
concentration after a bolus intravenous injection is
largely determined by the fraction of cardiac output
being delivered to the region of the brain being measured. The flow-limited delivery of such drugs as indicated in the text, may be an important factor in
changing the amount of drug delivered to brain after
bolus injection in various physiological and pathological
circulatory states.

DISCUSSION

If one contrasts the anticipated distribution to brain of morphine and of heroin after injection it would be predicted that a great deal more heroin would appear in brain than morphine. Furthermore, the actual regional distribution should be significantly different. In the case of heroin, which is very rapidly cleared by brain, one would expect the regional distribution to be dominated by the regional blood flow, since it is quite largely cleared during a single brain circulatory passage (1). On the other hand, morphine, which is cleared only to a very slight degree during one circulatory passage, would be expected to accumulate more slowly in the entire brain but achieve quite high levels in regions with an especially high binding activity. This may explain the apparent incongruity between the amount of heroin actually delivered to brain and its relatively low analgesic potency. In rats we have shown that after intravenous injection, over ten times more heroin is delivered to brain than morphine. It is expected that a similar difference would be found in humans. However, the difference in analgesic potency is only some 3 to 4 times greater. This disparity would be explained if the morphine were selectively accumulating at opiate receptor sites since these presumably represent only a small fraction of brain volume and would not be reflected in our overall brain studies.

When a heroin addict injects a bolus of drug intravenously, a substantial fraction of it is delivered to brain and remains there. It has been shown by Way (15) that heroin which enters brain is rapidly deacetylated back to morphine and it probably is as morphine that it is pharmacologically active. This morphine will be distributed in brain largely as a function of blood flow and not particularly as a function of regional opiate receptors. On the other hand, morphine may accumulate relatively slowly in brain because of its relatively slow BBB penetration, but it may accumulate much more pharmacologically effectively at high affinity opiate receptor sites.

The amount of heroin which is delivered to brain should be considerably affected by the fraction of cardiac output going to brain. The average adult brain takes about 800 cc of cardiac output and because of excellent autoregulation, this is quite constant in a wide variety of physiological states other than acidosis and alkalosis. It can be approximately doubled by tolerable CO_2 inhalation and approximately halved by extreme hyperventilation. Assuming a normal blood pH, the amount of heroin which is delivered to brain after intravenous injection could be substantially altered by both an abnormal cardiac output due to disease or to excessive blood flow to non-neural organs. Thus, it could be expected that a subject with greatly reduced cardiac output due to cardiac failure would deliver an unusually large fraction of heroin to brain after intravenous injection. Conversely, an individual who had performed a great deal of physical work just prior to an intravenous injection, would be expected to deliver relatively little of the drug to his brain. An extremely obese person would similarly deliver a rather smaller amount of drug to brain because of the large fraction of cardiac output distributing to fat depots. Such factors may in part explain the apparent variability of response to narcotic agents. This source of pharmacokinetic variability must be added to the probably more important source of variability based upon the nearly totally unpredictable potency of street narcotics.

It is interesting to speculate about what fraction of an addict's purchased drug actually prevents his withdrawal symptoms. Under ideal circumstances, where muscular blood flow is at a minimum in complete relaxation, perhaps 15% of an intravenously injected dose of heroin would be deposited in brain within the first 15 seconds. This will be distributed rather indiscriminately, mostly through the gray matter of the brain. Perhaps only 1% of this material will be deposited in brain containing a significant concentration of opiate receptors. This suggests that the greater majority of heroin actually deposited in brain is wasted on areas containing relatively few receptor sites and that some 85% of the total administered dose is wasted on non-neural organs in which there presumably is no desired pharmacological effect. In a state of cardiac failure where there were perhaps two liters per minute of cardiac output it would be expected that more than twice the amount of heroin would be delivered to brain relative to a similar injection in a healthy individual with 5 liters of output. If a person were extremely obese and had just performed a great deal of work, such as running up several flights of stairs, immediately prior to administering an intravenous dose of heroin, it would be expected that perhaps only about 1/3 as much of the injected dose would be deposited in brain, and the rest would be wasted to some degree on depot fat but largely on muscle, because of its very large blood flow. This reasoning suggests that the ideal circumstance for taking an expensive narcotic agent would be to relax for perhaps 10 to 15 minutes before administering an intravenous injection, to reduce the muscle blood flow as far as possible, and to be in a cool environment in which skin blood flow would be minimized. The amount delivered to brain could be further doubled if the individual were made hypercapnic during the time of the intravenous injection. If an individual were spending 100 dollars a day to support a heroin habit, it is quite possible that only a few cents worth of this material would actually be used, during ordinary circumstances of injection, to obtain the opiate effect at specific receptors.

An unknown factor in the distribution of drugs to brain is the effect of those small areas in brain which have no BBB. In these area the capillaries have general capillary permeabilities. The most notable of these are in the floor (median eminence) and pre-optic recess of the hypothalamus (16), and the area postrema at the caudal extreme of the 4th ventricle (17). In these areas drugs which achieve low concentrations in the remainder of brain because the BBB is impermeable to them presumably reach relatively high concentrations in the regional ECF. From this ECF, diffusion can take place into adjacent plasma. It is quite possible that this may create some highly unpredictable local drug concentrations in and adjacent to these small barrier-deficient brain regions.

It is widely held that addiction to heroin is more easily established and more refractory to treatment than morphine. If this is indeed the case, it could be that the explanation is due to 1. the greater amount of heroin delivered to brain; 2. the different brain distribution of heroin vs. morphine or, 3. as has been suggested by us, to the immediacy of delivery of heroin to brain after I.V. injection. This immediacy would tend to more strongly associate the CNS effects with the act of administration, thus reinforcing the relationship between drug response and drug administration.

ACKNOWLEDGEMENTS

We wish to thank Dr. Eain M. Cornford and Stella Z. Oldendorf for their many suggestions. Technical assistance was provided by Leon D. Braun and James Glass. Support was provided by NIDA Grant #01146.

REFERENCES

1. Bradbury, M.W.B., Patlak, C., and Oldendorf, W.H. (1975) : Am. J. Physiol., 229:1110-1115.
2. Cornford, E.M., and Oldendorf, W.H. (1975) : Biochim. Biophys. Acta, 394:211-219.
3. Crone, C., and Thompson, A.M. (1970) : In : Capillary Permeability, edited by C. Crone and N. Lassen, p. 477, Academic Press, New York.

4. Landis, E.M., and Pappenheimer, J.R. (1963) : In :
   Handbook of Physiology, Circulation,Vol. II,edited
   by W.F. Hamilton, p. 961. American Physiological
   Society, Washington, D.C.
5. Oldendorf, W.H. (1970) : Brain Res., 24:372-376.
6. Oldendorf, W.H. (1971) : Am. J. Physiol., 221:1629-
   1639.
7. Oldendorf, W.H. (1973) : Am. J. Physiol., 224:967-
   969.
8. Oldendorf, W.H. (1973) : Am. J. Physiol., 224:1450-
   1453.
9. Oldendorf, W.H. (1974) : Proc. Soc. Exp. Biol.Med.,
   147:813-816.
10. Oldendorf, W.H., and Braun L. (1976) : Brain Res.,
    in press .
11. Oldendorf, W.H., Hyman, S., Braun, L., and Oldendorf,
    S.Z. (1972) : Science, 178:984-986.
12. Oldendorf, W.H., and Szabo, J. (1976) ; Am. J.
    Physiol., 230:94-98.
13. Pardridge, W.M., and Oldendorf, W.H. (1975) :
    Biochim. Biophys. Acta, 382:377-392.
14. Pardridge, W.M., and Oldendorf, W.H. (1975) :
    Biochim. Biophys. Acta, 401:128-136.
15. Way, E.L. (1968): In : The Addictive States, Res.
    Publ. Assn. Res. Nerv. and Ment. Dis. vol. 46,
    edited by A. Wickler, p. 13. Williams and Wilkins,
    Baltimore.
16. Wislocki, G.B., and King, L.S. (1936) : Am. J.Anat.,
    58:421-472.
17. Wislocki, G.B., and Putnam, T.J. (1920) : Anat.
    Rec., 19:281-287.

Factors Affecting the Action of Narcotics, edited by
M.L. Adler, L. Manara, and R. Samanin.
Raven Press, New York©1978.

Pharmacokinetics of Morphine in Relation to Analgesia:
Effects of Routes of Administration

Bengt E. Dahlström and Lennart Paalzow

Department of Pharmacology, Pharmaceutical Faculty,
Biomedical Center, University of Uppsala
Box 573, S-751 23 Uppsala, Sweden

INTRODUCTION

The increasing knowledge of the pharmacokinetic
behavior of different drugs has opened new possibilities
of a more rational approach to drug therapy. Together
with studies on other drug-induced biochemical changes,
pharmacokinetic investigations can provide a deeper
insight into drug action.

The aim of pharmacokinetic investigations is to
study the time course of drug and metabolite levels in
different biological fluids, tissues, and excreta, and
also the time course of pharmacological response, and
to construct suitable models for interpreting such data
(34). Although investigations on the disposition and
metabolism of morphine and related compounds are numerous, very few studies have been performed on their
pharmacokinetic behavior according to the definition
given above. In the present article we will review
some of the pharmacokinetic properties of morphine,
with special emphasis on the effect of the route of
administration and its significance for analgesic
activity.

Pharmacokinetic Profiles of Morphine

Intravenous Administration

In describing the pharmacokinetic behavior of a
drug, the most suitable starting point is intravenous
administration. Data from such investigations are
necessary for a proper evaluation of factors that can
influence the time course of drug levels in the body.
Spector (31) found by radioimmunoassay that the serum
morphine concentration in rats after intravenous administration declined in a multi-exponential manner. Only
0.1% of the administered dose could be measured in
serum five minutes after injection, indicating a rapid
distribution to well-perfused tissues such as kidney,
lung, liver, spleen, and muscles (17,38). In humans,

233

a similar kinetic behavior has been found (1,32).
    Johannesson and Woods (14) found that minute amounts
of morphine entered the brain and only about 0.03% of
the administered dose was recovered. Since it is well
established that analgesia produced by morphine is
localized to the central nervous system, we have looked
in greater detail into the pharmacokinetic behavior of
morphine in discrete areas of the brain as well as in
plasma (4). In these studies we determined morphine
by a specific and sensitive gas-liquid chromatographic
procedure (5). After intravenous administration of
morphine in a low analgesic dose (2.5 mg/kg) the time
course of morphine concentration (C_p) in plasma (Fig. 1)
could be described by a three-exponential function
according to the general formula

$$C_p = A \cdot e^{-\alpha t} + B \cdot e^{-\beta t} + C \cdot e^{-\gamma t}$$

which can be interpreted as a three-compartment open

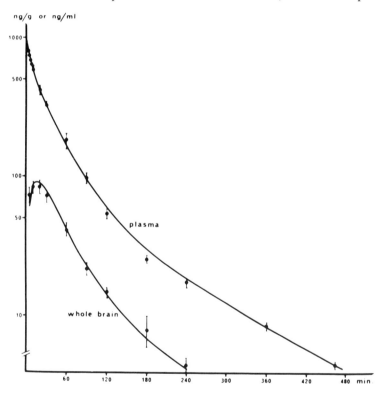

FIG. 1. Plasma and whole brain concentration of morphine after
intravenous administration of 2.5 mg/kg. Each point represents
the mean ± S.E. from 15-20 rats in the plasma curve and 5-10 rats
in the brain curve (4).

model connected with first-order rate constants. The
time course of morphine concentrations in four regions
of the brain can be seen in Fig. 2. As is apparent,
the same kinetic behavior was found in all areas, with
a maximal level of the drug 15-20 minutes after administration. The distribution of morphine was fairly
even in the brain with the highest concentration in
the cortical structures and hypothalamus, which probably
is a consequence of a high content of gray matter and
a more effective blood flow in these regions, a conclusion which concurs with earlier reports (19,21).
The half-life of the three phases of fall of plasma
morphine concentrations were 2.5, 25.3, and 128 minutes,
respectively (α, β, and γ phases).

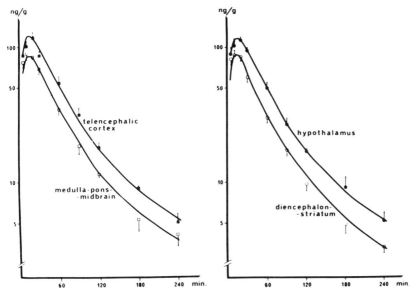

FIG. 2. Regional brain concentrations of morphine
after intravenous administration of 2.5 mg/kg. Each
point represents the mean ± S.E. from 5-10 rats (4).

By using different computer programs (SAAM-25; BMDX-
85), the data from the plasma and brain were simultaneously fitted to a three-compartment model, as given
in Fig. 3, in which the computed least-square estimates
of the transfer constants are also given.

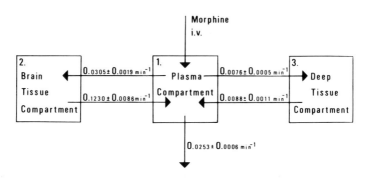

FIG. 3. Components of the three-compartment open model and the calculated rate constants ± S.D. of morphine given intravenously.

In this model, compartment 1.represents volume in equilibrium with plasma, 2.represents rapidly accessible tissues including the brain, and 3., slowly accessible tissues. It is assumed that morphine is excreted and metabolized only in the central compartment. As a consequence of these multicompartmental characteristics of morphine, a plasma-to-brain ratio is not constant with respect to time until the last phase of the kinetic profile of morphine is attained, i.e., about 4 hours after i.v. administration. This fact may explain the different ratios described in the literature (14,36).

When in possession of the data from the time course of morphine concentrations in the plasma, it is possible to calculate the mean plasma clearance or the systemic clearance according to the formula

$$Clearance_{sys} = Dose / \int_{o}^{\infty} C_p \cdot dt$$

(C_p = plasma concentration of morphine)

and this was found to be 12.2 ml/min, which is close to the blood flow to the liver (27), a consequence that will be discussed later.

Oral Administration

Rats were given morphine intravenously and orally, in doses of 7.6 mg/kg, and the plasma concentration-time profiles were determined. As can be seen in Fig.4, the intravenous curve showed the same exponential appearance of the three initial phases as earlier (Fig. 1). By comparing the areas under the curves, the

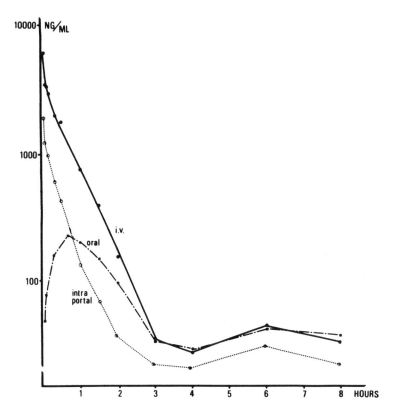

FIG. 4.   Plasma concentration of morphine after intravenous, intraportal, and oral administration of 7.6
mg/kg, respectively.   Each point represents the mean
from 5-7   rats.

oral availability can be determined, i.e., the fraction
of the administered dose that reaches the systemic
circulation.   This availability was found to be 20%
and thus, about 80% of the given oral dose of morphine
is lost during the passage from the intestinal tract to
the system circulation, an effect which is often   called
the "first-pass effect".   Since morphine has been found
to be completely absorbed from the gastrointestinal
tract (1,35), an extensive first-pass metabolism must
take place in the intestinal mucosa and/or in the liver.
By bypassing the intestinal muscosa through an intramesenterial vein (intraportal) administration of morphine, it was found in a subsequent experiment, with
the same dose of morphine, that the availability was

increased to 25%. The time-concentration profile of
morphine after intramesenterial vein administration can
also be seen in Fig. 4.

First-Pass Metabolism of Morphine in the Liver

In another study (3) we investigated the first-pass
metabolism of morphine in a perfused rat liver in situ,
according to the technique described by Hems, Ross,
Berry, and Krebs (9). The only modification was that
fresh bovine erythrocytes were used in the perfusion
medium. The flow of this medium was continuously recorded and the content of CO_2 as well as O_2 regularly
checked. Three types of experiments were performed:
1) Morphine was sampled in the reservoir of the recirculating perfusion medium (Fig. 5).
2) Morphine concentration was measured in the recirculating perfusion medium at the inflow and outflow from
the liver.
3) Morphine levels were determined in the outflow from
the liver using a steady-state concentration of morphine
in the inflow of the single passage of the perfusate.

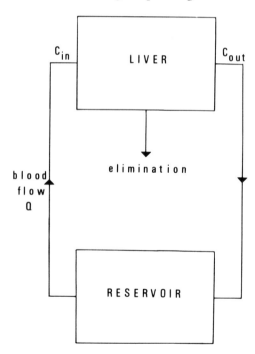

FIG. 5. Model depicting the isolated perfused liver
preparation.

In an isolated organ system as depicted in Fig. 5,
it is assumed that distribution into the eliminating
organ is perfusion rate-limited, the drug in the organ
being in equilibrium with that in the emergent venous
blood. It is also assumed that the drug concentration
in blood entering the organ equals that in the reservoir
and, similarly, concentrations in blood leaving the
organ and entering the reservoir are equal (28). Morphine was found to be rapidly eliminated from the
perfusate in a monoexponential manner with a half-life
of 5.3 minutes (Fig. 6). This monoexponential decline
is probably due to a relatively high extraction of
morphine in the liver, a large fraction of the drug
being removed as soon as it enters the liver. Another
possible reason for the first-order kinetics might be
that the liver acts as a sink for a significant time,
but this is probably not the case since the liver does
not accumulate morphine to any significant degree (16,
19).

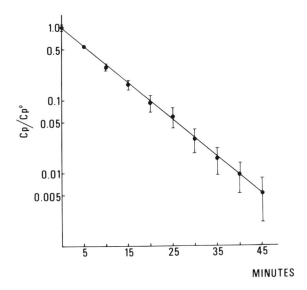

FIG. 6. The elimination of morphine from the perfusate
in the perfused rat liver in situ. Each point represents
the mean ± S.E. from 8 rats (Experiment 1). C_p = concentration of morphine in the perfusate. C_p^o = Initial
concentration of morphine in the perfusate (3).

The efficiency of the liver in irreversibly removing
morphine from the perfusing blood is called clearance,

the volume of blood from which drug is completely removed per unit time . The mean hepatic clearance can be estimated from the ratio Dose/Area under the morphine concentration-time curve, which was found in experiment 1 to be 13.1 ml/min (Table 1). After equilibrium (pseudo-steady state), the hepatic clearance (Cl_H) was also estimated in experiments 2 and 3 from the organ blood flow (Q) and the arterial-venous concentration difference across the organ (37), as given in the expression

$$Cl_H = Q \cdot E.R. = Q \cdot \frac{C_{in} - C_{out}}{C_{in}}$$

(E.R. = Extraction ratio; C_{in} = concentration of drug in the inflow to the liver and C_{out} in the outflow from this organ).

By registering the blood flow (approximately 17.3 ml/min), the three types of experiments yielded the following results (Table 1).

TABLE 1. Mean hepatic clearance and extraction ratio in three separate liver perfusion experiments with morphine.

	Hepatic clearance ±S.E.	Extraction ratio ±S.E.
Experiment 1[a]	13.1 + 1.0 ml/min	0.76 + 0.02
Experiment 2[b]	13.3 + 0.7 ml/min	0.77 + 0.03
Experiment 3[c]	13.6 + 0.5 ml/min	0.75 + 0.03

a) Recirculating perfusion with sampling in the reservoir; b) Recirculating perfusion with sampling of perfusion medium going in and out from the liver; c) One-way perfusion with constant infusion of morphine and sampling the perfusion medium coming out from the liver.

Furthermore, the hepatic clearance was found to be constant in the whole concentration range studied (800 ng/ml - 1.0 ng/ml). On the average, an extraction ratio (E.R.) of 0.76 was obtained, indicating that the hepatic clearance is about 76% of the liver blood flow and thus a fraction of 24% of the morphine doses is available after passage through the liver. Thus, the high first-pass degradation of morphine in the liver and the intestinal mucosa can most probably explain the low availability (20%) obtained in the previous experiment, in which areas of the oral and intravenous plasma concentration-time curves (Fig. 4) were compared. Since the experiments with the liver perfusion and the intraportal administration showed a 75% extraction in the liver, these results suggest that about 20% of the administered dose is lost in the intestinal mucosa, yielding a total oral availability of 20%. An important implication of the present finding is that the blood flow to the liver can be a factor infuencing the pharmacokinetics of the administered morphine.

General hemodynamic changes can affect drug disposition dynamics, and there is every reason to remember that such changes should be taken into account in the use of morphine. In the study mentioned above, we found from the plasma concentration-time profile in vivo that the total plasma clearance was about 12.2 ml/min. If we calculate that the in vivo blood flow to the liver is 1.2 ml/g liver/min (7) and that 5% of the body weight is liver tissue (8), this will yield a blood flow to the liver of 10.2 ml/min in a 170-g rat. Taking into account a 75% hepatic extraction of morphine, the in vivo hepatic clearance should be 7.6 ml/min. In the perfusion experiments, an average blood flow of 17.3 ml was used, yielding hepatic clearance of 13.3 ml/min (Table 1). If we had used a perfusion flow of 10.2 ml/min, this should have given a clearance of 7.8 ml/min, which is thus in good agreement with the results obtained in vivo. Consequently, we have obtained convincing evidence that the hepatic clearance is about

62% of the total body clearance in vivo ($\frac{7.6}{12.2} \cdot 100$), which is close to the reported values of 63% of the morphine dose excreted in the bile (16). Recently, Walsh and Levine (35) have found that approximately half of the subcutaneous dose of morphine was excreted via the bile after 3.5 hours, largely as morphine glucuronide. The glucuronide conjugated in the bile was poorly absorbed from the small intestine where its hydrolysis occurred slowly. In contrast, hydrolysis was rapid in the cecum where the rate of absorption was similar to that of free morphine.

Fig. 4 shows a second peak in the plasma concentration curve of morphine 6 hr after administration, which most probably derives from the enterohepatic circulation of morphine.

Relation of Pharmacokinetics to Analgesia

A current concept in pharmacology is that a direct and reversible pharmacological effect is associated

with a particular drug concentration at the site of
action. After a bolus dose of morphine, the drug concentration profile in plasma and in different parts of
the brain exhibits a three-exponential pattern (Fig. 1
and 2) and it can be expected that a given tissue level
of morphine at the site of action would always yield
the same pharmacological response during phases of
distribution (rising tissue levels), and also when the
tissue levels are on the decline. It was therefore of
interest to investigate the time course of analgesia
after the same doses used to characterize the pharmacokinetics of the drug in plasma and brain tissues.

The analgesic activity of morphine was determined by
a technique previously described (23,24). By applying
a standardized electrical stimulation to the tail of
the animal, two graded responses to nociceptive stimulation were followed in each rat. Increasing the intensity of stimulation causes the animal to respond at a
certain threshold with a vocalization response. When
the voltage is further increased, the rat responds with
a vocalization which persists after withdrawal of the
stimulus (vocalization afterdischarge). The vocalization response is considered to be mediated from structures within the medulla oblongata, while vocalization
afterdischarge is involved in the emotional component
of the pain reactions and includes brain structures
such as the thalamus-hypothalamus and the rhinence-
phalon (2,11).

After investigation of the logarithmic relationship
between dose and effect (Fig. 7), all time-effect data
were transformed according to this relationship to
yield values that are a function of the true "biophase
concentrations" (29,30). These transformed effect data
can then be regarded as concentration data and treated
as those obtained from chemical analyses.

The high degree of first-pass metabolism of morphine
is apparent from Fig. 8, showing the effect of morphine
administered per os and intravenously, each in a dose
of 7.6 mg/kg. After transformation to "biophase concentration", the pharmacologic experiments yielded an
oral availability of 20% from the areas under the
curves, a result which is the same as that obtained
using chemical analyses.

For morphine administered intravenously in doses
from 1.7 to 5.6 mg/kg, the correlation between the time
course of morphine concentrations in the brain and the
effect on the threshold for vocalization and vocalization afterdischarge was investigated. As apparent from
Fig. 9, the time course of morphine at the site of
action (biophase concentration obtained from pharmacologic data) declines much more slowly than the

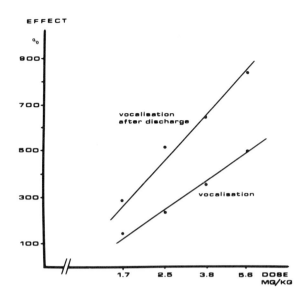

FIG. 7. The dose-dependent increase of the threshold for vocalization and vocalization afterdischarge after intravenous administration of morphine to rats (100 % = unchanged threshold). Each point represents the mean of 18-20 rats.

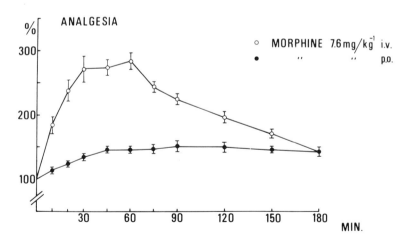

FIG. 8. The effect of morphine on the threshold for vocalization after intravenous and oral administration of 7.6 mg/kg, respectively. Each point represents the mean ± S.E. from 20 rats.

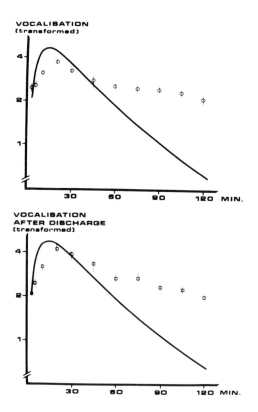

FIG. 9.   The effect of morphine (2.5 mg/kg i.v.) on the
threshold for vocalization and vocalization afterdischarge (circles and squares are experimentally registered data ± S.E. from 18-20 rats) and the computed
effect data from brain concentration data obtained by
the model given in Fig. 3 (solid line).

actually chemically found morphine concentrations. These
results indicate that morphine does not produce its
analgesic effect by a direct mechanism (6), a conclusion which also was drawn earlier from studies in mice
(25).
    It has been found in different species, using various
nociceptive tests, that a clear dose-response relationship exists for the analgesic activity of morphine,
also   reflected in the brain concentrations (10,25,
26). However, concerning the correlation between the
time course of morphine concentration in the brain

(and plasma) and analgesia, some authors have found a direct relationship (10,14,19,26), while others have failed to find such a correlation (6,13,20,25). When considering these contradictory results some pharmaco- kinetic and pharmacologic features have to be recalled, features which may explain the discrepancies in results.

Firstly, when evaluating correlations of time courses of drug concentration and pharmacologic activity, one has to bear in mind that changes of drug level are exponential (first order) for most drugs, while phar- macologic activity changes with a constant rate (0 order) in 20-80% of the maximal response range (15,33). To be able to make correlations, one therefore has to trans- form either of the data to the other as described above, or to prove that there is a linear relationship between the dose and effect (not log dose).

Secondly, the type of test for analgesia may produce different time courses of effect, and finally, the mode of administration can be important. The time course of the drug concentration in brain, for example, is among several factors a function of the rate of input and output from the brain. The input rate (dC/dt) is the product of the rate constant of entry and the drug con- centration in the plasma compartment, which in turn is dependent on other pharmacokinetic processes such as drug absorption. Such a process affects the time course of drug in plasma and, consequently, also in the brain. To overcome influences of the absorption when evaluat- ing correlations between drug level and pharmacologic activity, the drug levels should be determined in the potential target organ, and not in the plasma.

Considering these features, we have come to the con- clusion, as mentioned above, that there is no direct relationship between the decline of analgesia and the brain morphine concentration. Three possible explana- tions for this lack of correlation can be suggested (6):

1) The biophase might have a different kinetics from the whole or parts of the brain. However, because of the small size of the pool of stereospecific bound mor- phine, the kinetics of this pool will be difficult to evaluate.
2) The registered sustained analgesia might be a con- sequence of some pharmacologically active metabolite of morphine, which is slowly eliminated from the brain. Such an explanation does not seem attractive since mor- phine is primarily metabolized in the liver, and the metabolites formed are far less able to gain access to the brain than the parent compound (12).
3) The pharmacologic response that we observe and quan- tify is an indirect response of several events underlying

the analgesic action of morphine.

The latter conclusion seems plausible and is supported by studies showing that a sustained analgesic activity also can be obtained after selective stimulation of
certain brain areas (18). Furthermore, several neurotransmitter system in the CNS have been suggested to be
connected with the analgesic activity of morphine (for
review, 22). Moreover, the endogenous morphine factor
discovered may, of course, also be kinetically tied
to the time course of analgesia, and this will be a
matter of future experiments.

CONCLUSION

The mode of administration of morphine has a profound influence on its analgesic activity. Morphine
administered per os is subjected to about 80% degradation before reaching the systemic circulation. This is
most probably caused by a 20% degradation of the dose
in the intestinal mucosa followed by a 75% extraction
in the liver. After intravenous administration, morphine behaves pharmacokinetically as a three-compartment open model. The time course of analgesia and
morphine concentrations in discrete areas of the brain
after this mode of administration have revealed that
the analgesia produced by morphine can be described by
an indirect mechanism. The pitfalls when using other
modes of administration as well as not considering
different pharmacokinetic principles when evaluating
correlations of drug level and pharmacologic activity
are pointed out.

REFERENCES

1. Brunk, S.F., and Delle, M. (1974): Clin. Pharmacol.
   Ther., 16: 51
2. Carrol, M.N., and Lim, R.K.S. (1960): Arch. Int.
   Pharmacodyn. Ther., 125: 383
3. Dahlström, B.E., Jonsson, J., and Paalzow, L.K.
   (1976): Acta Pharmacol. Toxicol., 39: 46
4. Dahlström, B.E., and Paalzow, L.K. (1975): J.
   Pharmacokinet. Biopharm., 3: 293
5. Dahlström, B.E., and Paalzow, L.K. (1975): J.Pharm.
   Pharmacol., 27: 172
6. Dahlström, B.E., Paalzow, G., and Paalzow, L.
   (1975): Life Sci., 17: 11
7. Dobson, E.L., and Jones, H.B. (1952): Acta Med.
   Scand., 144 Suppl. 273: 34
8. Donaldson, H.H. (1924): The Rat Data and Reference
   Tables. 2nd edition, Wistar Institute of Anatomy,
   Philadelphia.

9. Hems, R., Ross, B.D., Berry, M.N., and Krebs, H.A. (1966): Biochem. J., 101: 284

10. Hipps, P.P., Eveland, M.R., Meyer, E.R., Sherman, W.R., and Cicero, T.J. (1976): J. Pharmacol. Exp. Ther., 196: 642

11. Hoffmeister, F., and Kroneberg. G. (1966): In: Methods in Drug Evaluation, edited by P. Mantegazza and F. Piccinini, p. 270. North Holland, Amsterdam

12. Johannesson, T. (1967): Acta Pharmacol. Toxicol., 25, Suppl. 3

13. Johannesson, T., and Schou, J. (1963): Acta Pharmacol. Toxicol., 20: 165

14. Johannesson, T., and Woods, L.A. (1964): Acta Pharmacol. Toxicol., 21: 381

15. Levy, G., Gibaldi, M., and Jusko, W.J. (1969): J. Pharm. Sci., 58: 422

16. March, C.H., and Elliott, H.W. (1954): Proc. Soc. Exp. Biol. Med., 86: 494

17. Mellet, L.B., and Woods, L.A. (1956): J. Pharmacol. Exp. Ther., 116: 77

18. Melzack, R., and Melinkoff, D.F. (1974): Exp. Neurol., 43: 369

19. Miller, J.W., and Elliott, H.W. (1955): J. Pharmacol. Exp. Ther., 113: 283

20. Mulé, S.J., Clements, T.H., Layson, R.C., and Hertzon, C. (1968): Arch. Int. Pharmacodyn. Thér., 173: 201

21. Mulé, S.J., and Woods, L.A. (1962): J. Pharmacol. Exp. Ther., 136: 232

22. Paalzow, G. (1976): Acta Univ. Upsaliensis, 9: 1

23. Paalzow, G., and Paalzow, L. (1973): Acta Pharmacol. Toxicol., 32: 22

24. Paalzow, G., Paalzow, L., and Stalby, B. (1974): Eur. J. Pharmacol., 27: 78

25. Paalzow, L., and Paalzow, G. (1971): Acta Pharmaceutica Suecica, 8: 329

26. Patrick, G.A., Dewey, W.L., Spaulding, T.C., and Harris, L.S. (1975): J. Pharmacol. Exp. Ther., 193: 876

27. Rowland, M. (1972): Eur. J. Pharmacol., 17: 352

28. Rowland, M., Benet, L.Z., and Graham, G.G. (1973): J. Pharmacokin. Biopharm., 1: 123

29. Smolen, V.F., Barile, R.G., and Theophanous, T.G. (1972): J. Pharm. Sci., 61: 467

30. Smolen, V.F., and Schoenwald, R.D. (1971): J. Pharm. Sci., 60: 96

31. Spector, S. (1971): J. Pharmacol. Exp. Ther., 178: 253

32. Spector, S., and Vesell, E.S. (1971): Science, 174:421

33. Wagner, J.G. (1971): J. Mondial Pharmacie, 14: 279
34. Wagner, J.G. (1975): Fundamentals of Clinical
    Pharmacokinetics, 1st edition, p. 1. Drug
    Intelligence Publ., Illinois.
35. Walsh, C.T., and Levine, R.R. (1975): J. Pharmacol.
    Exp. Ther., 195: 303
36. Way, E.L. (1967): Arch.Biol.Med.Exp. (Santiago),
    4: 92
37. Wilkenson, G.R., and Shand, D.G. (1975): Clin.
    Pharmacol. Ther., 18: 377
38. Woods, L.A. (1954): J. Pharmacol. Exp. Ther., 112:
    158

Factors Affecting the Action of Narcotics, edited by
M.L. Adler, L. Manara, and R. Samanin.
Raven Press, New York ©1978.

Pharmacokinetics of Naloxone in Rats

S. Spector, S.H. Ngai, J. Hempstead & B.A. Berkowitz

Roche Institute of Molecular Biology
Nutley, New Jersey
and

Department of Anesthesiology & Pharmacology
Columbia University
College of Physicians and Surgeons, New York
U.S.A.

In many circumstances, one of the rate-limiting factors that confront the pharmacologist in assessing the pharmacological properties of a drug is methodology. We have developed a radioimmunoassay (RIA) technique to measure naloxone in both serum and tissue which is both sensitive and specific so that many of its metabolites do not interfere with the determination of naloxone. Blumberg et al. (1), Hansbrouck (3), Evans et al. (2), Johnstone et al. (4) have reported on naloxone's ability to antagonize narcotic analgesics and its short duration of activity. Misra and coworkers (5) have calculated the half-life for naloxone in rat plasma. In our laboratory, we have used the RIA procedure to follow the pharmacokinetics of the drug following various routes of administration to rats and also to follow the serum concentration of the drug when given to man.

Initially, naloxone had to be conjugated to carrier protein : the chemical reactions used to couple the drug to bovine serum albumin (BSA), are illustrated in Fig. 1.

Rabbits were immunized with the immunogen obtained by coupling naloxone to BSA. Blood was taken after the third booster injection. Standard curves indicated that naloxone could be analyzed in serum and brain tissue and that the curves obtained were similar to a standard curve performed with a buffered saline solution. Also,the variability of the method was less than 10% and the limit of sensitivity of the method was about 0.1 ng, and one could measure 2 ng/g of naloxone in brain tissue and 0.5 ng/ml in serum (Fig. 2).

The specificity of the method is shown in Table 1. A 50% displacement of ^{3}H-naloxone from the antibody binding sites can be obtained with 2 ng of naloxone and in order to get that same degree of displacement with

249

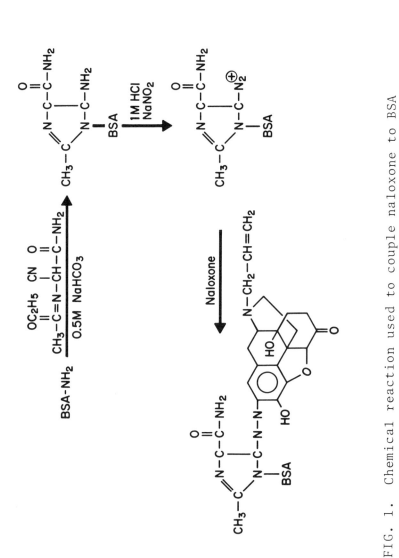

FIG. 1. Chemical reaction used to couple naloxone to BSA

TABLE 1.   Naloxone antibody specificity

DRUG	STRUCTURE	CONCENTRATION INHIBITING NALOXONE-H^3 BINDING TO Ab by 50% (NANOGRAMS)
NALOXONE		2
EN-2265		4
EN-3169		>40,000
NALOXONE GLUCURONIDE		240
NALTREXONE		4
MORPHINE		>40,000

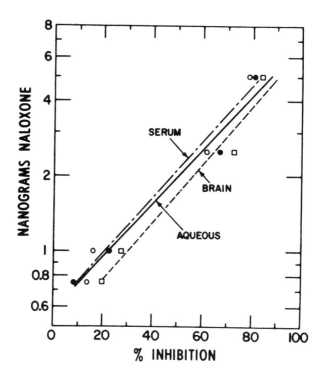

FIG. 2.   Inhibition of binding of naloxone-^{3}H to rabbit antiserum by nonradioactive naloxone in different fluids

Antisera was diluted 1:75 with phosphate-buffered saline. The lines were fitted by the method of least squares.

---

the major metabolite of naloxone, namely the 3-mono-glucuronide, approximately 120 times the concentration of naloxone is necessary. The N-dealkylated naloxone, noroxymorphine (EN 3169) cannot interfere with the assay since it would have to be present in excess of 2,000 fold. The reduced form of naloxone, EN 2265, is not a major metabolite in any species except chickens and pigeons;although small amounts have been reported in man it was found as the glucuronide conjugate. The antibody did bind naltrexone, the cyclopropylmethyl analogue of naloxone, and failed to bind morphine. A comparison of the ability of the antibody to bind EN 2265 vs EN 3169 indicates that the alkyl group   on

the N is a determinant group which influences binding
to the antibody.

Fig. 3 and 4 indicate the levels of naloxone and
morphine in brain and serum of rats following the intravenous injection of 5 mg/kg of each drug. Peak
serum concentrations are achieved within 15 minutes
indicating that both compounds are rapidly absorbed.
Serum half-life for both morphine and naloxone in the
first four hours was about forty minutes. However, there
was a marked difference in the brain/serum ratio of the
two drugs. At peak serum concentrations for morphine,
the ratio was 0.1 whereas for naloxone it was 15 times
greater. As the serum levels for morphine decline, the
brain/serum ratio approaches 0.5 while for naloxone it
remains 1.5 and 2.0. Thus, at equivalent serum levels
for both drugs one finds 3 to 4 times more naloxone in
the brain. It is also interesting to note that brain
concentrations of morphine were sustained for longer
periods than naloxone. These studies show that naloxone
gets into the brain rapidly and leaves rapidly, which
would explain why naloxone is both potent and short
acting.

Rats given 5 mg/kg of naloxone subcutaneously attain
peak brain levels of the drug within 5 minutes and the
brain/serum ratio ranged from 2.5-3.2 The serum T $\frac{1}{2}$
was about 30 minutes. When rats were injected with the
same dose of morphine by the same route the serum level
at 5 minutes was 1 μg/ml and showed a half-life of 40
minutes, similar to naloxone. But in contrast to
naloxone, brain concentrations of morphine were sustained
for about an hour. Thus, with comparable serum levels
and serum half-lives, naloxone and morphine achieve
different brain concentrations and different rates of
decline which could account for the differences in onset
of action and potency observed between naloxone and
morphine.

It becomes increasingly apparent that because of the
potency of many drugs, analytical methods are needed
which possess great sensitivity in order to relate
pharmacological effects to concentrations of the drug
in various biological fluids in tissues.

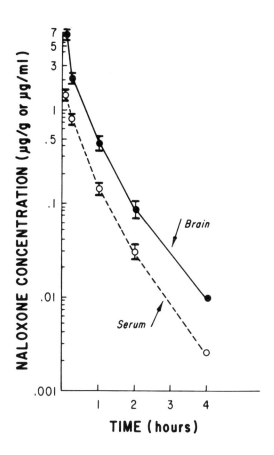

FIG. 3. Serum and brain concentrations of naloxone in rats at intervals following i.v. injection, 5 mg/kg

Each point represents the mean for 3-5 animals. Vertical bars are S.E.

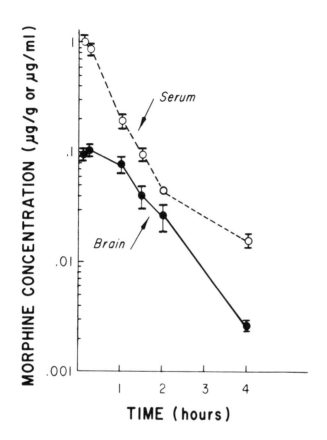

FIG. 4. Serum and brain concentrations of morphine in
rats at intervals following i.v. injection, 5 mg/kg

Each point represents the mean for 3-5 animals.
Vertical bars are S.E.

REFERENCES

1. Blumberg, H., Wolf, P., and Dayton, H. (1965) :
   Proc. Soc. Exp. Biol. Med., 118:763-766.
2. Evans, J.M., Hoff, M., Lunn, J., and Rosen, M.
   (1974) : Brit. Med. J., 2:589-591.
3. Hansbrouck, J.D. (1971) : Anesth. Analg. Curr. Res.,
   50:954-959.
4. Johnstone, R.E., Jobes, D.R., Kennell, E.M., Behar,
   M.G., and Smith, T.C. (1974) : Anesthesiology, 41:
   361-367.
5. Misra, A.L., Pontani, R.B., and Mule, S.J. (1974):
   Pharmacologist, 16:225.

Factors Affecting the Action of Narcotics, edited by
M.L. Adler, L. Manara, and R. Samanin.
Raven Press, New York©1978.

The Relationship Between Pharmacokinetics and Pharmacodynamic Data in Regard to Morphine Action

Ronald J. Tallarida

Department of Pharmacology
Temple University School of Medicine
Philadelphia, Pennsylvania, U.S.A.

INTRODUCTION

Although there have been relatively few studies of the pharmacokinetics of morphine and naloxone using compartmental analysis, several recent reports have provided us with valuable pharmacokinetic information on these agents in several species (4,8,14). These studies have used sophisticated and sensitive methods such as radioimmunoassay and gas-liquid chromatography, yet the relationship between the pharmacological effects and the kinetics is far from clear, perhaps owing to the fact that not every binding site is a pharmacological receptor in the sense that it can initiate a stimulus to produce a pharmacodynamic response. Thus, studies using measures which are related to some observable response are desirable. Such measures do exist; one such measure is E_{max}, the maximum effect elicited. Another measure obtained from response data is the dissociation constant, or its reciprocal, the affinity constant, of the drug-receptor complex. In this report we shall discuss and use the dissociation constant obtained from measurements at times of peak effect and at subsequent times in a way that permits us to determine the kinetics of an antagonist drug. The method is then applied to the combination morphine-naloxone in the rat.

The determination of the dissociation constant of both agonist and antagonist drugs is usually accomplished from experiments conducted on isolated tissue preparations. A frequently used concept is the pA_2 value (9), defined as the negative logarithm of the dissociation constant, K_B, of the antagonist-receptor complex:

$$pA_2 = -\log_{10} K_B \qquad /\overline{1}\_/$$

The value of K_B is determined from the equation

$$\frac{A'}{A} - 1 = \frac{B}{K_B} \qquad \underline{/2\_7}$$

where A' is the agonist concentration which produces a given effect, and A is the agonist concentration which produces the same effect in the presence of a pure competitive antagonist in concentration B (Fig. 1). The values of A, A', and B, used in equation 2 refer to the concentrations in the active (receptor) compartment at the time of appearance of the effect. In experiments on isolated preparations these concentrations are known or are controlled. It is for this reason that such experiments are usually carried out in vitro.

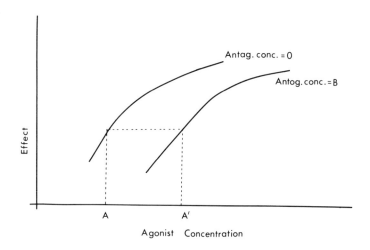

$$\frac{A'}{A} - 1 = \frac{B}{K_B}$$

$$pA_2 = - \log K_B$$

FIG. 1. The dose-ratio method for determining K_B

Several investigators (1,3,5,11) have applied this method to experiments conducted on intact animals using administered doses for A, A', and B on the assumption that, in such situations, the concentrations at the receptor site are proportional to the administered doses. This extension to the in vivo condition is certainly advantageous since knowledge of the K_B in vivo (also called "apparent" K_B) provides a means of summarizing quantitative data on competitive antagonism as well as a standard method to compare antagonists. Because the concentrations are time-dependent functions, however, the assumption of proportionality between dose and receptor concentration may lead to errors, depending on the kinetics of the agents studied. The present report is a more detailed analysis of the in vivo determination of pA_2 which takes into account several different kinetic assumptions. We have applied this time-dependent method to the analysis of data obtained in the rat, utilizing morphine and naloxone with the tail-compression test as an analgesic endpoint.

METHODS

1. Experimental

The details of the experimental protocol are those of Harakal et al. (6) and Tallarida et al. (13) in which Sprague-Dawley male rats (325-350 g) were used. They were held in an adjustable plastic restrainer and were allowed to adapt for 1/2 hour before testing. The nociceptive stimulus consisted of compression of the tail in the jaws of a micrometer, with vocalization by the animal taken as the endpoint. Control thresholds were determined prior to subcutaneous drug administration. Readings were made at 30,60,90,120 and 180 minutes after administration of morphine. To control for possible effects of injection trauma, some animals were given equal volumes of physiological saline and were tested at the same times as the experimental animals. Analgesia was recorded as per cent of maximum possible response for each animal, N being the number of turns of the micrometer for the test reading and C, the number of turns for the corresponding control reading[1]. Thus, each animal serves as its own control and per cent analgesia is given by E:

$$E = \frac{N-C}{21-C} \times 100$$

2. Theory

The dose-ratio method for determining K_B utilizes

[1]The number 21 appears in the formula since it represents the upper limit beyond which permanent tail damage results.

measurement of the effect usually taken at the instant
of peak effect, a time at which the agonist would most
likely be in equilibrium with the receptor. The importance of making measurements at peak effects has been
stressed by Takemori et al. (11). At subsequent times,
the concentration of drugs in the receptor compartment
decreases. Both the agonist and the antagonist concentrations change, so that the pair of dose-response
curves, without and with antagonist, would appear as
shown in figure 2 for two different times. Two observations should be made from this figure. First, the
effect diminishes at time t because the agonist concentration has decreased. Secondly, the magnitude of the
shift and, hence, the dose ratio, decreases with time
since concentration of antagonist has decreased.

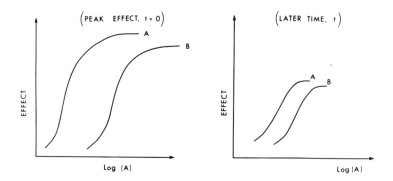

FIG. 2. Theoretical dose response curves in the absence
of (curve A) and in the presence of (curve B) a competitive antagonist at the time of peak effect (t = o)
and at time t

The concentrations at the receptor site are not
precisely known but are assumed to be proportional to
the doses administered[2]. Such an assumption is quite

---

[2]This same assumption is made even in isolated tissue
preparations.

reasonable at maximum drug concentration but, at later times, as concentrations decrease as a result of metabolism and/or excretion, correction must be made in accordance with the kinetics of disappearance. Prior to considering several cases for the agonist and antagonist, we will examine the time-independent form of equation 2, obtained at the time (t = o) of peak concentration of the agonist. The agonist concentration at t = o, denoted by A_o is some fraction (f) of the administered dose (D):

$$A_o = fD$$

In the presence of the antagonist, the concentration of agonist (A'_o) at t = o resulting from administered dose D is

$$A'_o = fD',$$

so that the ratio r = A'_o/A_o = D'/D. The antagonist concentration (B_o) at this time (of peak agonist concentration) is some fraction (g) of the administered dose (I), so that B_o = gI. Hence, using r-1 = I/(K_B) app instead of r - 1 = B_o/K_B means that (K_B)app = (1/g) K_B, a factor times K_B. These relations are summarized in figure 3.

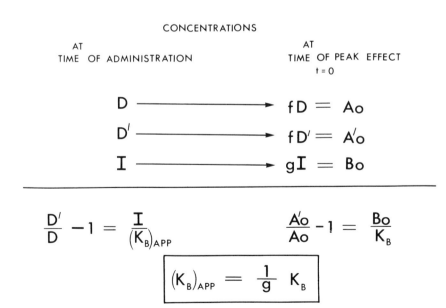

CONCENTRATIONS

AT
TIME OF ADMINISTRATION

AT
TIME OF PEAK EFFECT
t = 0

$$D \longrightarrow fD = A_o$$

$$D' \longrightarrow fD' = A'_o$$

$$I \longrightarrow gI = B_o$$

$$\frac{D'}{D} - 1 = \frac{I}{(K_B)_{APP}} \qquad\qquad \frac{A'_o}{A_o} - 1 = \frac{B_o}{K_B}$$

$$\boxed{(K_B)_{APP} = \frac{1}{g}\, K_B}$$

FIG. 3.   Comparison of K_B and (K_B)app

Thus, at times of peak effect the dose-ratio method yields a value of K_B, the apparent K_B, denoted (K_B)app, that is a meaningful constant which characterizes an agonist-antagonist pair. We now extend the analysis to times (t) subsequent to the time of peak effect.

Time Dependence

In the following analysis, we take t=o to be the time of peak concentration (or effect) of the agonist. At this time the concentrations of the agonist and antagonist will be denoted by A_o and B_o, respectively, and at a later time t, by $A(t)$ and $B(t)$. Thus we obtain the time-dependent form[3] of equation 2

$$\frac{A'(t)}{A(t)} - 1 = \frac{B(t)}{K_B} \qquad \underline{/3\_/}$$

Taking the administered dose ratio and the apparent K_B, we obtain

$$\frac{D'}{D} - 1 = \frac{I}{(K_B)app} \qquad \underline{/4\_/}$$

Dividing $\underline{/3\_/}$ by $\underline{/4\_/}$, rearranging and using $I = B_o/g$, we have

$$\frac{(K_B)app}{K_B} = \frac{B_o}{gB(t)} \cdot \frac{\frac{A'(t)}{A(t)} - 1}{\frac{D'}{D} - 1} \qquad \underline{/5\_/}$$

A salient feature of equation 5 is that (K_B) app is a constant factor $(1/g)$ times K_B only at t=o and may become very different from K_B depending upon the functions $A(t)$ and $B(t)$. There are numerous possibilities for $A(t)$ and $B(t)$. We shall examine only zero-order (linear) and first-order (exponential) disappearance as possible functions for the agonist and the antagonist, leading to four kinetic models.

Case 1. Agonist and antagonist - both zero order

When the agonist disappears linearly (at rate α), the ratio in equation 5

$$\frac{A'(t)}{A(t)} = \frac{A'_o - \alpha t}{A_o - \alpha t}$$

---

[3] Strictly speaking this form of equation 2 is invalid in that the conditions of equation 2 hold only at steady state which exists at the time of maximum effect. However, if the changes in concentration are slow as compared to the rates of chemical reaction, we have approximately steady state conditions.

may become very large. With $B(t) = B_O - \beta t$, where β is the rate of antagonist disappearance, the difference between pA_2 and $(pA_2)app$ is given by

$$pA_2 - (pA_2)app = \log\left[\frac{B_O}{g(B_O-\beta t)}\right] + \log\left[\frac{A_O}{A_O-\alpha t}\right] \quad \underline{/6\_7}$$

Case 2. Agonist, zero order and antagonist, first order

Again using $A = A_O - \alpha t$, and taking $B = B_O e-\gamma t$, where γ is a first-order rate constant,

$$\frac{(K_B)app}{K_B} = \frac{e^{\gamma t}}{g} \cdot \frac{\dfrac{A'_O \cdot \alpha t}{A_O - \alpha t} - 1}{\dfrac{A'_O}{A_O} - 1}$$

and the difference in pA_2 values is

$$pA_2 - (pA_2)app = \log\left[\frac{e^{\gamma t}}{g}\right] + \log\left[\frac{A_O}{A_O-\alpha t}\right] \quad \underline{/7\_7}$$

Case 3. Agonist, first order; antagonist, zero order

In this case $A'(t)/A(t) = A'_O/A_O$ and equation 5 becomes

$$\frac{(K_B)app}{K_B} = \frac{B_O}{g(B_O-\beta t)}$$

Thus,

$$pA_2 - (pA_2)app = \log\left[\frac{B_O}{g(B_O-\beta t)}\right] \quad \underline{/8\_7}$$

Case 4. Agonist, first order; antagonist, first order

In this case equation 5 becomes

$$\frac{(K_B)app}{K_B} = \frac{e^{\gamma t}}{g}$$

and

$$pA_2 - (pA_2)app = (\log e)\gamma t - \log g \quad \underline{/9\_7}$$

This case is of great interest, since many drugs obey these kinetics and one can readily use dose ratios at times other than at peak effect, in order to evaluate the constancy of the apparent pA_2 and to determine the rate constant, γ, for the antagonist. We have $\frac{A'(t)}{A(t)} - 1 = \frac{B(t)}{K_B}$ and, in this case,

$A'(t)/A(t) = D'/D$ and $B(t)/K_B = \frac{gI}{K_B} e^{-\gamma t}$. Thus from equation 3

$$\log (D'/D -1) = -\gamma t \log e + \log g + \log I - \log K_B \quad /\overline{10}/$$

If one plots $\log \left[\frac{D'}{D} - 1 \right]$ against t, a straight line results with slope $= -\gamma \log e \ (= -0.43\gamma)$ and intercept$= \log g + \log I - \log K_B$. Hence,

$$- \log K_B + \log g = \text{Intercept} - \log I \quad\quad /\overline{11}/$$

But the left hand side of equation 11 $= - \log (K_B/g) = - \log (K_B)$app. Thus,

$$(pA_2)\text{app} = \text{Intercept} - \log I \quad\quad /\overline{12}/$$

It follows, therefore, that if several different doses (I) of antagonist are used, one obtains a set of parallel lines of slope $- 0.43\gamma$, and for each the difference between the intercept and $\log I$ is a constant equal to (pA_2)app. (See Figure 4).

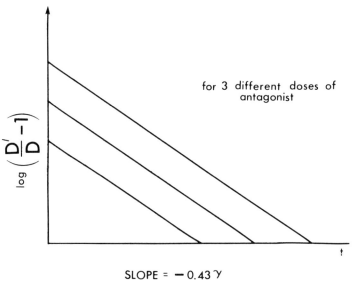

SLOPE $= -0.43\,\gamma$

INTERCEPT $= \left(pA_2 \right)_{APP} + LOG\ I$.

FIG. 4. Theoretical plots of $\log (D'/D - 1)$ vs time for several different doses of antagonist (I) for the case in which both agonist and antagonist are first-order. The apparent pA_2 = intercept - $\log I$. Time is measured after time of peak effect

This method is applied to data obtained for the combination morphine-naloxone in the rat, using the tail
compression test of analgesia.

3. Morphine-Analgesia in the Rat: Effects of Naloxone

The theory for case 4 is assumed for the combination
morphine-naloxone in the rat. The assumption of exponential decay for both agonist and antagonist is
reasonable, as shown by Dahlstrom and Paalzow (4);
Cerletti et al. (2); Weinstein et al. (14) and Ngai et
al. (8).

RESULTS

Figure 5 illustrates plots of log (ratio - 1) vs
time for the combination morphine-naloxone for four
different doses of naloxone, 0.01, 0.05, 0.10, and 0.25
mg/kg, yielding four parallel lines. The intercept at
peak effect (t = 30) is determined for each line. For
each naloxone concentration, the difference (Intercept
- log I) is given in Table 1, and is seen to be approximately constant with mean 2.57. Thus log (K_B)app =
-2.57 corresponding to 2.69 x 10^{-3} mg/kg or pA_2 = 8.1.
The slope (= -0.43γ) is 0.015/min, from which γ= 0.034/
min, corresponding to a half-life of 20 min for naloxone.

TABLE 1. Computation of (intercept - log I) from
graphs of log (ratio - 1) vs time for four doses of
naloxone

Naloxone dose (I)	(Intercept - log I)
0.25	2.54
0.10	2.56
0.05	2.60
0.01	2.57

DISCUSSION

There are several compelling reasons for extending
the analysis to times after the time of maximum effect.
First, the time of peak effect may vary among animals
or among different species, thus yielding different

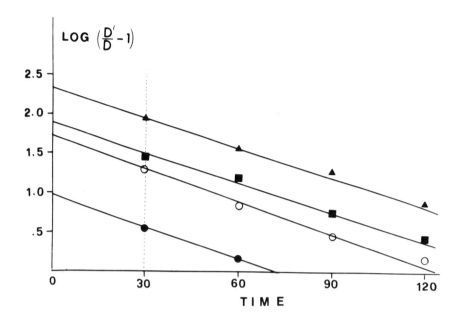

FIG. 5. Actual plots of log (D'/D - 1) vs time (min) after morphine at four doses of naloxone using the tail compression test in the rat. Naloxone doses: (●) 0.01, (o) 0.05, (■) 0.10, and (▲) 0.25 mg/kg

values for (pA_2) app which can possibly be accounted for by this analysis. Secondly, there may be any number of reasons for measuring effects at times after the peak, in which case the equations derived provide a method for determining the apparent pA_2 from such data. Finally, the application of the time course of the response may permit a bio-assay for the antagonist concentration and further provide a test for the kinetic assumptions. This application is especially important in the study of new antagonists for which chemical assays might not yet be available.

We have applied the time-dependent equations to the data obtained in our laboratories for morphine and naloxone on the rat. As predicted by equation 10, the plots of log (ratio - 1) vs time yield different but parallel straight lines for each of the naloxone doses. The agreement in the values of (intercept - log I) supports the validity of the use of first-order kinetics for both agents and yields reproducible values of the apparent pA_2. Such a finding supports the contention of Takemori (12) that the pA_2 value derived in vivo is a useful and reproducible pharmacological constant.

The half-time for disappearance of naloxone was 20 minutes, a value which agrees closely with that reported in guinea pig (7), namely, 19 minutes but is greater than its disappearance from plasma, $t_{\frac{1}{2}}$ = 16 min. in the rat (14). Such agreement lends additional support to the analysis from time-dependent data and provides a bio-assay for naloxone transference.

Two cases resulting from equation 5 are especially noteworthy in the use of time-dependent data in the determination of in vivo pA_2 values. These are cases 1 and 2 in which the rate of disappearance of the agonist is zero-order (linear). In such situations, the use of the administered dose ratio can lead to significant errors since the ratio at later times t may become very large. On the other hand, when the agonist obeys first-order kinetics, the dose ratio is at all times equal to the in vivo ratio. The use of a single exponential disappearance for morphine yielded consistent results in the present analysis. Yet Dahlstrom and Paalzow (4) have determined from a sensitive gas - liquid chromatographic procedure that the brain concentration curves appear to be composed of three exponential terms. The use of a single exponential, however, is a sufficiently good approximation over a limited time interval.

The value for the in vivo pA_2 obtained for morphine-naloxone in the rat was 8.1 using this time-dependent analysis. The standard method, in which pA_2 is determined from the intercept of a plot of log (ratio-1) vs log (naloxone), yields a value in the range 7.6-8.4, using the same data. Hence, there is good agreement in the two theoretical methods. These values are somewhat higher than those reported in other species: 7.07 in the mouse (11) using the writhing assay for analgesia; 6.60 in the mouse (10) using intestinal inhibition. However, Kosterlitz and Watt (7) reported a pA_2 of 8.73 using electrically stimulated guinea-pig ileum. Table 2 summarizes some pA_2 values obtained in various experimental situations. The value derived through our analysis may be indicative of an enhanced affinity for naloxone in the rat. Additional experiments with these agents, utilizing different effects in the rat are under way in our laboratories and may provide further confirmation of the in vivo pA_2 value.

TABLE 2.   Summary of pA_2 values

Species	Test	(pA_2)	References
Mouse	Writhing	7.07	(11)
Mouse	Intestinal Inhib.	6.60	(10)
Guinea-pig	Ileum	8.73	(7)
Rat	Tail Compression	8.10	This study

ACKNOWLEDGEMENT

This study was supported in part by USPHS grants DA 00049 and DA 00376 from NIDA.

REFERENCES

1. Blane, G.F., Boura, A.L.A., Fitzgerald, A.E., and Lister, R.E. (1967): Br. J. Pharmacol., 30: 11
2. Cerletti, C., Keinath, S., Reidenberg, M., and Adler, M.W. (1976) (in preparation)
3. Cox, B.M. and Weinstock, M. (1964): Br.J.Pharmacol., 22: 289
4. Dahlstrom, B.E., and Paalzow, L.K. (1975): J. Pharmacokinet. Biopharm., 3: 293
5. Green, R.D., III, and Fleming, W.W. (1967): J. Pharmacol. Exp. Ther., 156: 207
6. Harakal, C., Tallarida, R.J., Geller, E.B., Biunno, I., and Adler, M.W. (1976): Pharmacologist
7. Kosterlitz, H.W., and Watt, A.J. (1968): Br. J. Pharmacol. Chemother., 33: 266
8. Ngai, S.H., Berkowitz, B.A., Yang, J.C., Hempstead, J., and Spector, S. (1976): Anesthesiology, 44:398
9. Schild, H.O. (1947): Br. J. Pharmacol., 2: 189
10. Takemori, A.E., Kupferberg, H.J., and Miller, J.W. (1969): J. Pharmacol. Exp. Ther., 169: 39
11. Takemori, A.E., Hayashi, G. and Smits, S.E. (1972): Eur. J. Pharmacol., 20: 85
12. Takemori, A.E. (1974): In: Narcotic Antagonists edited by M.C. Braude, L.S. Harris, E.L. May, J.P. Smith, and J.E. Villarreal. Advances in Bio-chemical Psychopharmacology, 8: 335. Raven Press, New York.
13. Tallarida, R.J., Harakal, C., Geller, E.B., Maslow, J., and Adler, M.W. (1976): Pharmacologist

14. Weinstein, S.H., Pfeffer, M., and Schor, J.M. (1974): In: _Narcotic Antagonists_ edited by M.C. Braude, L.S. Harris, E.L. May, J.P. Smith, and J.E. Villarreal. _Advances in Biochemical Psychopharmacology_, 8: 525. Raven Press, New York

Factors Affecting the Action of Narcotics, edited by
M.L. Adler, L. Manara, and R. Samanin.
Raven Press, New York © 1978.

In Vivo Tissue Levels and Subcellular Distribution of Opiates with Reference to Pharmacological Action

L. Manara, C. Aldinio, C. Cerletti, P. Coccia, A.Luini
and G. Serra

Istituto di Ricerche Farmacologiche " Mario Negri "
Via Eritrea 62 - 20157 Milano, Italy

INTRODUCTION

The action of opiates, as of most other drugs, is determined essentially by the amount of pharmacologically active compound combining in vivo with the appropriate receptors. Thus the factors affecting narcotic action can be broadly divided into those depending, at least in part, on altered drug levels at receptor sites and those operating through mechanisms other than changes in such levels.

In vivo assays of the concentration of narcotics reached in target tissues of experimental animals under different conditions (e.g. dose and time schedule, concurrent administration of a specific antagonist or any interacting drug, tolerance and dependence), ideally should provide information on the availability of these drugs to receptors under the test situation. However, the diffuse distribution in tissues and non-specific binding of the majority of drugs is likely, as a general rule, to mask possible differences in their levels at receptor sites. Conversely, differences may be apparent in in vivo drug concentrations in tissue, which merely reflect non-specific factors inherent in the pharmacological response (e.g. altered blood flow through critical organs), without in any way causing it.

Combination of cell fractionation techniques with drug assay in order to evaluate the in vivo concentration of an opiate in specific subcellular components, supposedly closer to receptors, gives rise to further

271

complications. The artifacts of redistribution which
may occur during the subcellular separation process
create additional difficulties for critical appraisal
of apparent in vivo drug binding to given cellular
constituents. Despite these drawbacks, in vivo
measurement of opiates in tissues and subcellular
preparations remains the only approach by which
chemical determinations can be matched with simultaneous
functional appraisal of the narcotic action. Only
in vivo investigation of this type takes full account
of the pharmacokinetic and biotransformation factors
known to be relevant in determining drug effects.

In considering data available in the literature and
presenting some recent results illustrating the work
in progress in our laboratory, this short review
recognizes the advantages of in vivo determination of
tissue levels and subcellular distribution of opiates,
while admitting all the present limitations. The
discussion is confined to two conditions entailing an
altered response to narcotics, i.e. tolerance and the
concurrent administration of a narcotic antagonist.

TOLERANCE

Several reports have appeared in the literature on
comparative evaluation of in vivo levels of opiates
in tissues, with special reference to the CNS, in naive
animals and in animals rendered tolerant to these drugs.
Although the significance of the finding has not been
generally established, in most instances administration
of the same dose of an opiate to naive and tolerant a
animals resulted in lower drug levels in the brain of
the latter. Table 1 contains a summary from the
literature and shows that the most consistent finding,
i.e. lower brain levels of opiates in tolerant animals,
does not seem to depend on any particular compound
among those selected for study. In preliminary experiments performed in our laboratory, a single administration, either subcutaneously or intravenously, of the
powerful morphine-like agent etorphine labelled with
tritium, produced lower drug concentrations in brain
and spinal cord of rats rendered tolerant by daily
injections of non-labelled etorphine than in the same

tissues of naive rats (17).

Since pretreatment with non-labelled etorphine even at large doses does not result in diminished CNS levels of radiolabelled etorphine injected afterwards (4,20), the lower concentrations of ^{3}H-etorphine found by us in specimens from tolerant rats cannot be the result of non-labelled etorphine which might be expected to prevent further drug binding persisting in their tissue. Thus the data we obtained with etorphine (17) is consistent with findings by other investigators who used different, less powerful opiates and still found reduced drug levels in tissues of tolerant animals (Table 1).

TABLE 1. Brain levels of opiates : tolerant animals versus controls.

Opiate	Dose & route (mg/kg)	Tolerant animal	Brain levels (a)	Reference
Morphine	30 s.c.	dog	=	40
	30 i.v.	rat	–	38
	20 i.p.	rabbit	=	36
	2 s.c.	dog	–	30
	10 i.p.	rat	=	14
	5 s.c.	rat	=	15
	2 i.v.	mouse	–	16
	10 s.c.	guinea pig	=	29
	10 s.c.	guinea pig	+	27
1-Methadone	15 s.c.	rat	–	35
	20 i.p.	rat	–	37
	10 s.c.	rat	–	24
Levorphanol	2 s.c.	monkey	=	41
	50 s.c.	mouse	–	34
	40 s.c.	mouse	–	8
Cyclazocine	1.25 s.c.	dog	+	28

(a) Key : - lower; + higher; = no difference

TABLE 2. Etorphine levels in tissues of control and tolerant rats

		Minutes after etorphine							
		5		15		30		60	
		Control	Tolerant	Control	Tolerant	Control	Tolerant	Control	Tolerant
Brain	Hemispheres	1408±956	730±257	1005±403	628±106	479±303	343±21	237±20	155±42[a]
	Stem	1493±1024	655±253	1156±502	707±108	627±331	401±40	281±39	178±40[b]
	Cerebellum	566±328	297±133	264±70	259±94	170±73	118±10	79±11	50±22
Heart		1492±398	1146±239	747±130	670±65	441±155	352±37	247±23	229±41
Skeletal muscle		793±307	539±153	474±76	479±46	303±92	254±36	178±19	131±18[a]
Ileum		137±29	142±47	162±37	153±15	129±11	121±12	80±16	68±17
Epididymal fat		74±37	87±42	130±16	228±48[b]	220±33	419±55[b]	328±100	314±58
Plasma		395±242	282±85	217±58	169±10	118±45	93±7	72±11	39±8[b]

Male Sprague Dawley rats (180-200 g) were rendered tolerant by two subcutaneous implantations, 72 hr apart, of 75 mg morphine pellets (7) and 72 hr after the 2nd pellet by 2 daily injections of morphine HCl (30 mg/kg s.c.) for 3 days; controls received placebo pellets and morphine vehicle. Twelve hours after the last injection, all of the animals received, into a tail vein, 2 μg/kg radiolabelled etorphine HCl (courtesy of Reckitt and Colman, Tritium in positions 15 and 16, S.A. 28 Ci/mM, found to be over 60% radiochemically pure in our laboratory) diluted with non labelled etorphine to a final S.A. of 10 μCi/μg (for animals to be killed at 5,15 and 30 min) and of 25 μCi/μg (for animals to be killed at 60 min). When tested for catatonia on administration of etorphine, most controls but none of the tolerant rats were positive. Animals were decapitated at the specified intervals and ³H-etorphine was assayed as described in the legend to Table 6. Figures are means ± S.D. (n = 4). a and b denote significance of the difference from corresponding controls (p < 0.05 and p < 0.01 respectively) by Student's t test.

The results of our more recent experiments to determine the time course of etorphine in different tissues after a single administration to naive and tolerant rats are summarized in Table 2.

Tolerant animals show similarly lower etorphine levels, compared to controls, in the three main brain sections as well as in plasma and skeletal muscle.

In neither the heart nor the ileum are there any significant differences in drug concentrations between tolerant and naive rats, although under the test conditions etorphine was definitely less effective in tolerant animals in decreasing the distance travelled by a charcoal meal in the ileum. The picture is different in the epididymal fat where the time course of the drug peaks at late intervals and the drug level ratio between tolerant and naive rats is the opposite to that in brain, plasma and muscle (i.e. tolerant animals had more etorphine in the epididymal fat than controls).

The overall picture in tolerant rats (Table 2) suggests that the general metabolic disposition of etorphine changes in the body as tolerance develops. The different pharmacological responses to etorphine following tolerance, may lead to differences between control and tolerant animals in blood supply to critical organs (the data on the adipose tissue in Table 2 could be readily explained on such grounds); this in turn could at least contribute to a different metabolic disposition of the drug. Therefore it is difficult to establish cause- and -effect relationships in these studies, an aspect discussed in greater detail in the next section (see 'NARCOTIC ANTAGONISTS')

In conclusion, the lower concentrations of etorphine in the brain of tolerant rats (see Table 2) seem to depend more on general factors, i.e. drug metabolism and/or disposition, than on altered binding to cerebral tissue constituents, as also suggested by the results of studies of the subcellular distribution of etorphine under the heading 'SUBCELLULAR DISTRIBUTION'.

NARCOTIC ANTAGONISTS

The concurrent administration of compounds with specific antagonist properties alters or abolishes the pharmacological response to narcotics by a mechanism supposedly involving interactions at receptors. Indeed, opiate receptors have been recently character- ized on the basis of in vitro binding studies and such interactions are known to occur under in vitro conditions (see the review by Simon in this volume).

A summary from the literature on in vivo measure- ments of opiates in the brain of animals treated concurrently with a narcotic antagonist appears in Table 3. The most consistent finding of decreased opiate levels in animals also receiving a specific antagonist, compared to control animals, seems related to the choice of a potent narcotic such as etorphine. This may indicate that the diffuse distribution in the brain of the less powerful opiates at relatively high concentrations, with only a small proportion of the total drug molecules combining with receptors, is likely to obscure changes in the levels in proximity of the receptors, when whole tissue levels are assayed. Conversely, the low total brain levels of etorphine could reflect close enough receptor occupancy.

Etorphine Brain Levels

The decrease in brain etorphine concentration induced by a narcotic antagonist (4,6,11,12,20) has been ascribed to in vivo displacement from receptors (12). In support of this view (12), it is reported that up to 75% of total radioactivity in the mouse brain after administration of a labelled narcotic antagonist was lost when the administered dose was increased, thereby reducing the specific activity(with a ratio of 1 to 1 x 10^{-4} between the highest and lowest specific activity);it was concluded that this provided evidence of in vivo displacement from receptors (12). We believe this conclusion is open to question because it implies a discrimination between labelled and non- labelled molecules, otherwise identical, injected in the same solution, therefore conflicting with the basic principle of the tracer method (18); in addition no 'chemical identification' is provided of the total radioactivity measured in vivo, which is nonetheless assumed to represent unmetabolized drug in all instances.

TABLE 3. Brain levels of opiates : Animals concurrently receiving a narcotic antagonist versus controls

Opiate	Dose and Route (mg/kg)	Animal	Antagonist	Brain Levels[a]	Reference
Morphine	2 s.c.	dog	Nalorphine	+ =	31
Dihydromorphine	87 i.p.	rat	"	=	39
Levorphanol	2 s.c.	dog	"	-	42
	2 s.c.	dog	Levallorphan	-	42
	2 s.c.	rat	Nalorphine	=	10
1-Methadone	2×10^{-1} i.c.	rat	Naloxone	+	25
Etorphine	5.6×10^{-4} i.c.	rat	"	=	25
	4.9×10^{-3} i.m.	rat	Cyprenorphine	-	6
	2×10^{-2} i.v.	rat	"	-	4
	2×10^{-3} i.v.	rat	"	-	4
	2×10^{-2} i.v.	rat	"	-	20
	2×10^{-3} i.v.	rat	Nalorphine	-	20
	2×10^{-3} i.v.	rat	Naloxone	-	20
	4.5×10^{-4} i.v.	mouse	Naltrexone	-	11
	1×10^{-2} i.v.	mouse	Naltrexone	-	12

[a]Key : - lower; + higher; = no difference

In our laboratory,prior to radioassay each specimen
from animals given radiolabelled compounds is subjected to an appropriate separation procedure to identify
radioactivity (see legends to Table 6 and Fig.1).
We believe this approach (a) is the most reliable,
also as regards possible pitfalls that could invalidate
radioassay (3).

Comparison of the results obtained in different
laboratories should accordingly make allowance for
relevant methodological differences. We have confirmed
by more dependable assay, the early observations by
Dobbs based on gross radioactivity estimates (6), and
provided adequate evidence that etorphine brain levels
are lower in rats concurrently receiving an opiate
antagonist (4,20). The mechanism of this reduction
must, however, be considered within the framework of
the complexity of an _in vivo_ drug interaction for any
sound assessment of whether it can be assigned exclusively if at all to an event at the receptors (12).

Compounds which only have opiate agonist properties
seem to lack the ability to reduce _in vivo_ measured
brain levels of etorphine (4,11,12,20); this has been
credited to the pharmacological action of the former
compounds especially at high doses, while narcotic
antagonists lack this action (12).

However,the point of concern remains that brain
etorphine levels are lower in animals treated with a
narcotic antagonist. These animals, depending on the
administered dose of etorphine,may even show obvious
differences in appearance (e.g. no apparent opiate
effects versus loss of righting reflex) from controls

(a) Different approaches followed in the literature
    include: combustion of tissues; radioassay of
    homogenates, solvent extracts or subcellular
    fractions. When the results of chromatography of
    occasional .samples are referred to in connection
    with radioactivity measurements, poor correspondence
    between the material used for the latter and that
    chromatographed may invalidate quantitative and quali-
    tative estimates(e.g.chromatography of a tissue sol-
    vent extract may give little information on the chem-
    ical nature of the total radioactivity in that tissue
    determined by combustion).

receiving etorphine alone. Indeed the consistency
between the degree of antagonism of the pharmacological
effects of etorphine and the extent to which etorphine
brain levels are decreased by narcotic antagonists,
has been considered in our and other laboratories as
an approach to establishing functional correlations (4,
12,22). The question is whether the reduced or
abolished effects of etorphine in animals receiving
a narcotic antagonist derive from the fall in brain
etorphine levels, which accordingly would closely
reflect dissociation from receptors, or whether this
fall is determined by more favorable conditions for
clearing etorphine from the brain (e.g.improved circulation) than in controls that are fully sensitive to
the opiate. We present evidence (Table 4) that the
latter may well be the case, at least at doses of
etorphine in the upper range of those adopted by us
(22) with a view to monitoring obvious pharmacological
effects in individual animals and establish correlations with drug levels (e.g. time of recovery or righting reflex versus etorphine concentration in brain and
spinal cord) (22).

Table 4 shows that etorphine levels are considerably
lower in the brain of naloxone-pretreated rats whereas
in the heart and plasma of the same animals the difference in hardly apparent, thus somehow supporting
the specificity of the results in the brain.

However, under comparable conditions in antagonist
pretreated animals the clearance from plasma of bromsulphalein, a dye reflecting hepatic blood flow, (1,
13) exceeds that of controls by a factor of about 4.

Accordingly, there may well be differences between
control and naloxone-pretreated animals in circulation
in other districts, including the brain.

Depending on the kinetics of etorphine in a particular district, because of alterations in blood supply,
the drug concentration in the same tissues taken at
a given interval from etorphine controls and narcotic
antagonist pretreated animals, may be different from
one, either exceeding or not reaching unity. This
seems to be the case with the data on epididymal fat
in Table 4; although there is no statistical difference
the trend is similar to the epididymal fat of control
and tolerant animals (see Table 2).

TABLE 4. Etorphine levels and bromsulphalein (BSP) excretion after etorphine administration to control and naloxone-pretreated rats

| | Etorphine levels | | | | BSP Excretion index |
	Brain	Heart	Plasma	Epididymal fat	
Control	6.9 ± 1.9	9.3 ± 2.1	2.2 ± 0.4	1.5 ± 0.3	0.27
Naloxone	3.5 ± 0.5^a	7.6 ± 1.4	1.9 ± 0.5	3.0 ± 1.4	0.96

For etorphine assays as indicated in the legend to Table 6, control rats and naloxone pretreated (400 µg/kg, s.c. 30 min before) animals received, into a tail vein, 10 µg/kg tritium labeled etorphine HCl (same source and specifications as in Table 2, found to be over 65% radiochemically pure in our laboratory) and were killed 15 min afterwards. None of the controls had recovered the righting reflex at 15 min, whereas it was constantly present in naloxone pretreated rats. BSP excretion index was calculated from the data in the last column of Table 5 (etorphine at 10 µg/kg) according to the formula :

$$\frac{1}{mg \ BSP/ml \ serum} \times 100$$

Etorphine levels are means (ng etorphine HCl/g or ml) $\pm$ S.D. each based on 4 individually assayed specimens.

a denotes significance of the difference from corresponding controls at $p < 0.01$ by Student's t test.

Further information on bromsulphalein clearance
from serum of rats given different doses of etorphine
alone or in combination with a narcotic antagonist appears in Table 5.   The dye test is negative up to 1
µg/kg etorphine,i.e.,no differences are evident between the bromsulphalein serum levels in animals treated with etorphine only and those receiving naloxone in
addition to etorphine.However differences in the magnitude of the experimental error cannot be excluded,and
it should also be borne in mind that bromsulphalein
assay provides no proof that blood flow is comparable
in organs other than the liver.

Table 6 shows the etorphine concentrations in different brain areas of control and naloxone pretreated
rats receiving 1 µg/kg etorphine.   Although the
experimental conditions(i.e.doses of drugs and observation time) are not necessarily the most suitable to
permit exhaustive conclusions in this context, except
for the cerebellum, there is no overwhelming evidence
that etorphine distributes unevenly or that naloxone
causes a different reduction depending on the area
considered. In vitro binding studies by other
investigators have shown the cerebellum to be

TABLE 5. Effect of etorphine on serum bromsulphalein
(BSP)levels in control and naloxone-pretreated rats

Dose of etorphine (µg/kg)	–	0.2	1	10
Control	113 ± 30	97 ± 13	105 ± 27	368 ± 38
Naloxone	98 ± 6	106 ± 24	87 ± 15	104 ± 17 a

BSP(50 mg/kg) alone or mixed with etorphine HCl (dose
as indicated) in the same solution, was administered
into a tail vein to control and naloxone pretreated
(500 µg/kg s.c.,30 min before)rats. Animals were decapitated 9 min afterwards and serum was assayed for
BSP according to the Bromthalein ® liver function test
(E.Merck,Darmstadt). Figures are means ± S.D.(n = 5).
a : significantly different from corresponding controls
    at p < 0.001 by Student's t test.

TABLE 6.   Etorphine distribution in encephalic areas
of control and naloxone-pretreated rats

	A: Control	B: Naloxone
Cerebellum	137 + 22	110 + 18
Corpora Quadrigemina	511 + 72	209 + 48[b]
Diencephalon	452 + 105	183 + 32[b]
Limbic System	279 + 32	184 + 40[a]
Mesencephalon	349 + 53	195 + 47[a]
Pons and Medulla Oblongata	305 + 81	187 + 27[a]
Striata	402 + 81	175 + 27[b]
Telencephalon	422 + 96	229 + 50[a]
Plasma	209 + 33	150 + 22[a]

Control and naloxone pretreated (500 µg/kg, s.c., 30 min before)
rats received 1 µg/kg tritiated etorphine HCl (same source and
specifications as in Table 2), diluted to a final S.A. of 20
µCi/µg, into a tail vein and were sacrified 5 min afterwards.
Tissues were homogenized in 10 volumes acetone containing
4 µg/ml non-labelled etorphine; centrifuged acetone was dried
by blowing with nitrogen, and dried material was redissolved in
2 ml 1.5 N H_2SO_4, washed with 17 ml ethyl ether (which was then
discarded), and 2 ml borate buffer pH 8.5 was added; pH was
adjusted to about 8.5 by dropwise addition of 5N NaOH, and the
solution was extracted into 25 ml chloroform; plasma, with 0.5
volumes borate buffer pH 8.5 added, was also extracted into
chloroform.   Chloroform was dried under nitrogen and redissolved in 100 µl ethanol for TLC chromatography; ethanol aliquots
were spotted each on a separate glass rod (6.2 mm diameter, 21
cm long, previously coated with silica gel by dipping in a
slurry) (21), developed in a solvent system consisting of
butanol: acetic acid: water (6 : 1.5: 2.5); silica gel at the
same Rf as authentic etorphine was scraped into liquid scintillation counting vials containing 15 ml of naphthalene-dioxane
scintillation fluid (21), obtaining complete elution of the
labelled material, thus permitting radioassay (Packard TriCarb
C 2425 liquid scintillation spectrometer) in solution with high
(40%) and constant counting efficiency and no interference as
the silica gel settled on the bottom of the vial.
Figures are means + S.D. (pg/g or ml etorphine HCl) each based
on 5 individually assayed specimens and not corrected for recovery, which was constantly 80 to 90%. a and b significantly different from corresponding controls (p< 0.01 and p < 0.001
respectively) by Student's t test.

poor in opiate receptors (32), and here it has the lowest concentration of etorphine, a negative tissue to
plasma ratio, and shows no significant reduction in
levels following naloxone pretreatment. A moderate
but significant decrease in etorphine plasma concentration was also found in naloxone pretreated animals.
It is thus questionable whether, under the conditions
stated, our results (in Table 6) exclusively reflect the
action of naloxone on etorphine binding in the brain,
possibly at specific receptors. We believe that the
correct approach to establishing the significance of
drug levels and changes therein in tissues, is to make
appropriate measurements in plasma concurrently.
Evidence that narcotic antagonists affect the in vivo
binding of etorphine to cerebral tissue is presented
in the section 'SUBCELLULAR DISTRIBUTION'.

Morphine Brain Levels

Since it is not clear from the limited information
available in the literature whether narcotic antagonists cause a visible reduction in opiate brain levels
when less powerful opiates than etorphine, such as
morphine, are administered (31), we reinvestigated this
aspect.

Fig. 1 shows the effects of a relatively large dose
of morphine (20 mg/kg,i.v.),producing a severe condition in controls, which is completely prevented in
naloxone pretreated rats; accordingly bromsulphalein
clearance from plasma is about double in the pretreated
animals (data not shown).

Thus the lower morphine levels in animals pretreated
with naloxone reach statistical significance in plasma
at 15 min (see Fig.1) despite the broad variability in
controls (presumably inherent in the individual response to a subtoxic dose of morphine); in all probability this difference depends solely on non specific
factors, as previously illustrated for high doses of
etorphine (Table 4).

Fig.2 gives the results obtained with a smaller dose
of morphine (0.4 mg/kg i.v.) producing no pharmacological effects that are obvious on inspection, or if
any, too small for the bromsulphalein test to distinguish between morphine controls and antagonist pre-

284

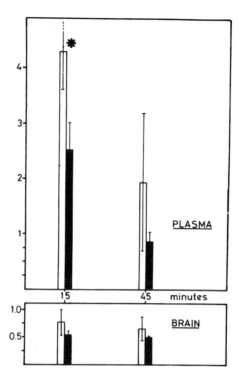

FIG. 1. <u>Drug levels in control and naloxone pretreated</u>
<u>rats after 20 mg/kg morphine</u>

Bars indicate means and S.D. (µg/g or ml,morphine HCl)
each based on 4 individually assayed specimens. The
asterisk denotes significance of the difference(naloxone
versus control at the same interval) at p < 0.01 by
Student's t test. Control rats(open bars) and naloxone
pretreated(400 µg/kg s.c.,30 min before)animals(dark
bars) received (N-methyl[14]C)-morphine HCl(Amersham
Searle,S.A. 60 mCi/mM,found to be over 80% radiochemically pure in our laboratory) diluted with non-
labelled morphine to a final S.A. of 1.1 µCi/mg, into
a tail vein, and were killed at the stated intervals.
For ^{14}C-morphine activity assays, brain was homogenized
in 5 volumes of 7% trichloroacetic acid (TCA) containing 20 µg/ml non-radiolabelled morphine, and plasma
was mixed with 2 volumes of this solution. To centrifuged TCA aliquots (6 and 1.5 ml for brain and plasma
respectively), depending on their size, proportional
volumes were added of 0.5 M borate buffer pH 10 (2 or
0.5 ml) and 40% K_2HPO_4 (4 or 1 ml); the pH was adjusted
to 9.2 - 9.7 by dropwise addition of 10 M NaOH, and the
solution was extracted into ethylene dichloride

(Legend to Fig.1 cont.)

containing 30% n-amyl alcohol (30 or 7.5 ml)which was then washed with 4% K_2HPO_4, dried under nitrogen and redissolved in 100 μl ethanol.Thereafter chromatographic (TLC)and radioassay procedures were the same as described for labelled etorphine,(see legend to Table 6) except for the solvent system for chromatography (butanol:acetic acid:H_2O,4:1:2). No correction was made for recovery which averaged 65 and 79% for brain and plasma respectively, with good reproducibility.

---

treated animals.

Under such experimental conditions, which are less subject to criticism regarding non specific factors arising from differences in pharmacological response, minor changes in morphine whole brain levels by the narcotic antagonist cannot be excluded. Indeed, at 45 min, i.e. when the tissue to plasma ratio has increased, the difference in brain morphine levels between control and naloxone pretreated rats (9.44 $\pm$ 0.97 and 7.83 $\pm$ 0.65 ng/g respectively, means and standard deviations),reaches statistical significance.

Although this difference appears small on a percentage basis (about 18%), it involves a total number of molecules (6.55 x 10^{-12} moles/g corrected for recovery) definitely larger than the more impressive percentage differences in etorphine levels reported in Table 6, yet falling within current estimates of the concentration of opiate receptors in rat brain (about 30 pico-moles/g)(33).

In view of the above considerations further experiments are in progress in our laboratory on the nature of the change in brain morphine levels induced by a narcotic antagonist, as reported in Fig.2

SUBCELLULAR DISTRIBUTION

Several reports in the literature have dealt with determination of the in vivo subcellular distribution of opiates in the brain by cell fractionation techniques (see Table 7). Although it was recognized over 20 years ago that artifacts inherent in such techniques should always be taken into account (9), studies

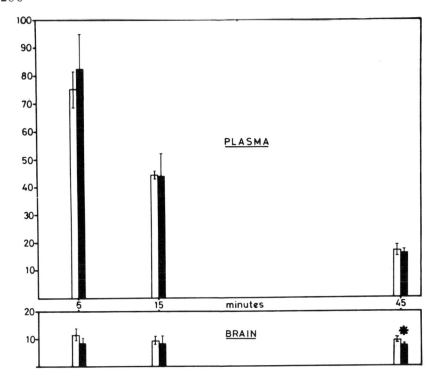

FIG. 2. <u>Drug levels in control and naloxone pretreated</u>
<u>rats after 0.4 mg/kg morphine</u>
Bars indicate means and S.D. (ng/g or ml, morphine HCl)
each based on 4 individually assayed specimens. The
asterisk denotes significance of the difference
(naloxone versus control at the same interval) at
$p < 0.05$ by Student's t test. Control rats (open bars)
and naloxone pretreated (same dose and schedule as in
Fig.1) animals (dark bars) received (N-methyl ^{14}C)-
morphine HCl (same source and specifications as in
Fig.1), diluted with non-labelled morphine to a final
S.A. of 78 μCi/mg, into a tail vein, and were killed
at the stated intervals. ^{14}C-morphine was assayed as
described in the legend to Fig.1.

of <u>in vivo</u> subcellular distribution of drugs are still
far from unanimous on any generally established criteria for critical evaluation of their results (22). The
reader is referred to another report by our laboratory
(3) for a more detailed discussion of the work by other

investigators indicated in Table 7, and of our own
results which follow.

We summarize here : <u>a</u> our approach for defining and
controlling the factors affecting the brain subcellular
distribution of etorphine; <u>b</u> evidence that the
etorphine subcellular distribution profiles may denote
differences in <u>in vivo</u> binding of the drug to brain
subcellular components, reflecting different pharmacological conditions; <u>c</u> a novel criterion for the
demonstration of <u>in vivo</u> opiate stereospecific binding.

<u>a</u>. For a critical appraisal of the factors affecting
the apparent <u>in vivo</u> subcellular distribution of
etorphine in the rat brain (19), we first determined
the patterns produced by adding different concentrations of the drug at 0°C to cerebral tissue from
drug-free animals. As shown in Fig.3, following
homogenization etorphine redistributes from the soluble to the particulate fractions, the extent among
these differing, depending on the total drug concentration in the system. Concentrations of 3.1×10^{-11}
and 2.1×10^{-9} closely approximate the levels established <u>in vivo</u> in the rat brain by a threshold, i.e.
0.2 µg/kg, the analgesic ED_{50} (2), and by a large
dose of etorphine (20 µg/kg i.v., $> ED_{100}$ for causing
loss of righting reflex). To overcome the problem
of concentration-dependent drug redistribution, in
a first set of experiments we operated constantly
with a high level of non-radiolabelled etorphine
'carrier' dissolved in the homogenizing medium, a
condition made possible by our assay method relying
on the use of tritium-labelled etorphine. The results
appear in Fig.4.

<u>b</u>. The subcellular distribution profiles of tritiated
etorphine observed either after adding the labelled
drug in the homogenizer, or when it was injected at
two dose levels to control and antagonist - pretreated
animals, were significantly different. These profiles as a whole reflect different pharmacological
conditions, also indicating that the underlying
mechanism results in differences in <u>in vivo</u> binding
of the drug to brain subcellular constituents. Thus
the data presented in Fig.4 may be taken as evidence
that the lowered brain etorphine concentration after

TABLE 7. Representative studies of the in vivo brain
         subcellular distribution of opiates

Opiate	Objective of the study and/or principal findings	Reference
Levorphanol	–Differences between in vivo and in vitro distribution	23
Dihydromorphine	–Distribution not altered by nalorphine	39
Morphine	–No differences between control and tolerant animals	29
Dihydromorphine, Morphine, 1–Methadone, Levorphanol, Naloxone,Nalorphine	–Distribution related to lipid solubility	5
1–Methadone, d–Methadone, Levorphanol, Dihydromorphine, Naloxone, Etorphine	–Localization in synaptic membranes	25
Etorphine	–Localization in synaptic membranes	26

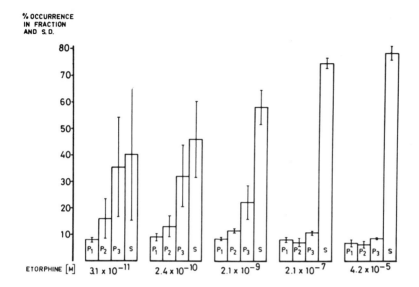

FIG. 3. <u>Distribution in rat brain subcellular fractions</u>
         <u>of etorphine added in the homogenizer</u>
The rat brain primary subcellular fractions were prepared by homogenization in isotonic sucrose and differential centrifugation (3,19). The molar concentration of etorphine added in the homogenizing sucrose is
given under each histogram. The bars represent means
and S.D., each based on 3 determinations, of the percentages of ^{3}H-etorphine activity found in each fraction (the sum of ^{3}H-etorphine activities of the four
fractions prepared from the same brain was made equal
to 100%). Etorphine assays were performed as indicated
in the legend to Table 6, with slight modifications to
extraction procedure (3).

---

concurrent administration of a narcotic antagonist
(see the previous section 'NARCOTIC ANTAGONISTS')
depends at least in part on altered binding of the drug
in the brain.
The mechanism whereby after administration of
etorphine, or of other opiates, lower concentrations
of the drug are found in the brain of animals
rendered tolerant than in controls (see the section

'TOLERANCE') may perhaps be interpreted more easily
through a similar approach based on comparison of
the subcellular distribution profiles. Preliminary
evidence from our laboratory did not disclose any
difference in such profiles (data not shown). This
supports the view that the lower etorphine levels
found in the brain of tolerant animals depend on
general 'metabolic' factors rather than on altered
binding to cerebral subcellular constituents, as
already discussed for rats given an opiate antagonist
concurrently with etorphine (Fig.4).

c. When radiolabelled etorphine was injected in vivo
at a threshold pharmacological dose, and the brain
was homogenized in unlabelled etorphine 'carrier'
free sucrose, the apparent distribution profile gave
peak presence in the microsomal (P_3) fraction (Fig.
5, profile A) and better reproducibility than the
profile obtained by adding a corresponding concentration of tritiated etorphine in the homogenizer
to brain tissue from drug-free animals (Fig.3
profile A). When the relative amount of the drug
found in a given fraction presumably depends solely
on physical-chemical factors (e.g.partition coefficient), prevailing localization is not apparent in
the P_3 fraction (Fig.3). Therefore the peak concentration of etorphine in the P_3 fraction of profile
A, fig.5,may be taken as evidence that this fraction
constitutes a major site for in vivo drug binding
(3).
In vivo binding of etorphine to the microsomal
fraction also appears to be largely stereospecific,
since homogenization of the brain in sucrose containing levorphanol, but not sucrose with added
dextrophan, results in significant release of the
labelled drug from the P_3 fraction (Fig.5). We
believe that these results are important since the
in vivo stereospecific binding shown by us in the
microsomal fractions involves a significant percentage (at least 15%) of the total drug present in the
brain. More refined fractionation techniques will
be required, however, to isolate the precise subcellular structures containing the stereospecific
binding sites.

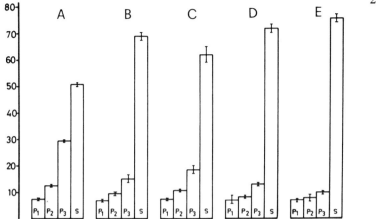

FIG. 4. Dependence of etorphine brain subcellular
distribution on injected dose and on pretreatment with a narcotic antagonist

The bars are means and S.D. (n=4) of the percentages
of ^{3}H-etorphine found in each fraction (see legend to
Fig.3). The letters on the histograms indicate the following experimental conditions. A and C: ^{3}H-etorphine
HCl (S.A. 63 μCi/μg, found to be over 70% radiochemically pure in our laboratory) was injected i.v. to rats at
doses of 0.2 and 20 μg/kg. B and D: ^{3}H-etorphine (0.2
and 20 μg/kg i.v.) was administered to cyprenorphine -
pretreated rats (100 μg/kg, i.p. 30 min prior to
etorphine). Animals were killed 15 minutes after ^{3}H-
etorphine administration. E: ^{3}H-etorphine was added
in the homogenizer to brain tissue from drug-free rats.
Tissue fractionation was performed in sucrose containing 4.2×10^{-5}M non-radiolabelled etorphine. Total brain
concentrations of ^{3}H-etorphine were 96±6 and 71±5 pg/g
(means±S.D.) respectively in conditions A and B,
13.2±4.0 and 6.2±0.3 ng/g (mean±S.D.) respectively in
conditions C and D. For comparison between fractions
of the same type, each under the influence of a different experimental condition, statistical analysis (3)
showed the following significant differences: P_2 , A ≠
B, A ≠ D, A ≠ E, C ≠ D, C ≠ E ($p < 0.01$);P_3 and S all
the conditions, except B versus D, different at p<0.01.
Comparison of the different fractions under one
particular experimental condition showed: A, B and C,
all the values significantly different from each other
at least at the 0.01 level; D and E all the values
significantly different from each other ($p < 0.01$)
except those of fractions P_1 and P_2.

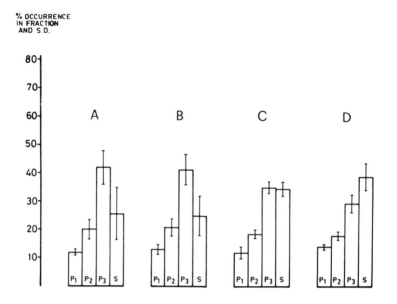

FIG. 5.   <u>Different influence of the enantiomers of an</u>
           <u>opiate added in the homogenizing medium on</u>
           <u>brain subcellular distribution of in vivo</u>
           <u>administered etorphine</u>

The bars represent mean values (n = 4) and S.D. of
the percentages of ^{3}H-etorphine found in each subcellular fraction prepared and assayed as per the
legend to Fig. 3.   Rats were administered ^{3}H-etorphine
HCl 0.2 µg/kg i.v. (same specifications as in Fig. 4)
and killed 15 minutes afterwards.   Each histogram
refers to the specific experimental condition indicated
by the letter above :

A : brain tissue homogenized in sucrose with non-
labelled opiate carrier;

B and C homogenizing sucrose containing 4.4×10^{-7}M and
4.4×10^{-5}M dextrorphan respectively;

D, sucrose containing 4.2×10^{-7} levorphanol.

For comparison between fractions of the same type,
each under the influence of a different experimental
condition, statistical analysis shows the following
significant differences : P_3, A ≠ D, B ≠ D (p < 0.01);
S, A ≠ D, B ≠ D (p < 0.01) and A ≠ C, B ≠ C (p < 0.05).
Comparison of the different fractions under one

                                            (cont.)

(Legend to Fig. 5 cont.)

particular experimental conditions showed : A and B, $P_1 \neq P_3$, $P_2 \neq P_3$, $P_3 \neq S$, $P_1 \neq S$ ($p < 0.01$) and $P_1 \neq P_2$ ($p < 0.05$); C, $P_1 \neq P_3$, $P_2 \neq P_3$, $P_1 \neq S$, $P_2 \neq S$ ($p < 0.01$); D, $P_1 \neq S$, $P_2 \neq S$, $P_1 \neq P_3$ ($p < 0.01$) and $P_2 \neq P_3$ ($p < 0.05$).

SUMMARY AND CONCLUSIONS

In vivo tissue levels and subcellular distribution of opiates are discussed for their potential ability to provide critical information on factors which affect narcotic action, partially if not entirely, by modifying drug availability at receptor sites.

In two conditions which entail an altered response to narcotics, i.e. tolerance and the concurrent administration of a narcotic antagonist, reduced brain concentrations of opiates can be detected in experimental animals. Present evidence indicated that a similar reduction in in vivo measured drug concentrations appears to denote primarily an altered general disposition of opiates in the body of tolerant animals, whereas in animals concurrently receiving an opiate antagonist it may reflect changes in drug binding, possibly to specific receptors, However, in both conditions, non specific factors such as altered blood flow through critical organs, which are inherent in the different pharmacological responses, may be the main causes of the lower drug tissue levels as compared to those in controls fully sensitive to opiates. Interpreting the results of brain subcellular distribution studies requires additional caution, but they seem likely to provide information on in vivo opiate binding and to indicate that it is modified by narcotic antagonists. Preferential release of etorphine bound in vivo to rat brain subcellular fractions by the pharmacologically active opiate enantiomer added in vitro, is presented as evidence for in vivo stereospecific binding. In view of the importance in assay of in vivo tissue levels of narcotics of analytical methods based on the use of high specific activity

radiolabelled opiates, attention is also called to the
problems of the different modes of application of these
tools.

ACKNOWLEDGEMENTS

The original work presented in this review was
partly supported through grants from WHO (N. A_2/181/19)
and from the Gustav and Louise Pfeiffer Research Fnd.,
New York, U.S.A.
The authors wish to thank Reckitt and Colman, Hull,
England, for kindly donating tritium labelled etorphine,
Mrs.Judy Baggott for stylistic revision of the
manuscript; Miss Alessandra Tavani for making available
the results on bromsulphalein, obtained in the preparation of her Biology thesis, for the University of Milan
and Mr. Sergio Bernasconi for dissecting rat brain
areas.

REFERENCES

1. Banaszak, E.F., Stekiel, W.J., Grace, R.A., and
     Smith, J.J. (1960): Am.J.Physiol., 198: 877-880.
2. Blane, G.F., Boura, A.L.A., Fitzgerald, A.E., and
     Lister, R.E. (1967): Br.J.Pharmacol.Chemother., 30:
     11-22.
3. Cerletti, C., Coccia, P., Manara, L., Mennini, T.,
     and Recchia, M. (1977): Br.J.Pharmacol. in press.
4. Cerletti, C., Manara, L., and Mennini, T. (1974):
     Br.J.Pharmacol., 52: 440P.
5. Clouet, D.H., and Williams, N. (1973): Biochem.
     Pharmacol., 22: 1283-1293.
6. Dobbs, H.E. (1968): J.Pharmacol.Exp.Ther., 160:
     407-414.
7. Gibson, R.D., and Tingstad, J.E. (1970): J.Pharm.
     Sci., 59: 426-427.
8. Goldstein, A., Judson, B.A., and Sheehan, P. (1973):
     Br.J.Pharmacol., 47: 138-140.
9. Harvey, S.C., and Pieper, G.R. (1955): J.Pharmacol.
     Exp. Ther., 114: 14-27.
10.Heng, J., and Woods, L.A. (1958): Fed.Proc.,17: 376.
11.Höllt, V., Dum, J., Bläsig, J., Schubert, P., and
     Herz, A. (1975): Life Sci., 16: 1823-1828.
12.Höllt, V., Haarmann, I., and Herz, A. (1976):

Arzneim.Forsch., 26: 1102-1104.

13.Klaassen, C.D., and Plaa, G.L. (1967): J.Appl.
Physiol., 22: 1151-1155.

14.Johannesson, T., and Schou, J. (1963): Acta
Pharmacol.Toxicol.(Kbh.), 20: 213-221.

15.Johannesson, T., and Woods, L.A. (1964): Acta
Pharmacol.Toxicol.(Kbh.), 21: 381-396.

16.Loh, H.H., Shen, F.H., and Way, E.L. (1969):
Biochem.Pharmacol., 18: 2711-2721.

17.Luini, A., and Manara, L. (1977): Res.Commun.Chem.
Pathol.Pharmacol., 17: 183-186.

18.Manara, L. (1971): In: Fundamentals of Biochemical
Pharmacology, edited by Z.M.Bacq, pp.29-34,Pergamon
Press, Oxford.

19.Manara, L., Cerletti, C., Coccia, P., and Mennini,
T. (1975): In: Sixth International Congress of
Pharmacology, Helsinki, July 20-25, p.438.

20.Manara, L., Cerletti, C., and Mennini, T. (1975):
Fed.Proc., 34: 815.

21.Manara, L., Mennini, T., and Carminati, P. (1972):
Eur.J.Pharmacol., 17: 183-185.

22.Manara, L., and Serra, G. (1977): In: Proceedings
of the 10th.CINP Congress, Quebec, Canada, July
1976, in press.

23.Mellet, L.B., and Woods, L.A. (1959): J.Pharmacol.
Exp.Ther., 125: 97-104.

24.Misra, A.L., Mulé, S.J., Bloch, R., and Vadlamani,
N.L. (1973): J.Pharmacol.Exp.Ther., 185: 287-299.

25.Mulé, S.J., Casella, G., and Clouet, D.H. (1974):
Res.Commun.Chem.Pathol.Pharmacol., 9: 55-77.

26.Mulé, S.J., Casella, G., and Clouet, D.H. (1975):
Psychopharmacologia, 44: 125-129.

27.Mulé, S.J., Clements, T.H., Layson, R.C., and
Haertzen, C.A. (1968): Arch.Int.Pharmacodyn.Ther.,
173: 201-212.

28.Mulé, S.J., and Gorodetzky, C.W. (1966):
J.Pharmacol.Exp.Ther., 154: 632-645.

29.Mulé, S.J., Redman, C.M., and Flesher, J.W. (1967):
J.Pharmacol.Exp.Ther., 157: 459-471.

30.Mulé, S.J., and Woods, L.A. (1962): J.Pharmacol.Exp.
Ther., 136: 232-241.

31.Mulé, S.J., Woods, L.A., and Mellett, L.B. (1962):
J.Pharmacol.Exp.Ther., 136: 242-249.

32.Pert, C.B., and Snyder, S.H. (1973): Science,179:

1011-1014.

33. Pert, C.B., and Snyder, S.H. (1975): Life Sci., 16: 1623-1634.

34. Richter, J.A., and Goldstein, A. (1970): Proc.Natl. Acad.Sci.USA, 66: 944-951.

35. Rickards, J.C., Boxer, G.E., and Smith, C.C. (1950): J.Pharmacol.Exp.Ther., 98: 380-391.

36. Siminoff, R., and Saunders, P.R. (1958): J.Pharmacol.Exp.Ther., 124: 252-254.

37. Sung, C.-Y., Way, E.L., and Scott, K.G. (1953): J.Pharmacol.Exp.Ther., 107: 12-23.

38. Szerb, J.C., and McCurdy, D.H. (1956): J.Pharmacol. Exp.Ther., 118: 446-450.

39. Van Praag, D., and Simon, E.J. (1966): Proc.Soc. Exp.Biol.Med., 122: 6-11.

40. Woods, L.A. (1954): J.Pharmacol.Exp.Ther., 112: 158-175.

41. Wuepper, K.D., and Woods, L.A. (1960): Fed.Proc., 19: 272.

42. Wuepper, K.D., Yeh, S.Y., and Woods, L.A. (1967): Proc.Soc.Exp.Biol.Med., 124: 1146-1150.

Factors Affecting the Action of Narcotics, edited by
M.L. Adler, L. Manara, and R. Samanin.
Raven Press, New York ©1978.

Metabolism of Opiates

Anand L. Misra

New York State Office of Drug Abuse Services
Research Laboratory
Brooklyn, New York , U.S.A.

INTRODUCTION

The duration and intensity of action of opiates in animals and man is chiefly limited by the extensive metabolism which these drugs undergo in the body.   In the last two decades, extensive work has been done on the sites of biotransformation of opiates and other drugs and the various physiological and environmental factors that affect their metabolism.   Concurrently,developments in analytical techniques and methodology, e.g. ultraviolet , fluorescence , infra-red , nuclear magnetic resonance spectro-photometry,gas chromatography-mass spectrometry,radioimmunoassay, radioisotope techniques,have progressively increased the potenti-ality for the determination of submicrogram quantities of drugs and metabolites in biofluids and tissues.   These developments have immensely contributed to an increase in our knowledge of pathways and mechanisms of biotransformation and various factors which control the level of opiates and their metabolites at receptor sites and thus to a better understanding of action of these drugs.

The objective of this review is to cover a general discussion of various aspects of the metabolism of opiates (Fig.1)and newer information on this subject (*).   Earlier literature on the biological disposition and metabolism of narcotic drugs cited in the reviews of Way and Adler (269), Mellett and Woods (168), Way (267), Mulé (195), Scrafani and Clouet (233), and Misra (171 , 172) has also been alluded to for the sake of continuity of discussion.

Metabolism of opiates in vivo represents a complex interplay among a variety of factors, including route of administration, absorption, degree of binding of drug to proteins, excretion and metabolism.

(*)Specific aspects of the metabolism of opiates are also discussed in this volume by Fishman and by Rance

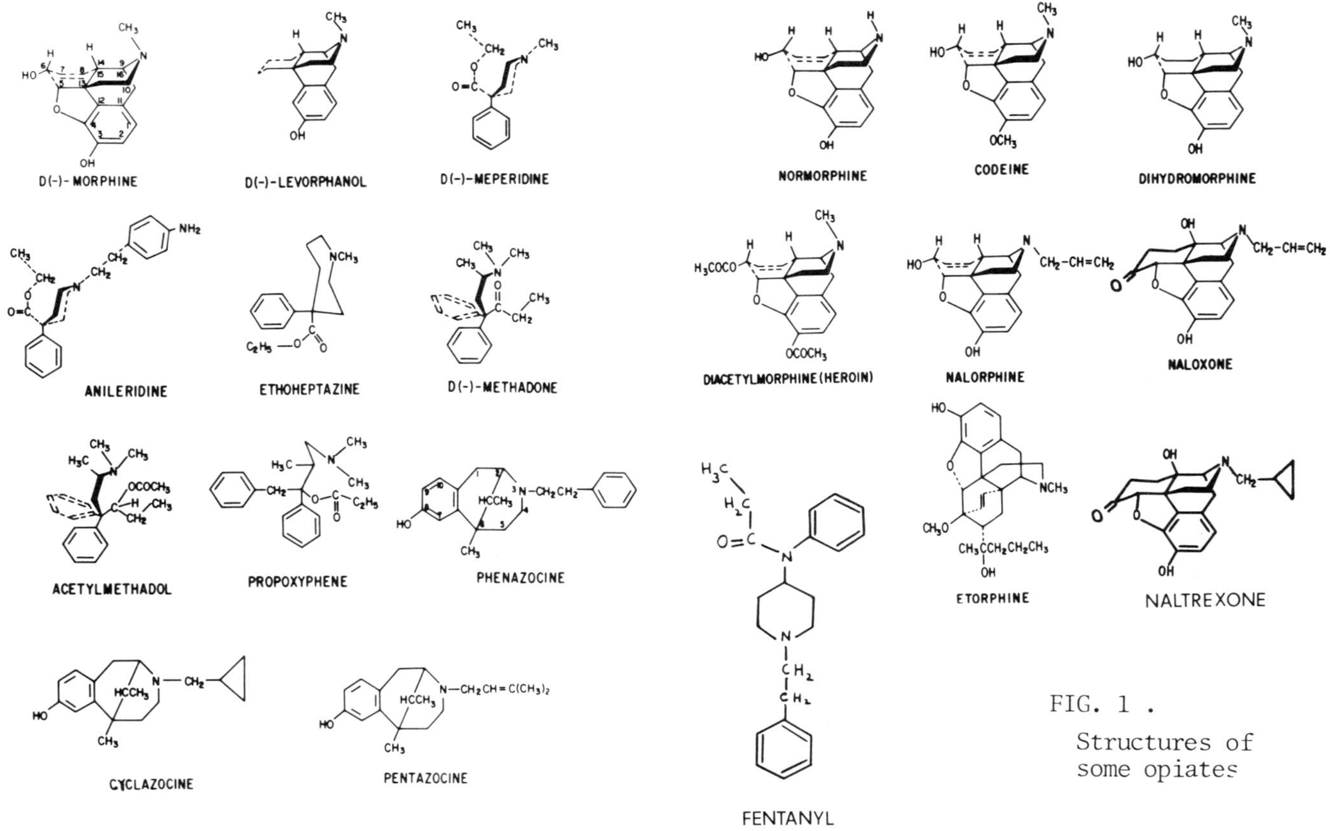

FIG. 1.
Structures of some opiates

Routes of Administration and Extent of Metabolism

This subject has recently been reviewed by Rowland (224) , Gibaldi and Feldman (105) and Gibaldi and Ferrier (106). The intravenous route gives a very rapid onset of action since the opiates reach the tissues in one circulation time (approximately 15 sec.). A sustained level of opiates in blood stream can be achieved by giving an intravenous infusion (72, 255). Opiates given by subcutaneous or intramuscular routes pass through the endothelium of the capillaries or lymphatic vessels before entering the systemic circulation and the area over which the solution spreads, the rate of capillary blood flow and diffusion determine the rate of entry into systemic circulation. By these routes, less than 30 percent of the dose of drug traverses the liver during the first passage in the body. Depot preparations of morphine (64, 111) obviate the need for repeated injections and give a prolonged action by slow release and a smoother control of opiate levels in blood. Pellets of morphine as sub- cutaneous implants (150) or morphine adsorbed on pellets of molecular sieves (123) have been used as sustained release preparations for rapid induction of tolerance to and physical dependence on opiate in experimental animals. A 75 mg morphine pellet s.c. implanted in rats gave sustained levels of 0.7 - 0.9 ug/ml from 5 - 96 hrs (29). The absorption of morphine from such a pellet continued for 6 days after implantation and decreased analgesia observed at later times was due to tolerance development and not to decreased absorption (211). Poly(lactic acid) composites and non-biodegradable polymers as subcutaneous implants have been utilized as long-acting delivery system for slow release of narcotic antagonists, naltrexone and naloxone , over a period of several weeks (3,92,153,232,299).

With intraperitoneal and oral routes, the opiate gains access to the peripheral circulation by hepatic portal system and in the event of extensive hepatic metabolism, only small amounts of drug appear in blood. With the oral route,factors such as solubility, crystalline form, particle size, rate of dissolution of solid dosage form, pH of the gastro-intestinal tract, rate of gastric emptying of contents into intestine, microbial flora and me- tabolising enzymes in gastro-intestinal tract determine the extent and rate of absorption (199, 224, 262). A large per- centage of dose of a drug after oral administration is metabolised during transport from gut into the systemic circulation. By sub- lingual or buccal administration, a drug enters the systemic circulation without passing through the portal circulation, thus avoiding the possibility of inactivation by the liver.

The gastric emptying of methadone appeared to be a rate - limiting step in its overall gastrointestinal absorption (265).

Burt and Beckett (52) observed that the percentage recovery of
pentazocine from human urine was greater after intravenous or
intramuscular injections than after oral route, despite complete
absorption of orally given drug. The greater amount of unchanged
drug after systemic administration may be the result of avoiding
the first passage through the liver occurring after absorption
into the portal circulation following oral administration. The
possibility of intestinal metabolism of pentazocine could also
contribute to observed differences in metabolism as functions of
the routes of administration (52). The toxicity of meperidine
was influenced by its rate of absorption,thus the administration
of meperidine by intramuscular route in the monkeys gave 2 : 1
ratio of meperidine and its metabolite normeperidine(with potent
convulsant activity)in plasma; with p.o. administration the
ratios of these compounds were reversed (76). For a comparison
of the analgesic potency of morphine and normorphine, these
opiates were administered to rats by three routes. After the
s.c. and i.p. injections of the same dose of these opiates, less
normorphine was found in rat brain 15 min. later, while after
i.v. injection the brain levels of two drugs were equal (129).In
a recent study on morphine metabolism in man (45), levels of free
morphine in plasma were significantly higher after s.c. and i.m.
injection than after intravenous injection and with the latter
route very rapid distribution, metabolism and excretion occurred.
Significant levels of free morphine were not observed in plasma
or urine with p.o. administration due to rapid conjugation in
gastrointestinal tract. N-demethylation of morphine was greater
after p.o. than after parenteral administration.Although routes
of administration altered the plasma levels of morphine,the
plasma t $\frac{1}{2}$ (2.1-2.6 hr) was not changed.Dobbs et al.(79) found
that the analgesic potencies of etorphine as measured by minimal
analgesic dose were 2 µg/kg i.v., 2.5 µg/kg i.m. and 5-10 µg/kg
sublingually. The levels of methadone in plasma and brain of
rats after 10 mg/kg subcutaneous injection were approximately
15-25 times those after the same dose by oral administration (183)
The average apparent availability of propoxyphene in man was only
18% as determined by comparing the total areas under the plasma
level-time curves of unmetabolised drug after oral and i.v. administration, despite the fact that the urinary recoveries after
p.o. administration suggested that the drug was well absorbed
(163,280).
    Intracisternal,intracerebral and intraventricular routes which
largely but not entirely obviate distribution differences between
the groups of opiates, have been used for localization of opiates
into brain particulate fractions (60,124,148) and for administration of polar compounds, e.g. N-methyl morphine and morphine-
2, 3-quinone which are not able to cross the blood-brain barrier
(96,190). Relative potencies of opiates, e.g. codeine and its
metabolites morphine and norcodeine,determined by the introduction of such drugs systemically and intraventricularly,provided
evidence that the pharmacological effects of codeine are mediated

primarily through these metabolites (6). Microinjections of
morphine in different areas of primate brain have been used for
the localization of anti-nociceptive action of morphine (213).
Administration of opiates in drinking water (139,154,165,200)and
intravenous self-administration of opiates in rodents and monkeys
(77,230,272) have been used by several groups of workers for the
induction of physical dependence on opiates .

Absorption of Opiates

The subject of absorption of drugs has been reviewed by
Schanker (228), Brodie (42) and Levine and Pelikan (145).   The
principal factors which determined the rate of absorption of
opiates are the extent of ionization (pKa), lipid-solubility and
molecular size.   These drugs diffuse across the lipoidal   biological   membranes as lipid soluble,nonionized molecules and the
rates of transfer are generally related to their lipid-water

TABLE 1 . Dissociation constants (pKa) and 1-octanol/water drug
distribution coefficients (P) of narcotic drugs [a]

Compound	pKa (37°C) [b]	P(pH 7.40) [c]
α-Acetyl methadol hydrochloride	8.61	1185.25
Codeine phosphate	8.10	2.28
Cyclazocine	9.38	21.54
Levallorphan tartrate	8.43	220.99
Levorphanol tartrate	9.37	13.68
Meperidine hydrochloride	8.50	38.82
Methadone hydrochloride	9.26	116.33
Morphine sulfate	7.93, 9.63	1.42
Nalorphine hydrochloride	7.59	28.16
Naloxone hydrochloride	7.82	33.55
Naltrexone hydrochloride	8.13	13.08
Oxymorphone hydrochloride	8.17, 9.54	0.98
Pentazocine	9.16	110.76

[a] Data from Kaufmann, et al.   (138)

[b] The relative proportions of ionised and unionised forms of
basic drugs are calculated from Henderson-Hasselbach equation:

$$pK_a = pH + \log \frac{(ionised)}{(unionised\ )}$$

[c] Drug distribution coefficient $P = \dfrac{(free\ base)lipid}{(free\ base\ +\ acid\ salt)\ aqueous}$

partition coefficients. The biological membranes are relatively
impermeable to the ionised species of these drugs. Active transport is not involved in disposition of these drugs but plays an
important role in excretion processes. The pK_a at 37°C and
distribution coefficients of some opiates in 1-octanol-water at
pH 7.4 are given in Table 1.

Distribution Aspects

After absorption, the opiates in blood stream diffuse rapidly
throughout the extracellular fluid and their entry into the intra
cellular fluid depends on their ability to cross lipid-like biological membranes e.g. blood-cerebrospinal fluid or blood-brain
barrier. The extent of transfer of opiates into the tissues
depends largely on the extent of binding of these drugs on either
side of the membrane barrier, the dissociation constant, pK_a
(which range between 7.6-9.6 for most opiates), lipid-solubility
and pH difference across the barriers. The vascularity of the
particular tissue also determines the tissue-plasma ratio attained
by these drugs. Rapidly perfused tissues like kidney,liver,lung,
brain attain higher values,muscle and skin intermediate values
and fat and skeleton,the poorly perfused tissues take a much
longer time for equilibration .

Penetration of Opiates Through the Blood-brain and Blood-cerebro-spinal Fluid Barriers (*)

The blood-brain barrier acts like a lipid membrane which is
preferentially permeable to nonionised lipid soluble opiates.The
importance of lipid solubility for permeation of opiates into the
brain has been outlined by Herz and Teschemacher (116). The rate
of entry of opiates through the blood-brain barrier also depends
on pK_a value, drug binding and pH difference on either side of
the barrier. The extra neuronal binding of opiates is extremely
important in regard to the amount which is available for passage
into the CSF. The pressure gradient from the CSF to the blood
capillaries and active transport of opiates by choroid plexus
favour the removal of these drugs from the CSF into plasma.
Details on permeation of narcotic drugs into brain and exit there
from have recently been discussed in a review by Misra (172).

(*)
    For a detailed discussion of this subject see the
    contribution by Oldendorf in this volume.

Binding of Opiates to Plasma and Tissue Proteins

Binding of drugs to plasma and tissue proteins has recently been reviewed by Mayer and Guttman (158) and Gillette (108,109). Reversible binding of opiates to plasma proteins involves ionic, hydrogen and van der Waals forces and is of immense pharmacologic significance. Although albumin is the major plasma protein which binds opiates, these drugs may also be bound to antibodies in the γ-globulin fraction. Treatment of rabbits e.g. with morphine covalently bound to serum albumin, has been shown by Spector and Parker (242) and Spector (241) to evoke the formation of antibodies that bind morphine and its analogues. The labile complexes of opiates with albumin are not antigenic. Binding of opiates to plasma proteins influences the distribution of these drugs to their site of action and retards their rate of movement. Extensive binding of methadone to plasma proteins (81,174,183) can also act as a reservoir to make this drug available over a long period of time. A correlation has been observed between binding of opiate drugs to plasma proteins and their lipid-solubility. Binding increased with increase in lipid-solubility, suggesting a hydrophobic interaction between narcotic drugs and plasma proteins (119). Data on the plasma protein binding of some narcotic drugs are given in Table 2.

TABLE 2. Binding of some opiates with plasma proteins _in vitro_

Drugs	Mean percentage of drug bound	References
Dihydromorphine	14	119
Morphine	34 – 37.5; 23	208, 119
Codeine	25	17
Naltrexone	21 – 29	176
Heroin	20 – 39	63
Pethidine	40	51
Levorphanol	50	236
Pentazocine	56 – 66	83
Nalorphine	57.3	176
Naloxone	68.3	187
Thebaine	66.7	186
Methadone	83.7-87.3	207
1-α-Acetylmethadol	76.2-82.2	Misra, unpublished
Etorphine	88	119
Fentanyl	70	119

Accumulation and longer retention of morphine (282), fentanyl (117), levorphanol (236), pentazocine (90), methadone (174,183, 221,251) and 1-α-acetylmethadol (162,252 and Misra, _et al._,

unpublished observations) in vivo in the lung of experimental
animals, implies binding with some structural component of this
tissue. The localization, metabolism and effects of other drugs
in lung has been reviewed by Brown (44). Accumulation and
persistence of certain narcotic drugs like morphine and methadone
and active metabolites of l- α-acetyl methadol in brain (179,
180 and Misra, et al. , unpublished observations), similarly
implies an interaction of these drugs with some specific anatomic
structure in the central nervous system or a metabolic conversion
to a nonpermeable form of the parent drug. The retention of some
drugs,e.g.pentazocine (90) and l-α-acetyl methadol (162) and
Misra, et al.,unpublished observations),in stomach and gastro-
intestinal tract long after the disappearance from other organs,
could possibly be due to the binding of such drugs with acidic
mucopolysaccharides present in mucosal wall. Accumulation of
certain drugs can also occur in skin, nucleoproteins, fat of
adipose tissue (which constitutes approximately 20% of the body
weight), melanin granules in eyes, phospholipids in intracellular organelles and plasma membranes.
    Extensive binding of drugs to proteins results in reduction
of their rates of metabolism and excretion and such binding
invariably increases the half-life of drugs. Significantly
higher amount of binding of morphine to 7S-γ-globulin in sera
of heroin addicts as compared to normal subjects could account
for the very slow phase of morphine excretion in addicts (225).
Berkowitz , et al. (28) have shown that the presence of
circulating antibodies which can sequester opiates, can have a
marked effect on their disposition.
    Species differences, genetic factors, the amount of protein
and pH, all play a role in the binding of drugs. Presence of
other drugs used in multi- drug therapy may also modify or alter
the binding of opiates by competition for binding sites. Sulfa-
pyridine (1.6 g/kg) administered to morphine-pretreated mice
long after morphine effect had worn off, produced analgesia 6
days after, by probable reversal of morphine binding to tissue
sites in brain (57). It is important to remember that tissue
binding and active transport have certain characteristics in
common, e.g. saturability and competition among the analogues of
the drug.

Excretion of Opiates

    The mechanisms of drug absorption and excretion (273) and
extra-renal excretion of drugs (244) have recently been reviewed.
The excretion of several narcotic drugs has been discussed in
earlier reviews by Way and Adler (269), Way (267) and Misra(171).
Renal and biliary excretion are prime pathways for several
opiates. The significance of pH-dependent excretion for these
drugs depends on four factors: the pK_a , the lipid-solubility,
the degree of binding and the extent of excretion of unchanged
drug. Promoting the ionization with acidifying agents(NH_4Cl)

could accelerate the excretion of opiates by reducing the proportion of free base available for tubular resorption.   Thus total
excretion of meperidine in man after NH_4Cl administration was
50% of the dose and less than 5% of dose after $NaHCO_3$ ingestion
(13). Excretion of other opiates, e.g. ethoheptazine,methadone
(22,25), levorphanol (41) has also been shown to be sensitive to
such pH changes. The primary mechanism of renal excretion of
morphine (19,266) and dihydromorphine (121) was by glomerular
filtration and tubular secretion respectively. Mammary excretion
(morphine), salivary excretion (pethidine and naltrexone) and
excretion through the sweat for morphine and methadone (115) ,
involve passive non-ionic diffusion of opiates into these secre-
tions. These and pulmonary excretion are minor routes for elimination of opiates. Species differences have been observed in the
pulmonary excretion of (^{14}C) levorphanol: the monkey, rat and
dog eliminated 20,5 and 1.5% of thedose respectively as $^{14}CO_2$
in the expired air (284).

Biliary Excretion

Excretion in bile is a relatively minor route for elimination
of unchanged opiates, but a major one for the polar glucuronide
conjugated metabolites which are excreted by a process of active
transport. It is an important pathway for morphine (152,282),
cyclazocine (196), methadone (21,85,174,175,270), 1 - α-acetyl
methadol (162 and Misra , et al. ,unpublished observations) ,
pentazocine (91) and etorphine (80). Biliary excretion of
morphine-3-glucuronide and morphine-3-sulfate proceeded along
different pathways in the rat (215). Chronic methadone treatment
stimulated the bile flow in the rat by some unknown mechanism
resulting in increased (58% of the dose in 4 hr and 84% of dose
in 24 hr) biliary excretion of methadone metabolites (20). Biliary
excretion is generally highest in the rat and dog.   In the rats,
the body temperature had a marked effect on the flow of bile and
as the rats lack gall bladder, the liberation of drugs from bile
into the gastro-intestinal contents is continuous in this species.
Detailed aspects of biliary excretion of drugs and species
differences in this connection have been reviewed by Abou-El-
Makarem, et al. (2). The cycle of biliary excretion of morphine
conjugates, intestinal reabsorption of morphine generated by the
hydrolysis of polar conjugate by hydrolytic enzymes in gut and
gastro-intestinal flora and re-excretion, is known as entero –
hepatic circulation and such a cycle can have a marked effect on
the persistence of such opiates in the body. The subject of
enterohepatic circulation has been covered in excellent reviews
(239,278).

Metabolism of Opiates

The majority of opiates undergo one or more metabolic conversion in the body. A feature characteristic of all these bio-

transformations is that the metabolic products are usually more polar than the parent drug, so that these cannot be readily re-sorbed through lipoidal biological membranes and can readily be eliminated by renal or biliary excretion. Although many me-tabolites are pharmacologically less active than the parent opiate, drug metabolism does not inevitably lead to a loss of pharmacological activity. The bioconversion of codeine to mor-phine, morphine to morphine-6-glucuronide, 1-α-acetyl methadol to acetyl normethadol and acetyl bisnormethadol,are some examples of formation of metabolites which have more pharmacological ac-tivity than the parent compound. The case of morphine-6-glucuro-nide is an unusual one (300) because this compound,although a minor metabolite of morphine in several species including man , was 45 times more potent as an analgesic compared to morphine after intracerebral injection and 3 - 4 times more potent after s.c. injection in mice (234). It produced prolonged analgesia in experimental animals.

Williams (277) , Gillette (107), Parke (210), Mellett (166)and Mandel (151) have presented a thorough discussion of individual mechanisms of biotransformation of various classes of drugs and physiological and environmental factors that influence these mechanisms. A convenient way of looking at the problem of drug metabolism is to think of it as occurring in two phases. Phase I involving oxidative, reductive and hydrolytic processes, which lead either to a decrease or increase in biological activity of the compound and Phase II synthetic processes involving conju-gations of drugs and metabolites with endogenous substrates such as glucuronic, sulfuric and acetic acids. These steps lead to the termination of the pharmacological activity of the parent drug. For conjugations to occur, there must be a group in the opiate molecule which can react with the conjugating agent.Heroin, meperidine, anileridine, methadone and 1-α-acetyl methadol , do not possess such a group and the purpose of Phase I reactions is to introduce such a group into these molecules. Both Phase I and II reactions usually lead to polar molecules and in some cases (meperidine to meperidinic acid) Phase I reaction itself produces a sufficiently polar metabolite for renal excretion. Very often, some drugs, e.g. thebaine (186), naltrexone (176) are subjected to several competing pathways simultaneously and the relative rates of various interactions determine the extent of formation of different metabolites. Although it is not yet possible to predict the pathways of opiate metabolism in different species, the major routes of metabolism can be anticipated .

Sites of Biotransformation of Opiates

The metabolic transformations of most drugs are catalyzed by enzymes that occur in cells of a wide variety of tissues including liver, small intestine, kidney,lung, brain, adrenal cortex , placenta, skin, testes and plasma (107,210). Of these, the liver is the most important organ for drug biotransformations. Phase I

oxidative metabolism of opiates is mediated by enzymes located
in the microsomal fraction of the mammalian liver and the enzyme
activity in this fraction is associated with the smooth endoplasmic reticulum,which has higher oxidation activity as compared
to the rough surfaced variety.The separation of these reticulums
can be achieved by sucrose density gradient centrifugation. The
microsomal fraction contains a hemoprotein or a family of closely
related hemoproteins,i.e.cytochromes P-450,which act as terminal
oxidase for a variety of oxidative biotransformations undergone
by opiates. Cytochrome P-450 is also found in the mitochondrial
fraction of the adrenal cortex. In vitro oxidation of opiates
can occur in a system containing liver microsomes,NADPH,molecular
oxygen and Mg^{2+} and this requirement of NADPH and molecular
oxygen categorizes this system as a mixed function oxidase.

$$NADPH + O_2 + \text{opiate substrate} + H^+ \longrightarrow NADP^+ + \text{oxidised opiate} + H_2O$$

The key enzymes of the mixed function oxidase are NADPH-cytochrome C-reductase, the flavin enzyme involved in the oxidation
of NADPH-Cytochrome P-450.

Other metabolic transformations, e.g. oxidation of alcoholic
group of morphine, reduction of keto group of methadone,naloxone
and naltrexone, hydrolysis of heroin, meperidine, anileridine,
1-α-acetyl methadol , α-prodine, etc. , are catalysed by non-
microsomal enzymes located in the mitochondria or the soluble
fraction of liver homogenates and in the plasma. The nature of
enzymes responsible for the reduction of 7,8-double bond in
morphine to dihydromorphinone are not known. A unique characteristic of these drug metabolising enzymes is that their specificity is generally directed towards certain functional groups attached
to the opiates rather than to their molecular conformation. Qualitative and quantitative differences in the metabolism of opiates
in different species arise due to the presence or absence of these
enzymes and variations in their amount .

Phase I   Oxidative Reactions

N-Dealkylation of opiates

The details of N-dealkylation of various drugs have been presented in a review by McMahon (161). The majority of opiates
which are tertiary amines undergo oxidative N-dealkylation of
N-methyl (morphine, codeine, heroin, dihydromorphine, thebaine ,
etc.) , N-ethyl (ethyl morphine), N-phenethyl (phenazocine), N-
allyl (nalorphine, naloxone,levallorphan), N-cyclopropyl methyl
(cyclazocine, naltrexone) groups to the corresponding norcompounds
(171,267,269).   A correlation was observed between lipid solubility and the rate of N-demethylation of dl-propoxyphene by an
in vitro liver microsomal enzyme system (160).   In the case of
1-α-acetyl methadol and propoxyphene, the tertiary amine was
N-demethylated more rapidly than the secondary amine metabolites

acetyl normethadol and norpropoxyphene (162,164).Narcotic antagonists e.g. nalorphine, naloxone, naltrexone were N-demethylated
somewhat faster than the agonists(16,176,187).The pharmacologically active levo-isomers of opiates,e.g. levorphanol, methadone,
were N-demethylated faster than the inactive isomers in vitro(15,
86) and in vivo (181,188). Oxidative N-dealkylation reactions
do not occur in vitro with whole homogenates of the liver, due
to the presence of thermolabile inhibitory factors in nuclei and
mitochondria.

Marked species differences in in vitro N-dealkylation of ethyl
morphine have been observed by Davies,et al. (75) by liver microsomal enzymes of mouse, rat, guinea pig and rabbit, the mouse
being the most and the rabbit the least active. Male rats were
more effective than females in N-dealkylation. Direct evidence
for N-demethylation of meperidine in vivo in the newborn on the
first day, has been observed by O'Donoghue (204) and normeperidine
and meperidinic acid were detected as urinary metabolites of
meperidine.

N-Dealkylation of opiates, e.g. morphine, codeine,nalorphine
and meperidine has also been shown to occur in the central
nervous system of rats but the process is comparatively much less
active than that in the liver (86,169).

Chronic treatment of rats with morphine, leads to a profound
reduction in the ability of liver microsomal enzymes to N-dealkyl-
ate morphine in vitro (15,61). This decrease has not been
observed in other species (53,137). Studies in vivo in other
animals and man showed no decrease in N-demethylation of morphine
and in some species an increased ability to demethylate narcotic
drugs, morphine and methadone has been observed (7,183). Administration of inducer drugs phenobarbital or chlorpromazine to rats,
resulted in an increase in the activity of microsomal enzymes
catalyzing the N-demethylation of morphine (231),meperidine (59),
dihydromorphine and codeine (130) and methadone (9).

O-Dealkylation

Codeine, thebaine, dextromethorphan are O-dealkylated to
corresponding phenolic compounds (135,185,186,279,295) by liver
microsomal enzymes. Takemori and Mannering (254) found that in
the case of codeine having both O-methyl and N-methyl groups in
the same molecule, N-demethylation was considerably greater than
the sum of that obtained by dealkylation of compounds having
only O-methyl or N-methyl groups.

Side chain oxidation

The oxidation of the side chain with keto group of methadone
to the corresponding carboxylic acid (245) and the methyl group
of dimethylallyl side chain of pentazocine to the corresponding
cis and trans alcohols (216), are catalyzed by enzymes in the
soluble fraction of the mammalian liver. The trans isomer was

approximately 5 - 10 times as much as cis in the mouse; in the rat 2 - 3 times more cis was formed than trans alcohol and the monkey gave predominantly the trans acid.

N-Oxidation

N-Oxidation of morphine (189,281), methadone (27,174) and meperidine (193) are probably brought about by a special amine oxidase, a flavoprotein distinct from NADPH-cytochrome C-reductase and cytochrome P-450 does not appear to be involved in this process. N-Oxide formation is an alternate pathway rather than an intermediate step in the oxidative N-dealkylation of opiates (161). The biotransformation of morphine-N-oxide to normorphine in vivo has been demonstrated by Misra and Mitchell (178).

Hydroxylation of opiates

Details on the nature of hydroxylation reaction and sites of biotransformation of a variety of compounds have been discussed by Gillette (107). The enzymes involved in the hydroxylation of opiates and other drugs are different from those that carry out the hydroxylation of phenylalanine,tyrosine and tryptophane. Several microsomal hydroxylases exist in different species and the nature of the hydroxylating intermediate is probably a super-oxide. Considerable species variation has been observed in hydroxylation reactions and it is usually a minor route in the monkey. Evidence for the oxidation of levallorphan at the 6 position (36), morphine at the 2 position (74,189), ethoheptazine (264) and meperidine in the para position of the aromatic ring (146), naltrexone and naloxone in the 2 position (176,257) and methadone (246), propoxyphene (164) and 1 -α-acetyl methadol in the aromatic ring (191) has been presented recently. Human neonate from day 1 has active enzyme systems for carrying out hydroxylation reactions characteristic of cytochrome P-450 system.

Hydrolysis of esters

Heroin, pethidine, α -prodine, anileridine, 1-α-acetyl methadol and propoxyphene are hydrolyzed by esterases present in blood plasma or liver, usually in the soluble fraction of the cell (269). 6-Monoacetyl morphine and 1-α-acetyl methadol are quite stable in the body for several hours. Homogenates of kidney and to a lesser extent brain also hydrolyse heroin. Species differences exist in hydrolysis reactions and active esterase is also present in neonatal tissues.

Oxidation of alcoholic group and reduction of double bond

Morphine has recently been shown to be biotransformed to a small extent in rat and other species but not in man, to dihydro-morphinone which is principally eliminated as a glucuronide conjugate (141,291). This biotransformation is not affected by chronic administration of morphine.

Reduction of keto group to an alcohol

This has been observed to be an important metabolic pathway in the case of methadone (174,183,247), naloxone (102,187,274) and naltrexone (56,65,103,176). A substantial species variation has been observed in the formation of 6α and 6β -epimeric alcohols in the case of naloxone and naltrexone (222).The chicken produced mainly the 6α -isomer and the rabbit and guinea pig the 6β -isomer (66).

Phase II Reactions

Glucuronide conjugation of opiates

This is one of the most common routes for the biotransformation of opiates having phenolic, alcoholic and carboxylic groups because of the availability of glucose in biological systems in most mammalian species except the cat and chicken. This route accounts for a major share of metabolism of opiates and leads to highly polar water-soluble glucuronides which are not resorbed by kidney tubules and are readily excreted. These are formed enzymatically by the transfer of glucuronic acid from uridine diphosphate D-glucosiduronic acid (UDPGA) to the opiates by glucuronyl transferases found in microsomes of liver and other tissues. UDPGA is synthesized in the soluble fraction of the liver cell. The exact substrate specificity of mammalian glucuronyl transferases is not clear (82). The glucuronyl transferases lack the ability to form N-glucuronides of amines. Excretion of glucuronides of opiates occurs by glomerular filtration,tubular secretion and elimination via bile for morphine. In general, glucuronide conjugation abolishes the pharmacologic activity of the opiate. A notable exception is morphine-6-glucuronide observed as a minor metabolite in rabbits,guinea pigs , mice,man and dog (192,301),which was several times more potent than morphine as an analgesic after intracerebral and systemic administration and had prolonged analgesic activity.Its pharmacological activity was not mediated by its conversion to morphine (300).The higher amount of glucuronide formation in male rats as compared to the females is mediated by testosterone and administration of estradiol to male rats reduces the amount of glucuronide formation. These observations do not apply to man. In addition to liver, kidney, gastro-intestinal tract and placenta also have the capacity to glucuronidate compounds. Glucuronide conjugation of morphine in rat intestinal loop (132), of etorphine and buprenorphine in intact gut wall (219) and by intestinal mucosa (114) has recently been described. Lipophilicity may be a determining factor with regard to the efficiency of gut UDP-glucuronyl transferase activity .

Cats can synthesize UDPGA but lack glucuronyl transferases used in conjugation reactions. Gunn strain of Wistar rats which is genetically incapable of forming glucuronide conjugates,lacks O-glucuronyl transferase activity even though the UDPGA levels are normal.

Short-term treatment of rats with pargylin, induced the glucuronyl transferase activity (294) and administration of inducer drugs such as phenobarbital to mother before delivery or to newborn,led to enhanced rate of formation of glucuronyl transferase. The levels of glucuronyl transferase and its coenzyme UDPGA are remarkably low in newborn of most species with the exception of the rat (82). Decreased liver function in old age may impair conjugation of opiates resulting in increased sensitivity to these drugs.

Sulfate conjugation of opiates

The sulfate conjugation of opiates having phenolic or alcoholic groups,occurs in the soluble fraction of the liver cell and also in the kidney and intestine by several sulfotransferases.   3'-phosphoadenosine-5'-phosphosulfate (PAPS) acts as a source of active sulfate.

R-OH + 3' - phosphoadenosine-5'-phosphosulfate $\longrightarrow$ R-OSO$_3$H + 3-phospho-adenosine-5' phosphate

Sulfate conjugation of opiates morphine (102,292) and nalorphine (297) and of naloxone (203) is a prime pathway in cat and chicken. Repeated administration of opiate in these species could lead to a depletion of the total pool of sulfate, making this pathway a zero order reaction. In man , sulfate conjugation is a minor pathway for morphine and 5 - 10% of the dose is eliminated as morphine-3-sulfate (288). Morphine-6- sulfate, although not a metabolite of morphine,possessed more and prolonged analgesic activity than morphine (194). Intestinal flora and placenta possess sulfatases which can cleave these conjugates to the corresponding opiate for resorption in intestine. Sulfate conjugation for endogenous substances (steroids)can also occur in adrenals, testes,ovaries and human fetal liver.

N- and O-methylation

N-methylation is a minor metabolic pathway for normorphine (58). S-Adenosylmethionine serves as a methyl donor for this biotransformation. Methyl transferase enzymes, e.g. catechol O-methyl transferase (COMT) are found in the soluble supernatant fraction of rat liver,in erythrocytes and other mammalian tissues such as brain. Another example of N-methylation is the conversion of methadone to N-methyl methadone in vitro (229). Gunn rats with an inherited deficiency of glucuronyl transferase , reportedly converted morphine to codeine (87). Evidence has also been presented (39,40) for the biotransformation of morphine to codeine and norcodeine, in addicts who had impaired hepatic function and disturbances of glucuronide conjugation pathway. Yeh (289),however, did not observe such a conversion in man.Tentative evidence has also been obtained for the formation of 3-methoxy-2-hydroxy naltrexol as a metabolite of naltrexone in man (257) and in the rat (176).

Acetylation

Acetylation is an important pathway for the metabolism of anileridine (218) and 1-α-methadol (247). The enzymes responsible for acetylation are located in the soluble fraction of the liver, kidney, spleen and gastro-intestinal mucosal cells of man, rat and rabbit and mainly involve a reaction with aliphatic or aromatic amino or hydroxy groups. Acetylation reactions also occur in the neonates. Genetic factors play an important role in controlling the levels of hepatic N-acetyl transferases in man.

Stereochemical Factors in Drug Metabolism

Stereochemical factors play an important role in metabolism of narcotic drugs which exist as two or more optically active enantiomorphs. Axelrod (15) and Elison, et al. (88) showed that the pharmacologically active levo isomers were demethylated faster in vitro by liver microsomal preparations as compared to dextro isomers.

TABLE 3. Comparative half-lives of levo and dextro methadone 1-^{3}H in rat brain and plasma and brain to plasma ratios after a 10 mg/kg (free base) dose by s.c. injection [a]

	Brain to plasma ratios at different times (hr)						Half-life (hr)	
	0.5	1	2	6	12	24	Brain	Plasma
Levo methadone	2.2	3.2	1.8	1.3	1.6	1.5	2.4	3.7
Dextromethadone	6.1	5.0	4.1	2.6	3.8	5.8	1.2	1.5

[a]Data from Misra, et al. (181,183).

Takemori and Mannering (254) did not observe such differences. Similarly, no differences in in vitro N-demethylation have been observed for enantiomorphs of prodine (1). The $t_{\frac{1}{2}}$ of pentazocine isomers in brain and plasma did not significantly differ in the rat (31). Our studies on the metabolism of levo and dextro

methadone in vivo in the rat (181) showed significant differences
in $t_\frac{1}{2}$ of l- and d-isomer in brain (2.4, 1.2 hr) and plasma (3.7,
1.5 hr) (Table 3).   The levo isomer was excreted in much higher
amounts (26.1% of the dose) as compared to the dextro isomer
(15.7% of the dose).   In addition, the formation of an apparently
active metabolite in brain was observed with l-isomer but not
with d-isomer and the brain to plasma ratios of dextro isomer
were consistently higher than those for the levo isomer. Some of
the discrepancies in in vitro and in vivo work on methadone
isomers could possibly arise due to a further metabolism of N-
dealkylated metabolites.   Our studies (188) on comparative
metabolism of levorphanol and dextrorphan in the rat, showed
significant differences in plasma levels of the two isomers,which
were consistently higher for the l-isomer as compared to the
d- isomer. Dextrorphan attained higher levels than l-isomer
initially in brain (0.5 and 1 hr), but disappeared much more rapidly from the CNS at subsequent times. Brain to plasma ratios
for the d-isomer were consistently higher than those of levorphanol up to 4 hr and $t_\frac{1}{2}$ of l and d isomers in rat brain were
2.1 and 1.2 hr and that in plasma 1.2 and 0.6 hr respectively
(Table 4). These differences in $t_\frac{1}{2}$ suggested differential rates

TABLE 4 . Comparative half-lives of (^{3}H)levorphanol and (N-Me-^{14}
C) dextrorphan in rat brain and plasma and brain to plasma ratios
after a 5 mg/kg (free base) dose by s.c. injection in male Wistar
rats [a].

	Brain to plasma ratios at different times (hr)					Half-life (hr)	
	0.5	1	2	4	6	Brain	Plasma
Levorphanol	0.4	1.1	1.2	2.8	2.6	2.1	1.2
Dextrorphan	2.4	3.9	5.4	3.8	3.0	1.2	0.6

[a]
   Data from Misra,et al. (188) .

of metabolism for the 2 isomers. Significant differences were
also observed in rates of elimination of 2 isomers due to a
faster metabolism of the d-isomer.Comparatively higher N-dealkylation for the l-isomer in vivo agreed with previous in vitro
findings of Axelrod (15).   There were,however,no significant
differences in plasma protein binding of the 2 isomers. Slower
biotransformation of the l-isomer accounted for its longer lasting
effects. The possibility exists that stereoselective differences
in metabolism of such enantiomorphs could be due to retarded

absorption or greater active secretion of one of the isomers into the gastro-enteric tract. These differences in distribution and metabolism,however, cannot account for the large potency ratios for these enantiomorphs,which are primarily related to the stereo-selective events at the receptor sites in the CNS (248). The influence of stereochemical factors on drug disposition has recently been reviewed by Jenner and Testa (128).

Effect of Age,Species,Strain,Sex,Hormonal Factors and Dose on Opiate Metabolism

Age is generally regarded as an experimental variable only when some of the experimental animals are immature,but recent work (227)has shown that age-related changes in responses of rats to morphine continued to occur after the animals have matured,the older animals (10 months old)being more sensitive than the younger ones(3 months old)and it was speculated that alterations in drug distribution,metabolism,elimination and target organ sensitivity may be involved in such differences in sensitivity to morphine.The disposition of morphine was actually shown to be altered in older rats and serum and brain levels of intravenously injected morphine were markedly higher in 20 month old rats as compared to 2 month old rats(29).Elderly patients over 50 years of age were also particularly sensitive to i.v. injected morphine and the serum levels in these patients were higher than those in younger patients.Age also influenced the rate of development of tolerance to morphine in the rat (202)and younger animals developed tolerance to morphine more readily than the older animals.Plasma levels of meperidine after intramuscular or intravenous injection in patients over 70 years of age,were about twice those in patients under 30 years and dosage of mepe-ridine in elderly patients has to be reduced because of higher sensitivity to respiratory depressant effects of this drug. Increasing age was also associated with increasing fraction of unbound meperidine in plasma (157). Age and exposure factors in drug metabolism have recently been reviewed by Hänninen(113).

The rate of metabolism and metabolic pathways of opiates also depend on the dose and the species. A 2 mg/kg s.c.injection of normorphine to monkeys and dogs resulted in higher blood levels of free and conjugated normorphine in a shorter time in the monkeys and in different patterns of urinary excretion of nor-morphine (177). The level of physical activity in the monkeys during the experimental period also played a role in metabolism and monkeys in restraining chair metabolized less of normorphine than unrestrained monkeys. N-Demethylation of [^{14}C] morphine was comparatively much more in the monkey as compared to the dog (167).Species-dependent differences in the identity of metaboli-tes of morphine have previously been discussed.Distinct diffe-rences in pharmacodynamics of propoxyphene in rat,dog and monkey have been observed by Sullivan,et al.(250)and plasma t$\frac{1}{2}$ of pro-poxyphene in rat and dog was 3.3 hr and in the monkey 7.2 hr; that of its metabolite norpropoxyphene in rat,dog and monkey 2.2,

14 and 15 hr respectively.Considerable species differences have been observed in the metabolism of codeine in dog,rabbit and cat (298).Dog converted little or no codeine to morphine and conjugation with glucuronic acid at the 6-position was the major pathway in the dog;in cats,N-demethylation was a major pathway, with little conjugation of codeine and no O-demethylation; in rabbits,both N- and O-demethylation occurred along with conjuga- tion at 3- and 6-hydroxy groups.Species differences in metabolism of several other drugs have been reviewed by Flynn,et al. (95).

Differences in rates of N-demethylation of ethyl morphine by liver microsomal preparations from male and female rats of 4 strains at two ages, have been described by Furner,et al. (104). Liver microsomal preparation from mature female rats, had less N-demethylating activity than those from male rats (15) for morphine, methadone and meperidine. Sex-related differences in metabolism of other drugs have been reviewed by Kato (136) and Sladek,et al. (237).

Recent work of Abrams and Elliott (4) has shown that,in spite of the abnormality of glucuronyl transferase activity in Gunn strain of Wistar rats, urinary excretion of morphine glucuronide and hepatic microsomal conjugation of morphine were not significantly different in the 2 groups of rats.

The size of experimental animals also gives rise to quantitative differences in drug excretion and metabolism and in general with some exceptions, excretion and metabolism of opiates occur more rapidly in smaller animals, which have a relatively larger surface area relative to body weight, than larger animals. Because of higher cardiac output per unit of body surface area, livers of smaller animals receive more blood and can metabolize more drug per unit time even if there are no differences in the action of metabolizing enzymes in certain animals. Meperidine was me- tabolized in man at a rate of 17% per hour, in dog 70% per hour and in rat and mouse at even higher rates (49). The use of body surface area as a criterion for inter and intra-species comparison derives support from the fact that a direct relationship exists between blood volume and body surface area in animals such as rabbit, guinea pig and mice and the ratio of kidney weight to body surface area is also identical for various species. The relationship between various animal species and man are more direct on the basis of mg of drug per square meter of body surface area . The equivalent surface area dosage conversion factors (98) are given in Table 5, and the representative surface area to weight ratios for various species are given in Table 6. The body surface area were estimated by the formula:

$$\frac{K \times W^{2/3}}{10^4}$$

where K is a value characteristic of the species and individual size and W is the body weight in grams. The conversion factors K_m were obtained by the formula:

316 OPIATE METABOLISM

TABLE 5. Approximate factors for converting doses as mg/kg from one species to an equivalent surface area dose as mg/kg in other species[a]

FROM	TO Mouse 20 g	Rat 150 g	Monkey 3.0 kg	Dog 8 kg	Man 60 kg
Mouse	1	1/2	1/4	1/6	1/12
Rat	2	1	1/2	1/4	1/7
Monkey	4	2	1	3/5	1/3
Dog	6	4	5/3	1	1/2
Man	12	7	3	2	1

[a] The assumptions and constants are based on Freireich, et al. (98).
Example : Given a dose of 50 mg/kg in the mouse , the approximate dose in the monkey assuming equivalency on basis of mg/square meter is 50 x 1/4 ~ 13 mg/kg.

TABLE 6. Representative surface area to weight ratios (K_m) for various species [a]

Species	Body Weight (kg.)	Surface Area (sq.m.)	K_m factor
Mouse	.02	.0066	3.0
Rat	.15	.025	5.9
Monkey	3.0	.24	12
Dog	8.0	.40	20
Human - Child	20	.80	25
Human - Adult	60	1.60	37

[a] The assumptions and constants are based on Freireich, et al. (98).
Example : To express a mg/kg dose in any given species as the equivalent mg/sq.m. dose, multiply the dose by appropriate K_m factor. In adult human 1 mg/kg is equivalent to 1 mg/kg. x 37 kg/sq.m. = 37 mg/sq.m.

$$K_m = \frac{10^2 \times (kg)^{1/3}}{K},$$ kg being the weight in kilograms.

Brodie and Reid (43) have objected to the use of body surface areas as a criterion for calculating safe dosage of a drug in man from animal data and proposed relating the drug effect to plasma levels,on the assumption that equal plasma levels in different species would produce similar pharmacological effects. Plasma levels of opiates are difficult to compare in various species because of differences in times for the attainment of peak levels and rates of decline of these levels. The area under the plasma-time curves calculated by the method of Wagner and Damiano (263) however,can be used for inter-species comparisons.

Effect of Enzyme Inducers and Inhibitors on Opiate Metabolism

The subject of enzyme induction and inhibition has been reviewed in detail by Conney (68) and Conney and Burns (70). Diazepam (Valium) was found to be an effective inhibitor of N-demethylation of methadone, which could explain in part the enhanced effect of methadone observed in addicts when such combinations of drugs are administered (240). Phenobarbital enhanced metabolism of methadone (223). The tricyclic antidepressant desipramine, potentiated and prolonged methadone analgesia in rats by increasing the brain concentration of methadone and inhibiting the metabolism of methadone by the liver (147).
Another interesting case of drug interaction concerns rifampin-induced methadone withdrawal in patients maintained on stabilized doses of methadone (142). Rifampin used in treatment of advanced tuberculosis, caused a lowering of plasma concentration of methadone and an increased urinary excretion of methadone metabolites, but the plasma $t\frac{1}{2}$ of methadone were not altered.
Brunk, et al. (46,47), have shown that propranolol did not affect morphine metabolism in man and ingestion of aspirin did not affect conjugation or N-demethylation of morphine.
Chronic alcohol intake did not impair the metabolism of meperidine in man,but increasing alcohol consumption was found to be associated with increasing volume of distribution of meperidine(lower initial plasma levels),possibly related to the generalised vasodilatation as a result of alcohol intake and this made heavy drinkers more refractory to this CNS depressant (157). The administration of β-diethylaminoethyl diphenyl propyl acetate (SKF-525A), an inhibitor of microsomal drug metabolising enzymes, shortly prior to meperidine, increased the in vivo $t\frac{1}{2}$ of meperidine and thus its duration of action (50). Men living in rural and urban environments differed in drug metabolising capacity. Individuals living in urban environments, required a larger dose of pentazocine to produce the same effect, as compared to those living in rural environments (71).
Endocrine factors markedly affected the action of opiates.

Adrenalectomy resulted in increased tissue levels of morphine
without impairing the conjugation ability of the animals (8,271).
Elliott and Elison (89) showed that the decreased pharmacological
effect of methadone observed after the administration of cortisone
or ACTH, was due to an enhancement of excretion of methadone .
Chronic administration of 1-thyroxine reduced the in vitro N-
demethylation of morphine (62).

Administration of alloxan to mature male rats,decreased the
activity of microsomal enzymes which metabolise codeine (78);the
activity in female rats, however, was not altered (107).
Irradiation of rats, decreased the ability of liver to metabolise
pethidine and resulted in its higher blood levels and greater
amounts in urine, as compared to untreated controls (112) .
Irradiation of rats,however, had no effect on tolerance development to morphine (197).

Disposition of meperidine is significantly impaired in patients
with either acute or chronic liver disease,thus both cirrhosis
(140) and viral hepatitis (159) impaired the elimination of this
drug to a similar extent. The prolongation in elimination $t\frac{1}{2}$
from 3.3 hr to 7.0 hr could be accounted for by a proportionate
decrease in plasma clearance. No significant differences were
observed in either the volumes of distribution or plasma binding
of meperidine. Patients with renal and hepatic failure are more
sensitive to clinical doses of morphine, at least in part due to
decreased binding to plasma proteins (209). Wilkinson and
Schenker (276) have recently reviewed the effect of liver disease
on drug disposition.

Effect of various physiological and environmental factors on
the activity of drug metabolizing enzymes, have been discussed in
detail in excellent reviews of Gillette (107,110), Parke (210),
Conney (69) and Mandel (151).

Maternal, Fetal and Neonatal Metabolism of Opiates

Opiates, e.g. morphine (18), dihydromorphine (226,296),heroin,
pethidine (11,24,206,235),etorphine (34),pentazocine (24,127)and
methadone (35,48,55,214), cross the placental barrier easily and
the rate of such a transfer and accumulation in fetal tissue
depend primarily on lipid solubility, pK_a, molecular size, pH
gradient across placental membrane, vascularity and uterine and
umbilical cord blood flow. In view of the differences in pH of
amniotic fluid (6.5 - 7.0) and maternal blood (7.35 - 7.40) basic
opiates pass into fetus in higher amounts. Thus, a higher ratio
of pethidine occurred in umbilical cord blood to that in maternal
blood (24). Several-fold higher concentrations of etorphine (34)
or methadone (214) occurred in fetal brain as compaired to the
maternal tissue. Respiratory depression, miosis, and moderate to
severe withdrawal syndrome have been observed in neonates of
mothers who either received opiates during labour or were dependent
on such drugs (143 , 220,256).

Placenta has actively metabolising enzymes and some of these opiates may be metabolised during their passage from maternal to fetal circulation. In laboratory animals, most of the hepatic microsomal enzymes were almost absent in fetus or newborn and adult levels of these enzymes were reached only slowly in the offspring (97,131). However Yaffe, et al. (286), Pelkonen, et al. (212) and Ackerman, et al. (5), have shown the presence of microsomal oxidative enzymes and UDP glucuronyl transferase activity in human fetus. Such differences in fetal development of enzyme activity in laboratory animals and man, probably arose due to continuous exposure of humans to enzyme inducers in the environment. Enzyme inducers in mother, e.g. cigarette smoke (26), barbiturates, tranquilizers, alcohol, etc., stimulate microsomal enzymes of fetus, neonate and newborn leading to increased oxidative N-demethylation of opiates.

Significance of fetal and neonatal metabolism of opiates

High permeability of the blood-brain barrier (144), low levels of metabolizing enzymes, depressed renal function, differences in plasma protein binding of opiates in fetus and newborn (84) may account for their higher sensitivity to opiates as compared to adults . In rats, the blood brain barrier to morphine developed about 16 days after birth (268). Breast feeding of the neonate by mothers who receive methadone or morphine, may prolong the exposure of infants to these opiates due to the mammary secretion. Phase I metabolic reactions could lead to the synthesis in developing fetal tissue of harmful agents (epoxides) or toxic N-demethylated metabolites, not only of opiates but of other drugs administered during pregnancy. Such metabolites may have an undesirable effect on embryonic and organogenesis processes leading to congenital abnormalities. Although no information is available on the effects of opiates and their metabolites on growth and development of fetal brain,fetal growth retardation, malformation and other long-lasting effects in experimental animals have been observed with morphine (12,99) and methadone(55,238).Placental transfer(14),maternal and neonatal metabolism of some opiates and other drugs have been covered in the recent reviews (23,120,170).

Effect of Chronic Administration of Opiates on Metabolism

Many opiates produce substantial decrease in the oxidative activity in vitro of liver microsomal enzymes of rats on chronic treatment (16) and the activity of hepatic glucuronyl transferase has also been reported to decrease in livers of male rats on chronic treatment with morphine (253). In vivo studies on the comparative distribution and excretion of several opiates, e.g. morphine, dihydromorphine,codeine,dextro methorphan,levorphanol, meperidine in acutely and chronically-treated animals, have not shown any marked differences in the metabolism of these opiates in the 2 groups; for review see Way and Adler (269) and Misra

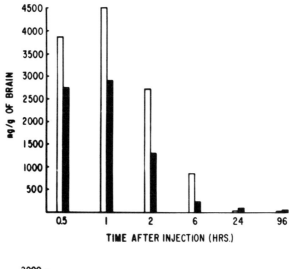

TIME AFTER INJECTION (HRS.)

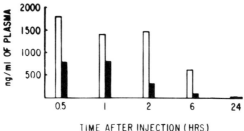

TIME AFTER INJECTION (HRS.)

FIG. 2. Comparative distribution of 1-methadone-1-^{3}H in brain
and plasma of nontolerant (white bar) and tolerant (black bar)
rats after s.c. injection of 10 mg/kg as free base. In the
chronic experiments, the rats were injected daily for 6 weeks
with a dose of 10 mg/kg of non-labeled methadone s.c.,followed by
one week with same dose of labeled drug before the terminal
injection and sacrifice .

(171). Unlike other opiates,however,methadone on chronic administration enhanced its own metabolism (10,155,260). Lower values
of methadone were consistently observed in brain and plasma of
methadone-tolerant as compared to the nontolerant rats at all
time periods, after 10 mg/kg s.c. injection (Fig. 2) and indicated
a clear differences in the penetration and egression of drug from
the CNS between the 2 groups. Lower $t\frac{1}{2}$ in brain and plasma of
tolerant as compared to nontolerant rats reflected a faster rate
of metabolism in tolerant animals (Table 7). Differences in
brain to plasma ratios suggested an altered distribution of

TABLE 7. The half-life of levo methadone-1-^{3}H in nontolerant and tolerant rats after either 10 mg/kg s.c. injection or 50 mg/kg oral administration [a]

Biological Material and route of administration	Half-life (hr)	
	Nontolerant	Tolerant
Brain (s.c.)	2.4	1.5
Plasma (s.c.)	3.7	1.7
Brain (oral)	14	3.1
Plasma (oral)	8	1.4

[a] Data from Misra, et al. (183)

methadone in the 2 groups (175,183).

Chronic administration of propoxyphene in man has also been reported to stimulate its own metabolism and/or elimination along with its metabolite norpropoxyphene (249). Our recent studies with 1-α-acetyl methadol (LAAM) in monkeys, indicate that chronic administration of LAAM enhances not only its own metabolism, but also the elimination of its persistent metabolites (Misra, et al. unpublished observations). Details on comparative metabolism of LAAM in acutely and chronically-treated monkeys are given later in this chapter.

Recent Work on the Distribution and Metabolism of Opiates

Earlier studies on the metabolism of various opiates have been discussed in the reviews of Way and Adler (269); Way (267); Scrafani and Clouet (233); Misra (171,172). Some recent work not covered in those reviews will be discussed briefly here.

Morphine

After a 10 mg i.v. injection of morphine in man (70 kg), the values in plasma (3.5 µg/ml) were attained within 5 minutes and declined to 0.0045 µg/ml 12 hr after injection (243). The $t_{\frac{1}{2}}$ in plasma was 1.9 - 3.1 hr and the elimination time in serum 10 - 44 hr. Long persistence of morphine in serum was attributed to the binding of morphine with serum albumin (243). After a 60 mg s.c. q.i.d. dose of morphine to morphine-dependent subjects, the excretion as percentage of dose was morphine 10, free normorphine 1, total normorphine (comprising free and conjugate) 4, total morphine 74 (comprising free drug, morphine 3-glucuronide and morphine-3-sulfate)(290). The values of total radioactivity (85%) excreted in urine and expired air observed in the studies of

Brunk and Delle (45) and Fishman, et al. (93) appeared to be in
agreement with the observations of Yeh (290).

Tolerance development in rats did not alter the plasma t ½ of
morphine (1 - 2 hr for the fast phase and 10 hr for the slower
phase) (29) and morphine could be detected in plasma 20 days after
the exposure to and removal of morphine pellets. Evidence has
also been obtained for the formation in vitro by rat brain and
liver homogenates of a 2,3-catechol type of metabolite of morphine
by aromatic hydroxylation, along with the formation of morphine-
N-oxide and normorphine (189). The norcompound was shown to be a
metabolite of morphine in vivo several years ago (184). Evidence
was also obtained for the formation in vivo of another metabolite
of morphine, tentatively assigned as a 2,3-dihydrodiol. Sequential
oxidation of morphine by alkaline ferricyanide and hydrogen
peroxide and copper ions gave a zwitterionic 2,3-quinone type of
compound , which appeared to be chromatographically similar to
the 2,3 -catechol type of metabolite of morphine formed in vitro
by brain and liver homogenates. The highly polar quinonoid
compound possessed no analgesic activity by systemic routes,but
had potent stimulant activity on intracisternal injection in the
rats (190).

The pharmacokinetics of morphine in plasma and discrete areas
of the brain in rats during 8 hr after i.v. injection indicated
a three-exponential function, which could be described by a
three-compartment model (73).

Heroin

Recent work of Yeh, et al. (293) showed that heroin was very
rapidly metabolised and eliminated in human urine. After a 10 mg
i.v. injection to 70 kg. human subjects, the percentages of dose
excreted as heroin, 6-monoacetyl morphine, conjugates of morphine
and 6-monoacetyl morphine and total normorphine, were 0.5 , 1.5 ,
7.2 , 52 and 4, respectively.   The conjugated morphine could be
detected in urine up to 96 hr.   The $t_{\frac{1}{2}}$ of urinary excretion of
free morphine, 6-monoacetyl morphine, conjugates of morphine and
6-monoacetyl morphine and total normorphine were 1.28 , 1.31 ,
2.76 and 2.72 hr , respectively (293).

Meperidine

N-Oxidation (193) and para aromatic hydroxylation (146) have recently been shown to be additional routes for the metabolism of
meperidine.Normeperidine,meperidinic and normeperidinic acids and
their conjugates were shown to be the metabolites of meperidine
in earlier studies. Highly sensitive and specific methods have
been developed for the determination of meperidine and nor -
meperidine in biofluids (54,156). The studies of O'Donoghue
(205,206) have shown that considerable distribution and conversion
of meperidine (30-70%) occurred in human fetal-maternal system
and that fetus itself can N-demethylate meperidine .

Thebaine

Thebaine is primarily a CNS stimulant with little or no
analgesic activity. In higher doses, it produces strychnine-like
convulsions in experimental animals.   Physical dependence and
tolerance to its convulsant effects, reportedly does not develop.
Studies of Misra, et al. (185,186) showed a comparatively faster
rate of penetration into and egress of thebaine from the CNS of
rats, as compared to morphine after a 5 mg/kg s.c.injection. The
levels of thebaine in the CNS were also not sustained as long as
those of morphine. Norcodeine, normorphine,morphine and codeine,
were observed to be the metabolites of thebaine in the CNS of the
rat 45 minutes after injection, but at this dosage these metabolites were cleared from the brain within 96 hours. Repeated
administration of thebaine,however,could lead to an accumulation
of some of these metabolites in the CNS and may be responsible
for the low grade physical dependence recently reported with
thebaine in the monkey (287). Thebaine was extensively
metabolized in the rat and in addition to the above metabolites,
evidence was obtained for the formation of O^3-desmethyl thebaine,
14-hydroxy codeinone and glucuronide conjugates of norcodeine,
normorphine, morphine and codeine.

Methadone

Studies on disposition of methadone after a single 15 mg oral
dose in man, showed that peak plasma levels (74 ng/ml) were
attained 4 hr after drug administration and these declined to
29 ng/ml 20 hr later with an apparent $t_\frac{1}{2}$ value of 15 hr. (126).
Excretion of methadone and metabolites was 52% of the dose in 96
hr. The peak plasma level in patients on methadone maintenance
given a 100 mg dose of methadone, was 860 ng/ml at 4 hr and the
levels declined to 460 ng/ml 24 hr after administration, with an
apparent $t_\frac{1}{2}$ value of 25 hr. The drug was partially reabsorbed
by kidney by a pH-dependent process (125).
Comparative disposition and metabolism studies with levo
methadone in non-tolerant and tolerant rats (183) and dogs (174,
175) showed a more rapid metabolism of this drug in tolerant
animals, which did not allow any marked accumulation of methadone in tissues and areas of the CNS, in spite of its persistence
in the brain after a single dose (180). In agreement with the
observations of Beckett, et al. (25), Pohland , et al. (217) ,
Beckett, et al. (27), Sullivan, et al. (246) , Lynn et al. (149),
methadone was extensively metabolised in the rat and dog by (a)
N-demethylation and cyclisation to substituted pyrrolidine and
pyrroline metabolites, (b) N-oxidation, (c) hydroxylation in the
para position of the aromatic nucleus, (d) keto group reduction
to an alcohol, (e) glucuronide conjugation of the resultant
hydroxyl groups, (f) minor conversion to secondary and primary
amines. The prolonged presence of methadone and its metabolites
in brain and binding of this metabolite to a specific brain
protein, could conceivably lead to a biochemical alteration of

the receptor site resulting in a reduced ability of this drug to initiate a pharmacological response. Our studies provided evidence that both dispositional and functional tolerance in the CNS, are involved in the genesis of pharmacological tolerance and protracted withdrawal syndrome with methadone.

Propoxyphene

Propoxyphene is widely used for symptomatic relief of mild or moderate pain.   Recent work by McMahon, et al. (164), Verebey and Inturrisi (258) and Nash, et al. (198) showed that after a single 130 mg oral dose in man, the $t\frac{1}{2}$ of propoxyphene in plasma was 4 - 6 hrs.   Norpropoxyphene, dinorpropoxyphene, cyclic dinor- propoxyphene, propoxyphene carbinol, dinorpropoxyphene carbinol, conjugates of p-hydroxy propoxyphene and p-hydroxynorpropoxy- phene, were observed to be the metabolites of propoxyphene. The excretion of persistent metabolites,i.e. norpropoxyphene and dinorpropoxyphene, continued for several days in man.

1-α-Acetylmethadol (LAAM)

Because of its properties of effective suppression of opiate withdrawal symptoms and longer duration of action, LAAM, a synthetic congener of methadone, has practical therapeutic ad- vantages over methadone in treatment and rehabilitation programs for heroin addicts. Thus, an oral dose of 80 mg three times a week has been suggested as a substitute for 100 mg of methadone daily.   Previous studies by Sung and Way (152), McMahon, et al. (162), Billings, et al. (32) ,Billings, et al. (33), Nickander, et al. (201) , Kaiko and Inturrisi (134), have shown that some of the pharmacological activity and long duration of action of LAAM may be due to its biotransformation to acetylnormethadol and acetylbisnormethadol.   Methadol and normethadol have also been reported as metabolites of LAAM (133).   The work on pharmaco - kinetics, metabolism and biological activity of these compounds has recently been reviewed by Misra and Mulè (182).

In our study (Misra, et al.,1971 : unpublished observations)a single 2 mg/kg oral dose of 1-α-(2-^{3}H) acetyl methadol was administered to the monkeys in the acutely-treated group. Chronic- ally-treated monkeys received 2 mg/kg oral dose of non-labeled LAAM on alternate days three times a week for approximately 30 weeks,followed by a 2 mg/kg oral dose of (^{3}H) LAAM. Data on the comparative distribution of free (^{3}H) LAAM and total radioactivity in plasma from 2 monkeys in each group appears in Fig.3.   The peak levels of free LAAM in plasma of acutely-treated monkeys occurred between 2-6 hrs and that in the chronically-treated monkeys at 6 hrs after administration and the levels of free drug in the chronic group were higher than those in the acute.   Free LAAM disappeared in both groups from plasma by 96 hrs after administration. Total radioactivity values,comprising free drug plus its metabolites,in the chronic group were consistently higher

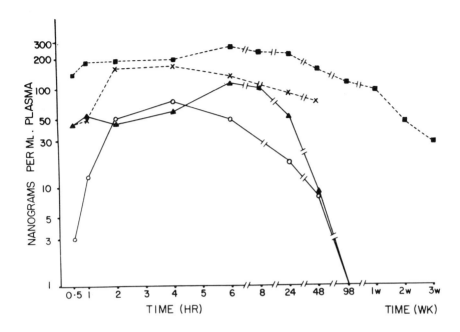

FIG. 3. Comparative distribution of 1-α-(2-³H) acetyl methadol
(LAAM) in plasma of acutely and chronically-treated monkeys
after a 2 mg/kg oral dose. In the chronic group, the monkeys
received an oral dose (2 mg/kg) of non-labeled LAAM on alternate
days 3 times a week for 30 weeks, followed by an oral dose of (³H)
LAAM.

■ - - - -■ Total radioactivity, chronically treated

✗ - - - -✗ Total radioactivity, acutely treated

○ ———— ○ Free LAAM, acutely treated

▲ ———— ▲ Free LAAM, chronically treated

than those in the acute at all times and significant amounts of
this radioactivity due to the metabolites acetyl bisnormethadol
and p-hydroxy acetyl bisnormethadol, persisted in plasma up to 3
weeks or longer. Acetylnormethadol constituted approximately 15-
20% of the values of free LAAM in plasma up to 6 hr and 65-70% at
later times. Acetyl bisnormethadol, p-hydroxy acetyl bisnormethadol and conjugated metabolites of methadol and normethadol, were
not extracted in significant amounts by our procedure (173).

The mean values of free LAAM in selected areas of the CNS, e.g.

temporal cortex, spinal cord,hypothalamus,thalamus,medulla,pons, mesencephalon,caudate nucleus,6 and 24 hrs after administration of a 2 mg/kg oral dose of (^{3}H) LAAM were 119-191 ; 36 - 84 ng/g in the acutely-treated monkey and 308-415 ; 33-100 ng/g in the chronically-treated monkeys respectively. The value (100 ng/g) in the spinal cord of chronically-treated monkeys 24 hrs after administration of LAAM were comparatively much higher than those in other areas of the CNS. Free LAAM was not detectable in brain one week after administration of LAAM,but significant total radio activity (25-32 ng/g) persisted in the areas of the CNS at this time. Chromatography of brain extracts on Amberlite XAD-2 and thin layer chromatography of the methanol eluate of adsorbed metabolites, provided suggestive evidence for the presence of p-hydroxy acetyl bisnormethadol and of small amounts of acetyl-bisnormethadol in brain, one week after administration of LAAM. At earlier times, evidence was obtained for the presence of LAAM, methadol, acetylnormethadol, normethadol,acetylbisnormethadol and p-hydroxy acetylbisnormethadol in brains of monkeys.The apparent $t_\frac{1}{2}$ of LAAM in areas of the CNS of the acutely and chronically - treated monkeys were 8.4 - 11.3 and 4.9 - 6.4 hr respectively.

Biliary excretion was an important route for the excretion of LAAM and its metabolites in the monkey and detectable levels of free LAAM and its metabolites (0.4-0.7 µg/ml) were still present in bile one week after administration .   Levels of LAAM were several-fold higher in lungs of chronically-treated monkeys at 6 hrs; duodenum and ileum had comparatively lower values as compared to the acute group at this time.

Stomach, duodenum, ileum , colon , liver and bile, in the chronically-treated monkeys, had significantly higher levels of radioactivity due to metabolites of LAAM one week after administration, as compared to the acutely-treated controls.

The t $\frac{1}{2}$ of LAAM in liver, kidney, spleen and lung, were lower   in the chronic as compared to the   acutely - treated monkeys .

Comparative excretion profiles of free LAAM and total radio - activity, in acutely and chronically-treated monkeys after a 2 mg/kg oral dose of (^{3}H) LAAM, appears in Fig. 4. Free LAAM , 3.3 and 17.6% of the dose,was excreted in 3 weeks in urine and feces respectively in the acutely-treated monkeys; 4.1 and 14.5% of the dose were the corresponding figures in the chronically treated monkeys. Fecal excretion was a major route for elimi-nation of LAAM and its metabolites. The mean percentage of dose excreted in 3 weeks as total radioactivity in urine and feces of acutely-treated monkeys was 22.4 , 28.0 respectively ; that in the chronically-treated monkeys 35.9, 35.8 respectively.

Comparative study on the urinary metabolic profile of LAAM in the two groups,showed several-fold higher excretion of free acetyl-normethadol and acetylbisnormethadol in the chronic group and lesser amounts of p-hydroxy acetylbisnormethadol, conjugates of methadol and normethadol as compared to the acute group.

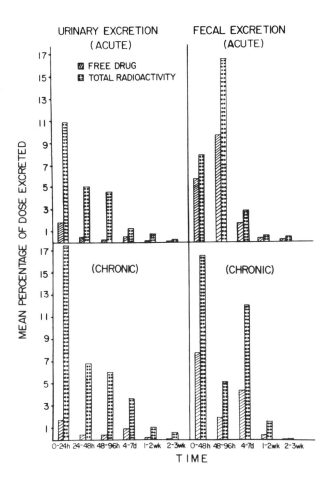

FIG. 4. Comparative urinary and fecal excretion of 1-∝-(2-³H) acetyl methadol in acutely and chronically-treated monkeys after 2 mg/kg oral dose. Other details as in legend to Fig. 3 .

p-Hydroxy acetylbisnormethadol was present in urine as free and conjugated metabolite.

In the course of chronic treatment of monkeys with LAAM, we observed a variable pharmacological response in the monkeys. Some monkeys were severely depressed, others not at all. Those severely depressed, did not respond promptly to a 1 mg/kg s.c. injection of nalorphine. This variable response is probably due to the differential rates of formation of acetylnormethadol, acetylbisnormethadol and p-hydroxy acetylbisnormethadol or some other metabolite in this species. Our studies show that chronic administration of LAAM in the monkey enhanced the metabolism of

LAAM and the elimination of its metabolites.

Fentanyl

Fentanyl (pK$_a$, 7.34) is a very short acting analgesic used in neuroleptanalgesia . After a 20 μg/kg i.v. injection in rabbits, the termination of analgesia occurred after 30 min.Within 5 min. of injection, high concentrations of fentanyl were attained in brain, lung, heart, kidney and comparatively lower concentrations in liver. The skeletal muscle and fat attained maximal concentrations only after a considerable time (117). A good parallelism was observed in the decline of drug concentration in brain and antinociceptive effect. Redistribution of fentanyl in tissues, metabolism and excretion led to a decrease in the effective concentration of this opiate at its site of action in the CNS. In man, the redistribution of fentanyl appeared to play a very important role in the termination of its action (118). Information on the metabolism of fentanyl is not available.

Narcotic Antagonists

Nalorphine and naloxone

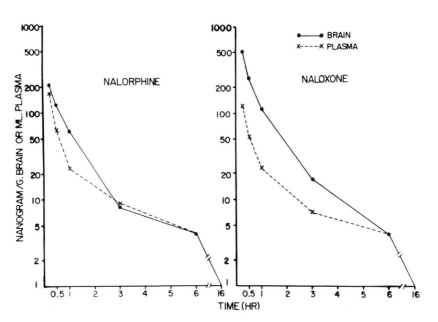

FIG. 5. Comparative distribution of (allyl-1',3'-^{14}C)naloxone and (allyl-1',3'-^{14}C)nalorphine in rat brain and plasma after a 1 mg/kg dose by s.c. injection

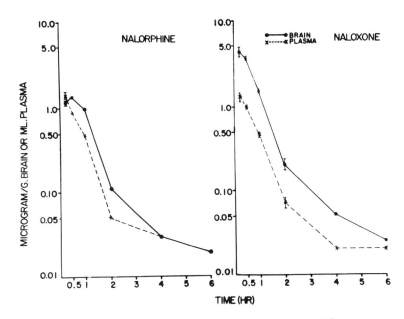

FIG. 6. Comparative distribution of (allyl-1',3'-^{14}C)naloxone and (allyl-1',3'-^{14}C)nalorphine in rat brain and plasma after a 10 mg/kg dose by s.c. injection.

Naloxone is a "pure opioid antagonist" which abolishes or prevents the pharmacological effects, not only of narcotic agonists but also of mixed agonist - antagonists such as nalorphine. Naloxone is 10 - 20 times more active than nalorphine in the rat (37). It has no abuse potential and no tolerance or physical dependence liability. Some information is available on its metabolism and distribution in normal and narcotic-dependent humans (94, 101,274) and experimental animals (100,203,275) . Earlier studies by Woods (283), Woods and Muehlenbeck (285) and Hug and Woods (122) on nalorphine,have provided much information on the disposition and metabolism of this compound.

Berkowitz, et al. (30) have shown that after a 0.4 mg i.v. injection of naloxone in man, serum levels (15 ng/ml) were attained within 2 min. after injection and declined with a t½ of 57 min.

Data (187) on the comparative uptake of (^{14}C) naloxone and (^{14}C) nalorphine in rat brain and plasma after a single 1 and 10 mg/kg s.c. dose,are given in Fig. 5 and 6. Rapid attainment of peak levels in brain and plasma occurred within 30 min and t ½ was approximately 24 min. with both doses. At equivalent doses, levels of naloxone 1.5 - 3.7 times higher than nalorphine were attained in brain,but plasma values were only 0.7 - 1.4 times those of nalorphine. The maximal values of naloxone in brain were approximately 11 times those of morphine with the same 10 mg/kg s.c. dose (179). The rate of disappearance of these antagonists from the CNS was much faster as compared to morphine. Significant differences were also observed in brain to plasma ratios of these 2 antagonists, the naloxone values (3.4 - 4.8) being consistently higher than those with nalorphine (0.8 - 2.7) and indicated an altered distribution for these 2 compounds. 7,8-Dihydro-14 hydroxy normorphinone and 2 other polar metabolites were shown to be present in brain along with free naloxone 0.5 hr after injection of 1 or 10 mg/kg s.c. dose of naloxone.

Comparatively higher excretion of free nalorphine (13% of the dose) compared to naloxone (8%) and higher excretion of total radioactivity in urine and feces for naloxone (64.2% of the dose) compared to nalorphine (54.0%),occurred after 10 mg/kg s.c. injection of these antagonists in the rat. The data on comparati ve amounts of conjugated drugs in plasma suggested a faster conjugation and excretion of naloxone as compared to nalorphine. Rapid metabolism and elimination rate of naloxone would appear to be the important factors in its short duration of action. Naloxone-3-glucuronide (major), 3-sulfate (minor), naloxol and conjugated naloxol (minor), free and conjugated 7,8-dihydro-14 hydroxynormorphinone, 7,8-dihydro-14-hydroxynormorphine and two polar hydroxylated compounds (with hydroxylation presumably in the 2-position or 17-side chain), were observed as urinary metabolites of naloxone.

Naltrexone

Naltrexone has therapeutic advantages over other opiate antagonists in ambulatory treatment of heroin addicts,because of the low incidence of side effects, lack of toxicity, oral effect-iveness and prolonged duration of action. It is about 8 times as active and 3 times as long acting as naloxone in the rat (38). In man, naltrexone was 17 times more potent than naloxone in precipitating acute abstinence.

Considerable work has been done in recent years on species-dependent stereoselective reduction of 6-keto group of naltrexone and naloxone in vivo to the corresponding diastereoisomeric 6α or 6β-alcohols, which are the important metabolites of these antagonists in several species. Naltrexone is metabolised to 6β-naltrexol in man (56,65,67), rabbit (103) and guinea pig (66). The relative narcotic antagonistic potency of 6β-naltrexol and naltrexone was 1/53 in the rat. Naltrexone and naloxone are bio transformed to the corresponding 6α-alcohols in the chicken (100). Current status of work on metabolism and pharmacology of these compounds has been reviewed by Verebey and Mulé (259).

Disposition of (15, 16-^{3}H) naltrexone in the CNS of the rats after a 10 mg/kg s.c. injection was studied by Misra, et al.(176) Distribution of naltrexone in brain and plasma after this dose is

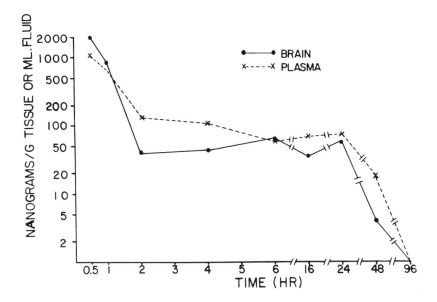

FIG. 7. Distribution of $(15,16-^3H)$ naltrexone in rat brain and plasma after a 10 mg/kg dose by s.c. injection .

given in Fig. 7 . Peak levels of naltrexone were attained in brain within 0.5 hr and naltrexone was not detectable 48 hr after administration. The naltrexone levels in brain were sustained between 2 to 24 hr and in plasma from 1 to 24 hr. The apparent $t\frac{1}{2}$ of naltrexone was 8 hr in brain and 11 hr in plasma. The brain to plasma ratios of naltrexone were lower than those for naloxone, but were in the range for nalorphine, possibly because of the lower lipid solubility of naltrexone as compared to naloxone. In addition to naltrexone, small amounts of 6β-naltrexol, 7,8 - dihydro-14-hydroxynormorphinone and 7,8-dihydro-14-hydroxynor-morphine and 3 other metabolites tentatively assigned as 2-hydroxy 3-methoxy, 2-methoxy-3-hydroxy and 2,3-dihydroxy naltrexol have been observed as metabolites in rat brain. Neither 6α nor 6β - naltrexol was detected as a metabolite in plasma, but the nor-compounds and hydroxylated-methoxylated metabolites were present in plasma as free and conjugated metabolites. Rapid N-dealkyl-ation of naltrexone and 6α naltrexol led to the formation of the norcompounds in significant amounts and the absence of 6α and 6β -naltrexol in rat plasma. The initial $t\frac{1}{2}$ of naltrexone in brain for the fast decay phase was in the range for nalorphine and naloxone (187), but the second much slower phase with a longer $t_{\frac{1}{2}}$ would imply that either the binding of naltrexone to some con- stituent in rat brain is particularly strong, or a slow release from some extravascular site into plasma may play a role in the prolonged duration of its antagonism.

Disposition and pharmacologic studies on acute and chronic treatment with 100 mg oral dose of naltrexone in man have recent- ly been done by Verebey et al. (261). After an acute dose, mean peak levels of naltrexone and 6 β-naltrexol in plasma were 43.6 and 87.2 ng/ml at 1 and 2 hr respectively and these values declined to 2.1 and 17.6 ng/ml respectively 24 hr after admini- stration. Following chronic administration, the mean peak plasma levels of naltrexone and 6 β-naltrexol were 46.4 and 158.4 ng/ml respectively at 1 hr, but by 24 hr these values declined to levels similar to those in the acute state. No accumulation of naltrexone and 6 β-naltrexol was observed in plasma with 100 mg oral dose during chronic treatment. The apparent $t_{\frac{1}{2}}$ of naltrexone in acute and chronic states were 10.3 , 9.7 hr respectively; that of 6 β-naltrexol 12.7 , 11.4 hr respectively. Renal clearance data indicated partial reabsorption of naltrexone and the active secretion of 6 β-naltrexol by the kidney. During acute and chronic treatments, the mean urinary excretion in 24 hr was 38 , 70% of the dose and fecal excretion 2.1 , 3.6% of the dose respectively. The opiate antagonism to 25 mg heroin challenges was nearly complete through 48 hr after naltrexone. 2-Hydroxy-3- methoxy naltrexol was the only other metabolite identified in this study (257). As in the case of the rat (176) , a substantial portion of naltrexone appeared to be sequestered in tissues, which gave rise to its slow release into plasma. The first pass hepatic biotransformation of naltrexone was indicated by the rapid appearance and attainment of substantially higher concentration of 6 β-naltrexol in plasma. These studies indicated that nal- trexone did not induce the rate of its own metabolism and in the chronic state, a steady state equilibrium is rapidly attained.

PERSPECTIVES FOR FURTHER WORK ON OPIATE METABOLISM

In view of the extensive and widespread use of opiate analgesics by women during pregnancy and paucity of our current knowledge on fetal pharmacology, there is a need for more work on factors which affect maternal, fetal and neonatal metabolism of opiates and also the possible effects of these drugs on the growth and development of brain in the fetus. Efforts should also be directed towards the development of more improved sensitive and specific methodology for the quantification of these drugs and their metabolites in the very small volume of blood, and urine available from the neonate. Although GC/MS/computer methods serve this need at the present time, there is further need for extension of their sensitivity in the pico and femtogram ranges. Further developments in high pressure liquid chromatographic technique will undoubtedly help in the speedy separation and identification of such drugs and their metabolites in biofluids.

The studies on the stimulatory and inhibitory effects of tranquilizers, alcohol, caffeine, aspirin, cigarette smoke, barbiturates, on opiate metabolism will continue to be an important area for further work.

The use of analog and digital computer techniques for the solution of potentially complex problems in absorption , distribution and metabolism of opiates has been very limited and it is hoped that computational methods involving the construction of suitable mathematical models will find increasing application to the solution of problems in the pharmacokinetics of opiates.

ACKNOWLEDGMENT

The work reported here was supported in part by USPHS grants MH-19004, DA-00061, NB-02928, NIDA Contract No. ADM-45-74-133. The author wishes to thank Dr. S.J. Mulè, Assistant Commissioner and Director, ODAS Testing and Research Laboratory , Mr.R.Bloch, Mr. R.B. Pontani, Mrs. J. Vardy and Mr.N.L.Vadlamani for their contribution to the work.

REFERENCES

1. Abdel-Monem,M.M., Larson,D.L., Kupferberg,H.J. and Porto-ghese,P.S. (1972): J.Med.Chem., 15: 494
2. Abou-El-Makarem, M.M., Millburn, P., Smith,R.L. and Williams, R.T. (1967) : Biochem.J. ,105 : 1289
3. Abrahams, R.A. and Ronel, S.H. (1976): J.Biomed. Materials Res. , 9:355
4. Abrams,L.S. and Elliott, H.W. (1974): J.Pharmac.Exp.Ther., 189: 285
5. Ackerman, E., Rane, A. and Ericsson, J.L.E. (1972): Clin. Pharmac. Ther., 13 : 652
6. Adler, T.K. (1963) : J.Pharmac. Exp.Ther.,140: 155
7. Adler, T.K. (1967) : J.Pharmac.Exp.Ther., 156 : 585
8. Adler T.K., Elliott, H.W. and George,R.(1957) : J.Pharmac.Exp. Ther. , 120 : 457
9. Alvares,A.P. and Kappas, A. (1972):   J.Lab.Clin.Med.,79:439
10. Ånggård, E., Gunne, L.M., Holmstrand, J., McMahon,R.E. , Sandburg, C.G. and Sullivan, H.R. (1975): Clin.Pharmac.Ther., 17 : 258
11. Apgar ,V., Burns, J.J., Brodie,B.B. and Papper, E.M. (1952): Amer.J.Obstet.Gynec. , 64 : 1368
12. Arcuri,P.A. and Gautieri, R.F. (1973) : J.Pharm.Sci., 62:1626
13. Asatoor, A.M., London , D.R., Milne, M.D. and Simenoff,M.L. (1963): Brit.J.Pharmac. 20 : 285
14. Asling,J. and Way,E.L. (1971): In : Fundamentals of Drug Metabolism and Drug Disposition, edited by B.N.LaDu, H.G. Mandel and E.L.Way,p.88.Williams and Wilkins,Baltimore .
15. Axelrod, J. (1956) : J.Pharmac. Exp.Ther.,117 :322

16. Axelrod , J. and Cochin, J. (1957) : J.Pharmac.Exp.Ther.,121: 107

17. Baggot,J.D. and Davis,L.E. : Amer.J.Vet.Res.,34: 571

18. Baker, J.B.E. (1960): Pharmac.Rev. , 12: 37

19. Baker W.P. and Woods, L.A. (1957) : J.Pharmac. Exp.Ther., 120: 371

20. Baselt, R.C., Bickel, M.H. (1974): Biochem.Pharmac., 23: 1405

21. Baselt, R.C. and Casarett,L.J.(1972): Biochem. Pharmac., 21: 2705

22. Baselt, R.C. and Casarett,L.J. (1972) : Clin.Pharmac. Ther. 13: 64

23. Beckett,A.H. (1973) : Brit.J.Anesthesiol., 45 suppl. : 770

24. Beckett, A.H. and Taylor, J.F. (1967) : J.Pharm.Pharmac.,19: 505

25. Beckett, A.H., Taylor, J.F., Casy, A.F. and Hassan, M.M.A. (1968) : J.Pharm.Pharmac.,20: 754

26. Beckett, A.H. and Triggs, E.J. (1967) : Nature(Lond.), 216 : 587

27. Beckett, A.H., Vaughan, D.P. and Essien,E.E. (1972) : J. Pharm. Pharmac. , 24: 244

28. Berkowitz, B.A., Ceretta,K.V. and Spector, S. (1974) : Life Sci., 15: 1017

29. Berkowitz, B.A., Ceretta,K.V. and Spector, S. (1974) : J. Pharmac. Exp.Ther., 191: 527

30. Berkowitz,B.A., Ngai, S.H., Hempstead, J. and Spector,S. (1975) : J.Pharmac.Exp.Ther., 195: 499

31. Berkowitz,B.A. and Way,E.L. (1971) : J.Pharmac.Exp.Ther. 177: 500

32. Billings, R.E., Booher, R., Smits,S., Pohland,A. and McMahon, R.E. (1973) : J.Med.Chem. , 16: 305

33. Billings, R.E., McMahon, R.E. and Blake, D.A. (1974) : Life Sci., 14: 1437

34. Blane,G.F. and Dobbs,H.E. (1967): Brit.J.Pharmac., 30: 166

35. Blinick, G., Inturrisi, C.E., Jerez,E. and Wallach,R.C. (1975): Amer.J.Obstet.Gynec., 121: 617

36. Blount, J.F., Mohacsi, E., Vane,F.M. and Mannering, G.J. (1973) : J.Med.Chem., 16: 352

37. Blumberg,H. and Dayton, H.B. (1973): In : Agonist-antagonist Actions of Narcotic Analgesic Drugs. Edited by H.W.Kosterlitz H.O.J.Collier, J.Villarreal, p.110,University Park Press, Baltimore .

38. Blumberg,H. and Dayton, H.B. (1974) : In "Narcotic Anta- gonists. Edited by M.C. Braude, L.S.Harris, E.L.May, J.P. Smith,J.E.Villareal. Adv. Biochem.Pharmac., 8: 33, Raven Press,New York.

39. Boerner,U. and Abbott, S. (1973) : Experientia, 29: 180

40. Boerner,U., Roe , R.L.and Becker, C.E. (1974) : J.Pharm. Pharmac., 26: 393

41. Braun, W., Hesse, I. and Malorney, G. (1963): Arch.Exp.Path. Pharmak., 245: 457

42. Brodie, B.B. (1964): In: Absorption and Distribution of Drugs

Edited by T.B.Binns, p.16, Williams and Wilkins, Baltimore
43. Brodie, B.B. and Reid, W.D. (1967) : Fed.Proc. , 26: 1062
44. Brown,E.A.B. (1974): Drug Metab.Rev., 3: 33
45. Brunk, S.F. and Delle, M. (1974): Clin.Pharmac.Ther., 16: 51
46. Brunk,S.F., Delle,M. and Wilson, W.R. (1974): Clin.Pharmac. Ther., 15: 283
47. Brunk,S.F.,Delle,M. and Wilson,W.R.(1974): Clin.Pharmac. Ther., 16:1039
48. Buchenauer,D., Turnbow, M. and Peters, M. (1974) : J.Pharmac. Exp.Ther., 189: 66
49. Burns, J.J. (1962) : In: Proc. First Intern. Pharmacology Meeting, Stockholm, 6: 227, The MacMillan Co., New York
50. Burns, J.J. (1971) : In: Fundamentals of Drug Metabolism and Drug Disposition. Edited by B.N. LaDu, H.G. Mandel and E.L. Way, p. 340, Williams and Wilkins, Baltimore
51. Burns,J.J., Berger,B.L., Lief, P.A., Wollack, A., Papper, E.M. and Brodie, B.B. (1955) : J.Pharmac.Exp.Ther., 114: 289
52. Burt,R.A.P. and Beckett,A.H. (1971) : Brit.J.Anesthesiol., 43: 427
53. Castro, J.A. and Gillette, J.R. (1967) : Biochem. Biophys.Res. Comm., 28: 426
54. Chan, K.K., Kendall, M.J. and Mitchard, M. (1974): J.Pharm. Pharmac. , 89: 169
55. Chandler, J.M., Robie, F.W., Schoolar, J.C. and Desmond, M.M. (1975) : J.Pharmac.Exp.Ther., 192: 549
56. Chatterjie,N., Fujimoto, J.M., Inturrisi , C.E., Roerig,S., Wang, R.I.H., Bowen, D.V.,Field, F.H. and Clarke, D.D. (1974): Drug Metab.Disp., 2: 401
57. Chryssanthou,C.P. (1973) : Proc.Soc.Exp.Biol.Med., 144: 770
58. Clouet, D.H. (1962) : Life Sci., 1: 31
59. Clouet, D.H. and Ratner, M. (1964) : J.Pharmac.Exp.Ther., 144: 362
60. Clouet, D.H. and Williams, N. (1973): Biochem.Pharmac., 22 : 1285
61. Cochin,J. and Axelrod,J. (1959) : J.Pharmac.Exp.Ther. ,125: 105
62. Cochin, J. and Sokoloff, L. (1960) : Proc.Soc.Exp.Biol.Med. : 104: 504
63. Cohn,G.L. and Cramer, J.A., McBride, W., Brown, R.C. and Klebber,H.D. (1974) : Proc.Soc.Exp.Biol.Med., 147: 664
64. Collier, H.O.J., Francis, D.L. and Schneider,C. (1972): Nature 237: 220
65. Cone,E.J. (1973): Tetrahedron Lett., 23: 2607
66. Cone, E.J. and Gorodetzky,C.W. (1976) : Fed.Proc., 35: 469
67. Cone, E.J. , Gorodetzky, C.W. and Yeh, S.Y. (1975): J.Pharm. Sci. , 64: 618
68. Conney, A.H. (1967) : Pharmac.Rev., 19: 317
69. Conney, A.H. (1971) : In : Fundamentals of Drug Metabolism and Drug Disposition. Edited by B.N. LaDu, H.G. Mandel, and E.L.Way, p.253, Williams and Wilkins, Baltimore
70. Conney, A.H. and Burns, J.J. (1972): Science, 178: 576

71. Conney, A.H., Craver,B., Kuntzman, R. and Pantuck,E.J.(1974):
    In : Pharmacology and Pharmacokinetics. Edited by T.Teorell,
    R.L.Dedrick and P.G.Condliffe, p.147, Plenum Press,New York
72. Cox, B.M., Ginsberg, M. and Osman, O.H. (1968): Brit. J.
    Pharmacol., 33: 245
73. Dahlström,B.E. and Paalzow,L.K. (1975): J.Pharmacokin. Bio-
    pharmac., 3: 293
74. Daly, J., Inscoe, J.K. and Axelrod,J. (1965) : J.Med.Chem.,
    8: 153
75. Davies,D.S., Gigon, P.L. and Gillette,J.R. (1969) : Life Sci.
    8: 85
76. Deneau,G.A. and Nakai, K. (1961) : In : Minutes of 23rd
    Meeting of Committee on Problem of Drug Addiction and Nar-
    cotics. Appendix 6, NAS-NRC, Washington, D.C.
77. Deneau, G.A., Yanagita, T. and Seevers, M.H. (1969): Psycho-
    pharmacologia, 16: 30
78. Dixon, R.L., Hart,L.C. and Fouts, J.R. (1961) : J.Pharmac.
    Exp.Ther., 133: 7
79. Dobbs,H.E., Blane, G.F. and Boura, A.L.A. (1969): Eur. J.
    Pharmac., 7:328
80. Dobbs,H.E. and Hall, J.M. (1969) : Proc.Eur.Soc.Study Drug
    Toxicity, 10: 77
81. Dole, V.P. and Kreek, M.J. (1973): Proc.Nat.Acad.Sci.(U.S.A.)
    70: 10
82. Dutton, G.J. (1966) : In : Glucuronic Acid, Free and Combined,
    Chemistry,Biochemistry ,Pharmacology and Medicine,p.185 .
    Academic Press, New York
83. Ehrnebo, M., Agurell, S., Boréus,L.O., Gordon, E. and Lönroth
    U. (1974) : Clin.Pharmac.Ther. , 16: 424
84. Ehrnebo, M., Agurell, S., Jalling,B. and Boréus,L.O. (1971):
    Eur.J.Clin.Pharmac., 3: 189
85. Eisenbrandt, L.L., Adler, T.K., Elliott, H.W. and Abdou,I.A.
    (1949): J.Pharmac.Exp.Ther., 98: 200
86. Elison , C. and Elliott,H.W. (1963): Biochem.Pharmac., 12:
    1363
87. Elison, C. and Elliott, H.W. (1964): J.Pharmac.Exp.Ther.,
    144: 265
88. Elison, C., Elliott, H.W., Look , M. and Rapaport, H. (1963):
    J.Med.Chem., 6: 237
89. Elliott, H.W. and Elison, C. (1961) : J.Pharmac.Exp.Ther. ,
    131 : 31
90. El-Mazati, A.M. and Way, E.L. (1971): J.Pharmac.Exp.Ther. ,
    177: 332
91. Ferrari, R.A. (1968): Toxic. Appl.Pharmac., 12: 404
92. Fishman, J., Hahn, E.F., Norton, B.I., Ronai, A. and Foldes
    F.F. (1975),Pharmacology , 13: 513
93. Fishman,J., Norton, B., Cotter,M. and Hahn,E.F.(1974) : J.
    Med.Chem., 17: 778
94. Fishman,J., Roffwarg,H. and Hellman,L. (1973): J.Pharmac.
    Exp.Ther., 187: 575
95. Flynn, E.J., Lynch, M. and Zannoni,V.G. (1972): Biochem .

Pharmac., 21: 2577
96. Foster, R.S., Jenden, D.J. and Lomax, P. (1967). J.Pharmac. Exp.Ther., 157: 185
97. Fouts, J.R. and Gram, T.E. (1969) : In : Microsomes and Drug Oxidations. Edited by J.R. Gillette, A.H.Conney , G.J. Cosmides, R.W. Estabrook, J.R. Fouts and G.J. Mannering, p.81, Academic Press, New York
98. Freireich, E.J., Gehan, E.A., Rall, D.P., Schmidt, L.H. and Skipper, H.E. (1966) : Cancer Chemotherapy Rep., 50: 219
99. Friedler, G. and Cochin, J. (1972) : Science, 175: 654
100. Fujimoto, J.M. (1969) : J.Pharmac.Exp.Ther., 168: 180
101. Fujimoto, J.M. (1970) : Proc.Soc.Exp.Biol.Med., 133: 317
102. Fujimoto, J.M. and Haarstad, V.B. (1969) : J.Pharmac.Exp. Ther. 165: 45
103. Fujimoto, J.M., Roerig, S., Wang, R.I.H., Chatterjie, N. and Inturrisi,C.E. (1975) : Proc.Soc.Exp.Biol.Med., 148: 443
104. Furner,R.L., Gram, T.E. and Stitzel,R.E. (1969): Biochem. Pharmac., 18: 1635
105. Gibaldi,M. and Feldman, S. (1972): Eur.J.Pharmac., 17: 323
106. Gibaldi, M. and Ferrier, D. (1974) : Drug Metab.Rev., 3 : 185
107. Gillette,J.R. (1963) : In : Progress in Drug Research, Edited by E. Jücker, 6, p.13, Birkhäuser Verlag,Basel.
108. Gillette,J.R. (1971) : Ann.N.Y. Acad.Sci., 177: 43
109. Gillette,J.R. (1973): J.Pharmacokin. Biopharm., 1: 497
110. Gillette, J.R. (1976): Fed.Proc., 35: 1142
111. Goode, P.G. (1971) : Brit.J.Pharmac., 41: 558
112. Grossman, V. and Chaloupka, Z. (1959) : Arch.Exp.Path. Pharmak., 236: 14
113. Hänninen, O. (1975) : Acta Pharmac.Toxic. , 36 Suppl.: 3
114. Hartiala, K. (1973) : Pharmac. Rev., 33: 496
115. Henderson, G.L. and Wilson, B.K. (1973) : Res.Comm.Chem. Path.Pharmac., 5: 1
116. Herz, A. and Teschemacher, H. (1971) : Adv.Drug Res., 6: 79
117. Hess,R., Herz, A. and Friedel, K. (1971): J.Pharmac.Exp. Ther., 179: 474
118. Hess , R., Stiebler, G. and Herz,A. (1972): Eur.J.Clin. Pharmac., 4: 37
119. Höllt,V. and Teschemacher, J. (1975) : Naunyn Schmiedeberg Arch.Pharmak., 288: 163
120. Horning, M.G., Butler, C.M., Nowlin, J. and Hill,R.M. (1975) Life Sci., 16: 651
121. Hug,C.C., Mellett,L.B. and Cafruny,E.J. (1965): J.Pharmac. Exp.Ther. , 150: 259
122. Hug,(Jr.),C.C. and Woods, L.A. (1963): J.Pharmac.Exp.Ther., 142: 248
123. Hui, K.S. and Roberts, M.B. (1975) : J.Pharm.Pharmac., 27: 569
124. Ingoglia, N.A. and Dole, V.P. (1970) : J.Pharmac.Exp.Ther., 175: 84
125. Inturrisi,C.E.and Verebey,K. (1972): Clin.Pharmac.Ther.,

13: 633

126. Inturrisi,C.E. and Verebey,K. (1972) : Clin.Pharmac. Ther., 13: 923

127. James, S.P., Pugh, G.C. and Wang, R.H. (1974) :Xenobiotica 4: 521

128. Jenner, P. and Testa,B. (1974) : Drug Metab.Rev.,2: 117

129. Jóhannesson, T. and Milthers,K. (1962) : Acta Pharmac. Toxicol.,29: 241

130. Jóhannesson, T., Rogers, L.A., Fouts, J.R. and Woods,L.A. (1965) : Acta Pharmac. Toxic., 22: 107

131. Jondorf,W.R., Maickel, R.P. and Brodie, B.B. (1959) : Biochem. Pharmac.,1: 353

132. Josting, D., Winne,D. and Bock, K.W. (1976): Biochem. Pharmac. , 25: 613

133. Kaiko,R.F. and Inturrisi,C.E. (1973): J.Chromat., 82:312

134. Kaiko,R.F. and Inturrisi,C.E. (1975): Clin.Pharmac.Ther., 18:96

135. Kamm,J.J., Taddeo, A.B. and Van Loon, E.J. (1967) : J. Pharmac.Exp.Ther., 158:437

136. Kato, R. (1974) : Drug Metab.Rev., 3: 1

137. Kato,R. and Gillette J.R. (1965) : J.Pharmac.Exp.Ther., 150:285

138. Kaufman, J.J., Semo, N.M. and Kosci, W.S. (1975): J.Med. Chem., 18: 647

139. Khavari,K.A. , Peters, T.C., Baity, P.L. and Wilson, A.S. (1975): Pharmac.Biochem.Behav., 3: 1093

140. Klotz,U., McHorse,T.S., Wilkinson,G.R. and Schenker,S. (1974) : Clin.Pharmac.Ther., 16: 667

141. Klutch,A. (1974): Drug Metab.Disp., 2: 23

142. Kreek,M.J., Garfield,J.W., Gutjahr,C.L. and Giusti,L.M. (1976) : New Eng.J.Med., 294: 1104

143. Kundstadter,R.H., Klein, R.I., Lundeen, E.G.,Witz ,W. and Morrison, M. (1958) : J.Amer.Med.Assoc., 168: 1008

144. Kupferberg,H.J. and Way, E.L. (1963) : J.Pharmac.Exp.Ther. 141: 105

145. Levine,R.R. and Pelikan,E.W. (1964) : Ann.Rev.Pharmac., 4: 69

146. Lindberg,C., Bogentoft,C., Bondesson,U. and Danielsson B. (1975) : J.Pharm.Pharmac., 27: 975

147. Liu, S.J. and Wang, R.I.H. (1975) : J.Pharmac.Exp.Ther. , 195: 94

148. Lomax,P. (1966) : Experientia, 22: 249

149. Lynn, R.K.,Smith,R.,Olsen, G.D., Leger, R.M. and Gerber,N. (1975): Fed.Proc.,34: 711

150. Maggiolo, C. and Huidobro, F. (1961) : Acta Physiol.Latino Amer.,11: 70

151. Mandel, H.G. (1971) : In : Drug Disposition and Drug Metabolism, p. 149,Williams and Wilkins, Baltimore

152. March, C.H. and Elliott,H.W. (1954) : Proc.Soc.Exp.Biol.Med. 86: 494

153. Martin, W.R. and Sandquist,V.L. (1974): Arch.Gen.Psychiat.

30: 31
154. Martin, W.R., Wikler,A., Eades, C.G. and Pescor,F.T.(1963): Psychopharmacologia, 4: 247
155. Masten,L.W., Peterson, G.R.,Burkhalter, A. and Way,E.L. (1975): Nature (Lond.),253: 200
156. Mather,L.E. and Tucker, G.T. (1974): J.Pharm.Sci., 63: 306
157. Mather,L.E., Tucker, G.T., Pflug,A.E., Lindop, M.J. and Wilkerson,C. (1975): Clin.Pharmac.Ther., 17: 21
158. Mayer, M.E. and Guttman, D.E. (1968) : J.Pharm.Sci., 57: 895
159. McHorse, T.S., Wilkinson, G.R.,Johnson,R.F. and Schenker,S. (1975): Gastroenterology, 68 : 775
160. McMahon, R.E.(1961) : J.Med.Pharm.Chem., 4: 67
161. McMahon, R.E. (1966) : J.Pharm.Sci., 55: 457
162. McMahon,R.E., Culp,H.W. and Marshall,F.J.(1965):J.Pharmac. Exp.Ther., 149: 436
163. McMahon, R.E., Ridolfo, A.S., Culp, H.W., Wolen, R.L. and Marshall, F.J. (1971) : Toxicol.Appl.Pharmac., 19: 427
164. McMahon,R.E., Sullivan, H.R., Due, S.L. and Marshall, F.J. (1973) : Life Sciences, 12: 463
165. McMillan, D.E., Waddell, F.B. and Cathcart, C.F. (1974) : J.Pharmac.Exp.Ther., 190 : 416
166. Mellett,L.B. (1969) : In : Progress in Drug Research, Edited by E.Jücker, 13: 136, Birkhäuser Verlag,Basel
167. Mellett,L.B. and Woods, L.A. (1961) : Proc.Soc.Exp.Biol.Med. 106: 221
168. Mellett,L.B. and Woods, L.A. (1963): In : Progress in Drug Research, Edited by E.Jücker, 5: 157,Birkhäuser Verlag, Basel
169. Milthers, K. (1962): Nature (Lond.), 195: 607
170. Mirkin,B.L. (1975) : Anesthesiology, 43: 156
171. Misra,A.L. (1972): In : Chemical and Biological Aspects of Drug Dependence . Edited by S.J.Mulé and H.Brill, p.219, CRC Press, Cleveland, Ohio
172. Misra,A.L. (1976): In : Tissue Responses to Addictive Drugs, Edited by D.H.Ford and D.H.Clouet , p.1, Halsted Press , New York
173. Misra, A.L., Bloch, R. and Mulé,S.J. (1975) : J.Chromat. , 106: 184
174. Misra, A.L., Bloch, R., Vadlamani, N.L. and Mulé, S.J.(1974) J.Pharmac.Exp.Ther., 188: 34
175. Misra,A.L., Bloch, R., Vadlamani,N.L. and Mulé,S.J. (1975): Xenobiotica, 5: 237
176. Misra, A.L., Bloch, R., Vardy,J., Mulé, S.J. and Verebey,K. (1976). Drug Metab.Disp., 4: 276
177. Misra,A.L., Jacoby,H.I. and Woods,L.A. (1961): J.Pharmac. Exp.Ther., 132: 311
178. Misra,A.L. and Mitchell, C.L.(1971) : Biochem.Med. ,5: 379
179. Misra, A.L., Mitchell, C.L. and Woods, L.A. (1971): Nature (Lond.) , 232: 48
180. Misra,A.L. and Mulé,S.J. (1972): Nature (Lond.),238: 155
181. Misra, A.L. and Mulé,S.J.(1973): Nature(Lond.),241: 281

182. Misra,A.L. and Mulé,S.J. (1975): Amer.J.Drug and Alc.Abuse, 2: 301
183. Misra,A.L.,Mulé,S.J., Bloch, R. and Vadlamani,N.L. (1973) : J.Pharmac.Exp.Ther., 185: 287
184. Misra,A.L. , Mulé, S.J. and Woods,L.A.(1961) : J.Pharm.Exp. Ther., 132: 317
185. Misra,A.L., Pontani, R.B. and Mulé,S.J. (1973): Experientia, 29: 1108
186. Misra, A.L., Pontani, R.B. and Mulé,S.J. (1974): Xenobiotica 4: 17
187. Misra,A.L., Pontani,R.B., Vadlamani,N.L. and Mulé, S.J.(1976) J.Pharmac.Exp.Ther., 196: 257
188. Misra,A.L., Vadlamani,N.L., Bloch, R. and Mulé, S.J. (1974): Res.Comm.Chem.Path.Pharmac., 7: 1
189. Misra, A.L., Vadlamani, N.L., Pontani, R.B. and Mulé,S.J. (1973) : Biochem.Pharmac., 22: 2129
190. Misra, A.L., Vadlamani, N.L.,Pontani, R.B. and Mulé,S.J. (1974). J.Pharm.Pharmac.,26: 990
191. Misra, A.L., Vardy,J.,Bloch, R.,Mulé,S.J. and Deneau,G.A. (1976); J.Pharm.Pharmac., 28: 316
192. Misra, A.L., Yeh,S.Y. and Woods,L.A.(1970): Biochem.Pharmac. 19: 1536
193. Mitchard,M., Kendall, M.J. and Chan, K. (1972). J.Pharm. Pharmac.,24: 915.
194. Mori,M., Oguri,K., Yoshimura, H., Shimomura,K., Kamata,O. and Ueki, S. (1972): Life Sci., 11: 525
195. Mulé, S.J. (1971) : In : Narcotic Drugs,Biochemical Pharmacology. Edited by D.H.Clouet, p.99. Plenum Press, New York
196. Mulé,S.J. and Gorodetzky,C.W. (1966) : J.Pharmac.Exp.Ther. 154 : 632
197. Mushlin,B. and Cochin, J. (1974): Fed.Proc. 33: 502
198. Nash,J.F., Bennett,I.F., Bopp, R.J., Brunson, M.K. and Sullivan, H.R. (1975): J.Pharm.Sci., 64: 429
199. Nelson, E. (1961) : J.Pharm.Sci., 50: 181
200. Nichols,J.R. (1968) : Res.Publ.Ass.Nerv.Ment.Dis.,46: 299
201. Nickander,R.,Booher,R. and Miles, H. (1974) : Life Sci., 14: 2011
202. Nozaki,M.,Akera, T.,Lee, C.Y. and Brody, T.M. (1975): J. Pharm.Exp.Ther., 192: 506
203. Ober,K.F. and Fujimoto,J.M. (1972): Proc.Soc.Exp.Biol.Med. 139: 1068
204. O'Donoghue, S.E.F. (1971): Nature (Lond.),229: 125
205. O'Donoghue,S.E.F. (1974): IRCS, 2: 1476
206. O'Donoghue, S.E.F. (1975): IRCS: 3: 395
207. Olsen,G.D. (1973): Clin.Pharmac.Ther., 14: 338
208. Olsen, G.D. (1975): Clin.Pharmac.Ther., 17: 31
209. Olsen, G.D.,Bennett,W.M. and Porter, G.A. (1975): Clin. Pharmac.Ther., 17:677
210. Parke, D.V. (1968): The Biochemistry of Foreign Compounds. Pergamon Press, Oxford
211. Patrick,G.A., Dewey, W.L., Spaulding,T.C. and Harris,L.S.

(1975): J.Pharmac.Exp.Ther., 193: 876

212. Pelkonen,O.,Vorne,M.,Arvela,P., Joupilla, P. and Kärki,N. T. (1971): Scand.J.Clin.Lab.Invest., 27 suppl.: 116

213. Pert,A. and Yaksh,T. (1975): Pharmac.Biochem.Behav., 3: 133

214. Peters,M. (1975): J.Pharmac.Exp.Ther., 192: 513

215. Peterson, R.E. and Fujimoto,J.M. (1973): J.Pharmac.Exp.Ther. 184: 409

216. Pittman, K.A., Rosi,D.,Cherniak,R.,Merola, A.J. and Conway, W.D. (1969): Biochem.Pharmac., 18: 1673

217. Pohland, A., Boaz,H.E. and Sullivan, H.R. (1971): J.Med. Chem., 14: 194

218. Porter, C.C. (1957): J.Pharmac.Exp.Ther., 120: 447

219. Rance, M.J. and Shillingford, J.S. (1976): Biochem.Pharmac. 25: 735

220. Reddy, A.M., Harper, P.G. and Stern,G. (1971): Pediatrics, 48: 353

221. Robinson,A.E. and Williams, F.M. (1971): J.Pharm.Pharmac., 23: 353

222. Roerig, S., Fujimoto, J.M., Wang,R.I.H.,Pollock,S.H. and Lange,D. (1976) : Drug.Metab.Disp.,4: 53

223. Roerig,D.L., Hasegawa,A.T. and Wang, R.I.H. (1975): Biochem. Pharmac., 24: 355

224. Rowland, M. (1972): J.Pharm.Sci., 61 : 70

225. Ryan, J.J., Parker, C.W. and Williams,(Jr.),R.C. (1972): J.Lab.Clin.Med., 80: 155

226. Sanner,J.H. and Woods, L.A. (1965) : J.Pharmac.Exp.Ther., 148: 176

227. Saunders,D.R.,Paolino,R.M., Bousquet,W.S. and Miya,T.S. (1974): Proc.Soc.Exp.Biol.Med., 147: 593

228. Schanker,L.S. (1962) : Pharmac.Rev., 14: 501

229. Schaumann,O. (1960): Arch.Exp.Path.Pharmak.,239: 311, 321

230. Schuster,C.R. (1970): Fed.Proc., 29: 2

231. Schuster,L. and Hannan, R.V. (1965) : Canad.J.Biochem.,43: 899.

232. Schwope, A.D., Wise, D.L. and Howes, J.F.(1975): Life Sci. , 17: 1877

233. Scrafani ,J.T. and Clouet, D.H. (1971) : In : Narcotic Drugs, Biochemical Pharmacology , Edited by D.H.Clouet, p.137 , Plenum Press, New York

234. Shimomura,K., Komata,O., Ueki,S., Ida,S., Oguri, K. , Yoshimura, H. and Tsukamoto, H. (1971) : Tohoku.J.Exp.Med., 105: 45

235. Schnider, S.H., Way,E.L. and Lord,M.J. (1966): Anesthesiol., 27: 227

236. Shore, P.A. ,Axelrod, J., Hogben,C.A.M. and Brodie,B.B. (1955): J.Pharmac.Exp.Ther., 113: 192

237. Sladek,N.E., Choplin,M.D. and Mannering, G.J. (1974): Drug Metab.Disp., 2: 293

238. Smith, A.A., Hui, F. and Glifford,M. (1974): Ann.N.Y.Acad. Sci., 228: 338

239. Smith,R.L. (1966): Prog.Drug.Res., 9: 299

240. Spaulding,T.C., Minium,L.,Kotake,A.N. and Takemori,A.E. (1974): Drug Metab.Disp., 2: 458
241. Spector,S. (1971): J.Pharmac.Exp.Ther.,178: 253
242. Spector,S. and Parker,C.W. (1970) : Science,168 : 1347
243. Spector,S. and Vessel, E.S. (1971): Science, 174: 421
244. Stowe, C.M. and Plaa, G.L. (1968): Ann.Rev.Pharmac., 8 :337
245. Sullivan, H.R. and Due, S.L. (1973): J.Med.Chem., 16: 909
246. Sullivan, H.R., Due, S.L. and McMahon, R.E. (1972) : J.Am. Chem.Soc., 94: 4050
247. Sullivan, H.R., Due, S.L. and McMahon, R.E. (1973): Res. Comm.Chem.Path.Pharmac., 6:1072
248. Sullivan,H.R., Due, S.L. and McMahon, R.E. (1975) : J.Pharm. Pharmac., 27: 728
249. Sullivan, H.R., Emerson, J.L., Marshall, F.J.,Wood, P.G. and McMahon,R.E. (1974): Drug Metab.Disp.,2: 526
250. Sullivan,H.R., Emerson, J.L. and Wolen,R.L. (1974): Fed . Proc., 33: 537
251. Sung, C.Y. and Way, E.L. (1953) : J.Pharmac.Exp.Ther., 190: 244
252. Sung, C.Y. and Way, E.L. (1954): J.Pharmac.Exp.Ther., 110: 260
253. Takemori, A.E.and Glowacki, G.A. (1962): Biochem.Pharmac. 11: 867
254. Takemori,A.E. and Mannering, G.J. (1958): J.Pharmac.Exp. Ther., 123: 171
255. Teiger ,D.G. (1974) : J.Pharmac.Exp.Ther., 190: 408
256. Van Reeuven,G., Buthrie,G. and Strange,F. (1965) : Pediatrics, 36: 635
257. Verebey,K., Chedekel, M.A., Mulé,S.J. and Rosenthal,D. (1975): Res.Comm.Chem.Path.Pharmac., 12: 67
258. Verebey,K. and Inturrisi,C.E. (1974): Clin.Pharm.Ther., 15: 302
259. Verebey,K. and Mulé,S.J. (1975): Amer.J.Drug and Alc.Abuse, 2: 357
260. Verebey,K., Volavka,J.,Mulé,S.J. and Resnick, R.B. (1975) : Clin.Pharmac.Ther., 18: 180
261. Verebey,K., Volavka, J., Mulé,S.J. and Resnick, R.B.(1976): Clin.Pharmac.Ther. ,20: 315
262. Wagner, J.G. (1971): J.Pharm.Sci., 50: 359
263. Wagner,J.G. and Damiano, R.E. (1969): J.Clin.Pharmac., 8 : 102
264. Walkenstein,S.S., MacMullen, J.A., Knebel,C. and Seifter, J.(1958) : J.Am.Pharm.Assoc., 47: 20
265. Walsh,C.T., Levine, R.R., and Squires, C. (1975): Drug Metab.Disp., 3: 525
266. Watrous, W.M., May,D.G. and Fujimoto,J.M. (1970): J.Pharmac. Exp.Ther., 172: 274
267. Way,E.L. (1968): Res.Publ.Ass.Nerv.Ment.Dis., 46: 13
268. Way,E.L. (1968) : Rep.Ross Pediat.Res.Conf.,58: 66
269. Way,E.L. and Adler,T.K. (1962): World Health Organization, Geneva

270. Way,E.L., Signorotti,B.T.,March,C.H. and Peng,C.T.(1951):
     J.Pharmac.Exp.Ther., 101: 249
271. Way,E.L., Sung, C.Y. and Fujimoto,J.M. (1954): J.Pharmac.
     Exp.Ther., 110: 51
272. Weeks,J.R. and Collins, R.J. (1968): Res.Publ.Ass.Nerv.Ment.
     Dis. 46:288
273. Weiner, I.M. (1967) : Ann.Rev.Pharmac., 7: 39
274. Weinstein,S.H., Pfeffer,M., Schor, J.M., Indindoli,L. and
     Mintz,M. (1971): J.Pharm.Sci., 60: 1567
275. Weinstein,S.H., Pfeffer,M.,Schor,J.M., Franklin,L.,Mintz,M.
     and Tutko,E.R. (1973): J.Pharm.Sci., 62: 1416
276. Wilkinson, G.R. and Schenker, S. (1975): Drug Metab.Rev.,4:
     139
277. Williams , R.T. (1959): Detoxication Mechanisms, Wiley,
     New York
278. Williams, R.T., Millburn,P., and Smith,R.L. (1965):Ann.N.Y.
     Acad.Sci., 123: 110
279. Willner, K. (1963): Arzneim.Forsch. 13: 26
280. Wolen, R.L., Gruber,C.M. (Jr.),Kiplinger,G.F. and Scholz,
     N.E. (1971): Toxicol.Appl.Pharmac., 19:480
281. Woo,J.T.C., Gaff,G.A. and Fennessy,M.R. (1968): J.Pharm.
     Pharmac., 20: 763
282. Woods, L.A. (1954): J.Pharmac.Exp.Ther., 112: 158
283. Woods,L.A. (1956): Pharmac. Rev., 84: 175
284. Woods,L.A., Mellett,L.B. and Anderson,K.A. (1958): J.
     Pharmac.Exp.Ther., 124: 1
285. Woods,L.A. and Muehlenbeck ,H.E. (1957):J.Pharmac.Exp.Ther.,
     120: 52
286. Yaffe,S.J., Rane, A.,Sjöqvist,F., Boréus,L.O. and Orrenius,
     S. (1970) : Life Sci., 9: 1189
287. Yanagita, T. (1974) : Bull.Narcotics (U.N.), 25: 57
288. Yeh,S.Y. (1973): Fed.Proc., 32: 763
289. Yeh,S.Y. (1974): Experientia, 30: 265
290. Yeh,S.Y. (1975): J.Pharmac.Exp.Ther., 192: 201
291. Yeh,S.Y. (1976): Fed.Proc., 35: 469
292. Yeh,S.Y., Chernov,H.I. and Woods, L.A. (1971): J.Pharm.Sci.
     60: 469
293. Yeh,S.Y., Gorodetzky,C.W. and McQuinn,R.L. (1976): J.
     Pharmac.Exp.Ther., 196: 249
294. Yeh,S.Y. and Mitchell,C.L. (1972): Experientia, 28: 298
295. Yeh,S.Y. and Woods, L.A. (1969): J.Pharmac.Exp.Ther.,166:86
296. Yeh,S.Y. and Woods, L.A. (1970): J.Pharmac.Exp.Ther.,174: 9
297. Yeh,S.Y. and Woods,L.A. (1971): J.Pharm.Sci.,60: 148
298. Yeh,S.Y. and Woods,L.A. (1971): Arch.Int.Pharmacodyn.Ther.,
     191: 231
299. Yolles,S.,Leafe,T.D.,Woodland,J.H.R. and Meyer,F.J. (1975):
     J.Pharm.Sci.,64: 348
300. Yoshimura,H., Ida,S., Oguri,K. and Tsukamoto,H. (1973) :
     Biochem.Pharmac., 22: 1423
301. Yoshimura,H., Oguri K. and Tsukamoto,H. (1969) : Biochem.
     Pharmac.,18: 279

Factors Affecting the Action of Narcotics, edited by
M.L. Adler, L. Manara, and R. Samanin.
Raven Press, New York©1978.

N-Demethylation of Narcotics

Jack Fishman and Elliot F. Hahn

Institute for Steroid Research, Montefiore Hospital &
Medical Center, and Department of Biochemistry,Albert
Einstein College of Medicine, Bronx, N.Y.10467, U.S.A.

Excluding conjugation, N-demethylation is the
principal metabolic biotransformation of morphine and
other narcotic agents. Its presence has now been demonstrated both in vitro and in vivo in several species
including man (9,11,19,30,36,38,39,41,50).   The presence of the reaction in the latter was initially inferred from the pulmonary excretion of $^{14}CO_2$ after administration of morphine-N-$^{14}CH_3$ (15).   Actual isolation
of the product of the reaction, N-normorphine,however
was achieved only recently using new improvements in
analytical techniques (7,8,51).

The primary site of the reaction is the liver and
more specifically in the hepatic endoplasmic reticulum
(2,3).   The mechanism of N-demethylation follows the
scheme described by Gillette (20) in which a mixed
function oxygenase utilizing either cytochrome P-450
and/or cytochrome C is involved. Hydroxylation takes
place on the methyl group attached to the nitrogen and
cleavage of the aminocarbinol intermediate leads to
formaldeyde and normorphine formation (34).

$$>N-CH_3 \xrightarrow{[O]} >N-CH_2OH \longrightarrow >N-H + HCHO$$

This was clearly demonstrated by Axelrod (2,3) and
other investigators (19,47), who showed the formation
of formaldeyde during in vitro incubation with rat
liver.

The physiological and pharmacological significance
of the N-demethylation reaction and particularly its
role in the induction of tolerance and addiction has
been the subject of considerable theoretical and

experimental exploration (13,14,40,48,49). Axelrod
(3) reported that chronic morphine treatment of rats
impaired the ability of their liver microsomes to
demethylate the alkaloid. He proposed that this
reflects the mechanism of tolerance since the reduction
of the hepatic enzymatic N-demethylation in vitro
parallels the decreased pharmacological response in
vivo (4,11). This concept stimulated additional
research which produced conflicting results. Clouet
and Ratner (10) reported that there appeared to be no
relationship between the level of liver drug metabolizing enzyme and tolerance. Adler (1) also found no
difference in the pulmonary excretion of CO_2 after
chronic morphine-N-$^{14}CH_3$ administration to rats, and
the urinary excretion of normorphine metabolites in
humans both after chronic or acute morphine administration is similar (7,50).

The interest in N-demethylation as a pharmacologically important reaction stems from the hypothesis
of Beckett et al. (5). They proposed that analgesia
results when the drug binds to an appropriate receptor
surface in the CNS, and is then N-demethylated. The
presence of the N-nor compound at the receptor is an
essential requirement for analgesia and hence N-demethylation would be critical to the pharmacology of
the drug. The lower analgetic potency of normorphine
when given peripherally(35)was rationalized by its lipo-
phobic nature which does not permit ready crossing of
the blood brain barrier and indeed when given intracis-
ternally normorphine is a potent analgesic (22,25,32).
It should however be noted that the toxicity of the
nor-compound by this route shows a corresponding
increase (35). Extensive discussion of the pro and
con evidence for the above hypothesis are contained in
several review articles (40,48,49).

Recently Belleau and Morgan (6) have revived interest in the pharmacological significance of N-demethylation by presenting evidence supporting a concept of
clastic binding of narcotics to opiate receptors, in
which the process of N-demethylation participates in
conjunction with the receptor in the mechanism of
opiate action. They propose that the regiospecifically
oriented pair of electrons on the nitrogen interact
with the electrophilic receptor site leading to an

electron transfer with a resulting oxidation of the
N-methyl substituent. This concept requires that the
location of the sites of N-demethylation within the
CNS is proximal to or coincident with that of the
opiate receptor. The existence of N-demethylation in
the central nervous system has previously been inferred
by Milthers (37) who observed that in hepatectomized
rats normorphine constituted 5% of the alkaloid in the
brain while representing only 1% of the alkaloid
content in the blood. In vitro studies involving
incubation of morphine-N-$^{14}CH_3$ with rat brain slices
produced release of $^{14}CO_2$, further confirmed the presence of N-demethylation in central tissues (13).

To study N-demethylation in the CNS, and particularly to be able to detect its precise location we have
monitored the reaction by means of a novel and sensitive
double isotope technique (17). A mixture of 6-^3H
morphine (18) N-$^{14}CH_3$-morphine (Amersham/Searle) of
known isotope ratio is injected into rats, and after
sacrifice, the isotope ratio of selected tissues is
determined accurately by combustion in a tissue oxi-
dizer. N-demethylation of this mixture generates ^{14}C
containing fragments such as formaldeyde and ultimately
CO_2 originating from the N-methyl group, while the
N-nor products of the reaction contain only ^3H. The
former are dissipated from the site of reaction much
more rapidly than the latter, so that an increase in
the ratio of ^3H to ^{14}C in a specific tissue would serve
to indicate the presence, and also the extent, of any
in situ N-demethylation. The results of a series of
such experiments using various dosage levels and dura-
tions are listed in Table 1. The liver is known to be
a site of N-demethylation (2) and in each study this
organ exhibits a ^3H to ^{14}C isotope ratio significantly
greater than that found in the blood, and serves to
confirm the validity of the method. Of the other tissues examined, only the hypothalamus, medial thalamus,
and corpus striatum showed similar increases in isotope
ratio (i.e. contained a ^3H to ^{14}C ratio significantly
greater than that found in the blood), indicating that
some of the administered morphine had been N-demethylated at these sites. Conversely, none of the other
CNS tissues listed in Table 1 had a ^3H to ^{14}C ratio
greater than that in the blood, showing that they were

TABLE 1. Rat tissue isotope ratios following subcutaneous administration of morphine
-6^3H/morphine-N-^{14}C (normalized to dose ratio = 1)

Experiment	1	2	3	4	5	6
Blood	0.89±0.02	0.92±0.05	1.06±0.04	0.92±0.02	0.88±0.01	1.02±0.07
Cerebral Cortex	0.82±0.08	0.73±0.08	0.84±0.09	0.89±0.04	0.99±0.005 p 0.001	0.85±0.11
Hypothalamus	1.04±0.07 $p < 0.001$	0.83±0.12	0.96±0.10	1.00±0.07 $p < 0.02$	1.43±0.16 $p < 0.001$	1.22±0.13 $p < 0.01$
Medial Thalamus	1.24±0.25 $p < 0.001$	0.79±0.19	0.92±0.13	0.98±0.07 N.S.	1.55±0.11 $p < 0.001$	1.40±0.23 $p < 0.01$
Corpus Striatum	1.15±0.08 $p < 0.001$	0.84±0.10	0.95±0.16	0.99±0.06 $p < 0.02$	1.48±0.10 $p < 0.001$	1.20±0.07 $p < 0.001$
Midbrain	0.83±0.04	0.69±0.07	0.87±0.04	0.91±0.07	0.89±0.07	0.86±0.10
Cerebellum	0.82±0.06	0.77±0.03	0.92±0.12	0.88±0.04	0.97±0.05	0.93±0.08
Medulla	0.88±0.04	0.82±0.08	0.95±0.10	0.97±0.07	1.03±0.09 $p < 0.02$	0.97±0.11
Liver	1.20±0.07 $p < 0.001$	1.23±0.04 $p < 0.001$	1.45±0.16	1.25±0.09 $p < 0.001$	1.10±0.06 $p < 0.001$	1.21±0.05 $p < 0.001$

The recorded isotope ratios are the average of six male Sprague-Dawley rats weighing ~250 gm used in
each study. Significance (to blood) was calculated by Student's t test (46). Animals were sacrificed
by cervical fracture, and CNS dissection was carried out as described by Glowinski and Iversen(21).
In experiments 1,2,3 and 6 animals were sacrificed 30 min after injection;in 4 after 60 min;in 5 after
15 min. Doses : 1 -2.5 mg morphine/rat, 2-0.2 mg morphine/rat, 3-0.02 morphine/rat,4 and 5-2.5mg
morphine/rat,6-2.5mg morphine/rat +0.1 mg naloxone/rat.

not sites of N-demethylation. This evidence need not
be exclusive, since further dissection of other brain
areas might provide fraction(s) with disproportionate
isotope ratios which were masked by the isotope
contents of the larger section employed in this work.

The results in experiment 1 were obtained after
administration of a pharmacological dose of morphine
(10 mg/kg). In experiment 2 and 3, a tracer and a
subpharmacological dose respectively were used. The
liver continued to exhibit clear evidence of N-demethylation in both studies; however no indication of this
biotransformation was found in any area of the CNS.
The failure to observe isotope ratio differences in
the central tissues in these latter experiments is not
due to insufficient sensitivity of detection, since
the amount of radioactivity present in the various
brain areas is comparable with that in experiment 1
even though they may contain less morphine. This suggests that N-demethylation in the CNS occurs only
when a pharmacological concentration of substrate is
present, which tends to confirm the pharmacological
significance of the reaction. Alternatively, it is
possible that morphine is also demethylated centrally
when low doses are administered, but that the smaller
amounts of N-nor metabolites that result are lost from
the sites of reaction prior to sacrifice at 30 min.
The loss of both isotopes would of course produce no
change in the isotope ratio.

To assess the effect of time on N-demethylation in
specific tissues, experiments in which the animals were
killed 60 minutes (experiment 4) and 15 minutes
(experiment 5) after injection were carried out. In
experiment 4 there is considerably less evidence for
N-demethylation in the hypothalamus, medial thalamus,
and corpus striatum, presumably due to the greater loss
of the N-nor compounds containing tritium from the site
of the reaction during the longer time period. In
contrast, in experiment 5 after the shorter interval
these central areas show clear and undiminished
evidence of isotope disproportionation. In fact, both
the cerebral cortex and medulla now contain isotope
ratios significantly greater than that in the blood.
In both experiments however, the ^3H to ^{14}C ratios in
the liver are not affected by the change in time, sug-

gesting either a continuing reaction or a greater
retention time of the N-demethylated products in this
organ.

An alternative explanation may be suggested for the
observed isotope ratio changes in specific central
tissues. It is possible that they result from preferential uptake of N-demethylated compounds originating
in the liver and the changes may therefore not be due
to in situ N-demethylation of the $6-{}^3H$ morphine and
$N-{}^{14}CH_3$-morphine mixture in the brain. Several lines
of evidence argue against this interpretation.
Normorphine and presumably other N-demethylated metabolites cross the blood-brain barrier less effectively than the corresponding N-methyl compounds (23,42),
and this would lead to isotope ratio changes which
would be the reverse of those observed. Furthermore,
in studies to be discussed later in this review in
which N-demethylation in the liver is eliminated,
isotope ratio changes are still observed in the CNS.

The above provides proof that the N-demethylation
of morphine in the brain of the rat is localized in
specific areas which include the hypothalamus, medial
thalamus, and corpus striatum. Previous reports have
shown that these are sites that contain a relatively
high concentration of the opiate receptor (24,31,43,44).
Similarly, tissues that were described as deficient in
opiate receptors such as the cerebellum showed no
evidence of N-demethylation. Therefore, the sites of
this biotransformation examined in this work and the
areas which contain the opiate receptor appear to
coincide, and this tends to support the hypothesis
that the receptor-mediated mechanism of opiate action
involves N-demethylation.

The results of a study in which a pharmacological
dose of naloxone was co-administered with the morphine
are listed in experiment 6. The data show that neither
in the CNS nor in the liver were there any clear changes
in morphine N-demethylation which were induced by the
presence of the antagonist. This suggests that the
reaction is either not pharmacologically significant,
or that the antagonist interferes with the biological
processes subsequent to N-demethylation of the agonist.
Alternatively, the antagonist may affect either the
time scale or quantitative aspects of N-demethylation

in a manner which was not detected within the experimental conditions that were employed.

A modification of the above double isotope
technique was also used to study the N-demethylation
of morphine in vivo in man. A mixture of morphine-6^{3}H
(18) and morphine-N-^{14}CH$_3$ was administered to one male
opiate addict and to one normal male control. Urines
were collected at intervals and their isotope content
was determined, with an increase in the ^{3}H to ^{14}C ratio
considered evidence of N-demethylation. The principal
advantage of this method over the previously employed
monitoring of ^{14}CO$_2$ exhalation after morphine-N-^{14}CH$_3$
(1) administration is that the latter may include
transformations which are the result of other degrada-
tions of the molecule besides N-demethylation while in
the present method the ^{3}H labelled morphine serves as
a constant standard. Table 2 lists the isotope ratios
of the sequential urine collections and the calculated
percentage of N-demethylation. The data show that
there is only a slight difference in the total percentage of N-demethylation in the two subjects. The
pattern of urinary excretion of N-nor metabolites however differs in the two studies. In normal subject HS,
the first urine collection already shows an elevated
isotope ratio and these values remain higher than the
corresponding ones of opiate dependent subject AO
through the first 24 hr. After this time they drop
off more rapidly than those of the addicted subject.
In both cases though, the relative percentage of N-
nor metabolites is greatest in the 6-12 hr urine collections. Our results for the total percentage of
N-demethylation are slightly higher than those
previously reported (7,51), but this may arise from
the different sensitivities of the methods employed to
measure the demethylated compounds, or may be due to
metabolic variations in different subjects.

The earlier studies of Axelrod (3) and others (16,
28,29), already demonstrated a difference in the ability of liver microsomes from male and female rats to
N-demethylate morphine. These have been construed as
representing differences in the activities of liver
microsomal enzymes, which appear only after the animals
reach sexual maturity (12,26). These differences
reside primarily in higher binding capacity of the

TABLE 2. Urinary isotope ratios (^{3}H/^{14}C) following administration of morphine-6-^{3}H and morphine-N-^{14}CH$_3$

Subject	AO Ratio	% Difference from dose	HS Ratio	% Difference from dose
Dose	1.76		1.76	
Urine Collection				
0-6 hr	1.79	1.7	1.92	9.1
6-12	1.99	13.1	2.06	17.0
12-18	1.90	7.9	1.99	13.1
18-24	1.96	11.4	1.98	12.5
24-48	1.96	11.4	1.84	4.5
48-72	1.72	--	1.88	6.8
Combined	1.91	8.5	1.94	10.5

cytochrome P-450 in male rats which is then reflected in greater activity (27). Androgenic steroids have been reported to reverse the decrease in this binding capacity occasioned by castration (19,45), although the mechanism of this hormonal action is unknown. Prompted by these studies and by additional reports (33,52) that morphine metabolism is affected by sex and gonadotrophic hormones, we have investigated the problem using the double isotope N-demethylation procedure and have extended the investigation to include brain N-demethylation.

Previous studies (3,19,45) have focused mainly on the liver, where measurable amounts of HCHO of CO_2 (labelled or unlabelled) are formed. In the brain, the small number of these molecules produced could not be detected. Use of the double isotope procedure avoids this difficulty and permits a sensitive assessment of the effect of sex and endocrinological status on this biotransformation in the liver and CNS.

The observed isotope ratios in a series of such experiments are listed in Table 3. The liver is a known site of N-demethylation in sexually mature male rats (2), and in experiment 1 this tissue indeed contains a ^{3}H to ^{14}C ratio significantly greater ($p < 0.001$) than that of the blood. In contrast, the relative ^{3}H to ^{14}C content of the liver of castrated male rats (experiment 2) is not significantly higher than that of the blood, suggesting that castration in males markedly reduces N-demethylation of morphine by this organ. Similarly, using intact (experiment 3) and ovariectomized (experiment 4) female rats, the isotope ratios in the liver are not significantly different from those of the blood, suggesting that in general the ability of this tissue to N-demethylate morphine is greatly diminished in the female rat. The data in Table 1 also indicate that the value of the isotope ratio in the blood differs substantially from that of the dose only in experiment 1. Since the release of the ^{14}C containing fragment into the blood exceeds that of the ^{3}H-N-nor compounds, a decrease in the ^{3}H to ^{14}C ratio in the blood is consistent with extensive N-demethylation. The failure to observe this isotope ratio change in the other experiments, is then also a consequence of the absence of N-demethylation in the

TABLE 3. Rat tissue isotope ratios following subcutaneous administration of morphine-6-^{3}H and morphine-N-^{14}CH$_3$ (normalized to dose ratio = **1**)

Experiment	1	2	3	4
Blood	0.88	1.00	1.01	1.01
Cerebral Cortex	0.86	0.97	1.04	0.92
Hypothalamus	1.00	1.37	1.27	1.15
Medial Thalamus	1.12	1.95	1.47	1.34
Corpus Striatum	1.15	1.58	1.26	1.20
Midbrain	0.85	1.06	0.95	0.93
Cerebellum	0.80	0.96	0.96	0.95
Medulla	0.86	1.04	1.04	1.02
Liver	1.19	1.03	1.04	1.07

The isotope ratios are the average of six rats (200-250 gm) used in each study. The ratios are recorded as ^{3}H/^{14}C with 10 mg/**kg** morphine administered to each rat. Castrated rats were used 30 days post-castration. Exp.(**1**) Intact males. Exp.(**2**) Castrated males. Exp.(**3**) Intact females. Exp.(**4**) Castrated females.

livers of these animals within the time span of these
studies. The observed changes in the metabolism of
morphine in the liver produced by castration, and the
differences between the intact sexes suggest the
participation of male gonadal hormones in the biotransformation of morphine. Our data are in agreement
with in vitro reports that the ability of female rat
liver to N-demethylate morphine is lower than that of
males (16,26). These and other studies also support
the suggestion that the changes are androgen related,
since testosterone therapy has been shown to increase
N-demethylase activity in both castrated male and
female rats, and in intact females (19,45).

The increase in the liver ^{3}H to ^{14}C ratio in
experiment 1, is also apparent in specific areas of the
CNS of intact male rats. These tissues, which include
the hypothalamus, corpus striatum and medial thalamus,
have a ^{3}H to ^{14}C ratio significantly greater (p < 0.001)
than that of the blood, suggesting the occurrence of
N-demethylation at these sites. As previously noted,
even though none of the other central tissues examined
showed comparable changes in isotope ratio, further
dissociation of these areas may yield sites with
isotope disproportionation that was not evident in the
present study due to masking by the greater isotope
content of the larger brain sections. The present work
clearly demonstrates that the N-nor compounds formed in
the liver are not transferred into the brain, since in
experiments 2,3 and 4, the CNS isotope ratio changes
are still observed, while the liver shows virtually no
evidence of N-demethylation. Castration in fact appears to increase this biotransformation in the central
nervous system, while causing a diminution of N-
demethylation in the liver. Furthermore,the relative
amount of N-demethylation in specific CNS areas appears to be increased in intact females and castrated
animals of either sex, when compared to that occurring
in intact male rats.

The current state of knowledge of the N-demethylation of morphine and morphine-like compounds does not
allow for any firm conclusions as to its significance.
Recent results concerned with this biotransformation,
however, suggest strongly that the importance of this
reaction extends beyond normal metabolic considerations

and that the original hypotheses as to its pharmacological significance deserve reconsideration and reexamination.

ACKNOWLEDGEMENT

We thank the National Institute on Drug Abuse (Grant DA 00134) for financial support, and Mrs. B. Norton for expert technical assistance.

REFERENCES

1. Adler, T.K. (1967): J.Pharmacol. Exp. Ther., 156: 585.
2. Axelrod, J. (1956): Science, 124: 263.
3. Axelrod, J.,(1956): J.Pharmacol. Exp.Ther., 117: 322.
4. Axelrod, J., and Cochin, J. (1957): J. Pharmacol. Exp.Ther., 121: 107.
5. Beckett, A.H., Casy, A.F., and Harper, N.J. (1956): J. Pharm Pharmacol., 8: 874.
6. Belleau, B., and Morgan, P. (1974): J. Med. Chem., 17: 908.
7. Boerner, U., Abbott, S., and Roe, R.L. (1975): Drug Metab. Rev., 4: 39.
8. Boerner, U., Roe, R.L., and Becker, C.E. (1974): J.Pharm. Pharmacol., 26: 393.
9. Brunk, S.F., and Delle, M. (1974): Clin. Pharmacol. Ther., 16: 51.
10. Clouet, D.H., and Ratner, M. (1964): J. Pharmacol. Exp. Ther., 144: 362.
11. Cochin, J., and Axelrod, J. (1959): J. Pharmacol. Exp. Ther., 125: 105.
12. Conney, H.R. (1967): Pharmacol.Rev., 19: 317.
13. Elison, C., and Elliott, H.W. (1963): Biochem. Pharmacol., 12: 1363.
14. Elison, C., Elliott, H.W., Look, M., and Rapoport, H. (1963): J.Med.Chem., 6: 237.
15. Elliott, H.W., Tolbert, B.M., Adler, T.K., and Anderson, H.H. (1954): Proc.Soc.Exp.Biol.Med., 85: 77.
16. ElMasry, S.E.D., and Mannering, G.J. (1974): Drug Metab. Disposition, 2: 279.

17. Fishman, J., Hahn, E.F., and Norton, B.I. (1976):
    Nature, 261: 64.
18. Fishman, J., Norton, B.I., Cotter, M.L., and Hahn,
    E.F. (1974): J.Med.Chem., 17: 778.
19. Franklin, M. (1965): Can. J.Biochem., 43: 1053.
20. Gillette, J.R. (1971): Ann. N.Y. Acad. Sci.,179:43.
21. Glowinski, J. (1966): J. Neurochem., 13: 655.
22. Harlington, M., and Lockett, M.F. (1959):
    J.Pharm.Pharmacol., 11: 415.
23. Herz, A., and Teschemacher, H.J. (1971): Adv. Drug.
    Res., 6: 79.
24. Hiller, J.M., Pearson, J., and Simon, E.J. (1973):
    Res.Commun.Chem.Pathol.Pharmacol., 6: 1052.
25. Johannesson, T., and Milthers, K. (1962): Acta
    Pharmacol.Toxicol., 19: 241.
26. Kato, R. (1974): Drug. Metab. Rev., 3: 1.
27. Kato, R., Chiesara, E., and Frontino, G.(1962):
    Biochem. Pharmacol., 11: 221.
28. Kato, R., and Gillette, J.R. (1965): J. Pharmacol.
    Exp. Ther., 150: 285.
29. Kato, R., Takahashi, A., Ohshima, T., and Hosoya,
    E. (1970): J. Pharmacol. Exp. Ther., 174: 211.
30. Klutch, A. (1974): Drug Metab.Disposition, 2: 23.
31. Kuhar, M.J., Pert, C.B., and Snyder, S.H. (1973):
    Nature, 245: 447.
32. Lockett, M.F., and Davis, M.M. (1958): J.Pharm.
    Pharmacol., 10: 80.
33. March, C.H., and Elliott, H.W. (1954): Proc. Soc.
    Exp. Biol. Med., 86: 494.
34. McMahon, R.E. (1966): J. Pharm. Sci., 55: 457.
35. Miller, J.W., and Anderson, H.H. (1954):
    J.Pharmacol.Exp.Ther., 112: 191.
36. Milthers, K. (1962): Nature, 195: 607.
37. Milthers, K. (1962): Acta Pharmacol. Toxicol., 19:
    235.
38. Misra, A.L., Mule, S.J., and Wood, L.A. (1961):
    Nature, 190: 82.
39. Misra, A.L., Mule, S.J., and Woods, L.A. (1961):
    J. Pharmacol. Exp. Ther., 132: 317.
40. Mule, S.J. (1969): In: The Scientific Basis of Drug
    Dependence, edited by H. Steinberg, p. 97.
    Churchill, London.
41. Oguri, K., Ida, S., Yoshimura, H., and Tsukamoto,
    H. (1970): Chem.Pharm.Bull.(Japan), 18: 2414.

42. Oldendorf, W.H. (1974): In: Narcotics and the Hypothalamus, edited by E. Zimmerman and R. George, p. 213. Raven Press, New York.

43. Pert, C.B., and Snyder, S.H. (1973): Science, 179: 1011.

44. Simon, E.J., Hiller, J.M., and Edelman, I. (1973): Proc. Natl. Acad. Sci.U.S.A., 70: 1947.

45. Sladek, N.E., Chaplin, M.D., and Mannering, G.J. (1974): Drug Metab. Disposition, 2: 293.

46. Snedecor, G.W., and Cochran, W.G. (1967): Statistical Methods, 6th ed., Iowa University Press, Ames.

47. Thompson, J.A., and Holtzman, J.L. (1973): J. Pharmacol. Exp. Ther. 186: 640.

48. Way, E.L. (1968): Res. Publ. Assoc. Nerv. Ment.Dis. 46: 13.

49. Way, E.L., and Adler, T.K. (1960): Pharmacol. Rev. 12: 383.

50. Yeh, S.Y. (1975): J. Pharmacol. Exp. Ther., 192: 201.

51. Yeh, S.Y., Gorodetzky, C.W., and McQuinn, R.L. (1976): J. Pharmacol. Exp. Ther. 196: 249.

52. Yeh, S.Y., and Woods, L.A. (1971): Proc. Soc. Exp. Biol. Med. 150: 285.

Factors Affecting the Action of Narcotics, edited by
M.L. Adler, L. Manara, and R. Samanin.
Raven Press, New York©1978.

The Metabolism of Opiates by the Gut

Michael J. Rance and John S. Shillingford[*]

Drug Metabolism Department
Reckitt and Colman Pharmaceutical Division
Dansom Lane
Hull, HU8 7DS U.K.

INTRODUCTION

To interact with the receptors responsible for opiate
actions, an analgesic drug has to gain access to the
central nervous system by crossing the blood-brain
barrier. The availability of any such agent for entry
to the site of action is dependent upon the concentration of the drug which reaches the peripheral circulation,
which is, in turn, a function of the rate and comple-
teness of drug mobilisation from its site of administration. Hence, for any particular drug, intravenous
injection represents the most efficient means of
achieving the required receptor occupation in the clinical situation. In contrast, a drug administered orally
in a solid formulation has to overcome possible dissolution problems ,cross the intestinal barrier and survive
a passage through the liver before it becomes available
for entry into the central nervous system. In consequence,
oral administration of a drug often leads to a slower
onset and a lower peak level of activity than would have
been obtained with a similar dose given parenterally.
A relative lack of oral activity has often been a
problem associated with strong analgesics and has been
demonstrated in clinical, pharmacological and pharmacokinetic studies with many drugs. In pharmacokinetic
terms, the problem of lowered availability of morphine
after oral administration in man has been elegantly
illustrated by Brunk and Delle (4) who showed that plasma
levels of unmetabolised morphine following an oral dose
were an order of magnitude lower than those obtained
after the same dose administered by three different
parenteral routes (Fig.1). It has been postulated that
the low oral efficacy of morphine is due to poor absorption

[*] Present Address : Drug Metabolism Dept.,
                      Allen and Hanbury Research Ltd.,
                      Priory Road, WARE, Herts., U.K.

from the gastro-intestinal tract (24) but studies in both animals and man have shown this not to be so (4, 6) and it follows therefore that the low peripheral availability of morphine after oral administration is due largely to its metabolism during a "first pass" through gut wall and liver.

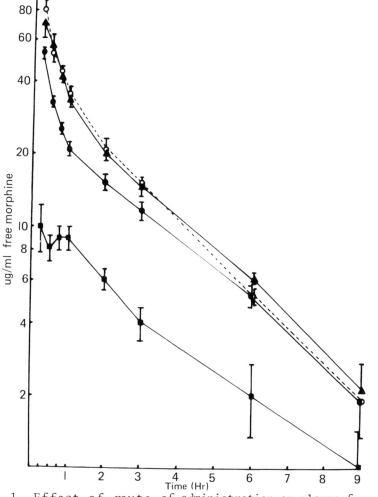

FIG. 1. Effect of route of administration on plasma free morphine levels in man. Dose for all routes was 5.75 mg/square metre body surface area. Results represent means ± S.E. (n= 6). ●——●, intravenous; ○-----○, intramuscular; ▲——▲ subcutaneous ; ■——■ oral. Reproduced with permission from Brunk and Delle (4).

The presence of a phenol function in morphine-like compounds appears to be beneficial to their activity. It is, however, this functional group which appears to be responsible for the observed first pass effect in many cases, since phase two metabolism at this site takes place very readily. In the past, the major organ of first pass metabolism has been assumed to be the liver and hepatic metabolism of opiates has been the subject of many studies which have been extensively reviewed (21, 23,24). Although the drug metabolising capacity of the intestinal mucosa has been known for many years(*), it is only recently that the role of the gut in the metabolism of opiates has been the subject of study.

Early work demonstrated the ability of the intestinal mucosa of many species to carry out a large range of biotransformations including hydroxylation (22) dealkylation (15) glucuronidation (10), sulphation (8) and acetylation (13). As conjugation reactions, together with N-dealkylation, comprise the most important metabolic processes undergone by phenolic morphine-like compounds, the extra-hepatic contribution to these processes is becoming the subject of an increasing amount of study.

CONJUGATION REACTIONS

Although Hartiala, Pulkkinen and Savola (12) carried out a full investigation of the distribution of UDP-glucuronyl transferase activity in rat using o-amino-phenol as substrate and were able to demonstrate the presence of the enzyme along the whole length of the gastrointestinal tract, it was not until recently that the synthesis of morphine-3-glucuronide by intestinal microsomes was reported (7). These workers demonstrated that though a rat intestinal microsomal preparation showed some UDP-glucuronyl transferase activity with morphine as substrate, this was considerably lower than the level found in liver (Table 1).
In contrast, p-nitrophenol was more rapidly conjugated in the intestinal preparation.

The above studies were carried out using in vitro techniques and the contribution that intestinal conjugation makes to the first pass metabolism of morphine and its surrogates in vivo remained to be determined. In 1974, Powell, Millar, Olavesen and Curtis (18) reported that phenol was subject to conjugation in rat intestine both in vivo and in an in vitro gut sac preparation, in such a way that all phenol reaching the

(*) Hartiala (11) has reviewed the early work in this area.

serosal side of the intestinal barrier was present in conjugated form. This observation prompted an examination in our laboratory of the role of the gut in the first pass metabolism of series of oripavine agonists and antagonists (Figure 2).

TABLE 1. Comparison of morphine and p-nitrophenol glucuronide synthesis by rat liver and intestinal microsomes.
Mean ± S.E. (n = 4). Data from Del Villar et al. (7).

Tissue	Rate of conjugation (nmol/mg protein/minute)	
	Morphine	p-nitrophenol
Liver	1.1 + 0.08	2.4 ± 0.4
Intestine	0.28+ 0.02	21.6 ± 1.2

Initial studies (19) showed that both ^{3}H-etorphine and ^{3}H-buprenorphine were efficiently conjugated by rat small intestine in vitro using an everted gut sac preparation (25). At low initial mucosal concentrations of drug, the efficiency of the conjugation was such that essentially all the drug-related material reaching the serosal fluid was present as glucuronide conjugates. The degree of conjugation decreased with increasing mucosal drug concentration, but remained significant at the highest concentration examined (10 μg/ml). ^{3}H-Dihydromorphine under similar conditions was subject to considerably less metabolism (Table 2).

In contrast to the oripavine derivatives (Fig. 2), dihydromorphine is hydrophilic in character and this led to speculation that lipophilicity might be an important factor in determining the efficiency with which phenols are conjugated by the intestinal mucosa. Further work (20) has yielded more evidence in support of this hypothesis. The degree of conjugation obtained in the rat small intestine everted sac preparation, was measured on the serosal side of the intestinal barrier for a total of five phenolic opiate agonists and antagonists.

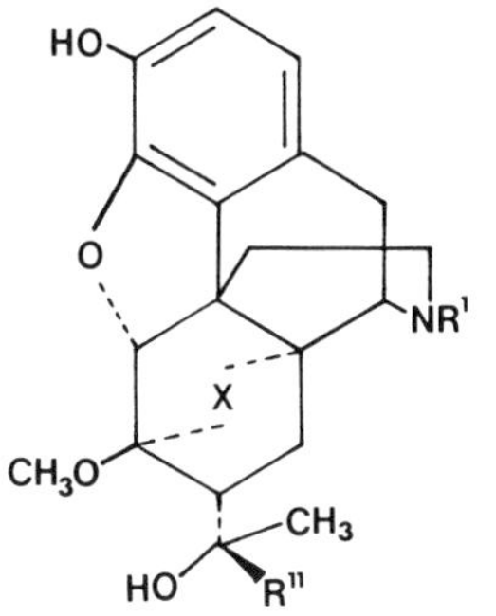

FIG. 2.

Buprenorphine	R^1= Cyclopropylmethyl, R^{11}= ^tBu,	X= $CH_2.CH_2$
Diprenorphine	R^1= Cyclopropylmethyl, R^{11}= Me,	X= $CH_2.CH_2$
Etorphine	R^1= Me, R^{11} =^nPr,	X = CH:CH

Fig. 3 demonstrates the relationship between the degree
of conjugation obtained and the partition coefficient
(N) between heptane and 0.1 M phosphate buffer (pH 7.4)
for each drug. A good correlation is found between the
degree of conjugation and Log N which is a measure of
lipophilicity. It appears therefore that the availability of opiates to the portal system is significantly
influenced by intestinal conjugation and that the
efficiency of the conjugation is a function of the lipophilicity of the drug in question.

The consequences of this detoxification system were
investigated in vivo by examination of the nature of
drug-related species found in portal blood after introduction of the labelled drugs into the in situ
cannulated small intestine of rat. As was found in
vitro, buprenorphine was efficiently metabolised at low
mucosal concentrations (1.0 µg/ml), all drug-related
material being recovered from portal blood as glucuronide

TABLE 2. In vitro absorption of $\sqrt{-3}H\sqrt{}$-buprenorphine, $\sqrt{-3}H\sqrt{}$-etorphine and $\sqrt{-3}H\sqrt{}$-dihydromorphine by a rat everted gut sac preparation. Results are means±S.E. (n = 4). Data from Rance and Shillingford (19).

D r u g	Drug luminal concentration (µg/ml)	Total drug related material absorbed (µg drug equiv/h)	Free drug absorbed %	% Dealkylation
Buprenorphine	1	0.32 + 0.04	3.4 + 0.3	11.5 + 1.8
	5	2.68 + 0.10	15.2 + 0.4	22.2 + 3.6
	10	4.25 + 0.31	20.0 + 1.9	24.6 + 1.7
Etorphine	1	0.39 + 0.07	3.3 + 0.2	-
	5	2.85 + 0.08	6.2 + 0.4	-
	10	4.25 + 0.26	30.1 + 4.3	-
Dihydromorphine	1	0.22 + 0.03	85.5 + 0.8	-
	5	1.60 + 0.11	86.8 + 2.4	-
	10	3.22 + 0.17	90.7 + 1.9	-

conjugates (Table 3). An increase in the initial mucosal drug concentration resulted in the appearance of low but detectable levels of free drug on the serosal side of the membrane. Dihydromorphine was conjugated to a greater extent in vivo than was found in the gut sac preparation, though considerable levels of free drug were detected even at low concentrations. It is interesting to note that overall absorption of the more lipophilic species, buprenorphine, was greater than that of dihydromorphine, which is consistent with classical theories of the absorption of molecules across lipid membranes.

In support of the above data, Josting, Winne and Bock (14), who had previously demonstrated the glucuronide conjugation of 1-naphthol by rat intestine (3), have shown that morphine is subjected to a considerable degree of conjugation in vivo in this organ (Table 4).

In summary, therefore, the results presented above supply good evidence for the existence of a major pathway in the gastro-intestinal tract for the metabolism of phenolic substrates and suggest that this system is

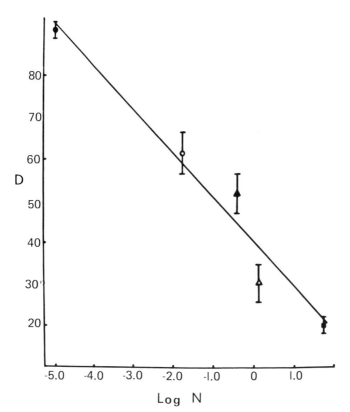

FIG. 3.   Relationship between the percentage of free —
drug absorbed   D   and partition coefficient N;(heptane/
0.1 M phosphate buffer, pH 7.4) in the rat everted gut
sac preparation at an initial luminal drug concentration
of 10 μg/ml.   Results represent means ± S.E. (n = 4).
●, dihydromorphine; ○, naloxone;   ▲, diprenorphine ;
Δ , etorphine;□, buprenorphine.
Regression equation D = 39.96 - 10.55 log N ;
r = -0.96 (p < 0.001), n= 25.
Reproduced with permission from Rance and Shillingford
(20).

TABLE 3. Portal vein plasma levels of $\sqrt{3}$H$\sqrt{\ }$-buprenorphine, $\sqrt{3}$H$\sqrt{\ }$-dihydromorphine and conjugates after absorption of the drugs from the rat isolated small intestine in situ. Results are means of 3 experiments. Ranges in parentheses. Data from Rance and Shillingford (20)

Drug concentration in small intestine [a] (μg/ml)	Time (min)	Buprenorphine		Dihydromorphine	
		Plasma level of total radioactivity (μg buprenorphine equivalent/ml)	% free drug	Plasma level of total radioactivity (μg dihydromorphine equivalent/ml)	% free drug
1.0	10	0.06 (0.04-0.07)	$-$[b]	0.014 (0.009-0.016)	41.2 (34.1-50.1)
	20	0.11 (0.09-0.14)	$-$	0.024 (0.021-0.027)	38.8 (36.4-43.4)
	30	0.12 (0.09-0.15)	$-$	0.043 (0.036-0.050)	36.7 (31.0-42.1)
	40	0.08 (0.06-0.09)	$-$	0.048 (0.039-0.052)	40.2 (33.1-42.0)
	50			0.036 (0.028-0.040)	39.9 (37.0-45.7)
10.0	10	0.37 (0.30-0.66)	10.1 (3.3-13.4)	0.034 (0.028-0.036)	41.8 (32.6-53.5)
	20	0.55 (0.45-0.73)	14.2 (8.2-20.2)	0.044 (0.040-0.048)	35.4 (27.3-42.9)
	30	0.54 (0.40-0.65)	13.5 (9.6-20.1)	0.079 (0.072-0.084)	39.9 (37.6-43.1)
	40	0.61 (0.42-0.73)	9.5 (7.8-15.0)	0.086 (0.082-0.094)	41.6 (38.0-46.7)
	50	0.55 (0.32-0.78)	9.3 (6.6-15.5)	0.094 (0.090-0.098)	40.2 (40.0-45.9)
	60				

a) Total volume introduced into the small intestine was 10.0 ml in each case

b) No free drug detected

responsible, at least in part, for the lower oral
efficacy observed with many phenolic opiate drugs.

TABLE 4.   Absorption and conjugation of morphine in the
rat in situ jejunal loop. Results are means of 3-6
experiments, ranges in parentheses.
Data from Josting, Winne and Bock (14).

Absorbed Species	% Recovery of morphine 30 min. after administration	
	Intestinal content	Venous blood[a]
Free morphine	73.9 (68.3 - 82.3)	6.9 (3.5 - 9.4)
Total conjugates[b]	5.1 (4.7 - 5.7)	6.1 (3.0 - 7.7)
Glucuronide	3.6 (3.4 - 4.1)	4.9 (2.3 - 5.8)

a)   Total venous output of isolated intestinal loop
     collected and analysed for drug and metabolites.

b)   Difference between total conjugates and glucuronide
     represents mainly sulphate ester conjugation.

N-DEALKYLATION

The N-demethylation of morphine in vivo was first
demonstrated directly by Misra, Mulé and Woods (17),
though the production of ^{14}C-carbon dioxide from morphine-
N-methyl-^{14}C had indirectly indicated this metabolic
reaction in several earlier studies. N-dealkylation
is now established as a significant route of metabolism
of narcotics and has been the subject of much study.
However, as with the conjugation reactions discussed
above, interest has been centred upon the role of the
hepatic drug metabolising systems, though dealkylations
have been demonstrated in the central nervous system
(9,16) and implicated as important to the mode of action
of narcotics (2).

Very little is known of the capacity of the intestinal mucosa for N-dealkylation of opiate substrates. The existence of ethylmorphine N-demethylase activity in intestinal microsomes from rabbit and guinea pig has been recently demonstrated (5), though these workers failed to find similar activity in rat, mouse or hamster. It was suggested, however, that the low levels of mixed-function oxidases found in rat intestinal microsomes in this study might have been due to an artefactual conversion of cytochrome P-450 to the in-active form P-420 during homogenisation.

Rance and Shillingford (19) showed the loss of the N-cyclopropylmethyl function from buprenorphine in the rat gut sac preparation discussed earlier (Table 2), though no N-demethylation of dihydromorphine or etorphine was detected. Significant N-dealkylation capacity in the gut would certainly contribute to any route depend-ency of biotransformation found with opiates and Brunk and Delle (4) have shown increased N-demethylation of morphine in man after oral administration. Evidence exists that oxidative N-dealkylation of narcotics with antagonist N-substituents, such as the allyl and cyclo-propylmethyl groups, is more facile than N-demethyla-tion. For instance, nalorphine is more rapidly deal-kylated than morphine in liver preparations (1). In-creased N-dealkylation, during a first pass through gut wall and liver after oral administration, may have particular significance with narcotic antagonist anal-gesics, as the N-alkyl function plays an important role in determining the pharmacological profile of this class of compounds.

CONCLUSIONS

It has not been the aim of this report to review exhaustively the literature with respect to metabolism of opiates by the gastro-intestinal tract. For example, the role of the intestinal flora has not been discussed. However, an attempt has been made to illustrate the important contribution made by the detoxification systems which exist in the intestinal mucosa, to the first pass metabolism of phenolic opiates.

In view of the paucity of information available concerning many areas of extra-hepatic metabolism of opiates, it is clear that this is a field in which there is considerable scope for further work. Species dif-ferences in the capacity of the gastro-intestinal tract to metabolise opiates remain to be fully elucidated and the implications of N-dealkylation, particularly of antagonist analgesics, in the gut and other extra-hepatic sites, should prove a fruitful area for further study.

REFERENCES

1. Axelrod, J., and Cochin, J. (1957):J. Pharmacol. Exp. Ther., 121:107.
2. Belleau, B., and Morgan, P. (1974) : J. Med. Chem., 17:908.
3. Bock, K.W., and Winne, D. (1975): Biochem.Pharmacol., 24:859.
4. Brunk, S.F., and Delle, M. (1975): Clin. Pharmacol. Ther., 16:51.
5. Chhabra, R.S., Pohl, R.J., and Fouts, J.R. (1974): Drug Metab. Disposition, 2:443.
6. Cochin, J., Haggart, J., Woods, L.A., and Seevers, M.H. (1954) : J. Pharmacol. Exp. Ther.,111:74.
7. Del Villar, E., Sanchez, E., and Tephly, T.R. (1974) : Drug Metab. Disposition, 2:370.
8. De Meio, R.H., and Arnoldt, R.I. (1944) : J. Biol. Chem., 156:577.
9. Fishman, J., Hahn, E.F., and Norton, B.I. (1976): Nature, 261:64.
10. Hartiala, K.J.W. (1961): Biochem. Pharmacol., 6: 82.
11. Hartiala, K.J.W. (1973): Physiol. Rev., 53:496.
12. Hartiala, K.J.W., Pulkkinen, M.O., and Savola, P. (1964) : Nature, 201:1036.
13. Hartiala, K.J.W., and Terho, T. (1965) : Nature, 205:809.
14. Josting, D., Winne, D., and Bock, K.W. (1976) : Biochem. Pharmacol., 25:613.
15. Miller, J.A., Miller, E.C., and Baumann, C.A. (1945) : Cancer. Res.,5:162.
16. Milthers, K. (1962) : Nature, 195:607.
17. Misra, A.L., Mulé, S.J.,and Woods, L.A. (1961) : Nature, 190:82.
18. Powell, G.M., Miller, J.J., Olavesen, A.H., and Curtis, C.G. (1974) : Nature, 252:234.
19. Rance, M.J., and Shillingford, J.S. (1976) : Biochem. Pharmacol., 25:735.
20. Rance, M.J., and Shillingford, J.S. (1976) : Xenobiotica, in the press.
21. Scrafani, J.T., and Clouet, D.H. (1971) : In : Narcotic Drugs-Biochemical Pharmacology, edited by D.H. Clouet, p. 137, Plenum Press, New York.
22. Wattenburg, L.W., Leong, J.L., and Strand, P.J. (1962) : Cancer Res. 22: 1120.
23. Way, E.L., and Adler, T.K. (1960) : Pharmacol. Rev., 12:383.
24. Way, E.L., and Adler, T.K. (1962): Bull. World Health Organisation, 27:359.
25. Wilson, T.H., and Wiseman, G. (1954) : J.Physiol., 123:116.

3. BIOCHEMICAL CONSIDERATIONS

Factors Affecting the Action of Narcotics, edited by
M.L. Adler, L. Manara, and R. Samanin.
Raven Press, New York©1978.

The Opioid Peptides (Endorphins):   A Progress Report

Avram Goldstein and Brian M. Cox

Addiction Research Foundation and Stanford University
Palo Alto, California 94304, U.S.A.

INTRODUCTION

Just a little over a year ago we reported the
discovery of morphine-like pharmacologic action in
peptide material obtained from pituitary extracts (4,
15). The search for an endogenous ligand for the
highly specific opiate receptors (8,13,14) had occupied
the attention of several laboratories, culminating in
the finding of two opioid pentapeptides in brain by
Hughes et al. (9,11). These peptides were eventually
identified as Tyr-Gly-Gly-Phe-Met (Met-enkephalin) and
Tyr-Gly-Gly-Phe-Leu (Leu-enkephalin) (10). Since the
sequence of Met-enkephalin is found uniquely as residues
61-65 of the pituitary peptide β-lipotropin (β-LPH)
(Fig. 1), it was supposed that enkephalin was in some
way derived from β-LPH. We showed, in collaboration
with Li (3), that the 91-residue β-LPH has no opioid
activity, whereas β-LPH-(61-91) and other fragments
starting with residue 61 have typical opioid actions
in a bioassay and in the opiate receptor binding assay.
A further line of logic led to the supposition that
the enkephalins were derived from β-LPH. No mechanisms
are known for synthesizing peptides larger than tri-
peptides in the animal kingdom, so our finding of
opioid activity in peptides of 1750 daltons and larger
suggested, a priori, that the enkephalins would prove
to be components of larger peptides.

PITUITARY ENDORPHINS

We now have a clear understanding concerning the
molecular weights of the pituitary opioid peptides (2).
These endorphins[*] exist in the native form, in beef,
pig, rat, and man, as peptides of about 3000 daltons,
i.e., approximately 30 residues. A cleavage to a
1750-dalton active fragment occurs during commercial
processing of porcine pituitary extracts (6), accompanied by a change in a critically placed Met residue,
so that although the opioid activity of the original

---

[*]Endorphin is a generic term to describe opioid peptides without designating any particular chemical
structure.

pituitary peptide is destroyed by cyanogen bromide
treatment, the residual activity in the 1750-dalton
fragment is cyanogen bromide resistant. Alternatively,
it is possible that processing concentrates a cyanogen
bromide resistant-endorphin present in the bulk extract in low concentration. The native 3000-dalton
size corresponds almost exactly to that of the
31-residue β-LPH-(61-91), and the cyanogen bromide
sensitivity is consistent with the idea that pituitary
endorphin contains Met-enkephalin. As we reported
initially (4), pituitary endorphin activity is sensitive to destruction by trypsin. Met-enkephalin has
about the same potency as the smallest active tryptic
fragment (residues 61-69). Degradation of biologic
activity by trypsin treatment means, simply, that
some residues to the right (i.e., toward the -COOH
terminus) of a basic residue must contribute to
potency, presumably by adding hydrophobic bulk in the
region of the receptor occupied by positions 6, 7,
and 8 in the morphine molecule.

We have found two major opioid components in
extracts of porcine pituitary. Both are very basic,
with isoelectric points (determined by isoelectric
focussing of the partially purified extract in sucrose)
of 10.1 and 10.6. The differing basicities of these
peaks were confirmed by chromatography on Amberlite
CG-50 cation exchange resin in sodium borate buffer.
Both of these peptides lost activity following incubation with trypsin, or after incubation with
cyanogen bromide, suggesting that they might well contain NH_2-terminal Met-enkephalin. The apparent molecular weight of the most basic of these peptides,
now almost pure, was about 3500 daltons. Thus this
peptide has many of the properties of β-LPH-(61-91),
and probably represents the major opioid peptide in
the gland. It is not yet clear whether the less basic
peptide is also related to β-LPH [perhaps β-LPH-(61-
87)], or whether it is a postmortem degradation
product of the more basic component.

The enkephalins are the smallest known peptides
with significant opioid activity. Although we think
that long peptides may mediate the physiologic
actions of the endorphins, the low potency of the
enkephalins compared with longer peptides when placed
in the cerebral ventricles or injected into the brain
(5,12) cannot be taken as evidence against a physiologic role of the pentapeptides. The good potency of
longer peptides containing enkephalin may simply reflect their protection against degradation.

BRAIN ENDORPHINS

There have also been surprises in our search for the brain endorphins. For all the reasons given above, we assumed that the native forms of the brain endorphins would prove to be peptides considerably larger than the five-residue enkephalins. In beef brain we attempted to demonstrate the presence of β-LPH, using the same fractionation procedure employed originally by Li (1) with pituitary. We treated the various peaks of ultraviolet-absorbing material with very low concentrations of trypsin, since in β-LPH, the Arg_{60}-Tyr_{61} bond can be cleaved in this way, yielding material [β-LPH-(61-91)] with opioid activity. But such treatment gave no evidence of the presence of β-LPH in brain extracts. It is not yet evident to us how the enkephalins come to be in brain, whether they are synthesized there as part of β-LPH-like longer peptides, whether they are cleaved to act on opiate receptors, or whether they are degradation artifacts produced during the isolation procedures.

We have identified an active opioid peptide of molecular weight 3000 or greater in beef and rat brain, as well as in pituitary. Chromatography on Amberlite CG-50 showed this peptide to be very basic; it also lost activity following incubation with trypsin or cyanogen bromide, and thus was similar and perhaps identical to β-LPH-(61-91). Other peptides with opioid activity have been partially purified from brain extracts. One of these, with an apparent molecular weight of 1200-1400 daltons did not lose activity following exposure to cyanogen bromide, and therefore cannot contain a critically placed methionine residue. From this standpoint, it could possibly contain Leu-enkephalin (which is known to predominate in beef brain, as contrasted to pig brain).

SUMMARY

It is clear now that the endorphins comprise a family of peptides with opioid activity (7). All interact with the opiate receptors of the guinea pig myenteric plexus to cause typical naloxone-reversible opioid effects. Peptides resembling β-LPH-(61-91) are present in porcine pituitary extracts, and in bovine and rat brain. We have shown that under some circumstances, processing of porcine pituitary extract can generate or concentrate an apparently smaller endorphin resistant to cyanogen bromide. An intermediate size, cyanogen bromide resistant endorphin was also

H-Glu—ʃʃ—Lys-Arg [-Tyr-Gly-Gly-Phe-Met] -Thr-Ser-Glu-Lys-Ser-Gln-Thr-Pro-Leu-Val-Thr— ʃʃ —Gln-OH

1   59 60   61 62 63 64 65   66 67 68 69 70 71 72 73 74 75 76   91

β-LPH

H [-Tyr-Gly-Gly-Phe-Met] -Thr-Ser-Glu-Lys-Ser-Gln-Thr-Pro-Leu-Val-Thr- ʃʃ -Gln-OH

61 62 63 64 65   66 67 68 69 70 71 72 73 74 75 76   91

β-endorphin [β-LPH-(61-91)]

H [-Tyr-Gly-Gly-Phe-Met] -Thr-Ser-Glu-Lys-Ser-Gln-Thr-Pro-Leu-Val-Thr-OH

61 62 63 64 65   66 67 68 69 70 71 72 73 74 75 76

α-endorphin [β-LPH-(61-76)]

H [-Tyr-Gly-Gly-Phe-Met] -Thr-Ser-Glu-Lys-OH   nonapeptide [β-LPH-(61-69)]

61 62 63 64 65   66 67 68 69

H [-Tyr-Gly-Gly-Phe-Met] -OH   Met-enkephalin

61 62 63 64 65

FIG. 1.   Endorphins derived from β-LPH.   The whole β-LPH molecule of 91 residues is without opioid activity.   All the fragments shown here are active endorphins.

extracted from bovine brain. The relationship of these endorphins to Leu-enkephalin remains to be established. It is intriguing to imagine that different endorphins interact in a specific manner with particular subclasses of opiate (endorphin) receptors, to mediate specific physiologic responses such as analgesia, euphoria, effects on release and inhibition of release of pituitary hormones, and so on, all of which are pharmacologic effects of the opiates.

ACKNOWLEDGEMENT

The investigations described here were supported by grants DA00972 and DA01199 from the National Institute on Drug Abuse. Significant contributions to the work were made by Drs. S. Gentleman, T.P. Su, and E. Baizman, and by M. Ross, L.I. Lowney, R. Padhya, P.J. Lowery, M. Rado, and A. Naidu.

REFERENCES

1. Birk, Y., and Li, C.H. (1964): J. Biol. Chem. 239: 1048-1052.
2. Cox, B.M., Gentleman, S., Su, T.P. and Goldstein, A. (1976): Brain Res., 115: 285-296.
3. Cox, B.M., Goldstein, A. and Li, C.H. (1976): Proc. Nat. Acad. Sci. U.S.A., 73: 1821-1823.
4. Cox, B.M., Opheim, K.E., Teschemacher, H. and Goldstein, A. (1975): Life Sci., 16: 1777-1782.
5. Feldberg, W.S. and Smyth, D.G. (1976): J. Physiol. (Lond.), 260: 30-31.
6. Gentleman, S., Ross, M., Lowney, L.I., Cox, B.M. and Goldstein, A. (1976): In: Opiates and Endogenous Opioid Peptides. edited by H.W. Kosterlitz, p. 27-34. North-Holland, Amsterdam.
7. Goldstein, A. (1976): Science, 193: 1081-1086.
8. Goldstein, A., Lowney, L.I. and Pal, B.K. (1971): Proc. Nat. Acad. Sci. U.S.A., 68: 1742-1747.
9. Hughes, J. (1975): Brain Res., 88: 295-308.
10. Hughes, J., Smith, T.W., Kosterlitz, H.W., Fothergill, L.A., Morgan, B.A. and Morris, H.R. (1975): Nature (Lond.), 258: 577-579.
11. Hughes, J., Smith, T., Morgan, B. and Fothergill, L. (1975): Life Sci., 16: 1753-1758.
12. Loh, H.H., Tseng, L.F., Wei, E. and Li, C.H. (1976): Proc. Nat. Acad. Sci. U.S.A., 73: 2895-2898.
13. Pert, C.B. and Snyder, S.H. (1973): Science, 179: 1011-1014.
14. Simon, E.J., Hiller, J.M. and Edelman, I. (1973): Proc. Nat. Acad. Sci. U.S.A., 70: 1947-1949.
15. Teschemacher, H., Opheim, K.E., Cox, B.M. and Goldstein, A. (1975): Life Sci., 16: 1771-1776.

Factors Affecting the Action of Narcotics, edited by
M.L. Adler, L. Manara, and R. Samanin.
Raven Press, New York©1978.

The Role of Brain Proteins and Peptides in Opiate Actions

Doris. H. Clouet

New York State Office of Drug Abuse Services, Testing & Research Laboratory, Brooklyn, New York, U.S.A.

HISTORICAL OVERVIEW

A requirement for protein synthesis in the central nervous system during the development of tolerance to chronic opiate exposure is suggested by the results of several diverse experimental approaches:

1) The administration of inhibitors of the synthesis of proteins or nucleic acids prolonged the time required for tolerance to develop (8 ,11 ,16,39,42, 50).

2) In morphine-treated animals, and in cells in culture, a major effect of opiate exposure was an inhibition of the rate of biosynthesis of macro-molecules (6,17,19,29,33,41,46).

3) 'Transfer factors'isolated from the brains of opiate-treated animals were able to affect opiate responses in naive animals (2,18,22,47).

4) An induction (i.e. an increase in enzyme levels) of some of the enzymes that catalyze the synthesis or metabolism of neurotransmitters has been demon-strated (5,24,25,37).

The nature of the protein synthesized during the development of tolerance has been pictured as a new species (transfer factors or antibodies) or as a protein already present (induced enzyme or 'expanded' opiate receptors in the neuronal membranes).

PRESENT STATUS

One hypothetical mechanism for the development of tolerance to chronic opiate exposure is that the number

of neuronal opiate receptors increases with drug
exposure (9,30). However, an alteration in the amount
or number of opiate receptors during the development
of tolerance has not been demonstrated experimentally
(43). The possibility that irreversible conformational
changes in receptor structure occur in tolerance is not
incompatible with the suggested receptor models (40).

The induction of enzymes involved in the regulation
of neurotransmitter availability clearly occurs during
the stress of opiate treatment. The induction of
tyrosine hydroxylase by morphine has been demonstrated
(37) as has its increase in the hypothalamus of
morphine-treated animals (5). A change in the levels
of tryptophan hydroxylase in brain synaptosomes is
produced by chronic morphine treatment (25). Adenylate
cyclase activity was increased in rat caudate nucleus
during the development of tolerance to morphine (31),
although this change in enzyme activity may reflect a
change in the sensitivity to neurohormonal influences
(24). The activity of such enzymes is modulated
constantly in a short time frame (seconds-minutes) by a
wide variety of regulators : ions, activators, end-
products, inhibitors, substrates etc. Long-term(hours-
days) changes in enzyme activity are accomplished by
such mechanisms as increased biosynthesis, decreased
catabolism, inactivation of inhibitors, sensitivity
changes, etc. These latter effects are seen in the CNS
during chronic morphine exposure and represent a part
of the biological adaptation to the continuing presence
of opiates.

An increased rate of biosynthesis in brain of the
proteins or peptides involved in the genesis of the
endorphins may play a role in the responses to acute or
chronic opiate treatment. The amino acid sequence of
the pentapeptide enkephalins (20), and of the larger
peptides isolated from hypothalamic-pituitary preparations (10,28) is found in the polypeptide hormone of
the anterior pituitary gland, β-lipotropin. In general,
the rate of biosynthesis of hypophyseal trophic
hormones is related to their release from the pituitary
(23,26), so that changes in the abundance of the
endorphins in brain might be expected to be related
to protein biosynthesis in the pituitary gland. We
offer some evidence that the rate of formation of

enkephalins in rat brain is altered by morphine treatment in the experimental section of this paper.

Effect of Peptides on the Actions of Opiates

Peptides are known to play a role in neuronal excitability (1,14,38). The possibility that some
peptides act as neurotransmitters in the CNS is supported by studies in which peptides such as TRH, somatostatin or substance P are localized in synaptosomes
(3,35) and released on nerve stimulation (12).
Enkephalin is also localized in nerve-ending particles
(34). However, there are differences between the
actions of neuropeptides and those of traditional
neurotransmitters, in particular, neuropeptides
produce long lasting effects.

Many behavioral parameters are altered by the administration of peptides, especially by the hypophyseal
trophic hormones and the hypothalamic releasing
factors. TSH produces euphoria on administration(3).
TRH and MIF have antisedative activity (32,36), while
vasopressin and some of its analogs antagonize the
amnesia induced in mice by puromycin (48). It is
pertinent to note that the administration of narcotic
analgesic drugs to man or laboratory animals has
significant effects on the release of trophic hormones
from the pituitary gland (15,51), possibly by way of
hypothalamic catecholamines (4).

Responses to morphine are altered by the simultaneous administration of peptides. An analog of vasopressin increases the analgesic response to morphine
in mice (27) while somatostatin antagonizes the
increased release of growth hormone induced by morph-
ine(13). β-MSH and ACTH $_{1-24}$ antagonize the actions of
morphine in spinal cats (51) and substance P abolishes
the abstinence syndrome (44). Some ACTH-like peptides
interact with rat brain opiate receptors in vitro (45).
It is interesting that the micro-injection of TRH into
brain areas produces shaking behavior in rats that is
similar to abstinent shaking, and that the brain areas
positive for TRH-shaking parallel the areas positive
for naloxone induced shaking in opiate tolerant
animals (49).

EXPERIMENTAL STUDIES

The incorporation in vivo of radiolabeled amino acids into enkephalin (ENK) was examined in the brains of rats treated with morphine (7). Tritiated glycine, leucine, tyrosine or methionine was injected into the CSF by way of the cisterna magna. After sacrifice by microwave irradiation, the brains of the rats were treated by batch ionic exchange chromatography, followed by high pressure liquid chromatography on cationic exchange resin (21). The amount of ENK was measured by the Fluram reaction with synthetic met-ENK as standard. Exposure to H^3-glycine for 30 minutes or 120 minutes resulted in radiolabeled ENK (Fig.1).

In the brains of rats killed two hours after H^3-glycine administration, the levels of ENK were the same as in control samples (Table 1). The specific

TABLE 1. The levels and rates of formation of enkephalin

Treatment	Levels (nmol ENK/g brain)	Rate of Formation (SR* = CPM/nmol ENK)
Control	21 ± 5	76 ± 10
Acute Morphine[a]	19 ± 4	53 ± 6
Chronic Morphine	10 ± 2	91 ± 7
Withdrawn	32 ± 4	44 ± 6

*SR = Specific Radioactivity

[a] The treatment of the animals is described in the text

radioactivity (SR) was decreased. Rats were made tolerant to morphine by the implantation of morphine pellets s.c. (75 mg morphine/pellet), followed by the injection s.c. of 60 mg/kg in the afternoon of day 4 and an injection s.c. of 100 mg/kg morphine on day 5 two hours before sacrifice of the rats. In the brains of these animals, both the levels and the SR of ENK

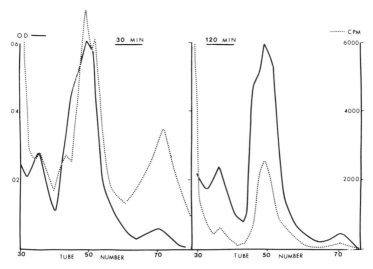

FIG. 1. The separation of a crude brain peptide
fraction by high pressure chromatography on AG-50W x4,
Na$^+$ cationic exchange resin. The solid line is the
optical density at 254 nm, the dotted line is the
radioactivity. The tube numbers for elution in 1 ml
samples are shown on the abscissa. On the left, the
rats were killed 30 minutes after the injection by way
of the cisterna magna of 100 μC of H^3-glycine/rat.
On the right, the animals were killed 120 minutes
after the injection of H^3-glycine.

were reduced. In rats made morphine-tolerant as
above, with an injection s.c. of 0.5 mg/kg of naloxone
instead of morphine on day 5, the levels of ENK were
significantly above control levels, although the SR
was lower than in control samples. Our interpretation
of these data is that the occupation of opiate
receptors (or endorphin receptors?) by morphine turns
off the formation of ENK, and that the dislodgement of
morphine by disassociation or by naloxone turns on ENK
formation. The mechanism by which ENK is synthesized
is not indicated in these experiments (i.e. whether
ENK is synthesized in brain cells on ribosomes, or
synthesized without ribosomes, or ENK is formed by
hydrolysis of prohormones synthesized in the hypo-
physis). However, these experiments do show that the
de novo biosynthesis of ENK from amino acids in the
free amino acid pool of brain is accomplished, by

whatever mechanism, in a two hour period.

ACKNOWLEDGEMENT

The experimental studies were undertaken in colla-
boration with K. Iwatsubo, M. Ratner and N.Williams.
They were supported, in part, by a research grant,
DA-00087, from the HEW National Institute on Drug
Abuse.

REFERENCES

1. Barker, J.L. (1976): Physiol.Rev., 56: 435.
2. Berkowitz, B.A., Cerretta, K.V., and Spector, S.
     (1974): Life Sci., 15: 1017.
3. Burt, D.R., and Snyder, S.H. (1975): Brain Res.,
     93: 309.
4. Clemens, J.A., and Sawyer, B.D. (1974): Endocr.
     Res.Commun., 1: 373.
5. Clouet, D.H., Johnson, J.C., Ratner, M., Williams,
     N., and Gold, G.J. (1973): In: Frontiers of
     Catecholamines Research, edited by E. Costa, and
     E. Usdin, p.1039. Pergamon Press, New York.
6. Clouet, D.H., and Ratner, M. (1967): Brain Res.,
     4: 33.
7. Clouet, D.H., and Ratner, M. (1976): In: Cellular
     Effects of Opiates, edited by H.W. Kosterlitz,
     North Holland, Amsterdam.
8. Cohen, M., Keats, A.S., Krivoy, W., and Ungar, G.
     (1965): Proc.Soc.Exp.Biol.Med., 119: 381.
9. Collier, H.O.J. (1968): Nature, 220: 228.
10.Cox, B.M., Goldstein, A., and Li, C.-H. (1976):
     Proc.Natl.Acad.Sci.USA, 73: 1821.
11.Cox, B.M., and Osman, O.H. (1969): Br.J.Pharmacol.,
     35: 373.
12.Edwardson, J.A., and Bennet, G.W. (1974): Nature,
     251: 425.
13.Ferland, L., Labrie, F., Coy, D.H., Arimura, A.,
     and Schally, A.V. (1976): Mol.Cell.Endocrinol.,
     4: 79.
14.Gent, J.P., and Wolstencroft, J.H. (1976): Nature,
     261: 426.
15.George, R. (1973): Prog. Brain Res., 39: 339.
16.Gispen, W.H., Krivoy, W.A., deWied, D., and

Zimmermann, E. (1975): <u>Life Sci.</u>, 17: 247.

17. Harris, R.A., Dunn, A., and Harris, L.S. (1974): <u>Res.Commun.Chem.Pathol.Pharmacol.</u>, 9: 299.

18. Hill, J.A., Wainer, B.H., Fitch, F.W., and Rothberg, R.M. (1973): <u>Clin.Exp.Immunol.</u>, 15: 213.

19. Hodgson, J.R., Bristow, R.L., and Castles, T.R. (1974): <u>Nature</u>, 248: 671.

20. Hughes, J., Smith, T.W., Kosterlitz, H.W., Fothergill, L.A., Morgan, B.A., and Morris, H.R. (1975): <u>Nature</u>, 258: 577.

21. Hughes, J., Smith, T., Morgan, B., and Fothergill, L. (1975): <u>Life Sci.</u>, 16: 1753.

22. Huidobro, F., and Miranda, H. (1968): <u>Biochem. Pharmacol.</u>, 17: 1099.

23. Ishikawa, H., and Goto, S. (1973): <u>Biochem.Biophys. Res.Commun.</u>, 52: 884.

24. Iwatsubo, K., and Clouet, D.H. (1975): <u>Biochem. Pharmacol.</u>, 24: 1499.

25. Knapp, S., and Mandell, A.J. (1972): <u>Science</u>, 177: 1209.

26. Koch, B., Bucher, B., and Mialhe, C. (1973): <u>Horm. Metab.Res.</u>, 5: 306.

27. Krivoy, W.A., Zimmermann, E., and Lande, S. (1974): <u>Proc.Natl.Acad.Sci. USA</u>, 71: 1852.

28. Lazarus, L.H., Ling, N., and Guillemin, R. (1976): <u>Proc.Natl.Acad.Sci.USA</u>, 73: 2156.

29. Lee, N.M., Ho, I.K., and Loh, H.H. (1975): <u>Biochem. Pharmacol.</u>, 24: 1983.

30. Martin, W.R. (1968): In: <u>The Addictive States</u>, edited by A. Wikler,, Williams and Wilkins, Baltimore.

31. Merali, Z., Tsang, B., Singhal, R.L., and Hrdina, P.D. (1976): <u>Res.Commun.Chem.Pathol.Pharmacol.</u>, 14: 29.

32. Nemeroff, C.B., Prange, A.J., Bisette, G., Lipton, M.A., and Breese, G.R. (1975): <u>Psychopharmacol. Commun.</u>, 1: 305.

33. Noteboom, W.D., and Mueller, G.C. (1969): <u>Molec. Pharmacol.</u>, 5: 38.

34. Pasternak, G.W., Goodman, R., and Snyder, S.H. (1975): <u>Life Sci.</u>, 16: 765.

35. Pelletier, G.F., Labrie, A., Arimura, A., and Schally, A.V. (1974): <u>Am.J.Anat.</u>, 140: 445.

36. Plotnikoff, N.P., and Kastin, A.J.(1976): <u>Biochem.</u>

    Pharmacol., 25: 363.

37. Reis, D.J., Rifkin, M., and Corvelli, A. (1969): Eur.J.Pharmacol., 8: 149.

38. Renaud, L.P., Martin, J.P., and Brazeau, P.(1975): Nature, 225: 233.

39. Ross, D.H., and Lynn, S.C. (1975): Biochem. Pharmacol., 24: 1135.

40. Simon,E.J., Hiller, J.M., and, Edelman, I. (1975): Science, 190: 389.

41. Simon, E.J., and Van Praag, D. (1964): Proc.Natl. Acad.Sci., 51: 877.

42. Smith, A.A., Karmin, M., and Gavitt, J. (1966): Biochem.Pharmacol., 15: 1977.

43. Snyder, S.H. (1975): Nature,257: 185.

44. Stern, P., and Hadzovic, S. (1973): Arch.Int. Pharmacodyn.Ther., 202: 259.

45. Terenius, L., Gispen, W.H., and deWied, D. (1975): Eur.J.Pharmacol., 33: 395.

46. Tulunay, F.C., and Takemori, A.K. (1975): Life Sci., 16: 551.

47. Ungar, G., and Galvan, L.(1969): Proc.Soc.Exp.Biol. Med., 130: 287.

48. Walter, R., Hoffman, P.L., Flexner, J.B., and Flexner, L.B. (1975):Proc.Natl.Acad.Sci.USA, 72: 4180.

49. Wei, E., Sigal, S., Loh, H.H., and Way, E.L.(1975): Nature, 253: 739.

50. Yamamoto, J., Inoki, R., Tamari, Y., and Iwatsubo, K. (1967): Jpn.J.Pharmacol., 17: 140.

51. Zimmermann, E., and Krivoy, W.A. (1973): Progr. Brain Res., 39: 391.

Factors Affecting the Action of Narcotics, edited by
M.L. Adler, L. Manara, and R. Samanin.
Raven Press, New York©1978.

Endogenous Peptides and Opiate Actions

H.H. Loh, L.F. Tseng, J.W. Holaday[o], and E. Wei[*]

Langley Porter Neuropsychiatric Institute
and
[o] Department of Pharmacology, University of
California, San Francisco,
Ca. 94143 USA

[*] School of Public Health, University of California
Berkeley, California 94708 USA

INTRODUCTION

The effects of a multitude of pharmacological agents
are dependent upon their physiochemical interaction with
specific receptor substances which mediate subsequent
cellular responses. This axiom holds true for endogenous compounds such as steroids, biogenic amines and
peptides. Likewise, since the turn of the century, it
has been generally recognized that many of the exogenously administered drugs also elicit their pharmacological responses through interaction with these
intrinsic receptors. Several investigators (33,37,41,
58) recently demonstrated that morphine and opiate-like
compounds are no exception to the above. These authors
have reported the presence of stereospecific binding
sites for opiates in the CNS which are possibly related
to the analgesic action of those compounds.
Since the presence of specific receptor substances
implies the existence of endogenous ligands with which
they interact, the discovery of opiate receptors has
recently evoked an exponentially increasing interest in
the presence of endogenous opiate-like compounds.
Predating this discovery, reports by Murray and Miller
(30) and Huidobro and Miranda (21) suggested that extracts from rat pituitaries and from tolerant mice
(respectively) potentiated narcotic effects. Later,
Davis and Walsh (10) suggested that in vivo condensation of biogenic amines with aldehydes may yield endogenous alkaloids that could play a role in alcohol
addiction. Collier (7), and later Goldstein (13),
proposed that a specific narcotic-like compound may
exist in neural tissue. Most recently, subsequent to
the discovery of opiate receptors in the CNS, several

investigators have reported that naloxone, a 'pure' narcotic antagonist, has an effect in opiate-naive in vitro and in vivo systems (1,22,52). Collectively, these observations strongly argue in favor of the presence of an endogenous opiate-like substance.

The search for such a substance has only recently culminated in the independent discovery of various morphine-like peptides in the CNS by several investigators. In this report, we will review the in vitro and in vivo evidence implicating enkephalins and α and β-endorphin in their role as candidates for the endogenous opiate ligand. Their relationship to β-lipotropic hormone (β-LPH), as well as other morphine-like peptides, will be discussed. The existence of endogenous antagonists to opiate effects will be reviewed to include the possible roles of adrenocorticotropic hormone (ACTH), melanocyte-stimulating hormone (MSH), thyrotropin-releasing hormone (TRH), and Substance P in modifying opiate responses. Lastly, we shall propose a possible mechanism for implicating these peptides in mechanisms of tolerance and dependence development.

I.   Endogenous Opiate Agonists

a. In Vitro Studies

Classic methods have evolved over the past few years which provide in vitro assay systems for testing substances with morphine-like activity. These include the displacement of stereospecifically bound radioactive opiates from synaptic plasma membrane (SPM) fragments (14) and bioassay in the mouse vas deferens and guinea pig ileum preparations as described by Henderson, Hughes, and Kosterlitz (17). In both procedures, steps must be taken to ensure that the effects of the putative narcotic-like compounds are opiate-specific. In particular, inhibition of ^{3}H-opiate binding to the SPM fractions must be sensitive to sodium ion (Na^+) concentration (decreased agonist binding). Also, in the case of the bioassay systems, inhibition of the electrically stimulated vas deferens or ileum by any prospective opiate substance must be reversible or blocked by the opiate antagonist, naloxone.

E. Simon first proposed the use of the term 'endorphin', a combination of endogenous and morphine, to signify any intrinsic substance with demonstrated opiate-like activity. This term is currently employed in descriptions of the endogenous peptides enkephalin, and β-endorphin.

Enkephalin was first purified from porcine brain by Hughes, Smith, Morgan, and Fothergill (20) and from bovine brain by Simantov and Snyder (35). The chemical structure of enkephalin was determined to be a mixture of 2 pentapeptides with the amino acid sequence of Tyr-Gly-Gly-Phe-Met-OH (Met-enkephalin) and Tyr-Gly-Gly-Phe-Leu-OH (Leu-enkephalin). In porcine brain, the ratio of Met-enkephalin to Leu-enkephalin is 4:1. The ratio is reversed in the bovine brain.

Both Met-enkephalin and Leu-enkephalin possess potent agonist-like activity in vitro. Enkephalin shows activity in competing for opiate binding in both SPM (44,45) and membrane preparations of rodent brains (18,32,36). A double-reciprocal analysis of the inhibition of ^{3}H-morphine binding by enkephalin indicated a classic competitive relationship (46). Also, the inhibition of ^{3}H-naloxone binding by enkephalin was influenced by cations. The IC_{50} for Met-enkephalin increased from 8 nM to 30 nM in the presence of 100 nM. In the presence of 1.0 nM Mn^{+2}, the IC_{50} decreased to 2.7 nM (35). Since enkephalin displaced ^{3}H-morphine binding 40 times better than ^{3}H-naloxone binding (3), and Na^+ and Mn^{+2} enhanced enkephalin binding, it is concluded that enkephalin has definite agonistic properties in these in vitro binding systems. Although Hughes, Smith, Kosterlitz, Fothergill, Morgan, and Morris (19) indicated that enkephalin is three times more potent than normorphine in binding studies, several other investigators report that enkephalin has only 0.2 to 0.3 times the activity of normorphine in this system (4,8,35,46).

In the bioassay systems, Hughes et al. (20) reported that both Met-enkephalin and Leu-enkephalin produced a dose-related inhibition of electrically stimulated contractions of mouse vas deferens and guinea pig ileum which could be stereospecifically reversed by opiate antagonists (19). However, others demonstrated that Met-enkephalin was only 1/3 as potent as normorphine in the guinea pig ileum (9).

Cox et al. (9) reported that a crude preparation of ACTH but not synthetic ACTH contained naloxone-reversible morphine-like activity. Hughes et al. (19) noted that the amino acid sequence of Met-enkephalin is present as residues 61-65 of β-lipotropin (β-LPH) as isolated from the pituitary gland (26). Guillemin, Ling and Burgus (15) isolated a hexadecaptide from porcine pituitary, named α-endorphin, which was observed to be identical to that of the residue 61-76 of β-LPH. Concurrently, Li and Chung (26) reported the isolation of an untriakontapeptide, named β-endorphin, also with opiate activity from camel pituirary glands. The peptide sequence of β-endorphin was determined to be identical to amino acid residues 61-91 of β-LPH.   In the guinea-pig ileum preparation, α- and β-endorphin were found to be 0.6 and 0.4 times as potent (respectively) as normorphine (8,15). β-MSH and β-LPH, at concentrations up to 10^{-6}M, were found to be inactive. Bradbury et al. (4) determined different residues of β-LPH which have opiate-like activity in the binding assay.   They found that β-endorphin was 10 times as potent as morphine or dihydromorphine in displacing specifically bound ^{3}H-naloxone, but only twice as potent as morphine in displacing ^{3}H-dihydromorphine. β-Endorphin exhibited a much smaller sodium effect. Thus β-endorphin may behave more like the antagonist naloxone than the potent agonists, morphine and levorphanol, in the binding assay.   On the other hand, the intermediate peptides of β-endorphin, sequences corresponding to residues 61-65 (Met-enkephalin),61-68, 61-69, 61-87, 61-89 of β-LPH, all had agonist-like activity, i.e. they exhibited higher potencies when assayed against ^{3}H - dihydromorphine than against ^{3}H-naloxone and had a positive sodium effect. No activity was observed with β-LPH, α-LPH (1-58), N-fragment (1-38), β-MSH (41-58 and 70-79) fragment. Generally, active fragments all contain the pentapeptide sequence of Met-enkephalin at their N-terminal. Met-enkephalin (61-65) and the intermediate peptides, 61-68, 61-69 and 61-87 were approximately 30 times less potent than β - endorphin.Moreover, potencies of two closely related peptides, β-LPH fragments 61-87 and 61-89, differed by a factor of 20, thus indicating the importance of the paired lysine residues (88 and 89) to binding affinity. It was demonstrated, in the guinea pig ileum by Sediah, Lis, Gianoulakis, Schiller and Chrétien (34) that fragment 61-82 was equipotent to Met-enkephalin, while 66-91 was completely devoid of activity.   The β-LPH (1-91) was active only at much higher concentrations (5 to 10 μM). The possibility that β-endorphin might be weakly active but requires proteolytic cleavage to yield a more active peptide is unlikely since β-LPH fragments 61-64, 61-65, 61-68, 61-69 and 66-91 were less active than β-endorphin.

b. In vivo Studies

Analgesia. Attempts to demonstrate any antinociceptive properties of enkephalin have been disappointing. Belluzzi, Grant, Garsky, Sarantakis, Wise, and Stein (2) reported that only a very high dose of Met-enkephalin (100-200 μg) injected intraventricularly produced a slight increase in the latency of the tail-

flick response in rats. The effect occurred 2-6
minutes after injection and dissipated within 10-12
minutes. A dose of 200 µg of Met-enkephalin was
required to produce an analgesic response equivalent
to 10 µg of morphine sulphate. Even so, the duration
of action was much shorter than morphine. The response
to Met-enkephalin appeared to be opiate-specific in
that it was blocked by naloxone. Similar results were
obtained by Loh, Tseng, Wei, and Li (28) in determining
the effect of Met-enkephalin on tail-flick, hot-plate,
and writing tests in mice. In those studies, 50 µg
of Met-enkephalin was only weakly analgesic upon intracerebral injection, with a duration of action of less
than 10 minutes.

Recently, the in vivo activity of β-endorphin and
some other residues of β-LPH have been studied by Loh
et al. (28). It was found that β-endorphin was a
potent antinociceptive agent when injected intracerebrally (28 and intravenously (47). β-Endorphin, at
doses of 0.2 to 1.0 µg administered centrally, produced
a dose-related increase of the tail-flick and hot-plate
latency for mice to these nociceptive stimuli, as
well as an inhibition of the writing response to
intraperitoneal injection of acetic acid. In these
three tests, the antinociceptive effects of β-endorphin
were completely blocked by the subcutaneous injection
of 1 mg/kg naloxone. The inhibitory effect of
β-endorphin on repetitive shaking movements induced
by immersion of anesthetized rats in ice water were
also studied. This experimental model, which has been
previously described in detail (55), is a sensitive
bioassay for detecting opiate activity in vivo .
β-Endorphin, injected into the periaqueductal gray
area, produced a dose-related inhibition of the shaking
response to ice water. This inhibitory effect was
readily antagonized by naloxone administration in a
dose of 5 mg/kg i.p. On a molar basis, β-endorphin was
18 to 33 times more potent than morphine sulfate.
Similar results were obtained with intravenous injection of β-endorphin in mice, with the exception that
β-endorphin was 3 to 4 times more potent than morphine
sulfate.

Since the molecular weight of β-endorphin is about
10 times higher than morphine, it is likely that the
lower potency ratio of β-endorphin as compared to
morphine when peripherally administered is due to the
relatively poorer penetration of β-endorphin into the
brain. Also, a different rate of degradation after
peripheral administration is a possible factor. It is
not likely that the β-endorphin is converted to an
active molecule which would result in the observed

antinociceptive activity, since β-LPH was at least 80 times less potent than β-endorphin. Also α-endorphin, β-LPH fragment 61-69, and the tryptic digest of β-endorphin, were found to be inactive when 40 μg, 20 μg and 10 μg per 25 g mouse were administered, respectively.

The pharmacological potencies of β-endorphin and related peptides in vivo are of interest when compared to the relative activities of these peptides in the in vitro bioassays. In the binding assay, β-endorphin was 2 to 3 times more potent, whereas enkephalin was 1/5 as potent as normorphine (8). In the in vivo study, β -endorphin was 18 to 33 times more potent than morphine, whereas Met-enkephalin was relatively inactive in the same test system.

Thus, the in vitro assays, although highly accurate in predicting the analgesic potencies of opiate alkaloids, do not appear to be quantitative estimators for the in vivo activities of opiate-like peptides.

Physical dependence. Physical dependence is generally characterized by abstinence behavior when opiate intake is abruptly terminated or when an opiate antagonist is administered (29). To find whether these opiate-like peptides can cause physical dependence, the osmotic minipump (manufactured by Alza Corp., Palo Alto, CA),a system capable of delivering a small volume of drug solution at a constant rate, was utilized to deliver β -endorphin, Met-enkephalin and morphine into the periaqueductal gray region of the rat brain for 70 hours (53). Upon challenge with naloxone, these animals infused with either β-endorphin or Met-enkephalin exhibited a withdrawal syndrome which was virtually indistinguishable from that observed with morphine.

β-Endorphin was much more potent on a molar basis than Met-enkephalin in these studies.

Cross-tolerance and the suppression of abstinence signs. The studies described previously show that β-endorphin possesses at least two classic pharmacologic properties of morphine, namely, analgesic activity and the ability to cause physical dependence. A third property is cross-tolerance with morphine and the ability to suppress the abstinence syndrome.

Waterfield, Hughes and Kosterlitz (51) were able to demonstrate cross-tolerance between morphine and Met-enkephalin in the mouse vas deferens and guinea pig ileum obtained from animals tolerant to morphine. The ID_{50} of Met-enkephalin increased from 3 to 400-fold in the guinea pig ileum from animals implanted with 2 or

TABLE 1.   Comparison of molar potency ratios among various opiate-like peptides
Potency ratio, opiate alkaloid = 1

Assay System	β-endorphin	α-endorphin	Met-enkephalin	β-LPH	Opiate alkaloid used for comparison
IN VITRO					
Binding assay:[a]					
³H-dihydromorphine	1.6	-	0.50	< 0.001	normorphine
³H-naloxone[b]	8.5	-	0.25	< 0.001	normorphine
³H-etorphine[b]	3.9	-	0.20	-	normorphine
guinea pig ileum	0.4[b]	0.600[c]	0.40[b],1.00[d]	< 0.100	normorphine
mouse vas deferens	-	-	20.00	-	normorphine
IN VIVO[e]					
Antinociception:					
Mice:					
hot plate test	17.5	< 0.045	< 0.012	-	morphine
tail flick test	33.0	< 0.056	< 0.015	-	morphine
writhing test	19.5	< 0.020	< 0.005	0.090	morphine
Rats:					
wet shake test	≤ 20.0	-	< 0.2	-	morphine
Physical dependence:					
Rats:					
chronic CNS infusion	≤ 1.0	< 0.05	< 0.05	-	morphine

a. Bradbury et al. (4); b. Cox et al. (8); c. Guillemin et al.(15); d. Hughes et al. (19) ; e. Loh et al. (28) ; Wei and Loh (53).

4 morphine pellets for 3 days. In in vivo studies, Tseng, Loh and Li (manuscript in preparation) demonstrated that the intracerebral AD_{50} of β-endorphin increased 8-fold in mice implanted with one morphine pellet for 3 days. A similar increase in the AD_{50} for morphine was also found in this study. The effects of β-endorphin on the withdrawal syndrome in morphine-dependent mice were also studied. β-Endorphin, in doses of 0.5 to 1 μg per mouse, blocked the abrupt withdrawal jumping in mice dependent on morphine. Met-enkephalin, in a dose of 200 μg per mouse, failed to affect the abrupt withdrawal jumping in this study. Collectively, these findings provide further support for a more significant in vivo role for β-endorphin than enkephalin as the true endogeneous opiate ligand.

II.   Endogenous   Opiate Antagonists

Although there is no direct demonstration of the existence of an endogenous opiate-antagonist, the discovery of such a compound could provide an attractive mechanism to explain the induction of tolerance and physical dependence by narcotic drugs. Indirect evidence which favors the existence of an antagonist-like-factor (ALF) included reports that protein synthesis inhibitors such as actinomycin D (6), puromycin (38), and cycloheximide (27) block the development of tolerance to morphine.

Ungar and Cohen (48), and later Ungar and Galvan (49), provided the first direct evidence of the existence of an ALF. These investigators described a heat stable chymotrypsin-sensitive factor which was extracted from the brains of tolerant rats. Intraperitoneal injection of this purified extract into opiate-naive animals rendered them tolerant to morphine. Biochemical evidence suggested that this 'tolerance factor' was a peptide. The significance of this finding remains unclear, however, since other workers have been unsuccessful in reproducing these results in similar animal models (39).

Substance P, a sialogogic undecapeptide present in the CNS, is also reported to modify the effects of narcotic drugs. Unfortunately, most of the available literature on the interaction between morphine and Substance P described the effects of a crude brain extract which contains a family of related peptides (see Zetler (59) for a review). At least one of these peptides antagonized morphine. In 1970, Chang and Leeman (5) isolated and characterized a single 'Substance P' from bovine hypothalami. In studies employing a synthetic version of this purified Substance P,

Stern and Hadzovic (40) found that it abolished the
abstinence syndrome in morphinized mice. However,
this result typifies the effect of an opiate agonist,
not antagonist.

In our own hands, utilizing a commercial source of
synthetic Substance P (Bachem, Inc.), we were unsuccessful in altering opiate analgesia by intracerebral or intravenous administration of doses between
0.2 and 0.8 mg/kg in mice. Furthermore, although Substance P in concentrations about 8×10^{-10}M effectively
reverses opiate induced depression of twitch height in
the stimulated guinea pig ileum preparation, we found
that those bath concentrations were equipotent in
reversing the same inhibitory effects produced by
norepinephrine and cyclic AMP. Hedqvist and von Euler
(16) also report that similar concentrations of Substance P in this assay system enhance the stimulated
concentrations of the guinea pig ileum in preparations
naive to inhibitory drugs. These arguments suggest
that if Substance P plays any role in antagonizing
narcotic effects, it is indirect and physiological.
This is further substantiated by the lack of Substance
P competition for opiate receptor binding sites (42).

The regional distribution of TRH in the brain
suggests a possible role in synaptic function (56) .
Microinjection of TRH into the periaqueductal grey area
of rat brains produced a shaking behavior similar to
that observed subsequent to naloxone precipitated withdrawal in dependent rats (54). Since this brain region
is also the principal area for morphine induced analgesia, TRH may be involved in modifying opiate action.

Krivoy, Zimmermann, and Lande (25) demonstrated that
desglycinamide[9]-Lysine vasopressin, a synthetic posterior pituitary cyclic nonapeptide which facilitates
retention of conditioned avoidance responses, also
facilitated the resistance to morphine analgesia.
Terenius, Gispen, and De Wied (43), however, found no
displacement of ^{3}H-dihydromorphine binding to synaptic
plasma membrane (SPM) fragments by this compound,
indicating little or no affinity for the opiate receptor. This result prompted them to postulate that
desglycinamide[9]-Lysine vasopressin may modulate opiate
effects by affecting some functional response of target
cells.

Early work by Winter and Flataker (57) suggested
that ACTH pretreatment antagonized the subsequent
analgesic effect of morphine. These findings were later
confirmed and refined by Paroli (31) Zimmermann and
Krivoy (60). In addition, the latter authors found
that β-MSH also antagonized morphine's effects on the
segmental reflex of the cat spinal cord (60). Recently,

Gispen, Greidanus, Ezrin, Zimmermann, Krivoy, and De
Wied (12) reported that ACTH 1-24 antagonized morphine
analgesia to electric foot-shock only in intact rats.
Adrenalectomy abolished this response; however, dexa-
methasone pretreatment in adrenalectomized animals also
antagonized morphine. They suggested that adrenal
integrity is essential for the antagonism.

The most intriguing finding in the search for an ALF
is the fact that ACTH, α-MSH, β-MSH, and β-LPH all
share a common heptapeptide sequence, namely Met-Glu-
His-Phe-Arg-Trp-Gly (subsequently referred to as ACTH
4-10). Of these four peptides,ACTH 1-24 and β-MSH
have been reported to antagonize morphine. It is
further noted that β-LPH, a 'pro' hormone for enkephalin and the more active agonist, β-endorphin, contains
the entire β-MSH peptide in β-LPH residues 41-58. This
may point to a role for β-LPH as a 'prohormone' for
both agonist and antagonist peptides and in part
explain the lack of significant effect of the intact
β-LPH peptide as an opiate agonist (28). Terenius et
al. (43) have recently demonstrated that ACTH 4-10 in
a concentration of 10^{-5} M displaces 50% of ^{3}H-dihydro-
morphine (0.8 x 10^{-9}M) from SPM opiate receptor sites,
thus adding evidence to the possible role of this
heptapeptide as an ALF.

In recent work, Ungar and Ungar (50) reported that
they had purified an antagonist factor and determined
its structure to be Arg-Tyr-Gly-Gly-Phe-Met. This
peptide, Arg-enkephalin or 'antendorphin', is likewise
found in β-LPH (amino acid 60-65). Although those
authors report in vivo antagonism of morphine by this
hexapeptide, they were unable to demonstrate in vitro
antagonism in the mouse vas deferens(50). In an
additional in vitro system, utilizing the guinea pig
ileum (our unpublished observations), Arg-enkephalin
also failed to show morphine antagonism. Furthermore,
this peptide did not precipitate an abstinence syndrome
when administered to morphine tolerant rats in our
studies. Additional work is required to see whether
this compound or modifications of this peptide may
reveal an opiate antagonist property.

DISCUSSION

In light of the in vitro and in vivo evidence
reviewed herein, the existence of an endogenous opiate
ligand seems certain. Of the several candidates reported, the family of peptides related to β-LPH is the
most thoroughly investigated. These include enkephalin,
α-endorphin, and β-endorphin, all of which have been
synthetically prepared. Furthermore, these three

TABLE 2. The amino acid sequence of ovine β –LPH

H-Glu-Leu-Thr-Gly-Glu-Arg-Leu-Glu-Gln-Ala-Arg-Gly-Pro-Glu-Ala-Gln-Ala-Glu-Ser-Ala
                                     5   10   15   20

Ala-Ala-Arg-Ala-Glu-Leu-Glu-Tyr-Gly-Leu-Val-Ala-Glu-Ala-Ala-Glu-Lys-Lys-
                25   30   35   40

β-MSH ————————————— ACTH 4-10 ——————————
Asp-Ser-Gly-Pro-Tyr-Lys-| Met-Glu-His-Phe-Arg-Trp-Gly- | Ser-Pro-Pro-Lys-Asp- | Lys-Arg-
            45   50   55   60

Enkephalin —————— α-Endorphin ———————————————————
| Tyr-Gly-Gly-Phe-Met- | Thr-Ser-Glu-Lys-Ser-Gln-Thr-Pro-Leu-Val-Thr- | Leu-Phe-Lys-Asn -
            65   70   75   80

β-Endorphin
Ala-Ile-Ile-Lys-Asn-Ala-His-Lys-Lys-Gly-Gln-OH
            85   90

related peptides subscribe to the requisite tests for opiate-like activity in the in vitro and in vivo systems yet studied, albeit with widely varying potencies.

Different potencies of these peptides have been ascribed to rapid degradation by peptidases in the in vivo preparation and bioassays. However, this explanation is untenable in view of the observed extreme in vivo potency of β-endorphin, a peptide with 31 amino acids which would presumably be more sensitive to exopeptidases, compared to enkephalin, a much smaller pentapeptide fragment (3,28). This may point to certain inadequacies of in vitro test systems presently employed as predictors of in vivo activity for these opiate-like peptides. An additional consideration is that differing secondary and tertiary structure among these endorphins could radically alter their biodisposition and explain why in vitro binding may not correlate with in vivo antinociception.

Although these peptides are reported to interact with opiate receptors, their relationship to a central issue in opiate research, namely the mechanism of tolerance and dependence induction, remains speculative.

Kosterlitz and Hughes (24), in their heuristic review on the significance of enkephalin, proposed that these endogenous peptide ligands play a role in inhibitory systems in the CNS, possibly as a neurotransmitter or modulator. Supplanting the intrinsic opiate with exogenously administered narcotic alkaloids for the purpose of enhancing this inhibition (e.g. analgesia) would de-emphasize intrinsic control in favor of the exogenous opiates. Tolerance would develop as a result of tachyphylaxis to alkaloid opiates, and increasing levels of these drugs would be required to prevent withdrawal. Furthermore, they speculated that continual stimulation of opiate receptors by exogenous ligands would result in a negative-feedback induced decrease in endogenous opiate synthesis. Lastly, withdrawal of exogenous opiates removes inhibitory dominance since endogenous opiates would be present in inadequate concentration. Excitatory systems would then be unopposed and the abstinence signs and symptoms would ensue.

The above model, however, offers no explanation for the acute tolerance phenomenon, e.g. tachyphylaxis, which is important for resolving the issue of tolerance and dependence. Simantov and Snyder (36) have also proposed that enkephalin is a putative neurotransmitter or modulator which controls inhibitory mechanisms in the CNS. In that report, they demonstrate an increase in enkephalin levels during tolerance induction, an

observation that is incompatible with the 'endogenous
agonist' hypothesis of Kosterlitz and Hughes (24), as
summarized above.

Since several peptides have been shown to antagonize
opiates, we believe that a viable alternative explanation for tolerance and dependence phenomena may be the
induction of such antagonist peptides by chronic
morphine administration. It is most tempting to speculate that β-LPH serves as a 'pro' hormone for both
agonist and antagonist peptides. The presence of ACTH
fragment 4-10 included in the β -MSH sequence of β -LPH
may serve to prevent morphine-like activity until
activation cleaves this antagonist portion from the
agonist-peptide at or near the opiate receptor. A
physiological precedence for this phenomenon is seen
with gastrointestinal peptides; e.g. trypsin converts
inactive chymotrypsinogen into the active endopeptidase,
chymotrypsin, in the intestinal lumen.

However, a pro-hormone role for β-LPH in this
proposed model would imply induction of the entire
peptide, to include both agonist and antagonist fractions, by chronic morphine administration. In this
regard, the agonist sequences appear to be unique to
β -LPH, whereas the heptapeptide antagonist-like
sequence is common to several peptides (ACTH,α-MSH,
β -MSH, and β-LPH). A non-specific induction of this
family of related antagonist sequences by chronic
morphine administration may result in a preponderance
of antagonist peptides. Withdrawal of alkaloid drugs
leaves antagonist peptides relatively unopposed in their
effects and, conversely, almost no expression of the
inhibitory tone usually provided by endorphin.

The role of opiate-antagonist peptides is, of course,
uncertain. In a recent review, George and Lomax (11)
allude to the interactions between narcotic drugs and
hypothalamo-adrenal hormones. They report that the
maximal rise in plasma glucocorticoid levels, an
indicator of ACTH secretion, temporally correlates well
with peak narcotic abstinence signs. Additionally,
plasma β-MSH was reported to be elevated by morphine
administration (23). These changes may be further
evidence to favor continued research on these interactions.

Another approach to the endogenous antagonist
issue relates to a structure-activity analysis of the
alkaloids. Addition of an allyl group on the nitrogen
of alkaloid drugs results in compounds with competitive
opiate-antagonist effects. Possibly this was the logic
behind the Arg-enkephalin antagonist reported by Ungar
and Ungar (50). We are currently pursuing the
hypothesis that such alterations of the N-terminus of

agonist peptides may result in antagonist effects.
We, like others, are most excited by the recent
advance in opiate research. The discovery of endogenous ligands has opened new vistas towards a better
understanding of the physiological mechanisms of
nociception and anti-nociception. Additionally, the
pharmacologist has been provided with a new tool with
which to attempt to shape analgesic agents with fewer
adverse effects. Ultimately, the quest for an explanation of narcotic tolerance and dependence phenomena may well be resolved as a consequence of research
brought about by this discovery.

ACKNOWLEDGEMENTS

This investigation was supported by NIDA Grant DA-
00564 and DA-00091. HHL is a recipient of a NIMH
Research Scientist Career Development Award, K2-DA-
70554.

REFERENCES

1. Akil, H., Mayer, D.J., and Liebeskind, J.C. (1975):
    Science , 191 : 961.
2. Belluzzi, J.D., Grant, N., Garsky, V., Sarantakis,
    D., Wise, C.D., and Stein, L. (1976) : Nature
    (Lond.) , 260 : 625.
3. Bradbury, A.F., Smyth, D.G., and Snell, C.R. (1976)
    Nature (Lond.),260 : 165.
4. Bradbury, A.F., Smyth, D.G., Snell, C.R., Birdsaell,
    N.J.M., and Hulme, E.C. (1976) : Nature (Lond.),
    260: 793.
5. Chang, M.M., and Leeman, S.E. (1970) : J.Biol.Chem.
    245 : 4784.
6. Cohen, M., Keats, A.S., Krivoy, W., and Ungar, G.
    (1965) : Proc. Soc. Exp. Biol. Med., 119 : 381.
7. Collier, H.O.J. (1973) : Proceedings of the 5th
    International Congress of Pharmacology, San
    Francisco, 1972, v. 1, edited by J. Cochin, p. 65,
    Karger, Basel.
8. Cox, B.M., Goldstein,A., and Li, C.H. (1976) : Proc.
    Natl. Acad. Sci. USA 73: 1821.
9. Cox, B.M., Opheim, K.E., Teschemacher, H., and
    Goldstein, A. (1975) : Life Sci. 16: 1777.
10. Davis, V.E., and Walsh, M.J. (1970) :Science , 167:
    1005.
11. George, R., and Lomax, P. (1972) : In : Chemical
    and Biological Aspects of Drug Dependence, edited
    by S.J. Mule, and H. Brill, p. 523, CRC Press,
    Cleveland.
12. Gispen, W.H., Van Wimersma Greidanus T.B.,
    Waters-Ezrin, C., Zimmermann, E., Krivoy, W.,and
    De Wied, D. (1975) : Eur .J.Pharmacol., 33 : 99.

13. Goldstein, A. (1973): In : Biological and
    Behavioral Approaches to Drug Dependence, edited
    by H. Cappel and A.E. LeBlanc, p. 217.
14. Goldstein, A., Lowney, L.I., and Pal, B.K. (1971):
    Proc. Natl. Acad. Sci. USA 68 : 1742.
15. Guillemin, R., Ling, N., and Burgus, R. (1976) :
    C.R. Acad. Sci. (Paris), 282 : 783.
16. Hedqvist, P., and von Euler, U.S. (1975) : Acta
    Physiol. Scand. 95 : 341.
17. Henderson, G., Hughes, J., and Kosterlitz, H.W.
    (1972) : Br. J. Pharmacol. , 45 : 764.
18. Hughes, J. (1975) : Brain Res., 88 : 295.

19. Hughes, J., Smith, T.W., Kosterlitz, H.W.,Fothergill,
    L.A., Morgan, B.A., and Morris, H.K. (1975) :
    Nature (Lond.) , 258 : 577.
20. Hughes, J., Smith, T., Morgan, B., and Fothergill,
    L. (1975) : Life Sci., 16 : 1753.
21. Huidobro, F., and Miranda, H. (1968) : Biochem.
    Pharmacol. , 17 : 1099.
22. Jacob, J.J., Tremblay, E.C., and Colombel, M.C.
    (1974) : Psychopharmacologia, 37 : 217.
23. Kastin, A.J., Schally, A.V., Viosea, S., and Miller,
    M.C. (1969) : Endocrinology, 84 : 20.
24. Kosterlitz, H.W., and Hughes, J. (1975) : Life Sci.
    17 : 91.
25. Krivoy, W.A., Zimmermann, E., and Lande, S. (1974):
    Proc. Natl. Acad. Sci. USA, 71 : 1852.
26. Li, C.H., and Chung, D. (1976) : Proc. Natl. Acad.
    Sci. USA, 73 : 1145.
27. Loh, H.H., Shen, F.H., and Way, E.L. (1969) :
    Biochem. Pharmacol. , 18 : 2711.
28. Loh, H.H., Tseng, L.F., Wei, E., and Li, C.H. (1976)
    Proc. Natl. Acad.Sci., 73 : 2895.
29. Martin, W.R. (1967): Pharmacol. Rev., 19 : 464.
30. Murray, W.J., and Miller, J.W. (1960) : J. Pharmacol.
    Exp. Ther., 128 : 380.
31. Paroli, E. (1967) : Arch. Ital. Sci. Farmacol. 13 :
    231.
32. Pasternak, G.W., Goodman, R., and Snyder, S.H.
    (1975) : Life Sci.,16 : 1765.
33. Pert, C.B., and Snyder, S.H. (1973) : Science ,
    179 : 1011.
34. Sediah, N.G., Lis, M., Gianoulakis, C., Schiller,
    P., and Chrétien, M. (1976) : Lancet , 1 : 1017.
35. Simantov, R., and Snyder, S.H. (1976) : Life Sci.,
    18 : 781-788.
36. Simantov, R., and Snyder, S.H. (1976) : Nature
    (Lond.), 262 : 505.
37. Simon, E.J., Hiller, J.M., and Edelman, I. (1973):
    Proc. Natl. Acad. Sci., 70 : 1947.
38. Smith, A.A., Karmin, M., and Gavitt, J. (1966) :

Biochem. Pharmacol.,15 : 1877.

39. Smits, S.E., and Takemori, A.E. (1968) : Proc. Soc.
    Exp. Biol. Med., 127 : 1167.
40. Stern, P., and Hadžović , J. (1973) : Arch. Int.
    Pharmacodyn., 202 : 259.
41. Terenius,L. (1973) : Acta Pharmacol. Toxicol.
    32 : 317.
42. Terenius, L. (1975) : J. Pharm. Pharmacol. 27 :
    450.
43. Terenius, L., Gispen, W.H., and De Wied, D. (1975):
    Eur. J. Pharmacol. 33 : 395.
44. Terenius, L., and Wahlström, A. (1974) : Acta
    Pharmacol. Toxicol., 35 (suppl. 1) : 55.
45. Terenius, L., and Wahlström A. (1975): Acta Physiol.
    Scand. , 94 : 74.
46. Terenius, L., and Wahlström, A. (1975) : Life Sci.
    16 : 1759.
47. Tseng, L.F., Loh, H.H., and Li, C.H. (1976) :
    Nature (Lond.) 263 : 239.
48. Ungar, G., and Cohen, M. (1965) : Int. J. Neuro-
    pharmacol. , 5 : 183.
49. Ungar, G., and Galvan, L. (1969) : Proc. Soc. Exp.
    Biol.,130 : 287.
50. Ungar, G., and Ungar, A.L. (1976) : Fed. Proc., 35:
    309.
51. Waterfield, A.A., Hughes, J., and Kosterlitz, H.W.
    (1976) : Nature (Lond.) , 260 : 624.
52. Waterfield, A.A., and Kosterlitz, H.W. (1975) :
    Life Sci., 16 : 1787.
53. Wei, E., and Loh, H. (1976) : Proceedings of the
    1976 International Narcotics Research Club Meeting,
    Aberdeen, Scotland, July 19-22, 1976. Elsevier/
    North Holland Biomedical Press, Amsterdam, in
    press.
54. Wei, E., Sigel, S., Loh, H., and Way, E.L. (1975):
    Nature (Lond.) 253 : 739.
55. Wei, E., Sigel, S., and Way, E. (1975): J.Pharmacol.
    Exp. Ther. , 193 : 56.
56. Winokur, A., and Utiger, R.D. (1974) : Science ,
    185 : 265.
57. Winter, C.A., and Flataker, L. (1951) : J.Pharmacol.
    Exp. Ther., 101 : 93.
58. Wong, D.T., and Horng, J.S. (1973) : Life Sci., 13:
    1543.
59. Zetler, G. (1970) : In : Handbook of Neurochemistry:
    vol. IV, edited by A. Lajtha, p. 135. Plenum
    Press, New York.
60. Zimmermann, E., and Krivoy, W. (1973) : In : Drug
    Effects on Neuroendocrine Regulation.Edited by
    E. Zimmermann, W.H. Gispen, B.H.,Marks , and D.
    De Wied. Progress in Brain Research 39 : 383.

Factors Affecting the Action of Narcotics, edited by
M.L. Adler, L. Manara, and R. Samanin.
Raven Press, New York©1978.

Inhibition of Protein Synthesis and Tolerance to
Opiates

D. Della Bella and V. Frigeni

ZAMBON, Research Laboratories, Bresso-Milan,Italy

INTRODUCTION

Several Authors have demonstrated that the onset of
tolerance to the analgesic effects of morphine (M) may
be prevented by protein synthesis inhibitors. Drugs
affecting both RNA transcription (actinomycin D
/ACT-D/ and 6-mercaptopurine) and peptide assembly
(puromycin and cycloheximide /CYH/) proved to be effective: no effect was found for chloramphenicol (CAP) or
5-fluoro-uracil (2,3,6). The experimental design generally adopted to obtain such evidence is illustrated
in Fig. 1: two groups of animals are treated with M
twice a day, usually for five days; one of the groups
is simultaneously treated with the protein synthesis
inhibitor. On the fifth day, the challenging dose of
M is administered and the magnitude of the pharmacological effect is evaluated. When the combined treatment is adopted, the analgesic activity of M appears
to be preserved, while tolerance to the same activity
is evident in the animals which received M alone.

Influence of Drugs on Onset of Tolerance:Experimental
Evidence

In Table 1 the results of the procedure described
are shown: the hot plate test as modified by Eddy,
Fuhrmeister Touchberry and Lieberman (8) was adopted
and separate groups of mice were used, so as to exclude
the influence of any learning experience acquired by
the animals through repetition of the testing procedures.
While repeated administration of M results in a
reduction of its analgesic effect, the simultaneous

403

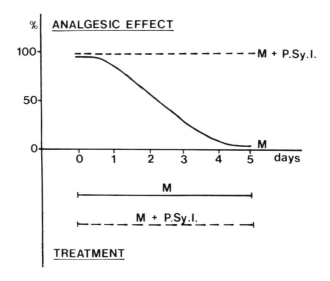

FIG. 1. Experimental design currently adopted in
tolerance studies. (M = morphine; P.Sy.I = Protein
synthesis inhibitors).

TABLE 1. Influence of actinomycin D (ACT-D) on the
onset of tolerance to morphine (M).

Treatment	Dose/kg/day (x 5 days)	Mice No.	Analgesia mean latency time (Sec ± S.E.)
SALINE	–	20	18.45 ± 0.39
M	5+5 mg s.c.	20	14.25 ± 0.99 $(P < 0.001)$
M + ACT-D	5+5 mg s.c. + 80 μg i.p.	20	18.85 ± 1.04

(Challenging dose: 5 mg/kg s.c.), Hot plate test.

$(P < 0.001)$ significance of the difference from saline.

injection of ACT-D markedly antagonizes the
onset of tolerance.   CYH   gave   the   same protective   effect as ACT-D. The results reported in
Table 2 show that CAP failed to affect the reduction
of the pharmacological activity of M.

TABLE 2. Influence of chloramphenicol (CAP) on the
onset of tolerance to morphine (M).

Treatment	Dose/kg/day (x 5 days)	Mice No.	Analgesia mean latency time (Sec $\pm$ S.E.)
SALINE	–	20	17.95 ± 0.93
M	5+5 mg s.c.	20	14.30 ± 0.51 (P $<$ 0.001)
M + CAP	5+5 mg s.c. + 100 mg os	20	13.85 ± 0.60 (n.s.)

(Challenging dose: 5 mg/kg s.c.). Hot plate test.

(P $<$0.001) significance of the difference from saline.

(n.s.) not statistically different from morphine.

Offset of Tolerance

In contrast to the data base available for the M
tolerance onset situation, no comparable detailed
studies appear to exist regarding the influence of
protein   synthesis inhibitors on M tolerance offset.
The few observations we were able to find in the literature show : a) that the rate of return to normal
responsiveness to M after repeated administration depends on the testing procedures adopted, and is very
rapid when the M effect on swimming (1) or running fit
(9) is studied but rather longer when its antinociceptive effect is measured; b) that the recovery
of analgesic responsiveness is biphasic, a first, fast
phase being followed by a slower phase whose mean half-

time is about 13 days in rats and 17 days in mice(5);
c) that the pure antagonist naloxone does not affect
recovery from tolerance (5); d) that ACT-D infusion
for 4 h after tolerance onset does not significantly
alter the reduced responses to a single, intravenous
infusion of M in rats (4).

Further experiments were therefore planned specifically to clarify to what extent the offset of M tolerance may also depend on active protein synthesis.
Differently from previous experiments, the protein
synthesis inhibitors were administered in this case
when the animals had already been made tolerant to M.
At that time M treatment was withdrawn and administration of drugs to be examined started. The new experimental design we adopted is illustrated in Fig.2

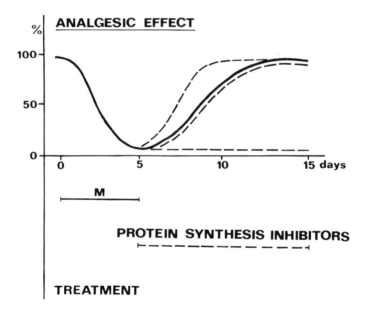

FIG. 2. Tolerance experimental design adopted in our
experiments. (M = morphine 5+5 mg/kg/day s.c.)

The kinetics of the offset of tolerance in these
experimental conditions were studied first. In the
absence of any drug treatment it appeared that about
10 days are needed for reappearance of normal sensitivity to M. In this set of experiments too, separate

groups of animals were used to exclude any risk of
conditioning by repeated testing. Following drug
treatment, started after M treatment was withdrawn,
three different events are theoretically predictable,
as shown in Fig. 2, depending on the mode of action of
the protein synthesis inhibitors : the first possibility is that the reversal time of M tolerance is shortened; the second is that on the contrary offset is
impaired; the third is that offset is not influenced
at all.

Experimental Evidence of Drug Influence

Fig. 3 illustrates the results obtained in this set
of experiments and shows the influence of administration of ACT-D after withdrawal of M. While the
reversal of M tolerance develops regularly in the group

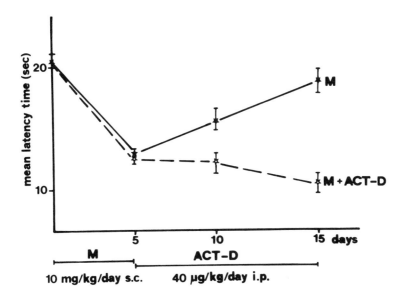

FIG. 3. Influence of actinomycin D(ACT-D) on the offset
of tolerance to morphine(M). (Challenging dose: 5 mg/kg
s.c.): Hot plate test in mice.
The morphine challenge at 5th,10th and 15th day was
performed on different mice groups (20 each) to avoid
any interaction between morphine effect and the test
procedure.

of untreated animals, mice treated with ACT-D at the
dose of 40 µg/kg/day/i.p. after withdrawal of M do
not show any change in their tolerance to the M
analgesic effect. It may thus be concluded that ACT-D
suppresses both the offset and onset of tolerance.

Fig. 4 depicts a similar experiment investigating
the effect of CYH.

It is clear that CYH has no influence; tolerance
offset occurs in both treated and untreated animals.
Unexpectedly, therefore, we have to note that the
impairment of protein synthesis processes exerted by
CYH, which is effective in antagonizing the tolerance
onset, does not appear to be of any consequence when
tested against tolerance offset.

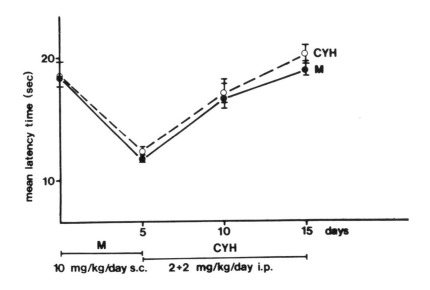

FIG. 4. Influence of cycloheximide (CYH) on the offset
of tolerance to morphine (M). (Challenging dose : 5mg/
kg s.c.): Hot plate test in mice.
The morphine challenge at 5th, 10th and 15th day was
performed on different mice groups (20 each) to avoid
any interaction between morphine effect and the test
procedure.

Quite unexpected results were also obtained in a
similar experiment to evaluate the effect of CAP
administered orally to mice at the dose of 50 mg/kg. As
it is evident from Fig. 5, tolerance to M remains unchanged. Thus, to our surprise, CAP treatment completely prevented the offset of M tolerance, just as
ACT-D did. Therefore, unlike CYH, CAP appears able
specifically to affect the processes of synthesis
involved in tolerance offset in mice.

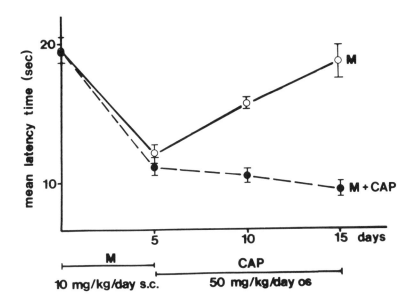

FIG. 5. Influence of chloramphenicol (CAP) on the offset of tolerance to morphine (M). (Challenging dose:
5 mg/kg s.c.): Hot plate test in mice.
The morphine challenge at 5th, 10th and 15th day was
performed on different mice groups (20 each) to avoid
any interaction between morphine effect and the test
procedure.

Similar findings were obtained in rats as well. In
the rat experiments analgesia was measured by the tail
flick test (7), and morphine was given daily for 8 days
before studying tolerance reversal. While prompt
recovery of M activity was observed in control animals,
in the CAP treated rats tolerance offset was abolished

and the marked reduction of M analgesia persisted to the same degree 30 days after narcotic withdrawal. Further, tolerance offset was observed after discontinuation of CAP treatment.

These results both in mice and rats strongly suggest that the repeated administration of M brings into play at least two adaptive mechanisms: one, responsible for the development of tolerance, is CYH sensitive but insensitive to CAP; the other, underlying the recovery from tolerance appears insensitive to CYH but specifically impaired by CAP. They show a similar degree of sensitivity to ACT-D.

CONCLUDING REMARKS

In Fig. 6 we summarize the results of these experiments. Repeated administration of M leads to tolerance to its analgesic effects. After M discontinuation, there is progressive recovery of sensitivity to its an-

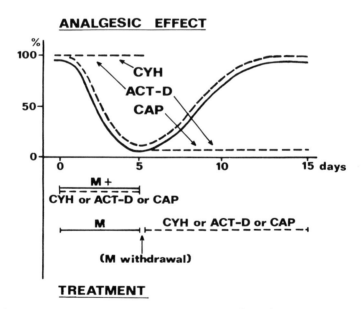

FIG. 6. Influence of cycloheximide (CYH), chloramphenicol (CAP) and actinomycin D (ACT-D) on the onset and offset of tolerance to morphine (M): Hot plate test in mice.

algesic action, and normal responses can be obtained
after 10-15 days. The onset of tolerance appears to be
related to an active synthesis process that both ACT-D
and CYH strongly inhibit; inhibition of this protein
synthesis antagonizes the development of tolerance. We
might assume that under the influence of the inhibitor,
M is no longer able to provoke the adaptive response
underlying the progressive lessening of its antinociceptive activity. To what extent this functional
response may resemble a supersensitivity condition following putative chemical denervation (10) produced by
M at the level of the neuronal synapses responsible for
the transmission and/or integration of the nociceptive
afferences may be a working hypothesis worth examining.
In contrast CAP, which is as active as CYH on the cellular peptide assembly, appears to be completely ineffective on the onset of tolerance.

The reversal of tolerance to M develops gradually
and it too seems to be dependent on active synthesis.
ACT-D, administered when tolerance is established,does
in fact antagonize its progressive reversal. Tolerance
offset, on the other hand, is not impaired by CYH,
while both CAP and ACT-D block it completely.

We are therefore led to the conclusion that the
onset and offset of M tolerance derive from independent
mechanisms, at least as regards their specific sensitivity to different drugs, whereas both are dependent
on active protein synthesis processes.

It may be relevant that while ACT-D, which antagonizes both the tolerance onset and offset, mainly affects RNA transcription, CYH and CAP mainly interfere
with peptide chain assembly. Our experimental evidence
leads us to suppose that the specific macromolecules
arising from ribosomal activity may be responsible for
tolerance onset in one case, sensitive to CYH treatment,
for tolerance offset in the other, sensitive to CAP.
Further experiments are needed to obtain evidence of
the underlying molecular mechanisms.

The very good general conditions of animals repeatedly treated with CAP in contrast to the irreversible
general toxicity produced by the protein synthesis
inhibitors such as ACT-D, CYH and others may, in our
opinion, permit more meaningful and wider investigations in this area.

REFERENCES

1. Cochin, J. and Kornetsky, C. (1964): J. Pharmacol. Exp. Ther., 145: 1.

2. Cohen, M., Keats, A.S., Krivoy , W. and Ungar, G. (1965): Proc. Soc. Exp. Biol. Med., 119: 381.

3. Cox, B.M. and Ginsburg, M. (1969): In: Scientific Basis of Drug Dependence, edited by H. Steinberg, p.77. Churchill, London.

4. Cox, B.M., Ginsburg, M. and Osman, O.H. (1968): Br. J.Pharmacol. Chemother., 33: 245.

5. Cox, B.M., Ginsburg, M. and Willis, J. (1975): Br.J. Pharmacol., 53: 383.

6. Cox, B.M. and Osman, O.H. (1970): Br. J. Pharmacol., 38: 157.

7. D'Amour, F.E. and Smith, D.L. (1941): J.Pharmacol. Exp.Ther., 72: 74.

8. Eddy, N.B., Fuhrmeister Touchberry, C. and Lieberman J.E. (1950): J.Pharmacol. Exp. Ther., 98: 121.

9. Goldstein, A. and Sheehan, P. (1969): J. Pharmacol. Exp. Ther., 169: 175.

10.Sharpless, S.K. (1964): Annu.Rev. Physiol., 26: 357.

Factors Affecting the Action of Narcotics, edited by
M.L. Adler, L. Manara, and R. Samanin.
Raven Press, New York©1978.

Relationships of Calcium to Morphine
Actions

E. Leong Way, R. Adron Harris and Horace H. Loh

Department of Pharmacology, School of Medicine
University of California at San Francisco,
San Francisco, CA 94143, U.S.A.

INTRODUCTION

Considerable evidence exists suggesting that calcium
may be important in the actions of morphine. The
ability of morphine to inhibit respiration in rat brain
slices was found to be dependent on low levels or the
absence of calcium (3, 20). The influx of Ca^{++} is
inhibited by morphine in brain slices (11) and in
synaptosomes (10). Morphine administration decreases
brain calcium levels (18) and the analgesic action of
morphine is reduced by exogenous calcium administra-
tion(11,12). The present communication summarizes
findings of some experiments performed in our laboratory to assess the interactions between calcium and
morphine (6,7,8).

Effect of Divalent Cations on Morphine Antinociception

The chloride salts of Ca^{++}, Mg^{++}, Mn^{++}, Ba^{++}, Sr^{++},
Cd^{++}, Hg^{++}, and Ni^{++} were each dissolved in 5 µl of
physiologic saline and administered intraventricularly
(i.vt.) in mice at a dose which was non-lethal but
large enough to affect motor activity (1/4 LD50).
Immediately thereafter, morphine sulfate at varying
doses was administered subcutaneously and the median
analgetic dose of morphine (AD50) was determined by the
tail-flick procedure. The morphine AD50 was increased
significantly by 15 µmol/kg of $CaCl_2$, $MgCl_2$, and $MnCl_2$,
but not by the chloride salts of the other cations. In
the case of Ca^{++}, the AD50 was increased 3-fold but no

413

increase was noted at a lower dose (4 μmol/kg). The antagonism of morphine analgesia by 15 μmol/kg of Ca^{++} lasted for about 6 h . Groups of 7-9 mice were used for each experiment. Statistical details are elaborated in Harris et al (8).

Effect of Chelators and an Ionophore on Morphine Analgesia

Two cation chelators, ethyleneglycol-bis (β -amino-ethyl ether)-N,N'tetraacetic acid (EGTA, 2 μmol/kg) and ethylenediaminetetraacetic acid (EDTA, 2 or 4 μmol/kg) in 5 μl 0.9% saline, were administered i.vt. and the morphine AD50 was determined as above. The results are shown in figure 1. EGTA, which has a much higher

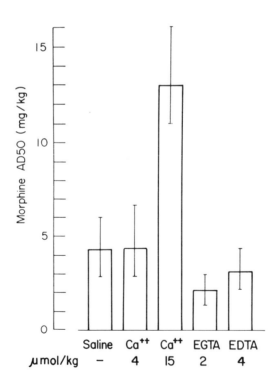

FIG. 1. Effect of Ca^{++}, EGTA and EDTA on morphine analgesia.

affinity for Ca^{++} than Mg^{++}, decreased the morphine
AD50 by 50 percent. On the other hand, EDTA, which has
similar affinities for Ca^{++} and Mg^{++}, decreased the
morphine AD50 slightly but the change was not statistically significant.

The influence of the ionophore X537A was investigated because it has been shown to increase the
permeability of membranes to Ca^{++} (17) and to promote
stimulus-secretion coupling (5). Estimations of the
morphine AD50 were made with X537A injected alone or in
combination with Ca^{++} (4 μmol/kg). For the i.vt. route
X537A was suspended in saline and the dose was 1 μmol/
kg; for subcutaneous administration it was dissolved
in 1:10 dimethylsulfoxide and the dose was 20 mg/kg.
As can be seen in Figure 2, X537A enhanced Ca^{++} antagonism of morphine antinociception. The combined

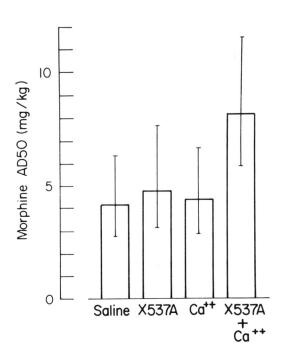

FIG 2. Effect of the ionophore X537A alone and in combination with Ca^{++} on morphine analgesia

i.vt. injection of Ca^{++} plus X537A produced a
morphine AD50 nearly 2-fold that of saline. It should
be noted that the administration of either Ca^{++} or
X537A alone did not modify the morphine AD50. Similar
results were obtained with subcutaneous administration
of X537A.

Effect of Lanthanum on Morphine Analgesia

Based on theoretical considerations it was hypothesized that specifically bound calcium could be
displaced by the rare earth element lanthanum (14).
It was of interest, therefore, to assess the effects of
lanthanum on the pharmacologic effects of morphine.
A low dose of La^{+++} (1 µmol/kg i.vt.), which itself had
little effect on the baseline response, increased the
analgesic effect of morphine. There was a parallel
shift of the morphine dose-response curve to the left
and the subcutaneous morphine AD50 was nearly doubled
from 2.6 to 5.1 mg/kg. Likewise, a low dose of
morphine increased the antinociceptive effect of La^{+++}.
The enhancement, however, was observed for low but not
high doses of La^{+++}. As a consequence, the slope of
the La^{+++} dose-response curve in the presence of
morphine was considerably flatter. Similar results
were observed by the hot-plate test.

Effect of Ca^{++} on Morphine Analgesia in Tolerant Mice and on Tolerance Development

The development of tolerance to morphine did not alter the antagonistic effect of Ca^{++} on morphine analgesia. After the implantation of a morphine pellet for
3 days, marked tolerance to morphine developed, as
judged by a large increase in the morphine AD50. In
tests performed at the same time on a group of non-
implanted mice, the morphine AD50 was 5 mg/kg, whereas
in the implanted group the AD50 increased 14-fold to
70 mg/kg. The i.vt. injection of Ca^{++} (15 µmol/kg) in
the tolerant animals increased the morphine AD50 an
additional 2-fold and this degree of antagonism of
morphine by Ca^{++} was similar to that observed in non-
tolerant mice.
     A single injection of Ca^{++} immediately before

morphine pellet implantation in another group of mice did not alter significantly the degree of tolerance that developed after 3 days; the AD50 and 95% confidence limits of the control group receiving saline was 108 (68-171) mg/kg and that of the Ca^{++} group was 122 (77-190) mg/kg.

Effects of Ca^{++} on the Antagonistic Actions of Naloxone

The morphine antagonist potency of naloxone was not altered by i.vt. injection of Ca^{++}. Administration of 0.04 mg/kg of naloxone increased the morphine AD50 5.3 fold in saline-treated animals and 6.0-fold in Ca^{++} - treated mice; 0.16 mg/kg of naloxone increased the AD50 11.9-fold in the saline group and 13.2-fold in the Ca^{++} group. Thus, the relative increase in the AD50 induced by two doses of naloxone was very similar for groups pretreated with either Ca^{++} or saline.

Ca^{++} treatment also failed to alter the antagonistic potency of naloxone against morphine in animals render-ed tolerant to morphine by pellet implantation. As can be seen in Figure 3, compared with saline, naloxone (55nmol/kg, i.e., 0.02 mg/kg) increased the morphine AD50 from 70 to 170 mg/kg (potency ratio of 2.43) and when combined with Ca^{++}, the AD50 increased from 150 to 360 mg/kg (potency ratio of 2.40). Thus, naloxone produced the same antagonism of morphine in tolerant animals treated with either Ca^{++} or saline, and this is similar to the finding in non-tolerant animals. This means that the morphine antagonist effects of Ca^{++} and naloxone are additive in both non-tolerant and tolerant animals, as neither potentiation nor antagonistic effects were observed when they were given in combination.

DISCUSSION

The possibility that neurotransmitter release might be involved in the antagonistic effects of Ca^{++} on morphine analgesia needs to be considered. In a vari-ety of systems in which elevated calcium levels have been found to result in the release of neurotransmit-ters, Sr^{++} and Ba^{++} also stimulated the release of neurotransmitters (4), whereas Mg^{++} and Mn^{++} inhibited

this release (2,15).   Because the antagonism of morphine effects was found with Ca^{++}, Mg^{++}, and Mn^{++},but
not with Sr^{++} or Ba^{++}, direct involvement of increased
neurotransmitter release seems an unlikely explanation
for the calcium antagonism of morphine.   This is supported by additional observations that calcium administration did not affect the ability of agents which
alter brain amine levels to influence morphine action.
Thus, the ability of pargyline to potentiate the effects of morphine or the ability of 6-OHDA to antagonize the effects of morphine were not affected by Ca^{++}
pretreatment.   An alteration of release of amine by
Ca^{++} would have changed the relative potency of
pargyline and 6-OHDA in potentiating or antagonizing
the action of morphine, but this effect was not seen.
    Although Ca^{++} produced the same relative degree of
antagonism of morphine in tolerant and non-tolerant

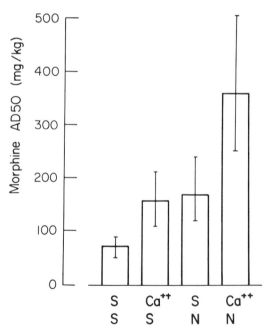

FIG.3 Antagonism of morphine analgesia by Ca^{++} and
naloxone (N) alone and in combination in morphine-
tolerant animals: Saline (S) controls.

animals on an absolute basis, it was able to antagoni-
nize the effects of more morphine in tolerant animals
than in non-tolerant animals. A possible explanation for
these findings is that Ca^{++} may be acting distal to
the site of tolerance development, thus the same number
of Ca^{++} ions are able to antagonize the effect of many
more morphine molecules because the effect produced by
the morphine has been reduced at a site proximal to
the site of action of Ca^{++}.

Despite the antagonizing effects of Ca^{++} on morphine
analgesia, the antagonist potency of naloxone, as
measured by pA_2 determinations, was not altered by Ca^{++}.
The failure of Ca^{++} to change the naloxone-morphine
pA_2 implies that Ca^{++} did not alter the apparent affinity of naloxone for the receptor. This finding
contrasts with the results of in vitro binding studies
(9,16) where Ca^{++} (as well as Mg^{++} and Mn^{++}) inhibited
the stereospecific binding of naloxone. It should also
be recognized that the in vitro binding of etorphine
is inhibited by p-chloromercuribenzoate and N-ethylmaleimide (19), whereas the binding of naloxone is
inhibited by Cd^{++} and Hg^{++} (unpublished observations),
indicating the involvement of sulfhydryl groups in this
binding; yet neither Cd^{++} nor Hg^{++} reduced the analgesic effect of morphine. In addition, Na^+ and K^+
have been found to reduce the binding of narcotic
agonists to brain homogenates (19), yet these ions do
not alter the analgesic effects of morphine (11).
Thus, there is incomplete agreement between the effects
of divalent cations on the in vivo actions of morphine
and naloxone and their effects on the in vitro binding
of narcotics to brain homogenates.

The antagonism of morphine analgesia by Ca^{++}, Mg^{++},
and Mn^{++} is probably competitive since parallel shifts
of the morphine dose-response curve were obtained with
each ion. On the other hand, cation chelators enhanced
morphine analgesia. Of the two cation chelators
studied, EGTA potentiated morphine analgesia to a more
significant degree than EDTA. Since EGTA has a much
higher affinity for Ca^{++} than Mg^{++}, the results suggest
that Ca^{++} is more important than Mg^{++} for modifying
morphine analgesia. Since these chelating agents probably remove the most loosely bound Ca^{++} on the outer
surface of the nerve membrane, the results with La^{+++}

may have greater relevance and significance.

It has been suggested that La^{+++} could replace Ca^{++} bound to specific high affinity sites (14) and, indeed, La^{+++} has been shown to inhibit Ca^{++} binding and transport in a number of biologic systems (21). It is of considerable interest, therefore, to find that La^{+++} not only enhances morphine analgesia per se but also possesses an antinociceptive action (8).

In brief, intracerebroventricularly administered lanthanum chloride was found to produce antinociceptive effects as measured by the mouse tail-flick and hot-plate tests and the rat tail-flick test. These anti-nociceptive effects were reduced by peripheral admin-istration of the narcotic antagonist naloxone or by i.vt. administration of calcium chloride. In addition, animals made tolerant to morphine were also tolerant to the effect of La^{+++}. In morphine-dependent mice, the incidence of both abrupt and naloxone-precipitated withdrawal jumping was reduced by La^{+++} administration. The active site for lanthanum analgesia was found to be similar to that for morphine in the peri-aqueductal gray region (6). In view of the known inhibitory ef-fects of La^{+++} on Ca^{++} binding and movement, these findings suggest that alterations in Ca^{++} localization may be involved in the analgetic action of narcotic drugs as well as the development of narcotic tolerance and dependence.

The possibility that an altered localization of Ca^{++} might be involved in the effects of chronic administra-tion of narcotic drugs prompted an examination of the binding of ^{45}Ca^{++} to brain membranes isolated from morphine tolerant-dependent animals (Yamamoto, Harris, Loh and Way, unpublished). Brain subcellular fractions were prepared by a modification of the method of Cotman and Matthews (1); binding was determined by filtration and scintillation spectrometry after incubating the membrane fractions at ambient temperature with ^{45}Ca^{++} solutions containing about 0.2 μCi ^{45}Ca^{++}. It was found that chronic morphine treatment decreased the amount of ^{45}Ca^{++} bound to synaptosomal plasma membranes (SPM) but not to any of the other subcellular fractions suggesting that the development of morphine tolerance is accompanied by a decrease in high-affinity Ca^{++} binding of SPM. The time course of the appearance of the decreased $^{45}Ca^{++}$ binding after morphine pellet implantation, parallelled the course of development of tolerance and physical dependence. It is particularly interesting that the Ca^{++} binding of intact synaptosomes was not altered by chronic morphine treatment, while the binding of the isolated SPM decreased. This decreased $^{45}Ca^{++}$ binding may be due to an increased binding of endogenous Ca^{++} to the tolerant SPM, thus decreasing the number of available binding sites for $^{45}Ca^{++}$. The site of the binding change is probably on the inner surface of the synaptosomal membrane, and thus would not be available for binding in the case of intact synaptosomes. It has been suggested by Hendrick and Blaustein (13) that the binding sites may be part of one of the Ca^{++} pumps which are responsible for maintaining very low intrasynaptosomal Ca^{++} concentrations. Thus alteration of Ca^{++} transport across the synaptic membrane represents another mechanism by which narcotic treatment may affect synaptosomal Ca^{++} homeostasis.

In summary, it appears that increasing brain Ca^{++} at intracellular sites antagonizes the effects of narcotic drugs as well as those of La^{+++}. This suggests that the increased synaptosomal Ca^{++} levels and the resultant decrease in available $^{45}Ca^{++}$ binding sites found after chronic morphine treatment might be involved in the development of tolerance to narcotic drugs as well as the cross-tolerance between morphine and La^{+++}. The specificity of this change is strengthened by additional preliminary observations that the decrease in Ca^{++} binding can be prevented by naloxone.

ACKNOWLEDGEMENTS

Supported in part by National Institute of Drug Abuse grants DA00037, DA00564 and DA02785.

REFERENCES

1. Cotman, C.W., and Matthews, D.A. (1971): Biochim. Biophys.Acta, 249: 380-394.
2. Douglas,W.W., and Rubin, R.P. (1964): J.Physiol. (Lond.), 175: 231-241.

3. Elliott, H.W., Kokka, N., and Way, E.L. (1963):Proc. Soc.Exp.Biol.Med., 113: 1049-1052.
4. Elmqvist, D., and Feldman, D.S. (1965): J.Physiol. (Lond.), 181: 487-497.
5. Foreman, J.C., Mongar, J.L., and Gompers, B.D.(1973): Nature(Lond.), 246: 249-251.
6. Harris, R.A., Iwamoto, E.T., Loh, H.H., and Way,E.L. (1975): Brain Res., 100: 221-225.
7. Harris, R.A., Loh, H.H., and Way, E.L. (1975): J. Pharmacol. Exp. Ther., 195: 488-498.
8. Harris, R.A., Loh, H.H., and Way, E.L. (1976): J. Pharmacol.Exp. Ther., 196: 288-297.
9. Hitzemann, R.J.,Hitzemann, B.A., and Loh, H.H.(1974): Life Sci.,pt.I, 14: 2393-2404.
10. Kaku, T., Kaneto, H., and Koida, M. (1974): Jap.J. Pharmacol., 24:suppl,123.
11. Kakunaga, T., Kaneto, H., and Hano, K. (1966): J. Pharmacol.Exp. Ther., 153: 134-141.
12. Kaneto, H. (1971): In: Narcotic Drugs: Biochemical Pharmacology, edited by D.H.Clouet, pp.300-309. Plenum Press, New York.
13. Kendrick, N.C., and Blaustein, M.P. (1975): Abstracts of Neurosciences Society, 1: 931.
14. Lettvin, J.Y., Pickard, W.F., McCulock, W.S., and Pitts, W. (1964): Nature(Lond.), 202: 1338-1339.
15. Meiri, V., and Rahaminoff, R. (1972): Science, 176: 308-309.
16. Pert, C., and Snyder, S.H. (1973): Science, 179: 1011-1014.
17. Pressman, B.C. (1973): Fed.Proc., 32: 1698.
18. Ross, D.H., Medina, M.A., and Cardenas, H.L. (1974): Science, 186: 63-64.
19. Simon, E., Hiller, J.M., and Edelman, I. (1973):Proc. Natl.Acad.Sci., 68: 1742-1748.
20. Takemori, A.E. (1962): J. Pharmacol. Exp. Ther., 135: 89-93.
21. Weiss, C.B. (1974): Annu.Rev.Pharmacol., 14: 343-354.

Factors Affecting the Action of Narcotics, edited by
M.L. Adler, L. Manara, and R. Samanin.
Raven Press, New York©1978.

Role of the Cyclic Nucleotide System in Opiate Actions

A. Carenzi

ZAMBON S.p.A. Research Laboratories, Bresso-Milano, Italy

INTRODUCTION

Over the past few years, evidence has been accumulated
suggesting that interaction of drug with receptors results in
variations of the cellular cyclic 3',5'-adenosine monophosphate
(cAMP) content, responsible for changes in the function of the
target cells, due to the action of cAMP on cAMP-dependent protein
kinase.

Different pharmacological and neurochemical findings suggest
that the molecular mechanisms responsible for the action of
morphine interfere with the function of the cyclic nucleotide
system. However, data implicating cAMP and cyclic 3',5'-guanosine
monophosphate (cGMP)   in the pharmacology of morphine is
compromised by contradictory findings. Our purpose is to summarize experimental results related to morphine's   action at the
receptor levels, obtained from pharmacological and neurochemical
studies.

Pharmacological Studies

It was reported in 1973 by Ho et al. (14) that the administration of cAMP intracerebrally or intravenously antagonized
morphine analgesia in non-tolerant and tolerant mice. Theophylline, a phosphodiesterase inhibitor, acted in a similar manner.
In contrast, the elevation of brain monoamines by pargyline
reversed the antagonistic effects of cAMP on morphine analgesia.

Increasing brain dopamine (DA) with L-DOPA did not prevent
cAMP antagonism of morphine analgesia. Increasing brain serotonin with tryptophan not only failed to reverse the effect of
cAMP, but appeared to enhance the cAMP response. However,
elevation of norepinephrine (NE) with dihydroxyphenylserine did
reverse the antagonistic effect of cAMP.

Figure 1 shows some results obtained a few years ago in our
laboratories: the experiments were performed in rats using the
tail flick test (11) for analgesia evaluation. Panel A reports
data on the antagonism of intravenously injected dibutyryl cAMP
on morphine analgesia; our results are in agreement with those
reported by Ho et al. (14) in a more extensive study.

Panel B illustrates the synergic action of d-amphetamine on
the analgesia elicited by morphine.   This seems to contradict

423

the previous result, because we have shown (1) that d-amphetamine increases cAMP content, at least in brain dopaminergic areas such as striatum and nucleus accumbens. Although it has been suggested by Ho et al. (14) that NE is more important for the reversal of the cAMP antagonism of morphine analgesia, it is still difficult to understand what is the real role of cAMP.

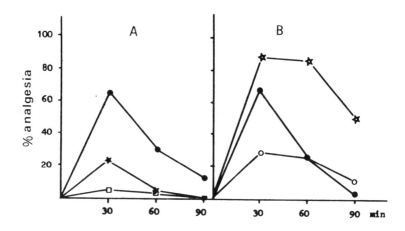

FIG. 1. Effects of dibutyryl cAMP (panel A) and of d-amphetamine (panel B) on the analgesia elicited by morphine in rats.
Panel A: ●—● morphine (1.5 mg/kg s.c. as base)
          □—□ dibutyryl cAMP (2 mg/kg i.v.)
          ★—★ dibutyryl cAMP (2 mg/kg i.v.) 5 min before
                             morphine (1.5 mg/kg s.c.)

Panel B: ●—● morphine (1.5 mg/kg s.c.)
          ○—○ d-amphetamine (2.5 mg/kg s.c.)
          ☆—☆ d-amphetamine (2.5 mg/kg s.c.) 5 min before
                             morphine (1.5 mg/kg s.c.)

NE, too, stimulates adenylate cyclase and produces accumulation of cAMP (16,34) and cAMP inhibits the firing rate of cortex pyramidal cells as well as NE does (30). Since an increase of brain biogenic amines leads to increased stimulation of the dependent adenylate cyclases, one would expect the increased activity of brain monoamines, induced by pargyline, to potentiate, not antagonize, the action of exogenously applied cAMP.

Systemically administered cAMP may have many pharmacological effects different from those produced by an increase of intracellular cAMP content in specific brain areas; it therefore seems impossible only by pharmacological studies to demonstrate a specific role for cAMP in the action of morphine.

In Vitro Neurochemical Studies

The in vitro neurochemical approach offers the possibility of studying the effects of morphine on the single components of the cyclic nucleotide system.

Effect of Morphine on Adenylate Cyclase Activity

Different authors have reported that adenylate cyclase, the enzyme that catalyzes formation of cAMP. functions in some tissues as a receptor for catecholamines (17,18). Moreover, it has been suggested (5) that the influence of drugs on the adenylate cyclase activity in vitro is related to the action of the same drugs at the receptor level in vivo. While apomorphine stimulates the adenylate cyclase activity of rat striatal homogenates (17) and neuroleptics antagonize the stimulation produced by DA or apomorphine (5), the addition of morphine to rat striatal homogenates changes neither basal adenylate cyclase activity nor the stimulation produced by DA (2). Our results are fully in agreement with those of Van Inwegen et al. (33) and of Tell et al. (31). Iwatsubo and Clouet (15) found that narcotic analgesics added in vitro did not inhibit DA sensitive adenylate cyclase activity in ruptured nerve-ending preparations from rat caudate nucleus.

Although opiates and neuroleptics are known to interfere with dopaminergic neurons in the central nervous system by increasing the striatal DA turnover rate (2,3,6,29), and catalepsy elicited in the rat by analgesics or neuroleptics has been related to an impairment of DA receptors (9,10,20), different authors (2,15,20) have supported the hypothesis that, while neuroleptics block the DA receptors directly, morphine inhibits dopaminergic transmission by some other mechanism. Collier and Roy (7) have reported that prostaglandin E (PGE) dependent cAMP synthesis is inhibited by narcotics in rat brain homogenates. Sharma et al. (26) found that narcotics reduce basal and PGE_1 stimulated cAMP levels in intact neuroblastoma x glioma hybrid cells and inhibit adenylate cyclase activity of homogenates. The inhibition of adenylate cyclase activity by narcotics is specific for the pharmacologically active stereoisomers. Studying different cell lines they found that the degree of sensitivity to morphine depends upon the abundance of narcotic receptors.

From the findings reported, we can conclude that morphine interferes with adenylate cyclase activity by a different mechanism from that of neuroleptics. The interaction of morphine with adenylate cyclase may be a consequence of morphine binding with the opiate receptors.

Effect of Morphine on Phosphodiesterase Activity

It was reported by Puri et al. (23) that high k_m phosphodiesterase (PDE) in rat striatum was inhibited by morphine both in vitro and by acute injection. In contrast, Chou et al. (4) and Singhal et al. (28) reported that in the mouse cerebellum, hypothalamus, cerebral cortex and brain stem PDE were not affected by morphine.

We obtained some results in 1973 (8) on cAMP content in different rat tissues after treating the animals with high doses of morphine, and these may be pertinent. Morphine (104 μmoles/kg i.p.) in rats increases the cAMP content in the striatum, pituitary, adrenal medulla and adrenal cortex. This increase lasts for several hours and is completely different from that obtained treating the animals with d-amphetamine or apomorphine. We reported (2) that d-amphetamine and apomorphine elicit an increase of cAMP concentrations in rat striatum lasting 10-15 min. Probably the cAMP increase leads to activation of PDE (12) which rapidly reduces the cAMP levels although synthesis is still increased. The cAMP increase after morphine, lasting more than 2 hours, suggests that PDE activity in vivo may be reduced by treatment with high doses of morphine. However in our opinion, this effect, cannot be considered the mechanism specifically responsible for the pharmacological action of morphine.

In Vivo Neurochemical Studies

Morphine injected in rats in doses increasing the striatal DA turnover rate fails to change the concentration of cAMP in striatum (2). We have compared the effects of morphine with those of d-amphetamine, which increases the striatal DA turnover rate by increasing the release of DA and by blocking reuptake of this amine. d-Amphetamine injected in rats produces a parallel increase of striatal DA turnover rate and cAMP concentration (2). Assuming the increase of cAMP as an index of an increased stimulation of the receptors, we can conclude that morphine increases striatal DA turnover rate, but fails to increase the release of DA in the striatum.

Some interesting results in this field have been recently obtained by Trabucchi et al. (32), studying the effect of morphine on the striatal cAMP content of two strains of inbred mice (C 57 and DBA). As described by Oliverio and Castellano (22), the predominant effect of morphine in C 57 mice is running activity and in DBA mice analgesia. Morphine injected at various doses induces an increase of striatal cAMP content only in the C 57 strain which gives the running response.

Assuming 3-methoxy-tyramine content in striatum as an index of DA release, Racagni et al.(24) demonstrated that in C 57 mice the release of DA is increased after morphine treatment whereas in DBA mice the same doses of morphine lead to a decrease of DA release in striatum.

On the basis of the in vivo neurochemical data reported we can conclude that morphine interferes with the function of striatal dopaminergic synapses by increasing or blocking the release of DA from presynaptic nerve terminals and not by direct action on the cyclic nucleotide system.

The molecular mechanism by which morphine regulates the release of DA is still unknown; prostaglandins, calcium ions, enkephaline or binding with opiate receptors may be involved in the earlier steps of morphine action.

As regards the influence of morphine on the cGMP system, Gullis et al. (13) have shown that the drug increases the cGMP content in neuroblastoma cell lines.   Recently Racagni et al. (25) reported that morphine, injected in rats, increases cGMP content in striatum and nucleus accumbens, but not in cerebellum. Since morphine fails to change the cGMP content of cerebellum direct action of the drug on guanylate cyclase cannot be the mechanism whereby this analgesic affects the cGMP content in striatum.   Various reports have correlated cGMP either with cholinergic (19,30) or with GABAergic (21) transmission. Morphine does affect the cholinergic system in different brain areas (9) and GABA has been indicated as a possible transmitter that may participate in morphine action (9,27). However our present understanding of the role of cGMP in cell function and of the interference of morphine with acetylcholine and GABA is still very poor and does not permit any firm conclusions.

REFERENCES

1. Carenzi, A., Cheney, D.L., Costa, E., Guidotti, A., and Racagni, G. (1975): Neuropharmacology, 14: 927-939.
2. Carenzi, A., Guidotti, A., Revuelta, A., and Costa, E. (1975): J. Pharmacol. Exp. Ther., 194: 311-318.
3. Carlsson, A., and Lindqvist, M. (1963): Acta Pharmacol. Toxicol., 2O: 140-144.
4. Chou, W.S., Ho, A.K.S., and Loh, H.H. (1971): Proc. West. Pharmacol. Soc., 14: 42-46.
5. Clement-Cormier, Y.C., Kebabian, J.W., Petzold, G.L., and Greengard, P. (1974): Proc. Natl. Acad. Sci. USA, 71: 1113-1117.
6. Clouet, D.H., and Ratner, M. (1970): Science, 168: 854-856.
7. Collier, H.O.J., and Roy, A.C. (1974): Nature, 248; 24-27.
8. Costa, E., Carenzi, A., Guidotti, A., and Revuelta, A. (1973): In: Frontiers in Catecholamine Research, edited by E. Usdin, and S. Snyder, pp.1003-1010. Pergamon Press, London.
9. Costa, E., Cheney, D.L., Racagni, G., and Zsilla, G. (1975): Life Sci., 17: 1-8.
10. Costa, E., Cheney, D., and Revuelta, A. (1974): Adv. Biochem Psychopharmacol., 8: 483-494.
11. D'Amour, F.E., and Smith, D.L. (1941): J. Pharmacol. Exp.Ther., 72: 74-79.
12. Gnegy, M.E., Costa, E., and Uzunov, P. (1976): Proc. Natl. Acad. Sci. USA, 73: 352-355.

13. Gullis, R., Traber, J., and Hamprecht, B. (1975): Nature, 256: 57-59.
14. Ho, I.K., Loh, H.H., and Way, E.L. (1973): J. Pharmacol. Exp. Ther., 185: 336-346.
15. Iwatsubo, K., and Clouet, D.H. (1975): Biochem. Pharmacol., 24: 1499-1503.
16. Kakiuchi, S., and Rall, T.W. (1968): Mol. Pharmacol., 4: 379-388.
17. Kebabian, J.W., Petzeld, G.L., and Greengard, P. (1972): Proc. Natl. Acad. Sci. USA, 69: 2145-2149.
18. Klainer, L.M., Chi, Y.M., Freidberg, S.L., Rall, T.W., and Sutherland, E.W. (1962): J. Biol. Chem., 237: 1239-1243.
19. Kuo, J.F., Lee, T.P., Reyes, P.L., Walton, K.G., Donnelly, T.E. Jr., and Greengard, P. (1972): J. Biol. Chem., 247: 16-22.
20. Kuschinsky, K., and Hornykiewicz, O. (1972): Eur. J. Pharmacol., 19: 119-122.
21. Mao, C.C., Guidotti, A., and Costa, E. (1974): Mol. Pharmacol., 10: 736-745.
22. Oliverio, A., and Castellano, C. (1974): Psychopharmacologia, 39: 13-22.
23. Puri, S.K., Cochin, J., and Volicer, L. (1975): Life Sci., 16: 759-768.
24. Racagni, G., Oliverio, A., Bruno, F., Maggi, A., and Cattabeni, F. (1977): Advances in Biochemical Psychopharmacology, 16: 565-570.
25. Racagni, G., Zsilla, G., Guidotti, A., and Costa, E. (1976): J. Pharm. Pharmacol., 28: 258-260.
26. Sharma, S.K., Nirenberg, M., and Klee, W.A. (1975): Proc. Natl. Acad. Sci. USA, 72: 590-594.
27. Sherman, A.D., and Gebbart, G.F. (1974): Neuropharmacology, 13: 673-675.
28. Singhal, R.L., Kacew, S., and Lafreniere, R. (1973): J. Pharm. Pharmacol., 25: 1022-1024.
29. Smith, C.B., Sheldon, M.I., Bednarczyk, J.H., and Villarreal, J.E. (1972): J. Pharmacol. Exp. Ther., 180: 547-557.
30. Stone, T.W., Taylor, D.A., and Bloom, F.E. (1975): Science, 187: 845-847.
31. Tell, G.P., Pasternak, G.W., and Cuatrecasas, P. (1975): FEBS Lett., 51: 242-245.
32. Trabucchi, M., Spano, P.F., Racagni, G., and Oliverio, A.: (1976): Brain Res., 114: 536-540.
33. Van Inwegen, R.G., Strada, S.J., and Robinson, G.A. (1975): Life Sci., 16: 1875-1876.
34. Weiss, B., and Costa, E. (1967): Science, 156: 1750-1752.

4. NEUROTRANSMITTER

MODIFICATION OF OPIATE

ACTIONS

Factors Affecting the Action of Narcotics, edited by
M.L. Adler, L. Manara, and R. Samanin.
Raven Press, New York©1978.

Opiate Action on Brain Acetylcholine Release : Role of
Monoamines

K. Jhamandas and J. Poulson

Department of Pharmacology, Faculty of Medicine, Queen's
University, Kingston, Ontario, Canada

INTRODUCTION

Following the demonstration of the inhibitory effect of morphine in the field stimulated guinea-pig
ileum (29,34) it was shown that this opiate could
depress the ventricular release of acetylcholine (ACh)
in the anesthetized cat (5), and the cortical release
of this substance in the unanesthetized rabbit (4).
Subsequent investigations of Jhamandas et al.(15,16)
showed that morphine and related opiate agonists could
inhibit the cortical ACh release in anesthetized cats,
and this effect could be specifically reversed by the
opiate antagonist naloxone. Comparable effects of
morphine on cortical ACh release have been observed on
the release of cortical or striatal ACh in brainstem
transected animals (20,39). In contrast to these
findings Mullin et al (27) reported that morphine
enhances the release of cortical ACh in unanesthetized
cats.

Many studies on the rat brain have shown that morphine elevates the ACh levels (11,13,21,25), an effect
which most likely reflects a depression of ACh release.
An inhibitory effect of morphine on cortical ACh
release has been directly demonstrated in the brainstem
transected or anesthetized rat (17,24). This inhibitory
effect of opiates on cortical ACh release in the rat is
specifically mediated through opiate receptors since
this action is antagonized by naloxone, exhibits stereospecificity and is diminished in opiate tolerant dependent animals (14,17).

Several attempts have been made to define the site

431

and mechanism of action of morphine on ACh release.
The failure to demonstrate a high sensitivity and
specificity of opiate action on ACh release from brain
slices has suggested that the primary site of action
may be subcortical (14,37). Electrolytic lesioning of
raphe nuclei (12), the septum (31) and the medial
thalamus (18), has been shown to abolish the morphine
effect on cortical ACh release thus supporting the possibility of a subcortical locus of action. The mechanism by which morphine influences the release of ACh is
not known. Morphine and other opiates could influence
ACh release by a direct action on the cholinergic
neurones, or they could do so indirectly by affecting
neuronal systems which modulate the release of ACh.
The monoamines such as norepinephrine (NE) and dopamine
(DA) have been proposed to modulate the release of ACh
in the cerebral cortex (2,3), and in the striatum (1,
9,26,36). Modulation of striatal ACh by 5-hydroxy-
tryptamine (5-HT) has also been proposed (6).

The present study was carried out to assess whether
monoamines such as NE, DA or 5-HT play a role in the
inhibitory actions of morphine on cortical ACh release.
To meet this objective we have examined the action of
morphine, and its reversal by naloxone, following
pretreatment of rats with either selective inhibitors
of catecholamine and 5-HT synthesis or their receptor
blocking agents. Furthermore, it was of interest to
determine whether a relationship exists between the
anti-release actions of morphine and its analgesic
action; we have therefore examined the influence these
treatments have on morphine induced analgesia.

METHODS

ACh Release Experiments

All experiments were carried out on Sprague Dawley
rats (250-300 g) which were lightly anesthetized with
pentobarbital (30 mg/kg) and urethane (400 mg/kg)
mixture. The release of endogenous cortical ACh was
investigated in the presence of an anti-cholinesterase,
neostigmine (5×10^{-5} g/ml) and atropine (5×10^{-7}
g/ml) using the cup technique of MacIntosh and Oborin
(23). Experimental details of this procedure, and

biological assay of the solutions containing ACh using the hearts of venus clam <u>Mercenaria</u> <u>mercenaria</u>, have been described in previous studies (15,17).

Analgesia Experiments

Analgesia produced by a fixed dose of morphine in control animals and those receiving drug treatments was evaluated by the hot-plate technique using the Analgesia Meter (Technilab Instrument, Peguannock, N.J.) maintained at 55°C. The latencies of response (paw-licking) to the thermal stimulus, pre and post-morphine, were recorded in groups of control and drug pre-treated animals. The percent change in the response latency after morphine was calculated, and the significance of differences between control animals and those receiving drug treatment was assessed by the Student's t test.

Drugs and Treatments

Drugs used in this study were atropine sulfate, DL-p-chlorophenylalanine (PCPA), haloperidol, meperidine hydrochloride, methysergide bimaleate, DL-α-methyl-p-tyrosine (AMPT), morphine sulfate, neostigmine bromide, naloxone hydrochloride, pentobarbital sodium, phenoxy-benzamine hydrochloride, propranolol hydrochloride and urethane. PCPA (316 mg/kg) suspended in saline and Tween 80 was administered i.p. 72 hours prior to the experiment (19). AMPT (250 mg/kg) was similarly administered 16-18 hours prior to the experiment (28). Other treatments were administered as described in the Results section.

RESULTS

A. Morphine Action on Cortical ACh Release

Effects of monoamine synthesis inhibitors

The results of three representative experiments showing morphine effects, and the antagonism by naloxone, in control, AMPT and PCPA pretreated animals are shown in Fig.1. The pooled results of several

434

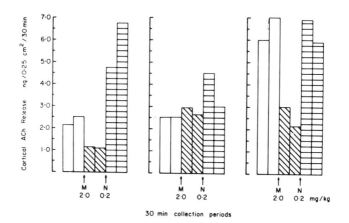

FIG. 1. <u>Effect of morphine (M) and naloxone (N) on the
cortical output of ACh in control, AMPT and PCPA pretreated animals.</u> Morphine and naloxone were injected
i.v. at the points indicated by arrows.
Each histogram is a single experiment.

tests of this type are shown in Fig.2 where the changes
in ACh output following morphine and naloxone have been
expressed on a percentage basis in order to standardize
the data obtained in different animals.   In control
animals morphine (2.0 mg/kg i.v.) depressed ACh output
by about 40%.   An injection of naloxone following
morphine reversed this depression and caused the release to exceed the pre-morphine value by nearly 200%.
In animals pretreated with AMPT, the same dose of
morphine did not inhibit the cortical ACh release and
in fact produced a significant enhancement.   Even
though there was no morphine induced depression,
naloxone administered after the agonist still enhanced
ACh output but the magnitude of this post-naloxone
release was smaller than in the control animals (Fig.
2).   In contrast to the AMPT treated animals, morphine
injection in PCPA treated animals depressed this
release and its effect in these animals was significantly greater ($p < 0.05$) than in control animals (Table
1).   Naloxone reversed the morphine induced inhibition
but in this case the post-naloxone increase did not

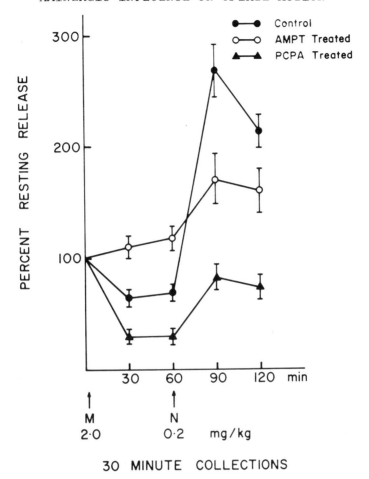

FIG. 2. <u>The comparative effects of morphine (M) and</u>
<u>naloxone (N) in the control, AMPT and PCPA pretreated</u>
<u>animals.</u> Results obtained from several experiments of
the type shown in Fig.1 have been standardized by
expressing post-morphine release as a percentage of
the pre-drug resting release. The average values for
resting release of ACh were 2.3 $\pm$ 0.4 (control), 2.4 $\pm$
0.3 (AMPT) and 6.8 $\pm$ 1.2 ng/0.25 cm^2/30 min (PCPA).

exceed the pre-morphine release of ACh (Fig.2). The
animals pretreated with PCPA exhibited a significantly
higher resting release of ACh than the control animals
or those given AMPT.
    To assess whether treatment with AMPT would block

the action of other agonists, the effect of the
synthetic opiate meperidine was tested in animals
receiving this treatment. The results of these tests
are shown in Fig.3. Injection of meperidine in control
animals (left histogram) depressed the release in the
first collection period but the release recovered to
the pre-drug level in the next collection period
indicating a shorter duration of action compared with

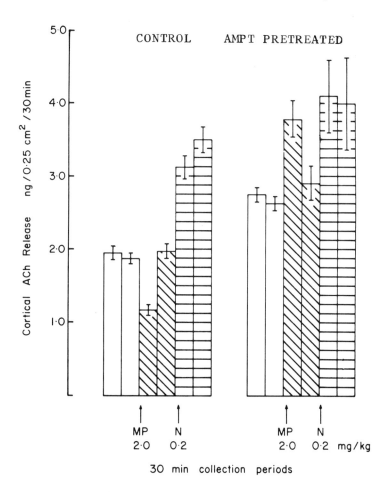

FIG. 3. Effect of meperidine(MP) and naloxone(N) on the
cortical output of ACh in control and AMPT pretreated
animals. Meperidine and naloxone were administered at
points indicated by arrows.AMPT(250 mg/kg i.p.)was administered 16-18 hours prior to the experiment.

that of morphine. Higher doses of meperidine (3.0 -
8.0 mg/kg)mainly evoked an increase in ACh release and
therefore these were not used. Naloxone given after
meperidine enhanced the ACh output over its resting
value. In the AMPT treated animals (right histogram)
meperidine did not depress ACh release and in fact
enhanced it. Naloxone given post-meperidine caused an
increase in ACh release, but as observed in the preceding tests, this effect was smaller than in the control animals.

Effect of monoamine receptor blocking agents

The effects of pretreatment with four receptor
blocking agents (methysergide, haloperidol, propranolol
and phenoxybenzamine) on the anti-release effects of
morphine are shown in Figs.4-7 and in Table 1.
    Figure 4   shows the results of experiments with
methysergide, a 5-HT receptor blocking agent. Injection of this drug in a low dose (0.5 mg/kg)produced a
100% increase in ACh output over its resting release
value and a subsequent injection (1.0 mg/kg) 60 min
later caused a 200% increase in this release. An injection of morphine given 60 min after the second
methysergide treatment reduced the release of ACh by
about 50%. This reduction in release was significantly
greater than that seen in the control animals (Table 1)
indicating that methysergide treatment facilitated the
anti-release action of morphine. Naloxone given post-
morphine reversed the opiate induced depression and
restored ACh output to pre-morphine levels.
    Fig.5 shows effects of two doses of haloperidol, a
dopamine receptor blocking agent, on cortical ACh output
and its influence on morphine action. The lower dose
(0.5 mg/kg) of the blocking agent enhanced ACh release
by about 30% (left histogram) but this effect of the
drug was not apparent after the administration of a
larger dose (right histogram) to another group of
animals. Morphine injected 30 min after either dose of
haloperidol depressed ACh release. When results of
these tests were compared with control tests the inhibitory effect of morphine following haloperidol was not
significantly different from its effect in the untreated animal. This indicated that haloperidol does not

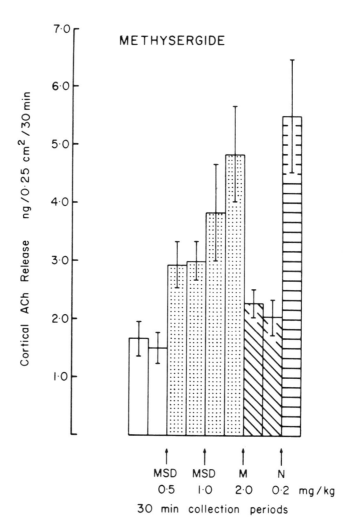

FIG. 4. Effect of methysergide (MSD) injection on the
cortical output of ACh and its influence on the action
of morphine on this release.
Drugs were injected (i.v.) at points indicated by the
arrows.

influence the inhibitory action of morphine on cortical
ACh release.

The effect of propranolol, a β -adrenergic receptor
blocking agent, on the ACh output and morphine effect
are shown in Fig. 6. This agent had no effect on the

resting release of ACh and also failed to affect the
inhibitory action of morphine in a significant manner
(Table 1).

   In contrast to the preceding tests, where each of
the three blocking agents was administered after starting the experiment, phenoxybenzamine, an irreversible
α -receptor blocking agent was administered to animals
three hours before starting the experiments. Initial
experiments in animals treated with phenoxybenzamine

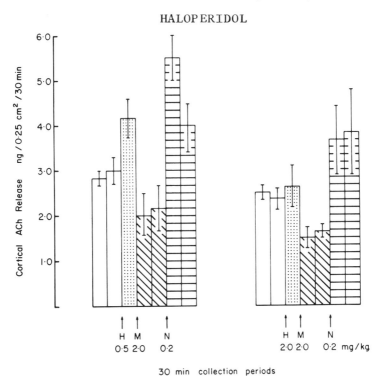

FIG. 5. Effects of haloperidol (H) treatment on the
cortical release of ACh and the effect of morphine following haloperidol. The histograms shown represent
two separate groups of animals.
Drugs were injected i.v. at the points indicated by
arrows.

TABLE 1. Morphine effect on cortical acetylcholine release after treatment with monoamine synthesis inhibitors and receptor blockers

Pretreatment (n)[a]	Dose (mg/kg)	% ACh release after morphine[b]	Significance (p)
Control	–	64.0 ± 4.0	–
PCPA (8)	316	30.6 ± 3.8	<0.001
AMPT (8)	250	107.2 ±11.4	<0.01
Methysergide(6)	1.5	48.8 ± 4.2	<0.05
Haloperidol(5)	0.5	55.6 ± 5.2	>0.05
Haloperidol(6)	2.0	62.5 ± 9.6	>0.05
Propranolol(5)	10.0	51.8 ± 5.8	>0.05
Phenoxybenzamine (6)	10.0	57.6 ± 3.3	>0.05
Phenoxybenzamine (6)	20.0	88.0 ± 7.5	<0.02
Phenoxybenzamine (6)	50.0	145.0 ± 2.3	<0.001

a   Number of observations

b Release is expressed as a percentage of output immediately prior to the injection of morphine (2 mg/kg).

(50 mg/kg) indicated a blockade of morphine effect on the cortical ACh release. In subsequent experiments morphine effect was evaluated in animals pretreated with lower doses (10, 20 mg/kg) of this blocking agent. The results of these tests are shown in Fig.7. The resting release of ACh in animals treated with phenoxy-benzamine, regardless of the doses used, was not significantly different from the control animals. In animals pretreated with the lowest dose of phenoxy-benzamine (10 mg/kg) morphine inhibited the release of cortical ACh and the magnitude of this effect was not significantly different from that in control tests (Table 1). Pretreatment with a dose of 20 mg/kg

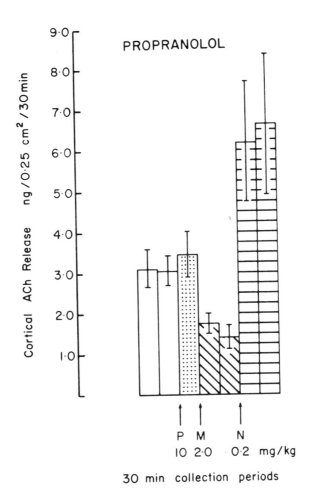

FIG. 6. Effect of propranolol (P) on the cortical ACh output and the action of morphine after propranolol. Drugs were injected i.v. at points indicated by arrows.

significantly enhanced the release of cortical ACh in response to morphine injection which normally depresses this release. An even greater enhancement of the morphine induced release was observed in animals that had been pretreated with a higher dose of phenoxybenzamine (50 mg/kg). Although there was no inhibition of ACh release by morphine in phenoxybenzamine treated animals (20, 50 mg/kg) administration of naloxone after morphine still evoked a very large increase in the cortical output of ACh. Previous work shows that the dose of naloxone used here has no significant effect on ACh release in the absence of morphine (17,18).

B. Morphine Analgesia:
Effects of Monoamine Synthesis Inhibitors and Receptor Blockers

To investigate whether agents which blocked or enhanced the anti-release action of morphine in preceding tests would also block or enhance morphine analgesia, their effect was tested on the analgesic response to a standard dose of morphine (10 mg/kg i.p.) using the hot-plate test. The interval between the drug pretreatments and morphine injection was adjusted to correspond as closely as possible to that in the

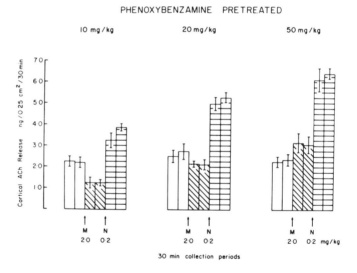

FIG.7. The effects of morphine (M) on the cortical release of ACh in animals pretreated with phenoxybenz-amine. The latter was administered i.p. 3 hours prior to each experiment. The histograms shown represent three separate groups of animals.
The drugs were injected at points indicated by the arrows.

release experiments. The effects of four treatments on
the latency of response (paw-licking) are shown in
Table 2. The treatment with AMPT had no significant
effect on the analgesic response to morphine whereas
pretreatment with PCPA produced a clear reduction
in the response as indicated by a smaller change in the
latency of response after the opiate. Phenoxybenzamine (20 mg/kg) markedly enhanced the analgesic
response to morphine as indicated by a large increase

TABLE 2. Morphine effect on the nociceptive response
after treatment with monoamine synthesis inhibitors
and receptor blockers

Treatment (n)[a]	Dose[b] (mg/kg)	% Change in latency[c]
Control (10)	–	134 ± 40
AMPT (8)	250	153 ± 61
PCPA (17)	316	44 ± 13[d]
Phenoxybenzamine (7)	10	126 ± 39
Phenoxybenzamine (6)	20	326 ± 31[d]
Methysergide (20)	2	150 ± 34

[a] n = no. of animals

[b] The interval between the treatment administered and
morphine (10 mg/kg i.p.) was the same as in the
release experiments

[c] Percent change in the latency of response (paw-lick)
after morphine

[d] Values significantly different from controls
(p < 0.05)

in the response latency. Methysergide (2.0 mg/kg) in these tests had no significant influence on morphine analgesia.

DISCUSSION

The results of this study show that the inhibitory effects of morphine and meperidine on the cortical release of ACh in the rat brain are blocked following pretreatment with AMPT which was used in a dose reported to reduce brain catecholamine levels (28). Similarly, treatment with phenoxybenzamine in doses shown by others to block the central effects of α-adrenergic receptor agonists (38) blocked the inhibitory morphine response. These findings indicate that the functional integrity of noradrenergic neurones is essential for the manifestation of morphine induced inhibition of cortical ACh output. These experiments also suggest that morphine may be causing a release of NE from these neurones which then acts to inhibit the output of cortical ACh. This explanation of morphine action is consistent with the report of Smith et al.(35) who showed that morphine specifically enhances the synthesis of brain DA and NE. It is also consistent with the studies of Beani et al.(3) and Beani and Bianchi (2) who demonstrated that NE inhibits the release of cortical ACh by acting on α-receptors. Pretreatment with AMPT has been found to reduce the EEG slowing produced by an injection of morphine (8). However, whether morphine causes a release of NE in vivo, and the site at which NE may act to inhibit the release of ACh is not known. Since subcortical lesioning of brain nuclei has been shown to block morphine effects on ACh release (18,31) it is conceivable that a subcortical site is involved in this interaction.

Administration of PCPA, in a dose that is known to deplete brain 5-HT (19), significantly enhanced the inhibitory effects of morphine on cortical ACh release. Methysergide, used here in doses similar to those reported to inhibit serotonergic transmission in vivo (7), also enhanced morphine induced inhibition of ACh release but to a lesser extent than PCPA pretreatment. These findings suggest that in contrast to catecholaminergic mechanisms, the integrity of the serotonergic mechanism is perhaps not essential for morphine induced depression of ACh release from the cortex. This observation is at variance with that of Garau et al.(12) who reported that surgical lesioning of the raphe nuclei abolished morphine effects on ACh release in the rat. The reason for this difference is not clear but it could be that lesioning destroys some component of the catecholaminergic system critical to the expression of the morphine effect. The reason why the morphine effect should be enhanced after the pharmacological blockade of the serotonergic system is not readily apparent. Recent studies of aminergic interaction indicate a reciprocal relationship between the central serotonergic and catecholaminergic systems (33). Destruction of the serotonergic system increases the turnover of cortical and cerebellar NE (32). Similarly the ability of amphetamine (which releases catecholamines) to increase locomotor activity in animals is augmented by pretreatment with PCPA, and on the basis of this observation a tonic inhibitory influence of 5-HT on the catecholaminergic neurones has been proposed (22). In view of these studies it is attractive to suggest that the morphine effect is enhanced following serotonergic blockade because the opiate is able to exert a greater action on the catecholaminergic system.

Pretreatment with PCPA and methysergide, was associated with a significant increase in the resting output of ACh, suggesting an inhibitory serotonergic tone on cortical ACh; removal of this tone by depletion, or by receptor blockade, leads to a rise in the ACh output. However, a previous study in which the release of ACh following PCPA treatment, or raphe lesioning was investigated did not reveal a significant change in the output of this substance (30). The difference between this and previous investigations could be related to factors such as the PCPA dosage, the addition of different agents to the collecting fluid in the cup, or the assay of ACh. The relationship between the serotonergic and the cholinergic mechanism in the cortex clearly deserves further study in view of the recent suggestion that 5-HT afferents may modulate striatal ACh (6).

Pretreatment with PCPA antagonized the analgesic

action of morphine whereas phenoxybenzamine enhanced this effect. If the inhibition of cortical ACh by morphine was directly related to its analgesic action PCPA should have antagonized the anti-release action of morphine and phenoxybenzamine should have enhanced it. In fact, opposite results were obtained in the ACh release experiments. These observations suggest that the inhibition of ACh release by morphine, at least at the cortical level, is not directly related to its ability to produce analgesia.

Both haloperidol and propranolol failed to influence the inhibitory actions of morphine on the release of cortical ACh suggesting that dopaminergic, or the β-adrenergic receptors, are not involved in this effect of morphine. In the striatum, where the cholinergic neurones are modulated by dopaminergic activity (see Introduction), dopamine appears to play a role in the narcotic action on the striatal cholinergic function (10). It is entirely possible that morphine effects on the cholinergic neurones in various regions of the CNS are manifested indirectly through its action on the neuronal system that modulate these cholinergic neurones. Since the nature of the modulatory system is likely to differ from region to region, the mechanism of morphine action on the regional cholinergic neurones may differ accordingly.

SUMMARY

Effects of morphine on the release of cortical ACh were investigated in animals treated with the monoamine synthesis inhibitors, PCPA and AMPT, or the monoamine receptor blocking agents methysergide, haloperidol, propranolol and phenoxybenzamine. Both AMPT and phenoxybenzamine blocked the morphine induced inhibition of ACh release. In contrast, PCPA and methysergide enhanced this effect of morphine. Haloperidol and propranolol had no effect on morphine action. Effects of PCPA, AMPT, methysergide and phenoxybenzamine were also evaluated on morphine analgesia. Treatment with PCPA antagonized morphine analgesia whereas phenoxybenzamine enhanced it. These observations suggest that noradrenergic mechanisms play an essential role in the inhibitory actions of morphine on cortical ACh release, and this effect is not directly related to its analgesic action.

ACKNOWLEDGEMENTS

The authors gratefully acknowledge gifts of naloxone (Endo Laboratories), methysergide (Sandoz), haloperidol (McNeil Laboratories), phenoxybenzamine (Smith, Kline & French), meperidine (Winthrop Laboratories), and propranolol (Ayerst Laboratories). This investigation was supported by the Medical Research Council of Canada and the Directorate for the Non-Medical Use of Drugs, Health and Welfare, Canada. We thank Dr.G.S. Marks for helpful discussion of the manuscript.

REFERENCES

1. Agid, Y., Guyenet, P., Glowinski, J., Beaujovan, J.C.,and Javoy, F. (1974): Brain Res., 86: 488.
2. Beani, L., and Bianchi, L. (1975): In: Abstracts Sixth International Congress of Pharmacology, p. 101, Sanomaprint, Helsinki.
3. Beani, L., Bianchi, C., and Castellucci, A. (1974): Eur.J.Pharmacol., 26: 63.
4. Beani, L., Bianchi, C., Santinoceto, L., and Marchetti, P. (1968): Int.J.Neuropharmacol., 7:469.
5. Beleslin, D., and Polak, L. (1965): J.Physiol. (Lond.), 177: 411.
6. Butcher, S.H., Butcher, L.L., and Cho, A.K. (1976): Life Sci., 18: 733.
7. Clineschmidt, B.V., and Anderson, E.G. (1970): Exp.Brain Res., 11: 175.
8. Colasanti, B., and Khazan, N. (1973): Neuropharmacology, 12: 463.
9. Consolo, S., Ladinsky, H., and Garattini, S. (1974): J.Pharm.Pharmacol., 26: 275.
10. Costa, E., Cheney, D.L., Racagni, G., and Zsilla,G. (1975): Life Sci., 17: 1.
11. Crossland, J., and Slater, P. (1968): Br.J.Pharmacol. Chemother., 32: 42.
12. Garau, L., Mulas, M.L., and Pepeu, G. (1975): Neuropharmacology, 14: 259.
13. Giarman, N.J., and Pepeu, G. (1962): Br.J.Pharmacol. Chemother., 19: 226.

14. Jhamandas, K., Hron, V., and Sutak, M. (1975):
Can.J.Physiol.Pharmacol., 53: 540.
15. Jhamandas, K., Phillis, J.W., and Pinsky, C. (1971):
Br.J.Pharmacol., 43: 53.
16. Jhamandas, K., Pinsky, C., and Phillis, J.W.(1970):
Nature, 228: 176.
17. Jhamandas, K., and Sutak, M. (1974): Br.J.
Pharmacol., 50: 57.
18. Jhamandas, K., and Sutak, M. (1976): Br.J.
Pharmacol., In press.
19. Koe, B., and Weissman, A. (1966): J.Pharmacol.Exp.
Ther., 154: 499.
20. Labrecque, G., and Domino, E.F. (1974): J.Pharmacol.
Exp.Ther., 191: 189.
21. Large, W.A., and Milton, A.S. (1970): Br.J.
Pharmacol., 38: 451P.
22. Mabry, P.D., and Campbell, B.R. (1973): Brain Res.,
49: 381.
23. MacIntosh, F.C., and Oborin, P.E. (1953): In:
Abstracts 19th International Physiological Congress
p.580.
24. Matthews, J.D., Labrecque, G., and Domino, E.F.
(1973): Psychopharmacologia, 29: 113.
25. Maynert, E.W. (1967): Arch.Biol.Med.Exp.(Santiago),
4: 36.
26. McGeer, P.L., Grewaal, D.S.,and McGeer, E.G.(1974):
Brain Res., 80: 211.
27. Mullin, W.J., Phillis, J.W., and Pinsky, C. (1973):
Eur.J.Pharmacol., 22: 117.
28. Papeschi, R., and Randrup, A. (1973):
Pharmacopsychiatr.Neuropsychopharmakol., 6: 137.
29. Paton, W.D.M. (1957): Br.J.Pharmacol.Chemother.,
12: 119.
30. Pepeu, G., Garau, L., and Mulas, M.L. (1974):
In: Serotonin:New Vistas.Histochemistry and
Pharmacology, edited by E.Costa, G.L.Gessa, and M.
Sandler, p.247. Raven Press, New York.
31. Pepeu, G., Garau, L., Mulas, M.L., and Marconcini-
Pepeu, I. (1975): Brain Res., 100: 677.
32. Pujol, J.F., Stein, D., Blondaux, C.H., Petitjean,
F., Froment, J.L., and Jouvet, M. (1974):
Biochem.Pharmacol., Suppl.2: 636.
33. Samanin, R., and Garattini, S. (1976): Life Sci.,
17: 1201.

34.Schaumann, W. (1957): Br.J.Pharmacol.Chemother.,
     12: 115.
35.Smith, C.B., Sheldon, M.I., Bednarczyk, J.H.,and
     Villarreal, J.E. (1972): J.Pharmacol.Exp.Ther.,
     180: 547.
36.Stadler, H., Lloyd, K.G., Gadea-Ciria, M. and
     Bartholini, G. (1973): Brain Res., 55: 476.
37.Szerb, J.C. (1974): Eur.J.Pharmacol., 29: 192.
38.Vaupel, D.B., and Martin, W.R. (1976): J.Pharmacol.
     Exp.Ther., 196: 87.
39.Yaksh, T.L., and Yamamura, H.I. (1975): Brain Res.,
     83: 520.

Factors Affecting the Action of Narcotics, edited by
M.L. Adler, L. Manara, and R. Samanin.
Raven Press, New York © 1978.

Acetylcholine Turnover Rate in Specific Brain Nuclei:
Effects of Narcotic Analgetics

G. Zsilla[*], D.L. Cheney and E. Costa

Laboratory of Preclinical Pharmacology,
National Institute of Mental Health,
Saint Elizabeths Hospital,
Washington, D.C. 20032, U.S.A.

INTRODUCTION

Several lines of independent investigation indicate
that morphine modifies cholinergic transmission; for
instance opiates can reduce the release of acetylcholine (ACh) from cortical synapses (2,23) and also
reduce the ACh released by coaxial stimulation of guinea
pig ileum (33,37). In rats made dependent on morphine,
the abstinence causes an excessive release of ACh (9)
which can be blocked by muscarinic receptor blockers
(11,22). An involvement in the action of morphine of
neuronal pathways other than cholinergic has been
proposed (10,17,35,36). To better understand how
opiates change the activity of cholinergic neurons, we
have developed a radiochromatographic method to measure
the turnover rate of acetylcholine (TR_{ACh}) in brain
parts (8,34) and, more recently, a mass fragmentographic
method to measure TR_{ACh} in brain nuclei (44). The
possibility that an endogenous morphine-like factor
(20) normally modulates the activity of various brain
neurons and that opiates mimic the action of this
endogenous modulator, suggests that morphine may change
the TR_{ACh} only in those brain areas in which the
endogenous morphine modulates the TR_{ACh}.
     Previously, we reported that during morphine analgesia
TR_{ACh} decreased in occipital cortex (8) but failed to
change in striatum. However in morphine dependent rats
TR_{ACh} was reduced in striatum but not in cortex. The
change of TR_{ACh} could be reversed by the opiate antagonist, naloxone. Hence, searching to establish a correlation between opiate analgesia and the modulation of
TR_{ACh} in brain areas containing different densities of

*Present address: Semmelweis University of Medicine,
                  Department of Pharmacology, Budapest,
                  Hungary

451

opiate receptors (39), we studied the analgesia elicited by various doses of morphine, meperidine, azidomorphine (24,25), viminol R_2 (14) and measured the TR_{ACh} in various areas of the brain. The correlation between analgetic doses and those that change TR_{ACh} was calculated statistically. In rats injected with morphine, the TR_{ACh} was also measured in brain nuclei containing low density of opiate receptors and cholinergic terminals which have their cell bodies in brain areas with abundant concentration of opiate receptors.

METHODS

Turnover of ACh

TR_{ACh} was measured in various brain areas following labeling of ACh stores with a constant rate infusion of phosphoryl-$^{14}CH_3$ choline. Phosphoryl-$^{14}CH_3$ choline/ sp. act. 49 μCi/μmole was infused i.v. 6 min through the tail vein (25 μCi/kg/min; 0.2 ml/min). ACh and Choline (Ch) were extracted using the method of Hanin, Cheney, Trabucchi, Massarelli, Wang and Costa (19) as modified by Cheney, Costa, Hanin, Trabucchi and Wang (6). In brain nuclei TR_{ACh} was measured by a mass fragmentographic technique following the infusion of deuterated phosphorylcholine (PhCh-D_4) for nine minutes (15 μmoles/kg/min; 0.1 ml/min); this infusion labels ACh stores at steady state as reported by Zsilla et al. (44)

Stereomicroscopic Dissection of Brain Nuclei

The rats were killed by focused microwave radiation (18) and their brain was mounted on a microtome stage of a cryostat. Sections (400 microns thick) were cut at -2°C. Coronal sections were cut perpendicular to the longitudinal plane of the brain until the genu corporis callosi appeared (27). Konig and Klippel (26) stereotaxic atlas was used as a general guide. The nuclei were punched out with steel tubing (0.8-1.2 mm i.d.) while the brain parts (striatum, cortex,hippocampus) were dissected according to Iversen and Glowinski (21). TR_{ACh} was calculated by multiplying the fractional rate constant of ACh efflux (k_b) by the steady state concentration of ACh ($TR_{ACh} = K_b\ ACh$) where

$$k_b = \frac{-1}{t_1}\ln\left(1 - \frac{k_B}{k_a} + \frac{k_B}{k_a}e^{-k_a t_1}\right) + \frac{1}{m}\left(\frac{k_B}{k_a} - 1\right)(1 - e^{-k_a t_1})$$

k_a = fractional rate constant of Ch, m = the ratio of Ch and ACh specific activities (34)

Estimation of Analgetic Activity

The ED_{50} for analgesia was determined by tail flick method (13). A drug was considered to exert an analgesic action if the time required to elicit the tail flick response was twice that recorded in rats injected with saline. Data were analyzed as a quantal response and the ED_{50} for analgesia was calculated according to Litchfield and Wilcoxon (31).

Statistical Calculation

Statistical significance was determined according to Dunnett's t-test (two tailed) corrected for unequal sample size (42). The dose that inhibits the TR_{ACh} by 50% for each of the drugs was calculated graphically, the correlation coefficient of the relationship between analgesia and the inhibition of TR_{ACh} was calculated by Fisher's method (15).

Animals and Materials

Male Sprague-Dawley rats (Zivic Miller Laboratory, Allison Park, Pa.) weighing 100-120 g were used throughout.
Morphine sulfate (S.B. Penick, N.Y., N.Y.), meperidine (Sterling-Winthrop, Rensselaer, N.Y.), azidomorphine (6-deoxy-6-azido-dihydroisomorphine bitartrate, Tiszavasvar, Hungary) and naltrexone (Endo Labs., Garden City, N.Y.) were dissolved in saline. Viminol R_2 (alpha-(N-o-chlorobenzyl)-pyrryl-2-di-sec-butylamine ethanol p-hydroxybenzoate) and viminol S_2 (Zambon Research Lab., Milan, Italy) were dissolved in acetic acid diluted with saline after adjusting the pH to 5. Phosphoryl-$^{14}CH_3$-choline was purchased from New England Nuclear Corp., Boston, Mass. Deuterated phosphoryl-choline was obtained from Merck, Sharp and Dohme, Quebec, Canada.

RESULTS

Maximal tolerated doses of morphine, azidomorphine, viminol R_2 and meperidine failed to change the steady state concentration of ACh and Ch in striatum (Table 1) in cortex and hippocampus (Table 2) 20 minutes after injection. Since the ACh steady state remained unchanged we could apply labeling with radioactive or stable isotope precursors and the principles of steady state kinetics to estimate the TR_{ACh}. The TR_{ACh} was unchanged in striatum of rats injected with high doses of the four analgetics (Table 1).but it was reduced

TABLE 1. Striatal TR_{ACh} after morphine, azidomorphine and viminol R_2 [a]

Drug (μmoles/kg)	ACh (nmoles/g)	Ch (nmoles/g)	TR_{ACh} (μmoles/g/hr)
Saline	52 + 3.4	24 + 3.4	0.83 + 0.071
Morphine, i.p. (70)	53 + 3.6	20 + 3.2	0.63 + 0.070
Azidomorphine, s.c. (0.64)	49 + 3.3	30 + 3.2	0.76 + 0.060
Meperidine, s.c. (607)	50 + 3.2	22 + 2.2	0.93 + 0.080
Viminol R_2, i.p. (20)	54 + 5.3	27 + 2.7	0.87 + 0.025
Naltrexone, i.p. (2.9)	53 + 3.6	20 + 2.5	0.80 + 0.070

[a]Data are the mean ± S.E.M. of at least five determinations. Rats were killed 20 minutes after injection of morphine, azidomorphine, meperidine and viminol R_2, and 15 minutes after naltrexone.

$TR_{ACh} = k_B$ (ACh).

TABLE 2. Naltrexone inhibition of the decrease in cortical and hippocampal TR_{ACh} elicited by azido-morphine, viminol R_2, morphine and meperidine[a]

Drug (μmol/kg)	CORTEX			HIPPOCAMPUS		
	ACh (nmol/g)	Ch (nmol/g)	TR_{ACh} (μmol/g/hr)	ACh (nmol/g)	Ch (nmol/g)	TR_{ACh} (μmol/g/hr)
Saline	14+0.40	25+3.7	0.20+0.020	29+4.2	38+3.6	0.58+0.030
Naltrexone (2.9)	15+1.6	30+2.7	0.23+0.090[b]	29+1.9	38+4.7	0.60+0.090
Morphine (52)	15+2.1	30+1.6	0.07+0.010[b]	29+1.7	38+4.8	0.19+0.010[c]
Morphine (52) + Naltrexone (2.9)	15+1.2	30+1.5	0.19+0.010[b]	27+1.7	39+3.2	0.45+0.18
Azidomorphine (0.32)	16+0.50	30+1.6	0.10+0.013[b]	28+3.9	39+4.8	0.17+0.040[c]
Azidomorphine (0.32) + Naltrexone (2.9)	15+1.4	30+1.9	0.17+0.040	28+3.0	38+4.8	0.34+0.13
Viminol R_2 (10)	12+1.3	29+2.1	0.070+0.010[b]	33+2.7	33+3.5	0.24+0.050[c]
Viminol R_2 (10) + Naltrexone (2.9)	15+1.2	30+3.0	0.14+0.010[d]	28+3.6	37+4.2	0.47+0.17
Meperidine (402)	15+1.3	25+4.1	0.11+0.011[d]	27+2.2	38+2.9	0.16+0.033[c]
Meperidine (402) + Naltrexone (2.9)	16+1.8	30+2.0	0.22+0.024	29+1.3	37+2.6	0.46+0.080

[a] Data are mean ± SEM of at least five determinations. Significance is indicated when treated group is compared to saline treated rats. Rats were killed 20 min after the administration of analgesics and 15 min after naltrexone injected intraperitoneally. The opiate antagonist was injected 5 min after the intraperitoneal injection of viminol R_2 or morphine and the subcutaneous injection of azidomorphine and meperidine.

$TR_{ACh} = k_B$ (ACh)

[b] $p < 0.01$ [c] $p < 0.005$ [d] $p < 0.05$

significantly in cortex and hippocampus 20 minutes after the injection of azidomorphine, viminol R_2, morphine and meperidine in doses of 0.20, 5, 35, 200 μmoles/kg, respectively. Table 3 shows the calculated ED_{50} of the various drugs for analgesia and to decrease the TR_{ACh}. Viminol S_2 a non-analgesic stereoisomer of viminol R_2 did not change the TR_{ACh} in the brain parts examined when injected in doses of 20 μmoles/kg i.p. Naltrexone opiate antagonist (2.9 μmoles/kg) decreased or antagonized the reduction of TR_{ACh} (Table 2) but when given alone it failed to change the TR_{ACh} of striatum (Table 1), cortex and hippocampus (Table 2). The data reported in Table 3 show that the ED_{50} for analgesia for each drug tested correlated with the ED_{50} for reducing TR_{ACh} in cortex and hippocampus. Moreover, the ED_{50} for analgesia and the ED_{50} for the reduction of TR_{ACh} were not statistically different. Morphine (70 μmoles/kg i.p.) decreased the TR_{ACh} in N. accumbens but not in N. raphe dorsalis, N. septi, N. interpeduncularis and substantia nigra (Table 4). Also in N. accumbens this reduction could be reversed by naltrexone (data not shown).

TABLE 3.   Correlation between ED_{50} to reduce TR_{ACh} in cortex and hippocampus and ED_{50} for analgesia: study of azidomorphine, viminol R_2, morphine and meperidine

Analgetic	ED_{50}[a] analgesia (y)	CORTEX		HIPPOCAMPUS	
		ED_{50}[a] TR_{ACh} (x)	Statistical[b] analysis	ED_{50}[a] TR_{ACh} (x)	Statistical[b] analysis
Azidomorphine	0.20	0.38	a=0.55$\pm$0.01	0.21	a=1.49$\pm$0.05
Viminol R_2	5.0	6.75	b=1.96$\pm$1.58	6.75	b=5.89$\pm$4.67
Morphine	35	55	r=0.999	33	r=0.998
Meperidine	220	200	t=31.61 P=0.001	150	t=22.33 P=0.002

[a] ED_{50} in μmoles/kg.   Five or six doses of each drug were used to calculate the ED_{50} for analgesia and the doses that reduce by 50% the TR_{ACh}.
[b] y = ax + b

DISCUSSION

The experiments reported show that morphine, meperidine azidomorphine, and viminol R_2, four analgetics with different chemical structures, inhibit the TR_{ACh} in cortex and hippocampus but fail to change that of striatum. Moreover, morphine inhibits TR_{ACh} in N. accumbens but not in other brain nuclei (interpeduncularis, N. septi, N. amygdalae, substantia nigra, N. raphe dorsalis). The action of morphine on TR_{ACh} of any given brain structure or nucleus does not appear to depend exclusively on its content in opiate receptors. Snyder (39) reported that the density of opiate receptors in striatum, amygdalae and substantia nigra is relatively high; our data show that the TR_{ACh} in these structures is not changed by doses of morphine that are twice or more the ED_{50} for analgesia (Table 4).

TABLE 4. TR_{ACh} in stereomicroscopically isolated rat brain nuclei: inhibition by morphine

		k_B hr^{-1}	TR_{ACh} (nmol/mg protein/ hr)
N. Caudatus	S	12 ± 1.5	6.7 ± 1.0
	M	12 ± 1.4	7.0 ± 1.1
N. Accumbens	S	13 ± 3.1	6.3 ± 1.0
	M	3.5 ± 0.88*	2.0 ± 0.75*
N. Septi	S	5.5 ± 0.87	1.1 ± 0.16
	M	3.9 ± 0.36	0.71 ± 0.065
N. Raphe Dorsalis	S	6.8 ± 1.6	2.4 ± 0.61
	M	4.7 ± 1.1	2.0 ± 0.66
N. Amygdalae	S	2.4 ± 0.63	0.92 ± 0.25
	M	2.1 ± 0.58	1.3 ± 0.26
Hippocampus	S	16 ± 2.6	3.7 ± 0.60
	M	7.2 ± 1.1*	1.8 ± 0.25*
Substantia Nigra	S	3.6 ± 1.4	0.59 ± 0.14
	M	3.7 ± 0.63	0.67 ± 0.009
N. Inter- peduncularis	S	1.9 ± 0.32	2.0 ± 0.33
	M	2.2 ± 0.36	3.3 ± 0.82

Each mean ± S.E.M. refers to 4 or 5 determinations.

S = pretreatment (20 minutes) with saline
M = morphine (70 μmoles/kg i.p.) 20 minutes before

Although striatum and N. accumbens have a similar
abundance of cholinergic interneurons (3,7) and important dopaminergic afferents (27,32,41), the action of
morphine on the TR_{ACh} of these nuclei is different.
Morphine decreases the TR_{ACh} in N. accumbens but not
in striatum (Table 4) although it increases the turnover
rate of dopamine (TR_{DA}) in both nuclei. Though morphine
and amphetamine increase the TR_{DA} in both nuclei only
amphetamine decreases the TR_{ACh} (4).   In contrast,
haloperidol increases both the TR_{DA} (43) and TR_{ACh} in
striatum and N. accumbens (40).   These results indicate
that the synaptic organization of cholinergic and
dopaminergic neurons in striatum and N. accumbens is
different. Hippocampus has low opiate receptor density
(39) but receives important cholinergic innervation
from cholinergic cell bodies located in septum (30).
Septal stimulation releases ACh from hippocampus (38),
lesions in septal area decrease ACh content and Ch
uptake in hippocampus (29). We infer that the decrease
in hippocampal TR_{ACh} reflects primarily a regulatory
action of cholinergic cell bodies on septum by opiate
receptors. If this mechanism were operative, it is
not reflected by changes in the TR_{ACh}, suggesting that
during trans synaptic stimulation, TR_{ACh} changes in
nerve terminals but not in cell bodies.
    Septum and hippocampus are innervated by serotonergic
pathways which originate in raphe nuclei (12,16).
Lesions of midbrain raphe decrease the analgesic and
antinociceptive effect of morphine (1) suggesting that
either serotonin transmission or axons of unknown
biochemical nature passing through the area may be
required for the action of centrally acting analgetics.
The dorsal raphe contains serotonergic cell bodies and
cholinergic terminals but doses which are ED_{50} for
analgesia fail to change the TR_{ACh} in dorsal raphe.
Morphine fails to change the TR_{ACh} in N. interpeduncularis
which receives cholinergic innervation from habenula
rich in opiate receptors (28,39) and in substantia
nigra which contains DA cell bodies and a high density
of opiate receptors and in amygdalae. This lack of
correlation between opiate receptor density and the
decrease of TR_{ACh} suggests that opiate receptors are
not universal modulators of cholinergic neurons; and
they may have a regulatory influence on cholinergic as
well as other kinds of neurons. Moreover, the conclusion that morphine does not primarily act on cholinergic
neurons is upheld although we have shown that analgetics
reduce TR_{ACh} in cortex, hippocampus and N. accumbens.
The correlation between ED_{50} for analgesia and the dose
that inhibits by 50% the TR_{ACh} of these structures is
highly significant.

REFERENCES

1. Adler, M., Kostowski, W., Recchia, M. and Samanin, R. (1975): Eur. J. Pharmacol. 32: 39
2. Beleslin, D. and Polak, R. (1965): J. Physiol. (Lond.), 117: 411
3. Butcher, S.G. and Butcher, L.L. (1974): Brain Res., 71: 167
4. Carenzi, A., Cheney, D.L., Costa, E., Guidotti, A. and Racagni, G. (1975): Neuropharmacology, 14:927
5. Carenzi, A., Guidotti, A., Revuelta, A. and Costa, E. (1975): J. Pharmacol. Exp. Ther., 194: 311
6. Cheney, D.L., Costa, E., Hanin, I., Trabucchi, M. and Wang, C.T. (1975): J. Pharmacol. Exp. Ther., 192: 288
7. Cheney, D.L., LeFevre, H.F. and Racagni, G. (1975): Neuropharmacology, 14: 801
8. Cheney, D.L., Trabucchi, M., Racagni, G., Wang, C. and Costa, E. (1975): Life Sci., 15: 1977
9. Collier, H.O.J., Francis, D.L. and Schneider, C. (1972): Nature (Lond.), 237: 220
10. Costa, E., Carenzi, A., Guidotti, A. and Revuelta, A. (1973): In: Frontiers in Catecholamine Research, edited by E. Usdin and S. Snyder, p. 1003. Pergamon Press, London
11. Crossland, J. (1970): In: Drugs and Cholinergic Mechanisms in the CNS, edited by E. Heilbronn and A. Winter, p. 355. Forsvarets Forskningsanstalt, Stockholm, Sweden
12. Dahlstrom, A. and Fuxe, K. (1964): Acta Physiol. Scand., 62 (suppl. 232): 1
13. D'Amour, F.E. and Smith, D.L. (1941): J. Pharmacol. Exp. Ther., 72: 74
14. Della Bella, D., Ferrari, V., Frigeni, V. and Lualdi, P. (1973): Nature (New Biol.), 241: 282
15. Fisher, R.A. (1958): Statistical Methods for Research Workers, p. 175. Hafner Publ. Co., New York.
16. Fuxe, K. (1965): Acta Physiol. Scand., 64 (suppl. 247): 37
17. Garau, L., Mulas, M.L. and Pepeu, G. (1975): Neuropharmacology, 14: 259
18. Guidotti, A., Cheney, D.L., Trabucchi, M., Doteuchi, M., Wang, C.T. and Hawkins, P. (1974): Neuropharmacology, 13: 1115
19. Hanin, I., Cheney, D.L., Trabucchi, M., Massarelli, M., Wang, C.T. and Costa, E. (1973): J. Pharmacol. Exp. Ther., 187: 68
20. Hughes, J. (1975): Brain Res., 88: 295
21. Iversen, L. and Glowinski, J. (1966): J. Neurochem., 13: 671
22. Jhamandas, K. and Dickinson, G. (1973): Nature (New Biol.), 245: 219

23. Jhamandas, K., Pinsky, C. and Phillis, J.W. (1970): Nature (Lond.), 228: 176
24. Knoll, J., Fürst, S. and Kelemen, K. (1973): J. Pharm. Pharmacol., 25: 929
25. Knoll, J. and Zsilla, G. (1974): Biochem. Pharmacol. 23: 745
26. Konig, J.F.R. and Klippel, R.A. (1963): The Rat Brain: A stereotaxic Atlas of the Forebrain and Lower Parts of the Brain Stem. R.E. Krieger Publ. Co., Huntingdon, New York.
27. Koslow, S.H., Racagni, G. and Costa, E. (1974): Neuropharmacology, 13: 1123
28. Kuhar, M.J., DeHaven, R.N., Yamamura, H.I., Rommelspacher, H. and Simon, J.R. (1975): Brain Res., 97: 265
29. Kuhar, M.J., Sethy, V.H., Roth, R.H. and Aghajanian, G.K. (1973): J. Neurochem., 20: 581
30. Lewis, P.R. and Shute, C.C.D. (1967): Brain, 90: 521
31. Litchfield, J.T. and Wilcoxon, F. (1949): J. Pharmacol. Exp. Ther., 96: 99
32. McGeer, E.G., McGeer, P.L., Darshan, S., Greewaal, V. and Singh, K. (1975): J. Pharmacol. (Paris), 6: 143
33. Paton, W.D.M. (1957): Br. J. Pharmacol., 12: 119
34. Racagni, G., Cheney, D.L., Trabucchi, M., Wang, C. and Costa, E. (1974): Life Sci., 15: 1961
35. Samanin, R. and Bernasconi, S. (1972): Psychopharmacologia (Berlin), 25: 175
36. Samanin, R., Gumulka, W. and Valzelli, L. (1970): Eur. J. Pharmacol., 10: 339
37. Schauman, W. (1957): Br. J. Pharmacol., 12: 115
38. Smith, C.M. (1972): Br. J. Pharmacol., 45: 172P
39. Snyder, S.H. (1975): Nature (Lond.), 257: 185
40. Trabucchi, M., Cheney, D.L., Racagni, G. and Costa, E. (1975): Brain Res., 85: 130
41. Ungerstedt, U. (1971): Acta Physiol. Scand., 367: 69
42. Winer, B.J. (1971): Statistical Principles in Experimental Design, p. 201. McGraw Hill Co., New York
43. Zivkovic, B., Guidotti, A., Revuelta, A. and Costa, E. (1975): J. Pharmacol. Exp. Ther., 194: 37
44. Zsilla, G., Racagni, G., Cheney, D.L. and Costa, E. (1977): Neuropharmacology, 16: 25

Factors Affecting the Action of Narcotics, edited by
M.L. Adler, L. Manara, and R. Samanin.
Raven Press, New York©1978.

Cholinergic-Dopaminergic Relationships During Antagonist-Precipitated Morphine Withdrawal

Edgar T.Iwamoto, Horace H.Loh and E. Leong Way

Department of Pharmacology, University of California
San Francisco, California 94143, U.S.A.

INTRODUCTION

There is considerable evidence suggesting that
brain dopamine may be involved in the manifestation of
withdrawal in morphine-dependent mice and rats.
Naloxone-precipitated withdrawal was accompanied by an
elevation of neostriatal dopamine levels (23).
Maruyama and Takemori (32) and Herz, Bläsig and
Papeschi (21) found that drug manipulations that compromised catecholaminergic mechanisms greatly hindered
the expression of morphine withdrawal. Other data
suggested that cholinergic regulation may also participate in withdrawal. Drug-induced elevation of brain
acetylcholine levels reduced the naloxone-precipitated
withdrawal jumping response in mice(5), whereas a
lowering of acetylcholine enhanced the response (6).
Since we have reported previously that contralateral
circling behavior was precipitated by naloxone in
morphine-dependent rats with unilateral lesions of the
substantia nigra zona compacta (SNC) (25), the following study was designed to examine the effect of
dopaminergic and cholinergic agonists and antagonists
on the naloxone-precipitated contralateral circling
and withdrawal behaviors in unilaterally SNC-lesioned,
morphine-dependent rats.

METHODS AND MATERIALS

Unilateral Electrolytic SNC Lesions

Male Sprague-Dawley rats weighing 95-105 g were
anesthetized with halothane-O_2 and unilateral

461

electrolytic lesions (0.5–0.6 mA for 10 seconds) were
made in the left SNC at +1.8 mm anterior, 1.8 mm
lateral and -2.3 mm vertical (29). The resulting
lesions 1.2–2 mm in diameter centered in the dorsolateral SNC and were histologically similar to those
previously described (24, 25) in which ipsilateral
neostriatal dopamine was depleted by 66 percent. Sham
operations were performed with the electrode at -1.8
mm vertical without the passage of current.

Chemicals

For intra-neostriatal administrations, arecoline
hydrochloride (K and K Laboratories, Plainview, N.Y.)
and atropine sulfate (Sigma Chemical Co., St.Louis,
Missouri) were delivered in 3 μl of artificial CSF
(36). Apomorphine hydrochloride (Merck, Sharp and
Dohme, Philadelphia, Pa.), d-amphetamine sulfate (K
and K Laboratories) and naloxone hydrochloride (Endo
Laboratories, Garden City, N.Y.) were dissolved in
saline. Haloperidol (McNeil Laboratories, Fort
Washington, Pa.) was dissolved according to Andén,
Butcher, Corrodi, Fuxe and Ungerstedt (1). All drug
doses refer to the free base.

Effect of Drug Treatments on Naloxone-Precipitated Withdrawal in Morphine - Dependent Rats

Two weeks after lesioning, animals were screened
for circling behavior after the administration of
4 mg/kg i.p. d-amphetamine. Circling movements were
scored according to Naylor and Olley (34) and Iwamoto
et al.(24,25).

The subcutaneous morphine pellet implantation
technique was used to render animals highly dependent
on morphine (22,41,43). One week after prescreening
for circling behavior, rats were surgically implanted
with one morphine pellet followed 24 hr later by two
additional pellets.

After 72 hr of pellet implantation, separate groups
of rats were administered i.p. saline, apomorphine or
haloperidol. Other groups were anesthetized with
halothane-O_2 and administered artificial CSF,
arecoline or atropine into the intact neostriatum of

the right side (CSF into all left neostriata) with the
aid of bilateral stereotaxically mounted Hamilton
microsyringes (24). 20 min after apomorphine or
arecoline and 30 min after haloperidol or atropine,
morphine withdrawal was precipitated by 20 mg/kg of
naloxone s.c., and the behavioral signs of precipitated ′
abstinence were evaluated for 10 min and scored according to Wei and Loh (42) using non parametric, rank-
scored methods. In all experiments, catalepsy (scored
according to ref.15), stereotypy (34), and circling
behavior were assessed during the 20- or 30 min periods
before and during the 10 min after the naloxone challenge. The Mann-Whitney U-test was used to evaluate
the behavioral responses (which were assessed using
ranking methods) by comparing the highest scores
achieved by each animal between groups.

RESULTS

Effect of Unilateral, Intraneostriatal Arecoline Administration on Naloxone-Precipitated Contralateral Circling in SNC-lesioned, Morphine-Dependent Rats

Arecoline, which was administered unilaterally into
the neostriatum, produced circling behavior towards
the injected side and did not modify the naloxone-
precipitated withdrawal signs. Table 1 shows circling
behavior after naloxone in both sham-operated and left-
SNC-lesioned rats 20 min after 0, 32.5, 65 or 130 μg
arecoline administered into the right, intact
neostriatum. In animals rendered dependent by morphine
pellet implantation, arecoline produced circling
behavior of mild intensity towards the side of drug administration in both sham-operated and left-lesioned
rats. The control group injected with artificial CSF
did not exhibit circling behavior. Naloxone precipitated circling behavior towards the contralateral side
in the left-SNC-lesioned, artificial CSF-injected
groups as previously observed. Increasing doses of
arecoline, which itself produced circling movements
contralateral to the SNC lesion, did not modify the
direction or the intensity of the contralateral
circling that was precipitated by naloxone. Additionally, intraneostriatal arecoline also failed to modify

naloxone-precipitated withdrawal signs in all groups
of animals.

TABLE 1, Intra-neostriatal arecoline effects on
circling and precipitated-withdrawal behaviors before
and after naloxone in morphine-dependent, unilaterally
SNC-lesioned rats[a]

Dose (μg)	Group (N)	Group Mean Scores		
		Before naloxone	After naloxone	
		Circling	Circling	Withdrawal
0	S(8)	0	0	3.0
	L(8)	0	2.8 R	3.0
32.5	S(6)	0.2 R	0	3.0
	L(6)	0.2 R	2.8 R	3.0
65	S(6)	0.8 R	0.3 R	3.0
	L(6)	0.7 R	2.5 R	3.0
130	S(6)	2.0 R[c]	1.0 R[b]	3.0
	L(10)	1.7 R[c]	2.6 R	3.0

[a]Arecoline, 0 to 130 μg, was administered into the
right neostriatum of sham-operated (S) and left-SNC-
lesioned (L) morphine-dependent rats 20 min before a
20 mg/kg naloxone challenge.

R = circling behavior to the right. Significant
  difference from the respective CSF-treated control
  groups : [b], $p < 0.05$; [c], $p < 0.01$.

Effect of Unilateral, Intraneostriatal Atropine Administration on Naloxone-Precipitated Contralateral Circling in SNC-Lesioned, Morphine-Dependent Rats

Atropine, administered unilaterally into the right,
intact neostriatum of rats with left-SNC lesions, produced circling behavior towards the opposite side
of injection and markedly diminished naloxone-precipi-

tated withdrawal signs. Table 2 shows circling behavior before and after naloxone in both sham-operated and left-SNC-lesioned animals 30 min after 0,32.5 65 or 130 µg atropine administered into the right intact neostriatum. In dependent animals, increasing doses of atropine produced dose-dependent circling behavior towards the left side in both sham-operated and left-SNC-lesioned animals. As observed previously, naloxone precipitated contralateral circling towards the intact neostriatum in the lesioned group of rats.

TABLE 2. Intra-neostriatal atropine effects on circling and precipitated-withdrawal behaviors before and after naloxone in morphine-dependent, unilaterally SNC-lesioned rats[a]

Dose (µg)	Group (N)	Group Mean Scores		
		Before naloxone	After naloxone	
		Circling	Circling	Withdrawal
0	S(8)	0	0	3.0
	L(8)	0	2.9 R	3.0
32.5	S(6)	0.5 L	0.2 L	3.0
	L(6)	0.3 L	2.0 R	3.0
65	S(6)	2.0 L[b]	1.7 L[b]	2.3[b]
	L(6)	1.7 L[b]	0.8 L[b]	2.2[b]
130	S(6)	3.0 L[b]	3.0 L[b]	0 [b]
	L(9)	3.0 L[b]	3.1 L[b]	0.2[b]

[a]Atropine, 0 to 130 µg, was administered into the right neostriatum of sham (S) or left-SNC(L) - lesioned morphine-dependent rats 30 min before a 20 mg/kg naloxone challenge. Circling behavior to the left (L) or right (R). Significant difference from the respective CSF-treated control groups: [b], p < 0.01.

In contrast to arecoline, unilateral atropine administration into the right neostriatum, which itself
produced circling to the left, not only diminished
naloxone-precipitated contralateral circling but also
reversed the direction of circling towards the side
ipsilateral to the lesion at the 65 and 130 µg
atropine dosages. Furthermore, atropine reduced
naloxone-precipitated withdrawal signs at the 65 µg
dose and virtually abolished them at the 130 µg
dose in both lesioned and sham-operated groups
of dependent rats. Indeed, of the total of 15 rats
given 130 µg atropine, the behavior observed after
naloxone was not that of precipitated withdrawal but a
continuation of pre-naloxone behavior after atropine,
namely, continuous circling behavior to the left.
However, 1 rat of 9 in the lesioned group given 130 µg
atropine did exhibit teeth-chattering for a score of 2.

Effect of Apomorphine on Naloxone-Precipitated Contralateral Circling in Morphine-Dependent Rats with unilateral SNC Lesions

Apomorphine reversed the direction of circling
precipitated by naloxone and also diminished precipitated withdrawal signs in both the lesioned and sham-
lesioned groups. Table 3 shows circling and stereotyped behavior before and after naloxone and precipitated withdrawal scores in both lesioned and sham-
operated groups pretreated with saline and 3 doses of
apomorphine. Apomorphine prior to naloxone produced
ipsilateral circling behavior in lesioned, morphine-
dependent animals which increased in intensity with
higher doses but not in the sham-operated controls.
Moreover, the contralateral circling induced by
naloxone in lesioned, dependent animals was blocked by
apomorphine. As can be seen in Table 3, naloxone
precipitated contralateral circling in lesioned, but
not in sham-operated, saline-treated animals as
previously observed (25). However, after pretreatment
with apomorphine, the naloxone-elicited contralateral
circling behavior gradually diminished in intensity
with increasing dose and was reversed to ipsilateral
circling with the highest apomorphine dose. It should
be noted that the naloxone-precipitated withdrawal

TABLE 3. Apomorphine effects on stereotyped circling and precipitated-withdrawal behaviors before and after naloxone in morphine-dependent, unilaterally SNC-lesioned rats[a]

Drug dose (mg/kg)	(Group) (N)	Group Mean Scores				
		Before naloxone		After naloxone		
		Stereotypy	Circling	Stereotypy	Circling	Withdrawal
0	S(8)	0	0	1.0	0	3.0
	L(8)	0	0	1.0	2.6R	3.0
1.5	S(6)	2.7c	0	2.5c,d	0	0.3c
	L(6)	0	0.8Lb	1.0	0.8Rc	3.0
3.0	S(6)	3.8c	0	3.7c,d	0	0c
	L(6)	1.3b	3.0Lc	1.0	0.3Lc	2.2b
6.0	S(6)	3.8c,d	0	3.7c	0	0c
	L(6)	1.8b	3.7Lc	2.8b	2.5Lc	0.3c

[a] Apomorphine, 0 to 6 mg/kg, was administered i.p. to sham(S) or left-SNC(L)-lesioned morphine-dependent rats 20 min before a 20 mg/kg naloxone challenge. Circling behavior to the left (L) or right (R). Significant difference from the respective saline-treated control groups   [d] (S) different from (L) at the same apomorphine

[b] $p < 0.05$,   [c] $p < 0.01$,   dose : $p < 0.01$

signs were significantly reduced by apomorphine pretreatment in both sham–operated and lesioned animals.
However, apomorphine was found to be more effective
in blocking withdrawal signs in sham–operated than in
lesioned rats.

Coincident with the ipsilateral circling induced by
apomorphine in morphine–dependent animals was the appearance of stereotyped behavior which also increased
in intensity with increasing dose. However, there
were qualitative differences in stereotypy between the
sham and lesioned groups of dependent animals. Administration of 3 mg/kg apomorphine consistently elicited
stereotypy scores of 3 or 4 in the sham–operated group
(mean score, 3.8). On the other hand, a lower degree
of stereotypy was observed in the SNC–lesioned animals
(mean score, 1.3) Thus, unilaterally, lesioned rats
appeared less responsive to apomorphine and this
observation, in part, is consistent with previous work
showing a reduction of apomorphine stereotypy after
chronic, bilateral electrolytic SNC lesions (13).

It was also apparent during the above observations
that the stereotyped behavior induced by apomorphine
may have been interfering with the expression of
withdrawal behavior precipitated by naloxone.
Apomorphine markedly reduced the precipitated withdrawal signs in sham–operated, dependent rats at all 3
doses used and diminished withdrawal intensity in the
lesioned group at the 6 mg/kg dose. As indicated in
Table 3, these groups of animals were exhibiting a
high degree of stereotypy which lasted for as long as
30 min after naloxone. Increased intensities of
stereotyped behavior with increasing doses of apomorphine in both sham and lesioned animals appeared to
be associated with a diminished appearance of naloxone
 precipitated withdrawal signs.

Effect of Haloperidol on Naloxone-Precipitated Contra-lateral Circling

Haloperidol, which invariably produced contralateral
circling and catalepsy in dependent and non–dependent
animals, did not modify naloxone–induced circling or
precipitated withdrawal in SNC–lesioned, morphine-
dependent animals. Table 4 shows circling and cata-

TABLE 4. Haloperidol effects on cataleptic, circling and precipitated-withdrawal behaviors before and after naloxone in morphine-dependent, unilaterally SNC-lesioned rats[a]

Drug dose (mg/kg)	Group (N)	Before naloxone		After naloxone		
		Catalepsy	Circling	Circling	Withdrawal	Catalepsy
0	S(7)	0	0	0	3.0	0
	L(7)	0	0	2.6 R	3.0	0
0.5	S(7)	0.9[c]	0	0	3.0	0
	L(7)	0.7[b]	0.7 R[c]	2.1 R	3.0	0
1.0	S(8)	1.8[c]	0	0	2.3	0.9 [b,d]
	L(8)	1.0[c]	1.0 R[c]	1.9 R	2.5[b]	0.5[d]
2.0	S(7)	2.3[c]	0	0	1.7[b]	1.6 [c,d]
	L(7)	1.4[c]	1.6 R[c]	1.7 R	2.6	0.4[d]

Group Mean Scores

[a] Haloperidol, 0 to 2 mg/kg, was administered i.p. to sham (S) or left-SNC(L)-lesioned morphine-dependent rats 30 min before a 20 mg/kg naloxone challenge. R = circling behavior to the right. Significant difference from the respective saline-treated control groups: [b], $p < 0.05$; [c], $p < 0.01$

[d] Naloxone precipitated the withdrawal behavior which was followed by cataleptic behavior appearing 1 to 10 min after naloxone administration.

leptic behavior before and after naloxone and the
withdrawal score precipitated by naloxone in lesioned
and sham-operated animals 30 min after saline, 0.5, 1
or 2 mg/kg haloperidol pretreatment. Administration
of haloperidol in morphine-dependent rats with SNC
lesions produced contralateral body asymmetry and
contralateral circling movements of low intensity
(mean score 1.6 after 2 mg/kg). However, the contralateral circling, precipitated by naloxone in the
lesioned but not the sham-operated group, was not
modified by increasing doses of haloperidol with
respect to either intensity or direction. Similarly,
the withdrawal behavior precipitated by naloxone remained unmodified after haloperidol pretreatment.

As previously mentioned, haloperidol produced dose-
dependent cataleptic behavior. Increasing doses of
haloperidol increased the intensity of catalepsy
observed in both sham and lesioned groups of rats. In
fact, some of the animals receiving the 1- and 2-mg/kg
doses of haloperidol were still cataleptic at the time
of naloxone administration, and as a consequence, the
intensity of catalepsy in these groups may have been
underestimated. Somewhat surprising was the elicitation of precipitated withdrawal by naloxone challenge
30 min after haloperidol injection since at this time
most of the animals appeared sedated and 3 rats were
still cataleptic. After naloxone administration, the
cataleptic rats exhibited locomotor activity and withdrawal behavior for 1-10 min before returning to a
milder cataleptic state (Table 4). It is conceivable
that the severe catalepsy observed in the sham-operated
group after the 2 mg/kg dose of haloperidol before the
naloxone injection may have interfered with the expression of certain precipitated withdrawal signs, such as
escape attempts. It should be noted, however, that
the predominant withdrawal signs that appeared after
naloxone in both the sham-operated and lesioned groups
of animals receiving the 2 mg/kg haloperidol pretreatment were wet shakes and teeth-chattering in addition to ptosis, abnormal posturing, ear blanching
and vocalization to touch. Additionally, escape attempts were manifested by both groups of rats receiving
0.5 and 1 mg/kg haloperidol. Thus, haloperidol pretreatment, at the doses administered in morphine-

dependent sham-operated or lesioned rats, did not modify appreciably either the withdrawal signs after naloxone or the precipitated contralateral circling.

DISCUSSION

The data presented in this communication indicate that naloxone-precipitated withdrawal in morphine-dependent rats may be accompanied by a diminution of dopaminergic activities or enhancement of cholinergic activities, or both, in the nigro-neostriatal pathway. Using unilaterally SNC-lesioned rats as the model, we found that the direction of circling (contralateral) observed after a naloxone challenge in morphine-dependent rats was the same as that observed in lesioned, non-dependent animals after haloperidol administration (2). This finding supports the hypothesis that a blockade of dopaminergic activity occurs in the nigro-neostriatal projection during naloxone-precipitated withdrawal (25). A decrease of dopaminergic transmission conceivably could lead to a diminished released with subsequent accumulation of dopamine in neostriatal terminals, which in fact was observed in morphine-dependent mice and rats during naloxone-precipitated withdrawal (23,25). Moreover, apomorphine reversed the direction of contralateral circling precipitated by naloxone in rats with unilateral electrolytic SNC lesions and markedly reduced the appearance of naloxone precipitated withdrawal signs. In contrast, both withdrawal behavior and naloxone-precipitated circling were unaffected by dopamine receptor blockade with haloperidol. Ary and Lomax(3) similarly have found that apomorphine reduced the incidence of certain signs of precipitated withdrawal in the rat when the drug was administered intraventricularly and also found that intraventricular pimozide did not appreciably alter withdrawal behavior.

Involvement of cholinergic neostriatal-paleostriatal activities is also suggested by these studies. Unilateral administration of arecoline into the intact neostriatum did not modify either the contralateral circling or the appearance of withdrawal signs precipitated by naloxone in morphine-dependent rats with unilateral SNC lesions. In contrast, both the circling

and withdrawal behaviors were markedly attenuated by
intraneostriatally administered atropine. These
results suggest that increased cholinergic activity
might occur at the level of the neo-paleostriatum
during naloxone-precipitated morphine withdrawal.

Recent evidence supports an hypothesis that the
dopaminergic neurons of the nigro-neostriatal pathway
may inhibit cholinergic interneurons in the neostriatum
(19, 33). Dopamine (DA) receptor stimulation should
then diminish acetylcholine (Ach) utilization (20,31,
39). Conversely, dopamine receptor antagonism would
be expected to enhance cholinergic activity (38).
Our recent results are in agreement with the notion of
an ACh-DA interaction at the level of the neostriatum
and extend previous findings to include the possibility
that the precipitated morphine withdrawal state may
involve such an interrelationship (40). That is, a
diminution of DA activity during precipitated withdrawal may result in an enhancement of cholinergic
mechanisms as evidenced by recent reports of increased
ACh utilization and/or decreased total brain ACh
content of morphine-dependent mice and rats during
abrupt withdrawal (17) and during naloxone-precipitated
withdrawal (6, 18).

Since intraneostriatal atropine diminished the
appearance of precipitated withdrawal signs (Table 2),
these data indicate that increased neostriatal cholinergic activity accompanies precipitated withdrawal.
The results on the effects of peripherally administered
anticholinergic drugs are less clear since both an
exacerbation (5,8) and an amelioration (28) of the
narcotic abstinence syndrome in mice have been reported. An explanation must await further experiments
in view of other findings which indicate that the varying effects on neostriatal dopamine turnover observed
after anticholinergic administration may depend on the
site of administration (4, 27). Cholinergic neurons
may exist in the SNC (9) as well as in the neostriatum
(12). These findings, therefore, may provide an
explanation for opposing effects of intraneostriatally
and peripherally administered anticholinergic agents on
precipitated withdrawal. Also, it cannot be stated at
this time whether the attenuation of withdrawal by
apomorphine is due to enhanced neostriatal DA activity

or to DA receptor stimulation of neostriatal or SNC cholinergic interneurons resulting in a decrease of ACh release at these sites. Additionally, a participatory role for gamma-hydroxybutyric acid should also be considered (33).

In similarity with our findings, Herz et al.(21) observed that a large dose of apomorphine, 5 mg/kg, interfered with levallorphan-induced withdrawal jumping behavior in morphine-dependent rats. Our results differ from theirs at the lower doses (1.5-3.0 mg/kg) of apomorphine in that we still observed a decrease in withdrawal intensity (Table 3), whereas a profound enhancement of withdrawal jumping behavior was observed by Herz at 2.5 mg/kg apomorphine. However, these workers did observe a diminution of other levallorphan-precipitated withdrawal signs after either d-amphetamine or apomorphine pretreatment, which is in agreement with our results. We can offer no reason for the discrepancy except to note that our animals were implanted with a lower dose of morphine and for a shorter period of time (1125 mg/kg morphine over 72 hr versus 2250 mg/kg morphine over 240 hr). Additionally, our sham-operated, morphine-dependent animals were observed to be quite stereotypic and almost all animals exhibited continuous sniffing and licking, biting or gnawing behavior before and after naloxone even at the lowest dose of apomorphine pretreatment, 1.5 mg/kg, and these data are similar to those previously reported in naive rats (25). It is conceivable, therefore, that drug-induced stereotyped behavior "occludes" naloxone-precipitated signs (21) and our results support this interpretation (Table 3). However, if increased dopaminergic transmission and dopamine release actually do occur during precipitated withdrawal, one might expect apomorphine and d-amphetamine to enhance the intensity of withdrawal signs. Since a reduction in withdrawal sign frequency was observed in our animals after those dopamine-mimetic agents, the results are more compatible with the interpretation that diminished dopaminergic transmission occurs during precipitated withdrawal.

If a diminution of dopaminergic transmission occurs during naloxone-precipitated withdrawal, one might expect that blockade of dopamine receptor with neuroleptic drugs should produce behavior similar to withdrawal. We have observed that certain withdrawal signs in the rat do bear at least superficial resemblance to some neuroleptic-induced behavioral signs such as ptosis, abnormal (hunched) posturing, vocalization to touch and blanching of the ears. These same signs generally occurred after the first 4-5 min of naloxone-precipitated withdrawal in morphine-dependent rats. However, such a simplification of the precipitated morphine-withdrawal syndrome does not seem complete since increased exploratory activity, wet shakes and escape attempts are observed during the first 4-5 min after naloxone (7,18,43).

A rather peculiar finding we have observed in morphine-dependent rats was the momentary disruption of haloperidol-induced cataleptic behavior shortly after a naloxone challenge (see present results, Table 4) during which animals exhibited withdrawal behavior lasting from 1 to 10 min. Since a reversal of cataleptic behavior was observed, this finding suggested that dopaminergic transmission may be enhanced. However, we believe that this is not the case since the 2 mg/kg dose of haloperidol used was more than adequate to block completely the stereotypy induced by 3 mg/kg apomorphine or 3.2 mg/kg d-amphetamine, doses of which produce profound stereotyped behavior alone (24). It is presently unknown how haloperidol catalepsy can be quickly reversed during naloxone-precipitated withdrawal. However, both neuroleptic-induced catalepsy and alterations of DA metabolism appear to require an intact nigro-neostriatal pathway (16, 35). Lesions of the nigro-neostriatal pathway at the level of the globus pallidus or SNC greatly diminish haloperidol-elicited catalepsy in rats (16). Thus, one possible explanation for the disruption of haloperidol-elicited catalepsy during naloxone-precipitated withdrawal may be a momentary presynaptic blockade of the nigro-neostriatal projection. Additionally, recent data suggest that haloperidol, narcotic agonists and antagonists may interact with the same tissue binding site of rat brain homogenates (10). However, this observation still does not explain the failure of narcotic antagonists to reverse neuroleptic-induced catalepsy in naive animals (26, 30).

It is thus apparent that the initial events of precipitated withdrawal, during which haloperidol catalepsy was disrupted by the naloxone challenge, differ both in character and in time sequence from withdrawal behavior appearing later. The sequence of neurochemical events during precipitated withdrawal cannot be determined at this time. However, our finding that naloxone disrupts haloperidol catalepsy only in morphine-dependent rats may provide a basis for further investigations of narcotic withdrawal.

In addition to a participation of both dopamine and acetylcholine, possible involvement of serotonin and noradrenaline in the circling behavior model has been suggested (11, 14, 37). Discussion of our present data has been limited to ACh-DA interactions in naloxone-precipitated circling behavior during morphine withdrawal in rats; the roles of serotonin and noradrenaline in this behavior must await additional experiments.

In summary, using the circling behavior model to differentiate dopamine agonistic and antagonistic effects, it was observed that the administration of apomorphine systematically and atropine intraneostriatally in morphine-dependent rats with unilateral, electrolytic SNC lesions either reversed the direction or decreased the intensity of the naloxone-precipitated contralateral circling behavior while concomitantly causing a diminution of the intensity of the precipitated withdrawal syndrome. It is proposed that naloxone-precipitated withdrawal may be accompanied by either a diminution of dopaminergic activities or an enhancement of cholinergic activities, or both, at the level of the neostriatum.

ACKNOWLEDGEMENTS

Supported in part by research grants from the National Institute of Drug Abuse, DA 0037 and DA 00564.

REFERENCES

1. Andén, N.E., Butcher, S.G., Corrodi, H., Fuxe, K.and Ungerstedt,U.(1970):Eur.J.Pharmacol.,11: 303.

2. Andén, N.-E., Dalhstrom, A., Fuxe, K. and Larsson, K. (1966): Acta Pharmacol.Toxicol., 24: 263.

3. Ary, M. and Lomax, P. (1976): Fed.Proc.,35: 470.

4. Bartholini, G. and Pletscher, A. (1971): Experientia, 27: 1302.

5. Bhargava, H.N. and Way, E.L. (1972): J.Pharmacol. Exp.Ther., 183: 31.

6. Bhargava, H.N. and Way, E.L. (1975): J.Pharmacol. Exp.Ther., 194: 65.

7. Blasig, J., Herz, A., Reinhold, R. and Zieglgansberger,S. (1973):Psychopharmacologia, 33: 19.

8. Brase, D.A., Tseng, L.-F., Loh, H.H. and Way, E.L. (1974): Eur.J.Pharmacol., 26: 1.

9. Butcher, L.L., Talbot, K. and Bilezikjian, L.(1975): Proc. West.Pharmacol. Soc., 18: 256.

10.Clay, G.A. and Brougham, L.R. (1975): Biochem. Pharmacol., 24: 1363.

11.Cools, A.R. and Janssen, H.-J. (1974): Eur. J. Pharmacol., 28: 266.

12.Corrodi, H., Fuxe, K. and Lidbrink, P. (1972):Brain Res., 43: 397.

13.Costall, B. and Naylor, R.J. (1973): Eur.J. Pharmacol.,21: 350.

14.Costall, B. and Naylor, R.J. (1974): Eur.J. Pharmacol., 29: 206.

15.Costall, B., Naylor, R.J. and Olley, J.E. (1972): Neuropharmacology, 11: 645.

16.Costall, B. and Olley, J.E. (1971): Neuro-pharmacology, 10: 581.

17.Domino, E.F. and Wilson, A.E. (1973): Nature(Lond), 243: 285.

18.Domino, E.F. and Wilson, A.E. (1975): Psychopharmacologia, 41: 19.

19.Groves, P.M., Wilson, C.J., Young, S.J. and Rebec, G.V. (1975): Science, 190: 522.

20.Guyenet, P.G., Agid, Y., Javoy, F., Beaujouan, J.C., Rossier, J. and Glowinski, J. (1975): Brain Res., 84: 227.

21.Herz, A., Blasig, J. and Papeschi, R. (1974): Psychopharmacologia, 39: 121.

22.Ho, I.K., Lu,S.E., Stolman, S., Loh, H.H. and Way, E.L. (1972): J.Pharmacol.Exp. Ther., 182: 155.

23. Iwamoto, E.T., Ho, I.K.,and Way, E.L. (1973):
J. Pharmacol. Exp.Ther., 187: 558.
24. Iwamoto, E.T., Loh, H.H. and Way, E.L. (1976):
Eur.J.Pharmacol., 37: 339.
25. Iwamoto, E.T., Loh, H.H. and Way, E.L. (1976):
J. Pharmacol. Exp. Ther., 197: 503.
26. Iwamoto, E.T., Loh, H.H. and Way, E.L. (1976):
Eur.J. Pharmacol., 38: 39.
27. Javoy, F., Agid, Y., Bouvet, D. and Glowinski, J.
(1974): Brain Res., 68: 253.
28. Jhamandas, R. and Dickinson, G. (1973): Nature
New Biology, 245: 219.
29. König, J.F.R. and Klippel, R.A. (1963): The Rat
Brain, Williams and Wilkins, Baltimore.
30. Kuschinsky, K. and Hornykiewicz, O. (1972): Eur. J.
Pharmacol., 19: 119.
31. Ladinsky, H., Consolo, S., Bianchi, S., Samanin, R.
and Ghezzi, D. (1975): Brain Res., 84: 221.
32. Maruyama, Y. and Takemori, A.E. (1973):
J.Pharmacol. Exp. Ther., 185: 602.
33. McGeer, P.L., Fibiger, H.C., Hattori, T., Singh,
V.K., McGeer, E.G. and Maler, L. (1974) : In:
Advances in Behavioral Biology, Vol.10, edited by
R.D. Myers and R.R. Drucker-Colin, p.27. Plenum
Press, New York.
34. Naylor, R.J. and Olley, J.E. (1972):
Neuropharmacology, 11: 91.
35. Nyback, H. and Sedvall, G. (1971): J. Pharm.
Pharmacol., 23: 322.
36. Palaic, D., Page, I. and Khairallah, P. (1967):
J. Neurochem., 14: 63.
37. Pycock, C.J., MacDonaldson, I.G. and Marsden, C.D.
(1975): Brain Res., 97: 317.
38. Stadler, H., Lloyd, K.G., Gadea-Ciria, M. and
Bartholini, G.(1973): Brain Res., 55: 476.
39. Trabucchi,N., Cheney,D.L., Racagni, G. and Costa,E.
(1975):Brain Res., 85: 130.
40. Way, E.L.,Iwamoto, E.T., Bhargava, H.N. and Loh,H.
H. (1975): In: Neurobiological Mechanisms of
Adaptation and Behavior, edited by A.J.Mandell,
p. 169, Raven Press, New York.
41. Way, E.L., Loh, H.H. and Shen, F.-H. (1969): J.
Pharmacol.Exp. Ther., 167: 1.

42.Wei, E. and Loh, H.H. (1972): Nature (Lond), 238:
   396.
43.Wei, E., Loh, H.H. and Way, E.L. (1973):
   J. Pharmacol. Exp. Ther., 184: 398.

Factors Affecting the Action of Narcotics, edited by
M.L. Adler, L. Manara, and R. Samanin.
Raven Press, New York©1978.

Effects of Drugs Affecting Extrapyramidal Motor Functions on Catalepsy and Stereotypies Induced
by Narcotic Analgesics

Liisa Ahtee

Department of Pharmacology, School of Pharmacy
University of Helsinki, Kirkkokatu 20
SF-00170 Helsinki 17 - Finland

INTRODUCTION

In laboratory animals neuroleptic and other drugs
which are thought to block striatal dopamine receptors
or which decrease the striatal dopamine concentration
induce a state of motor hypoactivity, the main feature
of which is akinesia (inability to start movement)
often associated with rigidity and tremor. Such a
condition is called catalepsy (43). In addition to
drugs that decrease dopaminergic activity in the
striatum, cholinomimetic compounds (20) and narcotic
analgesics (20,69) induce akinesia called either catalepsy or catatonia. Another disturbance of extrapyramidal motor function is stereotyped movements. In
rats stereotypy-inducing drugs cause continuous licking,
biting, or gnawing as well as repetitive movements of
head and legs. While catalepsy is often associated
with decreased striatal dopaminergic activity, stereotyped
behavior is induced by dopaminergic agonists (43,68,81).

I. Catalepsy and Stereotypies Produced by
Narcotic Analgesics

The cataleptic effect of narcotic analgesics,
accompanied by marked rigidity, seems to be specific
for these compounds. It is antagonized by nalorphine
and naloxone (7,53,69). The structural requirements
for the cataleptic and pain-relieving properties of
these drugs are closely related (5) and after repeated
administration tolerance develops towards the cataleptic
effect of methadone (1). In rats, repeated administration of the narcotic analgesics induces stereotyped
behavior (1,13,33), and implantation of morphine or
methadone into the ventral thalamus evokes compulsive
gnawing (17). The oripavine derivative M6007 induces
stereotypies which are preceded by a cataleptic phase

479

when the drug is administered for the first time (26).
Nalorphine and naloxone prevent or abolish the stereotypies produced by narcotic analgesics (1,13,17,33).
Recently, it was reported that naloxone prevents
apomorphine-induced stereotypies, too (31).

The cataleptic effect of narcotic analgesics, like
that of postsynaptic dopamine receptor blocking agents
(10,19), is accompanied by an increased concentration
of striatal homovanillic acid (HVA) and an increased
turnover of dopamine (for references, see 52). Nalorphine and naloxone antagonize the effects of narcotic
analgesics on dopamine metabolism (7,53). Moreover,
we found a close correlation between the cataleptogenic
and HVA-increasing properties of 10 narcotic analgesics
and related drugs; thebaine and cyclazocine, which do
not cause catalepsy, did not increase striatal HVA
content, and M99 was the most potent of the compounds
studied in both respects (5). The increased turnover
of dopamine in the striata of rats treated with narcotic
analgesics most probably occurs as a compensatory
mechanism when the organism tries to overcome the
catalepsy by increasing the production of dopamine.
This conclusion is supported by the findings that pretreatment of rats with the catecholamine synthesis
inhibitor α-methyl-p-tyrosine potentiated the cataleptic
effect of methadone (73,74). Furthermore, the findings
that the cataleptic effect of narcotic analgesics was
enhanced in rats after administration of 6-hydroxy-
dopamine into the caudatus-putamen areas (60) and after
electrolytic coagulation of caudate-putamen and globus
pallidus (26) indicate that the striatal dopamine
neurons "try to counteract" the cataleptic effect of
narcotic analgesics.

On the other hand, these two experiments (26,60)
suggest that the narcotic analgesics do not act primarily on the striatum when causing catalepsy. Drugs
should be able to increase the turnover of dopamine
without acting directly on the dopaminergic synapses.
For instance, the cholinomimetic compounds, which most
probably cause catalepsy by mechanisms other than
blockade of striatal dopamine receptors, increase
striatal HVA content and dopamine turnover (6,22). It
is to be noted that the maximum concentration of striatal
HVA produced by narcotic analgesics and cholinomimetic
compounds is only 2- to 3-fold the original concentration, whereas the neuroleptics and other drugs which
are supposed to block the striatal dopamine receptors
cause 4- to 6-fold increases in the HVA concentration
(2,4,6,37,47,54).

Several laboratories (18,37,44) recently found that
in contrast to the neuroleptic compounds, morphine and

related narcotic analgesics do not inhibit dopamine-sensitive adenylcyclase in rat striatum. This adenyl cyclase is thought to be closely connected with the postsynaptic dopamine receptors (38). Thus, these findings give further support for the suggestion that the mechanisms of action of neuroleptic compounds and narcotic analgesics are different and that the latter compounds do not act directly on the dopaminergic striatal systems.

Tolerance develops towards the enhancing effect of morphine on dopamine and HVA formation (34,77). In rats this tolerance seems to develop slowly, and Clouet and Ratner (21) have found that after administration of morphine to rats for 10 days, the formation of dopamine from tyrosine was accelerated even more than in control rats. In my experiments (1) methadone still increased striatal HVA content after the rats had been treated chronically with methadone for 8 weeks. Therefore, it is plausible that the primary effect of methadone is catalepsy, which induces a compensatory increase in the production of dopamine. Stereotyped behavior occurs when the rats become partially tolerant to the cataleptic effect; in such rats the additional dopamine causes the stereotypies. It is to be noted that in my experiment the maximum stereotyped response to methadone occurred after 5 to 6 weeks of chronic administration. It is possible that if the experiment had lasted longer than 8 weeks the rats would have developed tolerance both toward the stereotyped effect and toward the striatal HVA-increasing effect of methadone. The importance of striatal dopamine in the stereotypic effects of narcotic analgesics is demonstrated also by the findings that α-methyl-p-tyrosine and reserpine inhibit this behavior (1,13,17).

The effects of drugs on extrapyramidal motor functions can also be evaluated by studying whether they produce asymmetries and turning (rotation) in rats after unilateral lesions of nigro-neostriatal neurons (80). Morphine and other narcotic analgesics induce ipsilateral asymmetry and rotation in rats with unilateral degeneration of nigrostriatal dopamine neurons (30,35). This functional model will probably become useful in the pharmacological analysis of the extrapyramidal motor effects of narcotic analgesics. However, the following presentation, in which I shall try to characterize pharmacologically the extrapyramidal motor effects of narcotic analgesics, will be dealing only with the cataleptic and stereotypic effects of narcotic analgesics.

II. Effects of Dopaminergic Drugs

The catalepsy as well as the increased dopamine formation induced by morphine and methadone can be prevented by dopaminergic agonists, apomorphine, 1-DOPA, and amantadine (7,53,73,74). In fact, Kuschinsky and Hornykiewicz found that 1-DOPA and apomorphine inhibited the morphine-induced catalepsy much more effectively than the catalepsy induced by chlorpromazine. This fact supports their conclusion that morphine in contrast to chlorpromazine does not block dopamine receptors. In our laboratory (Table 1) it was found that amphetamine and theophylline also prevented the cataleptic effect of methadone in rats treated chronically with methadone. The effect of theophylline was very short and probably associated with its ability to inhibit phosphodiesterase and thereby induce a functional increase of dopamine receptor response (36).

On the other hand, the cataleptic effects of narcotic analgesics and neuroleptic compounds are additive, and their effects on the striatal HVA content are supra-additive, so that a combination of supramaximal doses of both groups of drugs increases the striatal HVA content more than either drug alone (37,54).

The suggestion that dopamine plays a role in the stereotyped behavior produced by narcotic analgesics is supported by the findings that neuroleptic drugs antagonize this behavior (13,17). Paradoxically, Fog (33) found that amphetamine prevented the stereotypies produced by morphine in rats treated chronically with morphine. Table 1 shows that in our experiments amphetamine and theophylline decrease the methadone-induced stereotyped gnawing in rats treated chronically with methadone. Apomorphine did not alter the total time the rats gnawed after injection of methadone. However, the apomorphine-pretreated rats started and also ceased the gnawing behavior earlier than the control rats which were treated only with methadone. The onset of gnawing was 11 ± 4 min in apomorphine + methadone-treated rats and 70 ± 10 min after injection in methadone-treated rats (means ± S.E.; $p < 0.001$). The early onset was most probably due to the strong stereotypy-producing effect of the 5 mg/kg dose of apomorphine, whereas the early discontinuation could be the result of a reduction of methadone-induced stereotypies.

The antagonistic effect of amphetamine on narcotic-induced stereotypies is most probably associated with the facts that the dopaminergic agonistic effect of amphetamine is mediated by released dopamine (67) and that the stereotypic effects of narcotic analgesics are

TABLE 1. Effect of apomorphine, d-amphetamine, and theophylline on the methadone-induced catalepsy and stereotyped gnawing in rats treated chronically with methadone*

Acute treatment [number of rats]	Cataleptic score (mean ± S.E.)				Proportion (mean ± S.E.) of 5-hr observation time when gnawing was observed
	10 min	30 min	1 hr	2 hr	
Methadone, exp.I [16]	2.1+0.8	6.6+0.6	6.2+0.6	2.5+0.8	51+5 %
Apomorphine + Methadone [15]	0 (a)	2.3+0.9 (d)	2.7+0.7 (c)	2.7+0.7	54+3 %
Methadone, exp.II [18]	2.7+0.9	6.4+0.7	7.1+0.6	2.7+0.6	56+7 %
d-Amphetamine + Methadone [17]	0 (c)	0 (d)	0 (d)	0 (d)	38+5 % (a)
Methadone, exp.III [10]	3.1+1.1	4.4+1.2	2.7+0.9	1.2+0.7	61+7 %
Theophylline + Methadone [13]	0.5+0.5 (a)	2.3+0.8	2.9+0.9	1.1+0.6	38+5 % (b)

Three different experiments were performed. In exp.I the rats had been treated chronically with methadone for 3 weeks; in exp.II, for 4 weeks; and in exp.III, for 5 weeks, respectively. In exp.I and II the acute dose of dl-methadone was 15 mg/kg s.c. and in exp.III, 10 mg/kg. Methadone was administered between 8 and 9 am. The penultimate injection was given at 3 pm on the preceding day. Apomorphine (5 mg/kg i.p.) was administered 10 min before, d-amphetamine (5 mg/kg s.c.) 5 min before, and theophylline (25 mg/kg s.c.) simultaneously with methadone. The times given were counted from the injection of methadone. The maximum cataleptic score in the method used was 8 (1).
The 5-hr observation time was divided into 10 subsequent half-hour periods during each of which gnawing was observed; if a rat gnawed during each half-hour period the proportion would have been 100%.
p-Values were calculated using Student's t-test. Compared to the corresponding group which was treated with methadone only: (a) $p < 0.05$, (b) $p < 0.02$, (c) $p < 0.01$, (d) $p < 0.001$
*(Ahtee, unpublished results)

also at least partially mediated via a release of
catecholamines as discussed in part I of this presentation. Another phosphodiesterase inhibitor, caffeine,
potentiates the stereotyped behavior induced by apomorphine and amphetamine (49). Therefore the antagonistic effect of theophylline on methadone-stereotypies
is surprising. It might be associated with the finding
that theophylline decreases the turnover of dopamine in
telencephalic cortex of rats (63). The earlier discontinuation of stereotyped gnawing in apomorphine +
methadone-treated rats than in rats treated only with
methadone could be explained by the fact that apomorphine
reduces the turnover of dopamine (11,70). Thus, when
apomorphine's own stereotypic effect wears off, methadone
stereotypies are reduced, because the amount of dopamine
available is reduced.

III. Effects of Cholinergic Drugs

The interactions of drugs acting on cholinergic
receptors with narcotic analgesics are interesting,
because there is evidence suggesting that in addition
to dopaminergic neurons, the cholinergic neurons regulate the extrapyramidal motor functions.
Muscarinic cholinomimetic compounds induce catalepsy and increase the turnover of striatal dopamine in
rodents (6,22,26,86). Antimuscarinic drugs prevent the
cataleptic effect in rodents of neuroleptic and other
drugs which are thought to block the dopamine receptors
as well as the catalepsy produced by muscarinic cholinomimetic compounds (2,29,59,86). In addition, antimuscarinic drugs diminish the increased disappearance
of striatal dopamine and increased striatal HVA concentration which the neuroleptic and the muscarinic drugs
produce (6,8,9,23,61).
The effects of the antimuscarinic compounds atropine
and scopolamine on morphine- and methadone-induced
catalepsy were opposite to their effects on the catalepsy produced by neuroleptic compounds (3,45). The
lowest dose of atropine required to potentiate the
cataleptic effect of morphine was 3 mg/kg, and in rats
pretreated with 30 mg/kg of atropine, 10 mg/kg of
morphine induced the maximum cataleptic score. The
corresponding doses of scopolamine were 0.3 and 10 mg/kg,
respectively. This potentiation is most probably a
central effect, because low doses of methylatropine or
methylscopolamine had no effect and 50 mg/kg of methylscopolamine was clearly less effective than 3 mg/kg of
scopolamine. Also, Herz (41,42) found that antimuscarinic
compounds prolonged the time that rats treated with
morphine would remain in an abnormal position with both

front limbs on a 12-cm-high wooden block. He concluded
that this prolongation resulted from a sedative effect
of the combination. However, in our experiments catalepsy was scored by using parallel bars and vertical
grid, in which tests a sedative effect could be expected
to decrease rather than increase the cataleptic score.
Moreover, we found that the muscarinic cholinomimetic
compounds RS86, arecoline, and pilocarpine reduced the
cataleptic effect of morphine and methadone. Thus,
they interacted with narcotic analgesics in a way
opposite that of antimuscarinic compounds.

That there are muscarine-sensitive brain structures
which regulate the extrapyramidal motor effects of
narcotic analgesics was further suggested by the findings that antimuscarinic compounds tended to diminish
and muscarinic compounds to potentiate stereotypies in
rats treated chronically with methadone (3). Antimuscarinic compounds potentiate and muscarinic compounds
reduce stereotyped behavior produced by apomorphine and
amphetamine (12,75). Thus, muscarinic cholinergic drugs
modify both catalepsy and stereotypies produced by
narcotic analgesics in a direction opposite that in
which they modify these effects of drugs acting on postsynaptic dopamine receptors. It should be remembered
that there are muscarine-sensitive brain structures whose
stimulation results in stereotyped behavior (76,84),
and that atropine, when injected into striatum or globus
pallidus, initially prevents amphetamine stereotypy (25).
Furthermore, the actions of neuroleptics and narcotic
analgesics on cholinergic neuronal pathways differ in
that the narcotic analgesics reduce whereas the neuroleptics increase the release of striatal acetylcholine
(78,85). Thus, it is understandable that drugs acting
on muscarinic cholinergic receptors can modify the
extrapyramidal motor effects of narcotic analgesics and
of drugs acting on postsynaptic dopamine receptors in
opposite directions.

However, the antimuscarinic and muscarinic drugs
tend to modify the morphine-induced changes in brain
dopamine metabolism in the same directions as they
modify those of neuroleptic compounds (45). The 10-
mg/kg dose of scopolamine clearly prevented the morphine-
induced increase in the rate of dopamine depletion
(Table 2). This finding agrees with that of Puri et al,
(66), who found that benztropine pretreatment blocked
the morphine-induced increase in cerebral dopamine
turnover. The combination of pilocarpine and morphine
accelerated the rate of dopamine depletion more than
either of the drugs alone (Table 2). Three muscarinic
compounds studied, RS86, pilocarpine, and arecoline,
increased the concentration of HVA in the striatum and

TABLE 2. Effect of morphine, pilocarpine, scopolamine, and α-methyl-p-tyrosine (αMT) on the concentration of dopamine in the brain of rats *

Treatment	Dopamine, μg/g $\pm$ S.E.
Saline	0.95 + 0.01
αMT	0.46 + 0.03
Morphine + αMT	0.37 + 0.04
Scopolamine + αMT	0.48 + 0.01
Scopolamine + Morphine + αMT	0.46 + 0.01
Pilocarpine + αMT	0.40 + 0.02
Pilocarpine + Morphine + αMT	0.32 + 0.02

Scopolamine (10 mg/kg) was injected 3 hr 25 min, pilocarpine (100 mg/kg) and morphine (10 mg/kg), 3 hr 5 min, and αMT (200 mg/kg) 3 hr before sacrifice. *From Kaakkola and Ahtee (45).

when combined with morphine, their effects were additive (45). Antimuscarinic compounds slightly reduced the increase in striatal HVA induced by narcotic analgesics (7,51). This slight reduction, which was clearly demonstrable only in probenecid-treated rats (45), was probably due to the fact that antimuscarinic compounds are known to decrease the concentration of striatal HVA (14,61). It could be argued that the antimuscarinic drugs reduce the synthesis of dopamine and consequently, the cataleptic effect of narcotic analgesics is enhanced because there is no dopamine available to counteract it. Analogous to this unlikely explanation is the contention that the cholinomimetics reduce the cataleptic effect of narcotic analgesics by increasing the formation of dopamine.

In addition to muscarinic cholinomimetic drugs, nicotine produces catalepsy in mice and in rats (26, 86). In rats treated chronically with methadone, nicotine caused a slight initial potentiation of methadone catalepsy (3). Mecamylamine, which blocks both central and peripheral nicotine receptors but does not prevent the cataleptic effect of neuroleptics in mice (87), clearly diminished the cataleptic effect of methadone. This was most probably a central effect, because hexamethonium, which blocks nicotine receptors but only poorly penetrates the blood-brain barrier, did not significantly alter the methadone-induced catalepsy (3). Mecamylamine significantly reduced the morphine-induced increase in striatal HVA concentration (Table 3), whereas hexamethonium (10 mg/kg) did not modify the morphine-induced increase in striatal HVA

concentration. Mecamylamine initially significantly
reduced but later tended to potentiate the methadone-
induced stereotypies (3). Thus, it seems that drugs
acting on central muscarinic and nicotinic cholinergic
receptors alter the extrapyramidal motor effects of
narcotic analgesics in opposite directions.

TABLE 3. Effect of mecamylamine on morphine-induced
increase in striatal homovanillic acid (HVA) concentration in rats *

Treatment	HVA, $\mu g/g \pm$ S.E.	
	1 hr	2 hr
Saline	0.65 ± 0.04	0.60 ± 0.03
Mecamylamine, 2 mg/kg	0.68 ± 0.22	0.57 ± 0.03
Morphine, 30 mg/kg	1.30 ± 0.12	1.62 ± 0.11
Mecamylamine + Morphine	0.93 ± 0.27 (b)	1.15 ± 0.11 (a)

Compared to morphine only group (a) $p < 0.05$, (b) $p < 0.01$
(Student's t-test).
*Kaakkola and Ahtee (unpublished results).

IV. Effects of Other Drugs

Of the putative neurotransmitters found in substantia nigra and striatum, γ-aminobutyric acid (GABA)
most probably exerts an inhibitory influence on
dopamine neurons in these brain regions (15). Amino-
oxyacetic acid (AOAA), a compound which increases the
cerebral GABA concentration, antagonizes the effects
of chlorpromazine and haloperidol on striatal dopamine
metabolism (46,55,83). Therefore it was not surprising
that AOAA potentiated the cataleptic effects of
metoclopramide (2) and haloperidol (46), which compounds
are thought to block postsynaptic dopamine receptors.
In addition, baclofen (p-chlorophenyl-GABA), a structural
analogue of GABA, potentiated haloperidol catalepsy in
rats (46). However, neither of these GABA-like compounds
altered the cataleptic effect of methadone, although
both compounds clearly potentiated the antinociceptive
effect of methadone (48). These results again suggest
that the effects of narcotic analgesics on extrapyramidal motor functions are different from those of
drugs which block the postsynaptic dopamine receptors.
Drugs and lesions which alter the cerebral concentration of 5-hydroxytryptamine (5HT) modify the effects
of dopaminergic drugs and narcotic analgesics on the
extrapyramidal motor functions. In rats,the cataleptic

activity of neuroleptic compounds is reduced by treatments which lower the cerebral 5HT concentration (24,
40,50). Likewise, lowering of cerebral 5HT content
reduced and the 5HT precursor, 5-hydroxytryptophan,
enhanced the cataleptic effect of narcotic analgesics
(28,39). However, lowering of brain 5HT by p-chloro-
phenylalanine reduced the haloperidol-induced increase
in striatal HVA content (83), whereas p-chloro-N-
methylamphetamine, another inhibitor of 5HT synthesis,
slightly enhanced the morphine-induced increase of HVA
content (39).

There is agreement that the stereotyped effects of
narcotic analgesics in rats are enhanced by treatments
which lower cerebral 5HT content (16,28). However, at
present there is no agreement about the effect of 5HT
on the stereotypies produced by dopaminergic agonists;
in some experiments lowering of cerebral 5HT content
enhances these stereotypies and in other experiments,
reduces them (16,27,40).

It is highly probable that in addition to the
neurotransmitter systems discussed above there are
other transmitters which are involved in the extrapyramidal motor effects of narcotic analgesics. For
instance, Da Silva and Rocha e Silva (32) reported
that in a dose which did not produce catatonia, morphine
significantly increased the duration of catatonia
induced by intracerebral injection of the nonapeptide
bradykinin. Furthermore, the results of Ayhan and
Randrup (13) suggest that noradrenaline plays an
important role in morphine-induced stereotyped behavior.
Their group (68) also found that when mice which are
stimulated by morphine are treated with the combination
of phenoxybenzamine and morphine, they become cataleptic.

V. Comparison of the Interactions of Dopaminergic,
    Cholinergic, Gabergic and Serotonergic Drugs
    with Narcotic Analgesics

Table 4, which summarizes the effects of dopaminergic,
cholinergic, GABAergic, and serotonergic drugs on the
catalepsy and stereotypies produced by narcotic
analgesics and dopaminergic drugs, shows that usually
the effects of an interacting agent on the catalepsy
and stereotypies are opposite to each other. However,
there are a few exceptions, e.g., amphetamine reduces
both the cataleptic and stereotypic effects of narcotic
analgesics and lowering of cerebral 5HT content in some
cases diminishes both catalepsy and stereotypies produced
by dopaminergic drugs. Dopaminergic agonists and
lowering of cerebral 5HT content reduce both the
catalepsy caused by narcotic analgesics and by dopamine

receptor blocking agents. The GABA agonists potentiated the cataleptic effect of the latter group of drugs but do not influence the cataleptic effect of methadone. On the other hand, the blockade of cerebral nicotinic receptors does not influence the cataleptic effect of neuroleptics in mice (87), but it diminishes the cataleptic effect of methadone in rats treated chronically with methadone. The muscarinic cholinergic drugs always modify the extrapyramidal motor effects of the two groups of drugs in opposite directions.

These findings show that the mechanism of action of narcotic analgesics in disturbing extrapyramidal motor functions is different from that of drugs which act on postsynaptic dopamine receptors. Such a difference can be anticipated from the differences in the catalepsy and stereotypies produced by these two groups of drugs. In contrast to that of neuroleptic drugs, the akinesia produced by narcotic analgesics is accompanied by a marked rigidity (20,82). Furthermore, the morphine-induced stereotyped behavior is more varied than the stereotyped behavior produced by amphetamine, which selectively stimulates certain items of behavior (68).

The effects of drugs acting on various neurotransmitter systems on the pain-relieving properties of narcotic analgesics have been widely studied and results from these studies are not in agreement. The main reasons for this incongruence seem to be the difficulties and differences in measuring the analgesic or hyperalgesic effect in experimental animals (for references, see 62,72). Therefore, the results collected in Table 4 are all from experiments in which the antinociceptive effect of narcotic analgesics was measured by testing the response of rats to electric foot-shock. Using other tests for measuring antinociceptive activity it has been found that apomorphine is antinociceptive and potentiates this effect of morphine (64,71), whereas some phenothiazine derivatives increase the amount of narcotic analgesic required to produce satisfactory relief from pain in humans (58). Furthermore, the dopamine receptor-blocking neuroleptic, pimozide, reduced the effect of morphine on the threshold for vocalization afterdischarge, which response is considered to reflect the emotional component of pain (65). Nicotine is antinociceptive in various tests and its action is antagonized by mecamylamine (56,57). Thus, in addition to modifying the effects of narcotic analgesics on the extrapyramidal motor function, the dopaminergic, cholinergic, GABAergic, and serotonergic drugs interfere with the antinociceptive actions of these compounds. However, even the few results in

TABLE 4. Modification of the cataleptic, stereotypic, and anti-nociceptive effects of narcotic analgesics and the cataleptic and stereotypic effects of drugs acting on dopamine receptors, by dopaminergic, cholinergic, GABAergic, and serotonergic drugs

Interacting agent	Modification of effects of:				
	Narcotic analgesics			Drugs acting on dopamine receptors	
	Cata-lepsy	Stereo-typies	Antinoci-ception f	Cata-lepsy	Stereo-typies
Apomorphine	↓a	○a		↓d	↑d
Amphetamine	↓a	↓a		↓d	↑d
Dopamine receptor blocking agent	↑a	↓a		↑d	↓d
Muscarine receptor blocking agent	↑b	↓b	○g	↓b	↑b
Muscarine receptor stimulating agent	↓b	↑b	↑g	↑b	↓b
Nicotine receptor blocking agent	↓b	1 ↓b 2 ↑		○b	
GABAergic agonist	○c		↑h	↑c	↓e
Lowering cerebral 5HT content	↓c	↑c	↓i	↓c	↑ or ↓ c

↑ = increase;   ↓ = decrease;   ○ = no alteration of effect

[1]initially; [2]later

Letters indicate references: a, b and c, see part II, III and IV of this presentation, respectively; d, (43,68); e, Ahtee and Auvinen (unpublished); f, only results from experiments in which antinociceptive effect was measured by testing the response of rats to electric foot-shock; g, (45); h, (48); i, (79).

Table 4 show that the drugs acting on various neurotransmitter systems do not produce parallel changes in
the cataleptic, stereotypic, or antinociceptive effects
of narcotic analgesics. For instance, antimuscarinic
drugs which clearly potentiate the cataleptic effect
do not modify the antinociceptive effect of narcotic
analgesics and on the other hand, GABAergic agonists
potentiate the antinociception but do not alter the
catalepsy caused by narcotic analgesics. Thus, it can
be concluded that, although the primary sites on which
the narcotic analgesics act to disturb extrapyramidal
motor function or to relieve pain, probably bear similarities or even might be the same, those neuronal
structures and pathways which mediate these two effects
are different and regulated by different neuronal
influences.

ACKNOWLEDGEMENTS

This work was supported by grants from the Medical
Research Council of the Academy of Finland, the Finnish
Foundation for Alcohol Studies and Sigrid Jusélius
Foundation.

REFERENCES

1. Ahtee, L. (1974): Eur. J. Pharmacol.,27: 221.
2. Ahtee, L. (1975): Br. J. Pharmacol.,55: 381.
3. Ahtee, L. (1976): Eur. J. Pharmacol., 39: 203
4. Ahtee, L. and Buncombe, G. (1974): Acta Pharmacol.
   Toxicol.,35: 429.
5. Ahtee, L. and Kääriäinen, I. (1973): Eur. J.
   Pharmacol.,22: 206.
6. Ahtee, L. and Kääriäinen, I. (1974): Naunyn-
   Schmiedeberg's Arch. Pharmacol.,284: 25.
7. Ahtee, L., Kääriäinen, I. and Paasonen, M.K. (1972):
   Ann. Med. Exp. Biol. Fenn.,50: 180.
8. Andén, N.-E. (1972): J. Pharm. Pharmacol.,24: 905.
9. Andén, N.-E. and Bédard, P. (1971): J. Pharm.
   Pharmacol.,23: 460.
10. Andén, N.-E., Roos, B.-E. and Werdinius, B. (1964):
    Life Sci.,3: 149.
11. Andén, N.-E., Rubenson, A., Fuxe, K. and Hökfelt, T.
    (1967): J. Pharm. Pharmacol.,19: 627.
12. Arnfred, T. and Randrup, A. (1968): Acta Pharmacol.
    Toxicol.,26: 384.
13. Ayhan, I.H. and Randrup, A. (1972): Psychopharmacologia
    27: 203.
14. Bartholini, G. and Pletscher, A. (1971): Experientia,
    27: 1302.
15. Bartholini, G. and Stadler, H. (1975): In: Chemical

Tools in Catecholamine Research II, edited by O.
Almgren, A. Carlsson and J. Engel, p. 235. North-
Holland Publishing Company, Amsterdam.
16. Bergmann, F., Chaimovitz, M. and Pasternak, V.
(1976): Psychopharmacologia,46: 87.
17. Bergmann, F., Chaimovitz, M., Pasternak, V. and
Ramu, A. (1974): Br. J. Pharmacol.,51: 197.
18. Carenzi, A., Guidotti, A., Revuelta, A. and Costa,
E. (1975): J. Pharmacol. Exp. Ther.,194: 311.
19. Carlsson, A.,and Lindqvist, M. (1963): Acta
Pharmacol. Toxicol., 20: 140.
20. Ciba Foundation Symposium (1964): In: Animal
Behaviour and Drug Action, edited by H. Steinberg,
A.V.S. de Reuck and J. Knight, p. 429. J. & A.
Churchill,   London.
21. Clouet, D.H. and Ratner, M. (1970): Science ,168:
854.
22. Corrodi, H., Fuxe, K., Hammer, W., Sjöqvist, F. and
Ungerstedt, U. (1967): Life Sci.,6: 2557.
23. Corrodi, H., Fuxe, K. and Lidbrink, P. (1972):
Brain Res., 43: 397.
24. Costall, B., Fortune, D.H., Naylor, R.J., Marsden,
C.D. and Pycock, C. (1975): Neuropharmacology,14:
859.
25. Costall, B. and Naylor, R.J. (1972): Life Sci.,11:
239.
26. Costall, B. and Naylor, R.J. (1973): Arzneim. Forsch.
(Drug Research) 23: 674.
27. Costall, B. and Naylor, R.J. (1974): Eur. J.
Pharmacol., 29: 206.
28. Costall, B. and Naylor, R.J. (1975): J. Pharm.
Pharmacol., 27, 67.
29. Costall, B. and Olley, J.E. (1971): Neuropharmacology, 10: 297.
30. Cowan, A., Dettmar, P.W. and Walter, D.S. (1975).
Br. J. Pharmacol., 55, 316P.
31. Cox, B., Ary, M. and Lomax, P. (1976): J. Pharmacol.
Exp. Ther.,196: 637.
32. Da Silva, G.R. and Rocha e Silva, M. (1971): Eur.
J. Pharmacol., 15: 180.
33. Fog, R. (1970): Psychopharmacologia, 16: 305.
34. Fukui, K. and Takagi, H. (1972): Br. J. Pharmacol.,
44: 45.
35. Fuxe, K. and Ungerstedt, U. (1970): In: Amphetamines
and Related Compounds, edited by E. Costa and S.
Garattini, p. 257. Raven Press, New York.
36. Fuxe, K. and Ungerstedt, U. (1974): Medical Biol.
52: 48.
37. Gessa, G.L. and Tagliamonte, A. (1975): Neuropharmacology, 14: 913.
38. Greengaard, P. (1976): Nature (Lond), 260: 101.

39. Groppe, G. and Kuschinsky, K. (1975): Neuropharmacology, 14: 659.
40. Gumulka, W., Kostowski, W. and Czlonkowski, A.
(1973): Pharmacology, 10: 363.
41. Herz, A. (1961): Naunyn-Schmiedeberg's Archiv. für
Exp. Pathol. Pharmakol., 241: 236.
42. Herz, A. (1963): Int. J. Neuropharmacol., 2: 205.
43. Hornykiewicz, O. (1973): Br. Med. Bull., 29: 172.
44. Iwatsubo, K. and Clouet, D.H. (1975): Biochem.
Pharmacol., 24: 1499.
45. Kaakkola, S. and Ahtee, L. (1977): Psychopharmacology, 52: 7.
46. Kääriäinen, I. (1976): Acta Pharmacol. Toxicol.,
39: 393.
47. Kääriäinen, I. and Ahtee, L. (1976): Medical Biol.,
54: 56.
48. Kääriäinen, I. and Vikberg, P. (1976): Acta
Pharmacol. Toxicol., 39: 536.
49. Klawans, H.L., Moses, H. and Beaulieu, D.M. (1974):
Life Sci., 14: 1493.
50. Kostowski, W., Gumulka, W. and Czlonkowski, A.
(1972): Brain Res., 48: 443.
51. Kuschinsky, K. (1974): Naunyn-Schmiedeberg's Arch.
Pharmacol., 281: 167.
52. Kuschinsky, K. (1976): Arzneim. Forsch., 26: 563.
53. Kuschinsky, K. and Hornykiewicz, O. (1972): Eur.
J. Pharmacol., 19: 119.
54. Kuschinsky, K. and Hornykiewicz, O. (1974): Eur.
J. Pharmacol., 26: 41.
55. Lahti, R.A. and Losey, E.G. (1974): Res. Commun.
Chem. Pathol. Pharmacol., 7: 31.
56. Mattila, M.J., Ahtee, L. and Saarnivaara, L. (1968):
Ann. Med. Exp. Biol. Fenn., 46: 78.
57. Mattila, M.J., Ahtee, L. and Vartiainen, A. (1965):
In: Tobacco Alkaloids and Related Compounds, p.321
Pergamon Press
58. Moore, J. and Dundee, J.W. (1961): Br. J. Anaesth.,
33: 422.
59. Morpurgo, C. (1962): Arch. Int. Pharmacodyn. Ther.,
137: 84.
60. Nakamura, K., Kuntzman, R., Maggio, A. and Conney,
A.H. (1973): Neuropharmacology, 12: 1153.
61. O'Keeffe, R., Sharman, D.F. and Vogt, M. (1970):
Br. J. Pharmacol., 38: 287.
62. Paalzow, G. (1976): Acta Universitatis Upsaliensis.
Almqvist and Wiksell, Stockholm.
63. Paalzow, G. and Paalzow, L. (1974): Acta Pharmacol.
Toxicol., 34: 157.
64. Paalzow, G. and Paalzow, L. (1975): Life Sci., 17:
1145.
65. Paalzow, G. and Paalzow, L. (1975): Psycho-

pharmacologia, 45: 9.

66. Puri, S.K., Reddy, C. and Lal, H. (1973): Res. Commun. Chem. Pathol. Pharmacol., 5: 389.

67. Randrup, A. and Munkvad, I. (1966): Nature (Lond.) 211: 540.

68. Randrup, A., Munkvad, I., Fog, R. and Ayhan, I.H. (1975): In: Catecholamines and Behavior. 1. Basic Neurobiology, edited by A.J. Friedhoff, p. 89. Plenum Press, New York.

69. Reynolds, A.K. and Randall, L.O. (1957): Morphine & Allied Drugs. University of Toronto Press, Canada.

70. Roos, B.-E. (1969): J. Pharm. Pharmacol., 21: 263.

71. Saarnivaara, L. (1969): Ann. Med. Exp. Biol. Fenn., 47: 180.

72. Saarnivaara, L. (1969): Thesis, University of Helsinki.

73. Sasame, H.A., Perez-Cruet, J., Di Chiara, G., Tagliamonte, A., Tagliamonte, P. and Gessa, G.L. (1971): Riv. Farmacol. Ter., 11: 99.

74. Sasame, H.A., Perez-Cruet, J., Di Chiara, G., Tagliamonte, A., Tagliamonte, P. and Gessa, G.L. (1972): J. Neurochem., 19: 1953.

75. Scheel-Krüger, J. (1970): Acta Pharmacol. Toxicol., 28: 1.

76. Smelik, P.G. and Ernst, A.M. (1966): Life Sci., 5: 1485.

77. Smith, C.B., Sheldon, M.I., Bednarczyk, J.H. and Villarreal, J.E. (1972): J. Pharmacol. Exp. Ther., 180: 547.

78. Stadler, H., Lloyd, K.G., Gadea-Ciria, M. and Bartholini, G. (1973): Brain Res., 55: 476.

79. Tenen, S.S. (1968): Psychopharmacologia, 12; 278.

80. Ungerstedt, U. (1971): Acta Physiol. Scand., 82, suppl. 367: 69.

81. Wallach, M.B. (1974): In: Neuropsychopharmacology of Monoamines and Their Regulatory Enzymes, Advances in Biochemical Psychopharmacology 12, edited by E. Usdin, p. 241. Raven Press, New York.

82. Wand, P., Kuschinsky, K. and Sontag, K.-H. (1973): Eur. J. Pharmacol., 24: 189.

83. Westerink, B.H.C. and Korf, J. (1975): Eur. J. Pharmacol., 33: 31.

84. Wolfarth, S., Dulska, E. and Lacki, M. (1974): Neuropharmacology, 13: 867

85. Yaksh, T.L. and Yamamura, H.I. (1975): Brain Res., 83, 520.

86. Zetler, G. (1968): Int. J. Neuropharmacol., 7: 325.

87. Zetler, G. (1971): Neuropharmacology, 10: 289

Factors Affecting the Action of Narcotics, edited by
M.L. Adler, L. Manara, and R. Samanin.
Raven Press, New York©1978.

Effect of Various Central Biogenic Amine-Modifiers and
Ambient Temperature on the Naloxone-Induced Jumping
in Morphine-Dependent Mice

J.T. Huang[1], Ichiro Yano[2] and A.E. Takemori

Department of Pharmacology, University of Minnesota
Health Sciences Center, Medical School
Minneapolis, Minnesota 55455, U.S.A.

INTRODUCTION

Nalorphine-induced jumping in morphine-dependent
mice was first described by Maggiolo and Huidobro (17).
Later Way, Loh, and Shen (23) used naloxone-induced
jumping behavior to quantify the degree of physical
dependence in morphinized mice. They reported an inverse
relationship between the degree of dependence and the
amount of naloxone needed to induce the jumping responses.
Since then many investigators have adopted the anta-
gonist-induced jumping test because it is simple,
objective, and quantitative. Although some investigators
have questioned jumping as a useful sign of abstinence
in mice (13) and others have produced similar jumping
in mice (16) and rats (6) by drugs unrelated to narcotics,
Smits (20) has recently shown that naloxone-induced
jumping is indeed a sensitive indicator of physical
dependence on the basis of the temporal dissociation
between the naloxone-induced jumping and the inhibition
of analgesia or locomotor activity by naloxone. It is
generally agreed that more than one sign of abstinence
should be monitored when one attempts to quantify
physical dependence in laboratory animals, but the
jumping response remains the most consistent and objective sign for quantifying physical dependence in mice.
    Previously, it has been reported that naloxone can
cause jumping in mice that had received only a single
injection of morphine (1,8,9,13,14,15,20) or levorphanol
(4). These results implied that a degree of physical

---

[1]Present address: New York State Research Institute for
Neurochemistry and Drug Addiction, Ward's Island, New
York, New York, USA.

[2]Visiting Research Fellow from the Department of
Pharmacology, Wakayama Medical College, Wakayama, Japan

dependence to narcotic drugs could develop within hours after an acute dose of the narcotic.

In this study, a comparison was made of the naloxone-induced withdrawal jumping between mice that had been injected with a single large dose of morphine and mice that had been chronically treated with morphine by means of subcutaneously implanted morphine pellets. The jumping incidence was altered by pretreatment of mice with various agents known to modify central biogenic amines to see whether or not the jumping incidence of acutely and chronically morphinized mice was modified in the same manner. The effect of different ambient temperatures on the naloxone-induced jumping is also described herein.

MATERIALS AND METHODS

Animals and Treatment

Male Swiss-Webster mice from Bio-Lab Corp. (St.Paul, Minn.) weighing 20 to 27 g were used. Acutely treated mice received 100 mg/kg morphine sulfate s.c. two hr before the naloxone-jumping test. Chronically treated mice were implanted s.c. with morphine pellets (50 or 75 mg free base) 72 hr before the injection of naloxone. The degree of tolerance and dependence did not differ between animals receiving morphine pellets of 50 and 75 mg. The various drugs used to modify the naloxone-induced jumping and the injection schedule of the drugs are indicated in the tables.

For the study of the effect of ambient temperature on jumping, the normal room temperature was $24 \pm 2°C$, the cold temperature was $2 \pm 1°C$ in a cold room, and the hot temperature was $35.5 \pm 0.5°C$, which was maintained by hanging a 250-watt infrared lamp over the Plexiglass observation cylinder.

Quantitation of Naloxone-Induced Jumping

Mice were placed singly into 30 x 30-cm Plexiglass cylinders immediately after the injection of various doses of naloxone. The number of jumps during the succeeding 15-min period was recorded. A response was considered a jump when all four extremities left the floor at the same time. Since a small percentage of control animals displayed spontaneous jumping responses when they were placed in the cylinder, the criterion for a positive jumping response was that a mouse had to jump more than 4 times during the 15-min observation period. The use of this criterion virtually eliminated all false positive responses because when a dependent mouse began jumping after the naloxone challenge, the

number of jumps invariably exceeded five. The ED_{50} of
naloxone-induced jumping was determined by the method
of Dixon (7) using 5 to 6 animals for each determination.

Chemicals and Drugs

The free base form of morphine was obtained from
Mallinckrodt Chemical Works and made into morphine
pellets containing 50 or 75 mg (18).   The drugs used
from commercial sources were atropine sulfate (KEK Lab.);
morphine sulfate and apomorphine hydrochloride (Merck
and Co.); pargyline hydrochloride (Abbott Lab.); sodium
diethyldithiocarbamate (DETC), L-β-3,4-dihydroxyphenyl-
alanine methyl ester hydrochloride (L-dopa), DL-α-methyl-
p-tyrosine methyl ester hydrochloride (α-MT), DL-
threodihydroxyphenylserine (DOPS), and physostigmine
sulfate (Sigma Chemical Co.); L(-)-tryptophan and DL-
tyrosine methyl ester hydrochloride (Aldrich Chemical
Co.); and DL-5-hydroxytryptophan (5-HTP), pargyline
hydrochloride, and DL-p-chloroamphetamine hydrochloride
(p-CA) (Regis Chemical Co.). Drugs which were received
as gifts were pimozide (Janssen Pharmaceutical), naloxone
hydrochloride (Endo Lab.), haloperidol (McNeil Lab.),
phenoxybenzamine hydrochloride (Smith, Kline and French),
propranolol (Ayerst Lab.) and tetrabenazine methane-
sulfonate (Hoffmann-LaRoche).
Most of the drugs were dissolved in saline solution.
Pimozide and haloperidol were dissolved in 3% citric
acid solution. Tryptophan and 5-HTP were dissolved in
1 part of 0.01 N HCl and diluted with 5 parts of
distilled water. Phenoxybenzamine was dissolved in 2
parts of acidified ethanol and diluted with 8 parts of
distilled water. DOPS was suspended in 1% poloxalene
(Pluronic) which was obtained from Wyandotte Chemicals.
None of the various vehicles altered the naloxone-
induced jumping response of acutely or chronically
morphinized mice.

RESULTS

Development of Acute Dependence

The time course for the development of the naloxone-
induced jumping behavior after an acute dose of morphine
was relatively short. One hr after the injection of
morphine, 50% of the mice displayed naloxone-induced
jumping and at 2 hr all mice exhibited jumping. The
maximum jumping behavior lasted until the fourth hr and
the jumping incidence subsided thereafter.

Effect of Catecholaminergic Modification (Table 1)

Depletion of the central stores of catecholamines by
α-MT or tetrabenazine inhibited the naloxone-induced
jumping in both the acutely and chronically morphinized
mice as evidenced by the 2- to 3-fold increase in the
naloxone ED_{50}. Repletion of norepinephrine (NE) or
dopamine (DA) stores by administration of DOPS or L-dopa
concomitantly with α-MT reversed the inhibitory effect
of α-MT in morphine-implanted mice. In acutely
morphinized mice, administration of DOPS along with
α-MT had no influence on the inhibitory effect of α-MT
whereas concomitant L-dopa administration not only
reversed the α-MT effect but markedly enhanced naloxone-
induced jumping. Reduction of central NE levels by
DETC inhibited jumping of acutely and chronically
morphinized animals as seen by the 3- to 4-fold increases
in the naloxone ED_{50}. Administration of DOPS had no
influence on the jumping of morphine-implanted mice
but resulted in a 67% decrease in the naloxone ED_{50} of
acutely morphinized mice.

Effect of α- and β-Adrenergic Blockers (Table 2)

Phenoxybenzamine markedly reduced naloxone-induced
jumping as seen by the 7- and 3-fold increase in the
naloxone ED_{50} of acutely and chronically morphinized
animals, respectively. Propranolol did not have any
influence on the naloxone-induced jumping of either
morphine-injected or morphine-pelleted mice.

Effect of Dopaminergic Modification (Table 3)

The administration of L-dopa markedly enhanced
naloxone-induced jumping in acutely morphinized mice
but had no effect on the jumping of morphine-implanted
mice. Apomorphine, at various doses, uniformly inhibited naloxone-induced jumping of chronically morphinized
mice. Low doses of apomorphine stimulated naloxone-
induced jumping of acutely morphinized mice while doses
above 0.5 mg/kg inhibited jumping. The dopaminergic
blockers, haloperidol and pimozide, inhibited naloxone-
induced jumping of both morphine-injected and implanted
mice as evidenced by the 2- to 4-fold increases in the
naloxone ED_{50}.

Effect of Cholinergic Modification (Table 4)

Whereas high doses of atropine exacerbated and physostigmine greatly inhibited naloxone-induced jumping in
morphine-implanted mice, both drugs inhibited the jumping in acutely morphinized mice.

TABLE 1. Effect of biogenic amine depletors on the naloxone-induced jumping of morphine-treated mice

Pretreatment	ED$_{50}$ of naloxone (mg/kg) $\pm$ S.E.	
	Acute[a]	Chronic[a]
Control	2.7 $\pm$ 0.5 (6)	0.037 $\pm$ 0.004 (6)
α-MT (100 mg/kg, i.p., 7 and 3 hr prior to N[b] doses)	4.9 $\pm$ 0.8 (4)[d]	0.074 $\pm$ 0.007 (5)[d]
Tetrabenazine (30 mg/kg, s.c. 30 min prior to N doses)	8.7 $\pm$ 1.6 (3)	0.096 $\pm$ 0.003 (3)
α-MT[c] + DOPS (300 mg/kg, i.p. 5 and 2 hr prior to N doses)	4.4 $\pm$ 0.8 (3)	0.042 $\pm$ 0.006 (4)
α-MT[c] + L-Dopa (200 mg/kg, s.c. 30 min prior to N doses)	0.3 $\pm$ 0.1 (3)	0.043 $\pm$ 0.004 (4)
DETC (300 mg/kg, i.p., 4 hr prior to N doses)	8.0 $\pm$ 1.9 (3)	0.141 $\pm$ 0.021 (4)
DOPS (300 mg/kg, i.p., 5 and 2 hr prior to N doses)	0.9 $\pm$ 0.2 (4)	0.032 $\pm$ 0.003 (4)

[a] Acutely treated animals received 100 mg/kg of morphine sulfate s.c. 2 hr prior to naloxone doses. The chronically treated animals received morphine free base pellets s.c. 72 hr prior to the naloxone challenges.

[b] N = naloxone hydrochloride

[c] Same dose as above

[d] Numbers in parentheses indicate the number of ED$_{50}$ values determined. Values are significantly different from their respective control values ($p < 0.05$)

TABLE 2. Effect of phenoxybenzamine and propranolol on the naloxone-induced jumping of morphine-treated mice

| Pretreatment | ED_{50} of naloxone (mg/kg) $\pm$ S.E. | |
	Acute[a]	Chronic[a]
Control	2.4 ± 0.9 (5)	0.037 ± 0.003 (8)
Phenoxybenzamine (10 mg/kg i.p., 2 hr prior to N[b] doses)	17.4 ± 3.3 (4)[c]	0.121 ± 0.012 (4)[c]
Propranolol (5 mg/kg, i.p., 1 hr prior to N doses)	3.1 ± 0.5 (4)	0.032 ± 0.113 (5)

[a] Acutely and chronically treated animals received morphine as indicated in the legend of Table 1.

[b] N = naloxone hydrochloride

[c] Numbers in parentheses indicate the number of ED_{50} values determined. Values are significantly different from their respective control values ($p < 0.05$).

TABLE 3. Effect of stimulators and blockers of dopaminergic receptors on the naloxone-induced jumping on morphine-treated mice.

Pretreatment	ED$_{50}$ of Naloxone (mg/kg)± S.E.	
	Acute [a]	Chronic [a]
Control	2.6 + 0.3 (8)	0.037 + 0.004 (6)
L-Dopa (200 mg/kg, s.c., 2 hr prior to N[b] doses)	0.3 + 0.3 (5) [c]	0.044 + 0.009 (6) [c]
Apomorphine (10 mg/kg,s.c., 15 min prior to N doses)	46.2 + 3.8 (3)	0.169 + 0.051 (4)
Apomorphine (4 mg/kg, s.c., 15 min prior to N doses)	16.0 + 3.2 (3)	0.208 + 0.008 (3)
Apomorphine (2 mg/kg, s.c., 15 min prior to N doses)	13.0 + 3.3 (3)	0.128 + 0.028 (3)
Apomorphine (1 mg/kg, s.c., 15 min prior to N doses)	5.5 + 0.9 (3)	0.091 + 0.013 (4)
Apomorphine (0.5 mg/kg, s.c., 15 min prior to N doses)	2.1 + 0.6 (5)	0.090 + 0.015 (3)
Apomorphine (0.1 mg/kg, s.c., 15 min prior to N doses)	1.3 + 0.3 (5)	0.087 + 0.026 (4)
Haloperidol (2.5 mg/kg, i.p., 35 min prior to N doses)	5.3 + 1.1 (3)	0.090 + 0.009 (3)
Pimozide (1.25 mg/kg, i.p., 2 hr prior to N doses)	7.0 + 0.6 (4)	0.150 + 0.024 (3)

[a] Acutely and chronically treated animals received morphine as indicated in the Legend of Table 1.

[b] N = naloxone hydroxhloride

[c] Numbers in parentheses indicate the number of ED$_{50}$ values determined. Values are significantly different from their respective control values.

TABLE 4. Effect of atropine and physostigmine on the naloxone-induced jumping of morphine-treated mice

| Pretreatment | ED_{50} of naloxone (mg/kg) $\pm$ S.E. | |
	Acute[a]	Chronic[a]
Control	2.6 $\pm$ 0.3 (8)	0.036 $\pm$ 0.003 (5)
Atropine (2 mg/kg, s.c., 30 min prior to N[b] doses)	5.1 $\pm$ 0.8 (4)[c]	0.033 $\pm$ 0.008 (4)[c]
Atropine (4 mg/kg, s.c., 30 min prior to N doses)	7.2 $\pm$ 0.8 (3)	0.022 $\pm$ 0.004 (8)
Physostigmine (0.05 mg/kg, s.c., 30 min prior to N doses)	1.9 $\pm$ 0.6 (6)	0.104 $\pm$ 0.028 (4)
Physostigmine (0.1 mg/kg, s.c., 30 min prior to N doses)	11.7 $\pm$ 3.8 (5)	0.196 $\pm$ 0.103 (4)

[a]Acutely and chronically treated mice received morphine as indicated in the legend of Table 1.

[b]N = naloxone hydrochloride

[c]Numbers in parentheses indicate the number of ED_{50} values determined. Values are significantly different from their respective control values ($p < 0.05$).

Effect of Serotonergic Modification (Table 5)

Although both tryptophan and 5-HTP inhibited naloxone-induced jumping in morphine-implanted mice, they had no influence on the jumping of acutely morphinized mice. The serotonergic depleting agent p-CA did not alter the naloxone ED_{50} of either acutely or chronically morphinized animals.

Effect of Ambient Temperature (Table 6)

In acutely morphinized mice, both hot and cold ambient temperatures potentiated naloxone-induced jumping when compared to the jumping behavior of the animals at normal room temperature. The hot atmosphere decreased the naloxone ED_{50} by over 95% and the cold environment decreased it by about 80%. On the other hand, in morphine-implanted mice, only the hot environment influenced the naloxone ED_{50} which was decreased by one-half when compared to the ED_{50} estimated at normal ambient temperature.

Effect of Ambient Temperature on the Jumping
of Naive Mice (Table 7)

The hot ambient temperature was not only conducive to enhancement of naloxone-induced jumping in morphinized mice but in naive mice as well. Relatively high doses of naloxone caused naive mice to jump under high ambient temperature but not under cold or normal room temperatures. Although some incidence of jumping among the control animals (saline-injected mice) was observed when they were placed in the hot atmosphere, the naloxone-treated mice always jumped sooner after injection and jumped many more times than the saline-treated mice.

TABLE 5. Effect of serotonin precursors and p-chloramphetamine on the naloxone-induced jumping of morphine-treated mice

| Pretreatment | ED_{50} of naloxone (mg/kg) ± S.E. | |
	Acute[a]	Chronic[a]
Control	2.4 ± 0.4 (5)	0.037 ± 0.004 (6)
Tryptophan (75 mg/kg, i.p. 4 and 1.5 hr prior to N[b] doses)	1.6 ± 0.4 (5)[c]	0.064 ± 0.010 (5)[c]
5-HTP (25 mg/kg, i.p. 4 and 1.5 hr prior to N doses)	1.4 ± 0.4 (3)	0.085 ± 0.012 (3)
p-CA (5 mg/kg, i.p., 24 hr prior to N doses)	3.8 ± 1.1 (3)	0.044 ± 0.006 (6)

[a]Acutely and chronically treated animals received morphine as indicated in the legend of Table 1.

[b]N = naloxone hydrochloride

[c]Numbers in parentheses indicate the number of ED_{50} values determined. Values are significantly different from the control value ($p < 0.05$).

TABLE 6. Effect of various ambient temperatures on the naloxone-induced jumping of morphine-treated mice

Ambient temperature (°C)	ED_{50} of naloxone (mg/kg)			
	Acute [a]		Chronic [a]	
	N [b]	m ± S.E.	N [b]	m ± S.E.
35 to 36°	5	0.097 ± 0.035 [c]	5	0.016 ± 0.002 [c]
22 to 26°	8	2.54 ± 0.51	7	0.032 ± 0.004
1 to 3°	5	0.51 ± 0.07 [c]	5	0.026 ± 0.004

[a] Acutely and chronically treated mice received morphine as indicated in the legend of Table 1 and in the Methods.

[b] Number of ED_{50} values determined using 5 animals for each determination.

[c] Values are significantly different from values obtained at normal room temperatures (22 to 26°C).

TABLE 7. Effect of various ambient temperatures on the naloxone-induced jumping of naive mice

Ambient Temperature (°C)	No. mice jumped/No. mice tested		
	Naloxone		Saline
	50 mg/kg	25 mg/kg	10 mg/kg
35 to 36°	15/18	4/8	3/18
22 to 26°	0/8	0/8	0/8
1 to 3°	0/8	1/8	0/8

DISCUSSION

Assuming that the naloxone-induced stereotyped jumping in narcotic-dependent mice is indeed a sensitive withdrawal sign in mice, the present data along with others in the literature do indicate that physical dependence can develop within a few hours after a single dose of morphine. However, the manifestation of the withdrawal jumping sign by mice made physically dependent acutely and by mice after continual exposure to morphine appears to differ in some respects. For example, the naloxone-induced jumping of acutely and chronically morphinized mice is modified differently by pretreatments with DOPS, L-dopa, apomorphine, atropine, tryptophan, 5-HTP or by a cold environment. This may be interpreted to mean that the dependence which develops over a relatively short period may differ from that which develops over days. However, we believe it is more likely that the withdrawal signs seen after a single exposure to a narcotic are the manifestations of the true initiating step which leads to physical dependence. On the other hand, the abstinence syndrome observed after chronic treatment with narcotics is complicated by the physical and physiological condition of the animals, stress, homeostatic mechanisms, and certain environmental factors. The latter interpretation implies that the naloxone-induced jumping which is observed in acutely morphinized mice is a truer sign of the actual dependence-producing process itself.

Accepting the above latter interpretation, our data suggest, as we previously concluded (19), that the expression of withdrawal jumping requires the integrity of the central stores of NE and DA. This is indicated by the fact that depletion of the stores of these catecholamines inhibited naloxone-induced jumping and increasing the stores potentiated it.

With regard to NE, α-adrenergic rather than β-adrenergic systems appear to be involved in the withdrawal since phenoxybenzamine greatly inhibited withdrawal jumping whereas propranolol did not. The involvement of the α-adrenergic system in abstinence of rats has also been suggested earlier by Cicero, Meyer, and Bell (5).

Stimulation of dopaminergic receptors with treatments of L-dopa or low doses of apomorphine enhanced naloxone-induced jumping while dopaminergic receptor blockers, haloperidol and pimozide, inhibited the jumping. These results are in contrast to those of Way, Loh, Tseng, and Wei (24). However, in agreement with the above authors, pretreatment of mice with large doses of apomorphine inhibited the naloxone-induced jumping. In this case apomorphine may be acting in a different manner, as suggested and reviewed by Tolosa and Sparber (21). Apomorphine may be acting as a partial antagonist at postsynaptic dopaminergic receptors which results in decreased impulse flow and decreased release of DA from presynaptic nerve terminals. The possibility also exists that the increased ED_{50} of naloxone after large doses of apomorphine may be due to stereotypy.

It was previously suggested that an increased release of brain acetylcholine may be associated with narcotic abstinence signs in narcotic-dependent animals (11,12, 24). The finding that atropine and mecamylamine greatly inhibited naloxone-induced jumping in morphine-dependent mice (11) would support the above suggestion. However, Brase et al. (3) reported that a number of cholinergic agonists inhibited and cholinergic antagonists potentiated the naloxone-induced jumping in morphine-implanted mice. Withdrawal jumping in mice has also been shown to be unaffected or inhibited by atropine in the same laboratory (2,10). The latter investigators reported that the time of naloxone injection after the atropine pretreatment was the determinant factor. Enhancement of jumping was observed when naloxone was given to mice 10 min after atropine but after 30 min jumping was inhibited, and at 2 hr jumping was unaffected. In our study with acutely morphinized mice, both atropine and physostigmine inhibited naloxone-induced jumping. However, atropine potentiated while physostigmine markedly inhibited naloxone-induced jumping in morphine-implanted mice. The potentiation with atropine was observed 30 min after atropine pretreatment, and pretreatment times shorter or longer resulted in no change in the naloxone ED_{50} (Yano and Takemori, unpublished data). The effects of cholinergic agents appear complicated and in view of the non-specific effect on the jumping of acutely morphinized mice, cholinergic mechanisms do not appear to be intimately tied to the dependence-related withdrawal jumping.

Regarding the serotonergic system, tryptophan and 5-HTP inhibited naloxone-induced jumping in morphine-implanted mice but had no effect on that of acutely morphinized mice. p-CA had no influence on the jumping of either acutely or chronically-treated mice. Thus, the serotonergic system also does not appear to be associated with the dependence-related withdrawal jumping.

There is the possibility that changes in the ED_{50} of naloxone which were observed in this study may be the result of an altered disposition of naloxone. It is unlikely that the drugs used to modify biogenic amines caused an altered distribution of naloxone to the brain since the modifiers did not alter the concentration of naloxone in brains of mice (22).

The effects of different ambient temperatures on the expression of withdrawal signs in rats has been studied by Way et al. (24). They found that high ambient temperature potentiated withdrawal jumping and low ambient temperature inhibited it. In contrast, low ambient temperature enhanced wet shake behavior and high ambient temperature inhibited it. They suggested that jumping and wet shakes may be related to heat loss and heat gain mechanisms, respectively, and drugs which make the

animals feel cold or hot would influence the appropriate withdrawal sign. In this study with mice, hot
ambient temperature also enhanced naloxone-induced
jumping in morphine-implanted animals. However, both
cold and hot ambient temperatures enhanced jumping in
acutely morphinized mice. Thus, in mice, the enhanced
jumping appears to be related to stressful factors
rather than the animal's adaptive mechanisms. It
should be mentioned that since temperature does affect
the jumping response, some of the drugs used in this
study may alter the jumping response by changing the
body temperature. We have not investigated systematically this possibility.

In conclusion, drugs which influence the naloxone-
induced jumping in chronically morphinized mice may or
may not influence that of acutely morphinized animals
in the same manner. We suggest that the naloxone-
induced jumping of mice acutely treated with morphine
is more intimately related to the dependence-producing
process and the jumping observed in animals chronically
treated with morphine is complicated by a number of
other factors which may or may not be related to the
dependence process.

ACKNOWLEDGEMENT

This investigation was supported by a U.S. Public
Health Grant DA00289.

REFERENCES

1. Barthelemy, C. and Jacobs, J. (1972): J. Pharmacol.
   (Paris), 3: 530-
2. Bhargava, H.N. and Way, E.L. (1976): Eur. J.
   Pharmacol., 36: 79.
3. Brase, D.A., Tseng, L.F., Loh, H.H. and Way, E.L.
   (1974): Eur. J. Pharmacol., 26: 1.
4. Cheney, D.L. and Goldstein, A. (1971): Nature, 232:
   477.
5. Cicero, T.J., Meyer, E.R. and Bell, R.D. (1974):
   Neuropharmacology, 13: 601.
6. Collier, H.O.J., Francis, D.L., Henderson, G. and
   Schneider, C. (1974): Nature, 249: 471.
7. Dixon, W.J. (1965): J.Am.Statist.Assoc., 60: 967
8. Eidelberg, E. and Erspamer, R. (1974): Arch. Int.
   Pharmacodyn. Ther., 211: 58.
9. Huidobro, F. (1971): Eur. J. Pharmacol., 15: 79
10. Iwamoto, E.T., Ho, I.K. and Way, E.L. (1973): J.
    Pharmacol. Exp. Ther., 187: 558.
11. Jhamandas, K. and Dickinson, G. (1973): Nature,
    245: 219.

12. Jhamandas, K., Phillis, J.W. and Pinsky, C. (1971): Br. J. Pharmacol.,43: 53.
13. Kamei, C., Shimomura, K. and Ueki, S. (1973): Jap. J. Pharmacol., 23, 421.
14. Kaneto, H., Koida, M. and Nakanishi, H. (1972): Jap. J. Pharmacol., 22: 755.
15. Kosersky, D.S., Harris, R.A. and Harris, L.S. (1974): Eur. J. Pharmacol., 26: 122.
16. Lal, H., Colpaert, F.C. and Laduron, P. (1975): Eur. J. Pharmacol., 30: 113.
17. Maggiolo, C. and Huidobro, F. (1961): Acta Physiol. Latinoamer., 11: 70.
18. Maruyama, Y., Hayashi, G., Smits, S.E. and Takemori, A.E. (1971): J. Pharmacol. Exp. Ther., 178: 20.
19. Maruyama, Y. and Takemori, A.E. (1973): J.Pharmacol. Exp. Ther., 185: 602.
20. Smits, S.E. (1975): Res. Commun. Chem. Pathol. Pharmacol., 10: 651.
21. Tolosa, E.S. and Sparber, S.B. (1975): Life Sci., 15: 1371.
22. Tulunay, F.C., Yano, I. and Takemori, A.E. (1976): Eur. J. Pharmacol., 35: 285.
23. Way, E.L., Loh, H.H. and Shen, F.H. (1969): J. Pharmacol. Exp. Ther., 167: 1.
24. Way, E.L., Loh, H.H., Tseng, L.F. and Wei, E.T. (1974): In: Narcotics and the Hypothalamus, edited by E. Zimmermann and R. George, p. 9. Raven Press, New York.

Factors Affecting the Action of Narcotics, edited by
M.L. Adler, L. Manara, and R. Samanin.
Raven Press, New York©1978.

On The Role of Dopamine in Precipitated
Morphine Withdrawal in Rats

E. Laschka, Ch. Gramsch, J. Bläsig and A. Herz

Dept. of Neuropharmacology, Max-Planck-Institut für
Psychiatrie, Kraepelinstrasse 2, 8000 München 40
Germany

INTRODUCTION

A series of investigations in the past few years have
dealt with the role of catecholamines in the development of morphine dependence and in the expression of
withdrawal. These two phenomena have to be clearly
differentiated. Whereas catecholamines do not seem to
be very important for the development of morphine
dependence (4), there is evidence that the integrity
of the central catecholamine stores is required for
the full expression of the withdrawal syndrome (24).
   Concerning the particular role of dopamine (DA)
there are results from different experimental approaches which are difficult to reconcile. Lal (22)
suggests that upon chronic exposure to opiates DA
receptors develop supersensitivity which manifests
itself when the opiate is withdrawn. Other findings
also seem to point to an increased activity of the DA
system during withdrawal. Thus results obtained from
in vitro studies with striatal slices of withdrawn
rats showed an accelerated K^+-induced release of DA
(7). On the other hand, biochemical results of Tseng
et al. (26) are interpreted in terms of reduced DA
activity within the striatum during withdrawal.
This suggestion was further supported by other experiments in which the turning of rats with unilateral
lesions of the substantia nigra was studied (27).
This conflicting data prompted us to investigate the
role of DA during withdrawal in more detail using

various experimental approaches.

1.BEHAVIOURAL EXPERIMENTS

The experiments were performed in rats in which a
medium degree of dependence was induced by the s.c.
implantation of morphine containing pellets (6/10
group, see (3)).When the effect of various substances,
supposed to have DA agonistic properties,on the withdrawal sign jumping was investigated, a significant
increase in the frequency of this sign was observed
with all substances used (Fig. 1.). This increase was
dose-dependent within dose ranges which did not induce
strong stereotypies.   When such stereotypies were
present (e.g. with 10 mg/kg i.p. apomorphine, see
Fig. 1) the opposite effect on jumping was observed.
From these results one might expect that DA antagonists
will decrease this sign.   However, the effects of the
DA receptor blockers haloperidol and pimozide (2) on
jumping were difficult to interpret .
As shown in Fig.2, haloperidol did not decrease jumping in a dose-dependent manner.   Also, with the rather
specific DA antagonist, pimozide, no clearly dose-
dependent effects were obtained.
The results best fit the concept that dopaminergic
mechanisms have only a facilitatory effect on jumping
but that they are not directly involved in the neural
pathway eliciting this sign.

2.BIOCHEMICAL STUDIES

The behavioural data does not permit any conclusions
as to which of the different dopaminergic structures
is mainly involved in the effects described.   To get
more detailed information on this question biochemical
changes occuring in striatal DA during withdrawal were
investigated.

As has been reported by Iwamoto et al (19) DA levels
within the striatum of mice and rats increase during
withdrawal.   Since this increase was observed only in
mice which jumped it was suggested to be causally related to this sign.   An increase in DA levels in the
striatum of rats during withdrawal was also reproduced

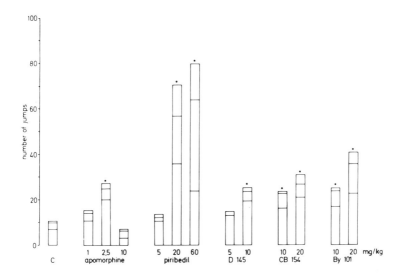

FIG. 1. Effect of various drugs with supposed dopamine
agonistic properties on jumping behaviour during
naloxone-precipitated morphine withdrawal in rats
which have been made dependent to morphine by repeated
implantation of morphine containing pellets. One
pellet was implanted on the 1st day, 2 pellets on the
4th day and 3 pellets on the 7th day, withdrawal was
precipitated on the 10th day (6/10 group).
C = controls : Jumping frequency within 30 min after
i.p. injection of 1 mg/kg naloxone (the vertical lines
in the columns indicate the three 10 min intervals of
the 30 min observation period). Apomorphine i.p.;
piribedil (ET 495) i.p.; D 145 (1,3-dimethyl-5-amino-
adamantan) i.p.; CB 154 (2-Br-ɑ-ergocryptine) s.c.;
By 101 (1-isopropyl-4,4-diphenyl-piperidin-hydrochlo-
ride) s.c.;
*= significance of difference to controls at $P < 0.05$.
For details of the method see Bläsig and Herz (6).

_____

by Gramsch et al.(16). However, the height of this
increase did not correlate with the frequency of jumps
This became evident from experiments in which two different compounds were used to precipitate withdrawal,
naloxone and the partial agonist, ZK 48491, a
benzomorphan derivative, which was shown to induce

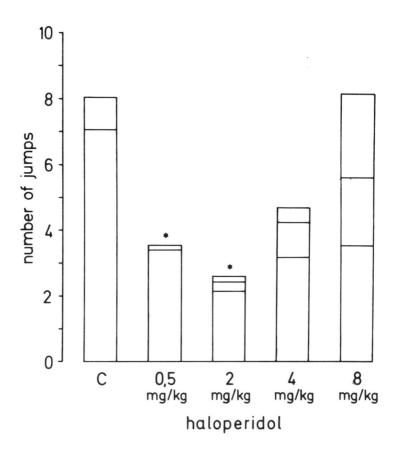

FIG. 2. Effect of the dopamine receptor blocking agent haloperidol on jumping behaviour during naloxone-precipitated withdrawal in morphine dependent rats (6/10 group, see Fig.1).
C = controls : Jumping frequency within 30 min after i.p. injection of 1 mg/kg naloxone (the vertical lines in the columns indicate the three 10 min intervals of the 30 min observation period).
* = significance of difference to controls at P< 0.01. Haloperidol was injected i.p. 60 min before naloxone. For details of the method see Bläsig and Herz (6).

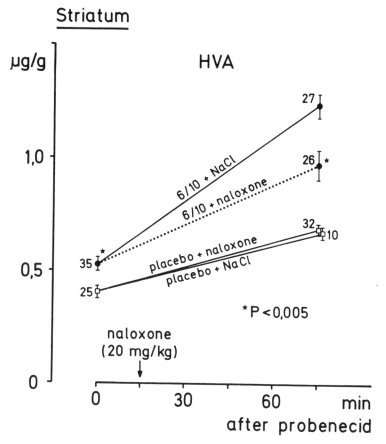

FIG. 3. Accumulation of homovanillic acid (HVA)after
probenecid during precipitated morphine withdrawal in
morphine dependent rats (6/10 group, see Fig.1).
Probenecid (200 mg/kg, i.p.) was injected 15 min before
withdrawal was precipitated by naloxone (20 mg/kg i.p.).
Ordinate: μg/g HVA; abscissa: min after injection of
probenecid. The numbers at each point indicate the
numbers of animals used.

●——● Dependent rats injected with 0.9% saline solu-
      tion instead of naloxone.
●·····● Dependent rats injected with naloxone
□——□ Above: rats implanted with placebo pellets
      instead of morphine containing pellets and
      injected with naloxone.
      Beneath: rats implanted with placebo pellets
      and injected with saline.

For details of the method see Gramsch et al.(16).

much higher frequencies of jumps than naloxone (5).
An increase in DA of similar extent was observed with
both of these substances, regardless of the differences
in the frequencies of jumps induced.

There are several possible explanations for the
increase in striatal DA during withdrawal: An increase
in biosynthesis, a decrease in utilization or release,
a block of catabolism or changes in the reuptake
mechanism. To help distinguish between these many
possibilities, the turnover of DA during withdrawal
was studied. It was found that the accumulation of
the main DA metabolite, homovanillic acid (HVA), was
significantly reduced after probenecid induced blockade
of its active transport out of the central nervous
system during naloxone precipitated withdrawal (Fig.3).
The same was true for the accumulation of another DA
metabolite after probenecid, dihydroxyphenylacetic
acid (DOPAC). The content in 3-methoxy-tyramine (3-MT)
estimated according to the method of Kehr (20)(pooling
8 striata for each estimation) was reduced in these
rats by 40%. This decrease in DA metabolites was not
due to a decreased activity of DA metabolizing enzymes
since the activity of catechol-0-methyltransferase
(COMT) or monoaminooxidase (MAO) proved to be normal
during withdrawal (for details see Gramsch et al.(16).

In principle, similar changes in the accumulation
of HVA and DOPAC after probenecid were found in
extrastriatal structures, such as the nucleus accumbens
and the tuberculum olfactorum, whereas in the remaining brain (without striatum, cortex, tuberculum
olfactorum and nucleus accumbens) a considerable
increase in HVA accumulation was observed. This latter
finding may point to differences in DA metabolism
between the nerve terminal areas and other non-terminal
DA areas, supposed to contribute mainly to the DA
metabolism in this remaining part of the brain.

The turnover studies indicate that the release of
DA from striatal nerve endings is reduced during
withdrawal. This is in line with the interpretations
of Way (27). On the other hand, the finding obtained
in vitro, showing that the K^+-induced release of DA
from striatal slices of withdrawn rats is increased
(7) apparently contradicts the above results. However,
it has to be considered that the in vivo studies

measure the integrated result of changes in neural
input into the striatum as well as changes originating
within the striatum itself whereas measurements made
in this in vitro experiment can only detect effects
originating within the detached, disafferentiated
slice under study.

Although the biochemical results indicate a reduced
release of DA from striatal terminals one cannot draw
any conclusions from these results on the functional
state of the striatum. The reduction of DA release
may be a secondary effect resulting from feed-back
inhibition, triggered by stimulation of super-
sensitive DA receptors.

3.TURNING EXPERIMENTS

Further inquiry into the functional state of the
striatum during withdrawal was made using the turning
model initially introduced by Andén et al. (1). This
model is based on the observation that animals with
unilateral striatal lesions show a typical motor
asymmetry following systemic injection of either DA
agonists or antagonists. This asymmetry manifests
itself in body torsion (turning) or running in circles
(circling), the direction of which depends on whether
the DA receptors of the intact striatum are activated
or blocked. In the experiments presented the striatum
was unilaterally inactivated by spreading depression
induced by the injection of 1 µl 25% w/v potassium
chloride (KCl) solution into the centre of the neostriatum (see 25).

a) Naive rats
Not chronically morphinized (naive) rats, unilaterally
injected with KCl (1-2 min before) showed transient
contralateral turning immediately after injection and
normal behaviour afterwards. When injected with DA
receptor blocking agents, like haloperidol or pimozide,
these animals performed strong turning contralateral
to the inactivated striatum. This turning behaviour
lasted for 20-30 min and could not be reversed by
manipulation. In contrast DA agonists like apomorphine or d-amphetamine (12) elicited long lasting
ipsilateral circling (> 30min) when given within a

dose range at which stereotypies were induced.
Ipsilateral circling was obtained, too, but much less
frequently, with the less strong agonist piribedil
(10) or with L-dopa. The weak DA agonist CB154 (11,14)
even when given at very high doses, did not induce any
significant asymmetry in naive rats. The same was
true for some other drugs,not primarily influencing
the DA system,like caffeine, desipramine, atropine,
and arecoline as well as for naloxone and morphine.

b) Dependent rats
When dependent animals were injected with naloxone
after unilateral administration of KCl, they showed
contralateral circling lasting for 20-30 min (Fig.4).
A high dose of apomorphine (3 mg/kg, s.c.) completely
reversed the contralateral withdrawal circling to
ipsilateral whereas a low dose (0.05 mg/kg, s.c.)
strongly enhanced contralateral circling. D-amphetamine
piribedil and L-dopa (with decreasing efficiency in
this order in the doses used) also induced ipsilateral
circling during withdrawal without, however, completely
abolishing the contralateral circling. CB 154 did not
convert the withdrawal circling to ipsilateral but
strongly enhanced the contralateral withdrawal
circling like the low dose of apomorphine. Haloperidol
and pimozide did not influence withdrawal circling.
Thus the power of the drugs to enhance withdrawal
jumping in non-striatal lesioned rats seems to parallel
their power to enhance contralateral circling during
withdrawal whereas their abilities to convert withdrawal circling into ipsilateral were not related to
their jumping increasing effects. This was further
supported by experiments in which the effects of the
high (2 mg/kg, s.c.) and the low dose (0.05 mg/kg,
s.c.) of apomorphine on withdrawal jumping were
compared. With the low dose, jumping (in the non-
lesioned rats) as well as contralateral withdrawal
circling (in the lesioned rats) was strongly enhanced,
whereas with the high dose jumping was suppressed and
the contralateral withdrawal circling was completely
reversed to ipsilateral.

Probably, the strong stereotypies induced by high
doses of apomorphine interfere with jumping and are
thus responsible for its suppression (18). As has

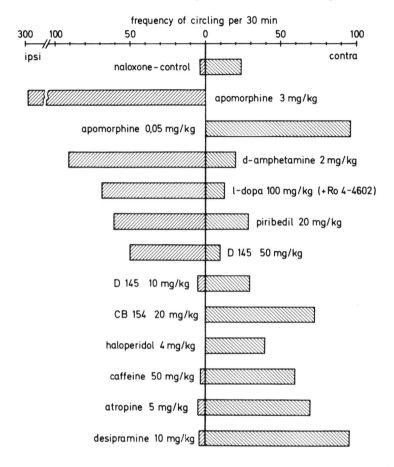

FIG. 4. Influence of various drugs on contralateral
circling during morphine withdrawal in morphine dependent rats with unilaterally inactivated striatum(6/10
group,see Fig.1). Left: Frequency of ipsilateral
circling; right: Frequency of contralateral circling.
Naloxone-control: Frequency of circling within 30 min
after i.p.injection of 1 mg/kg naloxone.
Dopamine agonists:Apomorphine s.c.; d-Amphetamine i.p.;
L-dopa i.p. 45 min after 50 mg/kg, s.c. of benserazide
(Ro 4-4602) (N'-/DL-seryl/N^2/2,3,4,trihydroxybenzyl/
hydrazine); piribedil (ET 495) i.p.; D 145(1,3-dimeth-
yl-5-aminoadamantan)i.p.;CB (2-Br- ⍺ -ergocryptine),
s.c. Dopamine antagonist: Haloperidol i.p. Other drugs:
Caffeine i.p.; atropine i.p.; desipramine i.p.
For details of the method see Laschka et al.(23).

been suggested by Kehr et al.(21) apomorphine in a low dose range mainly acts at presynaptic receptors resulting in reduced output of DA; it cannot be excluded, therefore, that the enhancement of jumping by low doses of apomorphine is due to stimulation of presynaptic DA receptors.

The finding showing that animals turn to the direction of DA receptor blockers during withdrawal suggests that DA activity within the striatum is reduced during withdrawal. Thus it seems improbable that the decreased turnover of DA seen during withdrawal is the result of feed-back inhibition (see above). The possibility that cholinergic, serotonergic or noradrenergic mechanisms are responsible for the turning seen during withdrawal also seems improbable. It has recently been suggested by Glick et al.(15) that these mechanisms may have a modulatory influence on turning behaviour. Nevertheless, these authors conclude that turning behaviour is primarily induced by the functional state of the striatum, which might be indirectly influenced under certain conditions by other transmitter systems than the dopaminergic nigro-striatal system.

CONCLUSIONS

In summary, the biochemical results together with those from the turning experiments clearly indicate that DA activity within the striatum is reduced during morphine withdrawal.

The question remains, however, why, in spite of an obviously reduced DA transmission within the striatum during withdrawal, is jumping enhanced by DA agonists. One possible answer to this question is that pre-synaptic receptors are involved as discussed in the case of apomorphine (see above); another explanation is offered by the concept of Cools and van Rossum (9) who postulate different kinds of DA receptors within the striatum. The role of extrastriatal structures is presently under further investigation.

REFERENCES

1. Andén, N.-E., Dahlström, A., Fuxe, K., and Larsson, K. (1966): Acta Pharmacol.Toxicol., 24: 263-274.
2. Andén, N.-E., Butcher, S.G., Corrodi, H., Fuxe, K., and Ungerstedt, U. (1970): Eur.J.Pharmacol., 11: 303-314.
3. Bläsig, J., Herz, A., Reinhold, K., and Zieglgänsberger, S. (1973): Psychopharmacologia, 33: 19-38.
4. Bläsig, J., Herz, A., and Gramsch, Ch. (1975): Naunyn Schmiedebergs Arch.Pharmacol., 286:325-336.
5. Bläsig, J., Höllt, V., Herz, A., and Paschelke, G. (1976): Psychopharmacologia, 46: 41-51.
6. Bläsig, J., and Herz, A. (1976): Submitted
7. Bosse, A., and Kuschinsky, K. (1976): Naunyn Schmiedebergs Arch.Pharmacol., Suppl.293: 36.
8. Brase, D.A., Tseng, L.-F., Loh, H.H., and Way, E.L. (1974): Eur.J.Pharmacol., 26: 1-9.
9. Cools, A.R., and van Rossum, J.M. (1976): Psychopharmacologia, 45: 243-254.
10. Corrodi, H., Fuxe, K., and Ungerstedt, U. (1971): Eur.J.Pharmacol., 23: 989-991.
11. Corrodi, H., Fuxe, K., Hökfelt, T., Lidbrink, P., and Ungerstedt, U. (1973): J.Pharm.Pharmacol., 25: 409-412.
12. Ernst, A.M. (1967): Psychopharmacologia, 10: 316-323.
13. Francis, D.L., Roy, A.C., and Collier, H.O.J.(1975): Life Sci., 16: 1901-1906.
14. Fuxe, K., Corrodi, H., Hökfelt, T., Lidbrink, P., and Ungerstedt, U. (1974): Med.Biol., 52: 121-132.
15. Glick, S.D., Jerussi, T.P., and Fleisher, L.N. (1976): Life Sci., 18: 889-896.
16. Gramsch, Ch., Herz, A., and Bläsig, J. (1977): Eur.J.Pharmacol., 44: 231-240.
17. Herz, A., Bläsig, J., and Papeschi, R. (1974): Psychopharmacologia, 39: 121-143.
18. Herz, A. (1975): In: Opiate Receptor Mechanisms, edited by S.H. Snyder, and S. Mathysse, Neuroscience Res.Progr.Bull., 13: 118-123.
19. Iwamoto, E.T., Ho, I.K., and Way, E.L. (1973): J.Pharmacol.Exp.Ther., 187: 558-567.

20.Kehr, W. (1974): Naunyn Schmiedebergs Arch.
  Pharmacol., 284: 143-158.
21.Kehr, W., Carlsson, A., and Lindquist, M. (1975):
  Adv.Neurol., 9: 185-195.
22.Lal, H. (1975): Life Sci., 17: 483-496.
23.Laschka, E., Herz, A., and Bläsig, J. (1976):
  Naunyn Schmiedebergs Arch.Pharmacol., 296:15-23.
24.Maruyama, Y., and Takemori, A.E. (1973):
  J.Pharmacol.Exp.Ther., 185: 602-608.
25.Stille, G., and Sayers, A.(1969): Int.J.
  Neuropharmacol., 8: 181-189.
26.Tseng, L.-F., Loh, H.H., Ho, I.K., and Way, E.L.
  (1974): Proc.West.Pharmacol.Soc., 17: 178-183.
27.Way, E.L. (1975): In: Opiate Receptor Mechanisms,
  edited by S.H.Snyder,and S. Mathysse, Neuroscience
  Res.Progr.Bull., 13: 112-118.

Factors Affecting the Action of Narcotics, edited by
M.L. Adler, L. Manara, and R. Samanin.
Raven Press, New York ©1978.

Serotonergic Mechanisms of Narcotic Action

Rosario Samanin, Franca Miranda and Tiziana Mennini

Istituto di Ricerche Farmacologiche Mario Negri
Via Eritrea 62, 20157 Milano, Italy

INTRODUCTION

Much research has been recently aimed at clarifying
the interaction of narcotic analgesics with serotonin
(5HT) in the central nervous system (CNS). Three types
of findings are frequently obtained : 1) both acute
and chronic administration of morphine increases the
rate of turnover of brain 5HT (20,25,26,36,38,58,61);
2) drugs believed to act specifically on serotonergic
mechanisms can modify the effects of narcotics,
particularly morphine (15,21,35,54,60); 3) electrolytic
or chemical lesions and stimulation of central serotonergic neurons, respectively, reduce or potentiate
morphine analgesia (17,19,40,44,45,58). However, the
complexity of the various methodologies and the
existence of some discrepancies between various authors
have made it difficult to draw any definite conclusions
on the role of 5HT in narcotic action.
This article briefly examines some studies made in our
and other laboratories in an attempt to clarify the
relation between brain 5HT and the analgesic effect of
narcotics, particularly morphine, in the rat. Close
consideration will be given to the experimental strat-
egies used to study the functional role of 5HT, with
a view to straightening out some of the apparent
discrepancies in the literature.

Effects of Narcotics on Serotonergic Mechanisms

The ability of narcotics to affect one or more
serotonergic mechanisms in the rat brain has been examined on several occasions. Steady-state levels of

523

TABLE 1. The effect of two doses of morphine hydrochloride on the levels of 5-hydroxyindoleacetic acid (5HIAA) in various brain areas of the rat

Dose of morphine(a) (mg/kg i.p.)	5HIAA levels (% control)			
	Mesencephalon	Diencephalon	Striatum	Telencephalon
10	115 ± 9	122 ± 7**	89 ± 4	116 ± 2*
20	125 ± 9**	127 ± 9**	121 ± 4**	108 ± 3*

Each figure is the mean of six animals. The animals were killed 90 minutes after drug administration.

5HIAA was estimated according to the method of Curzon and Green (11)

* p< 0.05 compared with control (Student's t test)
** p< 0.001 compared with control (Student's t test)

(a) calculated as base

Statistical analysis was performed on actual levels of 5HIAA

brain 5HT are not usually modified by morphine even
at doses higher than those required to cause analgesic
effect. A significant increase of brain 5-hydroxy-
indoleacetic acid (5HIAA) was observed by various
authors after relatively high doses (16-30 mg/kg) of
morphine (25,38,61), while doses of 4-8 mg/kg are
reported to be ineffective (61).

As shown in Table 1, we found a significant increase
of 5HIAA in the diencephalon and telencephalon of the
rat with 10 mg/kg i.p. of morphine, while 20 mg/kg
produced a significant effect in the striatum and
mesencephalon as well. We also found (Table 2) that
analgesic doses of etorphine, a potent morphine-like
compound (5), significantly increased brain levels of
5HIAA, the effect lasting for two hours, which corresponds to the duration of the analgesic effect.

TABLE 2. The effect of etorphine hydrochloride on
5-hydroxyindoleacetic acid (5HIAA) levels in the rat
brain

Dose of etorphine HCl(μg/kg s.c.)	Brain 5HIAA (% control)			
	30'	60'	120'	240'
0.5		115$\pm$1*		
1.0		142$\pm$8***		
2.0	126 $\pm$ 8**	138$\pm$4***	138$\pm$15*	111$\pm$4

Each figure is the mean of 6 animals. The animals were
killed 60 min after treatment. 5HIAA was estimated
according to Curzon and Green (11).
* $p < 0.05$ compared with control
** $p < 0.01$ compared with control
*** $p < 0.001$ compared with control
The data were statistically evaluated using
Duncan's new multiple range test.
Statistical analysis was performed on actual levels of
5HIAA.

The mechanism by which morphine increases brain 5HIAA levels is not completely clear. Some authors have found that an acute administration of morphine increases 5HT synthesis (25,61). Particularly interesting are the results of Goodlet and Sugrue (20) who found an increase of 5HT synthesis with morphine but not with other narcotics such as pethidine, pentazocine, and methadone. These authors found that morphine, but not the other narcotics, increases brain levels of tryptophan, an effect which could, by itself, explain the increase of 5HT synthesis, since brain tryptophan hydroxylase does not appear to be saturated by the concentrations of tryptophan normally present in the brain (22,33). However, tryptophan levels are increased by several other situations and drugs, such as fasting, a carbohydrate - rich diet, salicylate and clofibrate; this effect cannot therefore be considered a reliable basis for evaluating the role of 5HT in narcotic action.

A few in vitro experiments have been conducted to study the effects of narcotics on 5HT mechanisms such as re-uptake and release but, with the exception of methadone, which appears to be very active in blocking the uptake of 5HT in brain synaptosomes or slice preparations (9,37), drugs such as morphine and heroin show no activity of this type unless very high doses are used. We recently studied the effects of morphine and etorphine on synaptosomal accumulation of 5HT in the brain and spinal cord and found no effects except at concentrations so high that they are unlikely to be reached in vivo (Table 3). The release of 5HT from brain and spinal synaptosomes is not markedly affected either by morphine or etorphine at concentrations ranging from 10^{-6}M to 10^{-4}M. (Table 4).

It has been recently reported (39) that morphine can increase the tryptophan hydroxylase activity in the rat brain, and this would agree with the increase in 5HT synthesis and raised 5HIAA levels observed by various authors. However, there are several difficulties in interpreting these effects of morphine on brain 5HT. For instance, morphine has been reported to interact with other biogenic amines such as noradrenaline and dopamine (60). Moreover, it remains to be established whether the biochemical change is

TABLE 3. Percentage inhibition of C^{14}-5HT accumulation by rat synaptosomal preparations

Drug	Concentration $/\bar{M}_7$	% inhibition Brain	Spinal cord
Morphine	5×10^{-5}	8 ± 4	21 ± 19
	10^{-4}	13 ± 10	22 ± 15
	5×10^{-4}	26 ± 3	46 ± 18
	10^{-3}	42 ± 8	65 ± 9
Etorphine	5×10^{-5}	13 ± 4	31 ± 6
	10^{-4}	31 ± 17	55 ± 10
	5×10^{-4}	75 ± 6	91 ± 14
	10^{-3}	91 ± 6	94 ± 10

Synaptosomes were obtained according to the method described by Gray and Whittaker (23) and diluted with Krebs-Henseleit buffer, half Ca^{++}, containing 0.25 mM pargyline to obtain a final protein concentration of 0.5-1.0 mg/ml (34).
Aliquots of 0.6 ml were incubated for 5 min at 30°C (or 0°C, to determine passive diffusion) in the presence of C^{14}-5HT (55 mCi/mmol, 0.1 µM). Drugs were added to the incubation medium during a preincubation of 5 min. Samples were then filtered through Millipore filters, 0.65 u pore size; filters transferred into vials containing 10 ml of Bray's solution (7) and were counted in a Packard Tri-Carb Mod 3002 spectrometer. Results are expressed as follows :

$$\% \text{ inhibition accumulation} = \frac{CPM \text{ control} - CPM \text{ drugs}}{CPM \text{ control}}$$

Figures are mean values $\pm$ S.D. of 4 determinations.

---

strictly related to the effect under study or is the consequence of pharmacological events not necessarily related to the primary site of action. The biochemical approach has not, in general, contributed significantly to clarifying the role of 5HT in narcotic action.

Effects of Serotonergic Drugs on Narcotic Action

Another frequently used approach is to study the effect of morphine in animals pretreated with compounds known to interact with brain 5HT at various levels. These studies assume that if the analgesic effect of morphine is mediated by a serotonergic mechanism, then an alteration of brain 5HT should modify the effect of morphine. Thus, it has been reported by various authors that reserpine antagonizes morphine analgesia (15, 46,53,57), while others have found no effect (8) or even potentiation (18,56) in reserpinized animals.

Apart from these discrepancies, which may derive from various factors such as differences in dose, time of pretreatment, and animal species, the major problem in interpreting the results obtained with reserpine is that it markedly affects brain catecholamines as well as 5HT. Therefore, it has proved difficult to deter-

TABLE 4. Percentage release of C^{14}-5HT induced in synaptosomal preparation

Drug	Concentration $/\overline{M}7$	% release	
		Brain	Spinal cord
Morphine	10^{-6}	2.5 ± 2.5	9.3 ± 8.4
	10^{-5}	1.5 ± 1.5	1.6 ± 2.2
	10^{-4}	3.6 ± 2.4	5.1 ± 4.8
	10^{-3}	33.3 ± 2.2	24.7 ± 12.4
Etorphine	10^{-6}	4.3 ± 4.3	12.1 ± 10.2
	10^{-5}	6.1 ± 6.1	12.8 ± 12.4
	10^{-4}	10.8 ± 10.0	33.4 ± 10.2
	$10-3$	64.2 ± 12.4	66.9 ± 4.8

See legend to Table 3 for methodological details. Release was studied in synaptosomes pre-loaded with C^{14}-5HT, 0.1 μM, incubated at 37°C for 20 minutes with drugs, after a pre-incubation of 5 minutes (0 time). Release is expressed as follows:

$$\frac{\text{CPM control 20'-CPM drug 20'}}{\text{CPM control 0'}} \%$$

Figures are mean values $\pm$ S.D. of 4 determinations.

mine what relative role brain monoamines play in the
action of reserpine. Particularly interesting are the
results obtained by Sparkes and Spencer (50), who found
that reserpine pretreatment significantly antagonizes
the analgesic effect of morphine in rats and that this
antagonism is reversed by an intraventricular injection
of 5HT, but not NA.

Attempts have been made to use compounds which have
a more selective effect of 5HT mechanisms in the brain
but the results obtained appear to be equally conflicting. Thus, potentiation (49) or no effect (41) on
morphine analgesia has been found with 5-hydroxy-
tryptophan (5HTP). Antagonists such as methysergide
or cyproheptadine have been found to have no effect on
(15) or to antagonize (21) the analgesic effect of
morphine.

Another frequently used compound is parachloro-
phenylalanine (PCPA), a potent blocker of 5HT synthesis
in the brain at the level of tryptophan hydroxylase
(25). But this compound has also produced some discrepancies as shown in Table 5, which briefly sets out
some representative results obtained by several
authors. Various factors can contribute to the discrepancies, such as pretreatment doses and time schedule of PCPA, dose of morphine, sensitivity and variability of the test used to measure analgesia. Nevertheless, the lowest doses of morphine, 1.33 and 2 mg/kg
are antagonized by PCPA, in spite of all the differences in methodology. Vogt, though, found that in the
same conditions, doses of 1.33 and 2.25 mg/kg s.c. are,
respectively, antagonized or not affected by PCPA pretreatment. Our data (ref.43 and Table 8) confirm that
in animals with raphe lesions the dose can determine
the extent to which morphine activity is reduced.

Aside from these considerations, the following
points should be borne in mind in interpreting work
with PCPA: 1) PCPA can inhibit tyrosine hydroxylase to
some extent (29); 2) PCPA may form some p-chloro-
phenethylamine which can release 5HT and NA (29);
3) regional brain 5HT and tryptophan hydroxylase can be
affected differently by PCPA (2,28); 4) there are differences in species sensitivity to the effect of PCPA
on brain 5HT (29).

It is thus hardly surprising that this type of approach

TABLE 5. Some results obtained by various authors with p-chlorophenylalanine(PCPA)

Dose of PCPA (mg/kg)	Time	Dose of morphine (mg/kg)	Test to measure analgesia	Effect of morphine	Reference
100 x 3 p.o.	24 h	10 s.c.	flinch-jump	reduced	(54)
300 i.p.	48 h	10 s.c.	flinch-jump	reduced	(21)
300 p.o.	72 h	2 i.p.	Randall-Selitto	reduced	(8)
300 p.o.	48 h	8-16 i.p.	hot-plate	unchanged	
300 p.o.	48 h	8-16 i.p.	tail-flick	unchanged	
300 p.o.	72 h	10 s.c.	vocalization	unchanged	(41)
100 x 3 i.p.	48 h	9 s.c.	flinch-jump	reduced or / unchanged	(55)
320 i.p.	48 h	2.25 s.c.	foot pressure	unchanged	(58)
320 i.p.	48 h	1.33 s.c.	foot pressure	reduced	

has led to so much uncertainty about the role of brain
5HT in morphine analgesia.

Effects of Lesioning Serotonin-Containing Neurons on
Narcotic Activity

In an attempt to overcome some of the difficulties
inherent in the use of drugs believed to have a
specific effect on 5HT mechanisms, some years ago we
studied the analgesic effect of morphine in animals
with selective degeneration of brain 5HT-containing
neurons. This was achieved by placing electrolytic
lesions in the nucleus raphe medianus (MR), which is
known to be an important site of origin of 5HT neurons
in the brain (13). Fig.1 shows the exact location of
one lesion which is restricted to and destroys the en –
tire nucleus medianus. Since the test used to measure

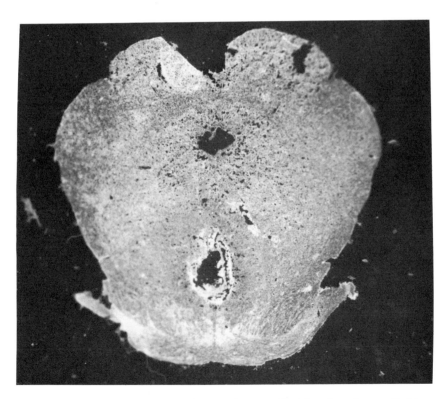

FIG. 1. One representative electrolytic lesion of the
        nucleus raphe medianus.

response of animals to painful stimuli can influence
the results, in our first experiments we used three
methods to measure antinociception in rats: the hot
plate, tail compression and electrical stimulation of
the tail (44). We found that the effect of morphine
was markedly less in the rats with lesions of the
nucleus raphe medianus, suggesting that integrity of
the serotonergic system could be important for morphine
analgesia in rats.

Some time after publication of these findings,
reports appeared showing that lesions placed in the
raphe area, although lowering brain 5HT, did not antagonize morphine analgesia. These have been quoted as
contradicting our data, but if one looks at the experimental conditions used, none attempted to repeat our
exact experiments. Thus, Lorens and Yunger (32) state
that their primary intent was to replicate our data,
but they published a photo of what they considered a
representative lesion in the median raphe nucleus which
is clearly different in size and location from that
used in our experiments. The difference is underlined
by the fact that these authors found only a 27% decrease of brain 5HT in the rats with this type of
lesion while our experiments gave a decrease between
50 and 60%. Another example is Buxbaum et al.(8),
who made three large lesions along the midline as
compared with our one and gave a relatively high (16
mg/kg i.p.) dose of morphine. It could be significant
that authors using experimental conditions much closer
to ours found a complete abolition of morphine analgesia in rats (17).

In an attempt to establish the precise reasons for
the apparently contradictory results, we made lesions
in separate parts of the raphe system and correlated
the lesion location with changes in 5HT levels and
morphine analgesia. We found that morphine had
significantly less analgesic effect in rats with lesions in the nucleus raphe medianus whereas no
significant differences were found between controls and
any of the remaining experimental groups (1). Since
brain 5HT was also reduced in rats with lesions placed
in the nucleus raphe dorsalis or in an area between the
two raphe nuclei, it is clear that a reduction of
brain 5HT does not necessarily imply a decreased effect

of morphine. This may explain why Blåsig et al. (6)
failed to find a correlation between brain 5HT levels
and morphine analgesia in animals with lesions in the
midbrain raphe area.

Recently, we have further explored the relationship
between the two raphe nuclei and morphine analgesia by
making separate lesions in these nuclei and attempting
to relate changes in morphine activity to changes in
5HT and 5HIAA levels in various brain areas and in the
spinal cord. Again we found a marked reduction in
morphine analgesia in the animals with lesions of MR,
while in the animals lesioned in the DR there was only
a slight and not significant reduction (Table 6). In
agreement with results obtained by other authors (27,
31), considerable differences in the reduction of 5HT
and 5HIAA levels were found in two brain areas following the MR or DR lesions. As shown in Table 7, both
indoles almost completely disappeared from the hippocampus of MR-lesioned rats, but no marked differences

TABLE 6. Analgesic effect of morphine in rats lesioned
either in the nucleus raphe medianus (MR) or in the
nucleus raphe dorsalis (DR)

Experimental Groups	Time after injection (Min)			
	30	60	120	180
Sham	0.62 ± 0.14	0.73 ± 0.05	0.53 ± 0.02	0.25 ± 0.01
MR	0.13 ± 0.04*	0.21 ± 0.04*	0.07 ± 0.04*	0.01 ± 0.01
DR	0.60 ± 0.15	0.62 ± 0.14	0.35 ± 0.16	0.08 ± 0.05

Each figure represents the mean $\pm$ S.E. of the analgesic
index, calculated according to Cox et al.(10).
Analgesia was evaluated by the tail compression test
(44) using morphine hydrochloride, 5 mg/kg s.c.,
calculated as base.

* $p < 0.01$ with respect to sham-lesioned animals
(Kruskal-Wallis test).

TABLE 7. Regional serotonin (5HT) and 5-hydroxyindolacetic acid (5HIAA) in the central nervous system of rats lesioned either in the nucleus raphe medianus (MR) or in the nucleus raphe dorsalis (DR)

Experimental Groups	Hippocampus (ng/g ± S.E.)		Diencephalon (ng/g ± S.E.)		Striatum (ng/g ± S.E.)		Cortex (ng/g ± S.E.)		Spinal cord (ng/g ± S.E.)	
	5HT	5HIAA	5HT	5HIAA	5HT	5HIAA	5HT	5HIAA	5HT	5HIAA
Sham	298±13	253±10	564±9	303±1	321±14	399±12	232±10	176±3	340±30	278±22
MR	36±5[*][+]	50±2[*][+]	374±34[*]	189±14[*]	206±19[*][+]	239±16[*][+]	97±7[*][+]	95±13[*]	350±13	320±13
DR	244±10	236±14	381±33[*]	199±19[*]	146±11[*]	187±20[*]	92±8[*]	80±5[*]	315±21	294±24

Indoles were estimated according to the Curzon and Green (11) method.
Each value is the mean ± S.E. of 6 determinations.
The data were statistically evaluated according to Duncan's new multiple range test

[*] p < 0.01 with respect to sham-lesioned animals.
[+] p < 0.01 between MR- and DR-lesioned animals

in hippocampal indoles were found between DR-lesioned rats and controls. On the other hand, the striatal indoles are much more affected in the animals with a lesion in the DR. Neither lesion significantly changes the levels of the two indoles in the spinal cord.

These findings can be interpreted in several ways. One possible explanation is that other than 5HT neurons are involved in the reduction of morphine analgesia observed in animals lesioned in the nucleus raphe medianus. However, that serotonin is specifically involved in this effect is indicated by the fact that 5-hydroxytryptophan restores 5HT levels and morphine analgesia in MR-lesioned animals (42). That 5HT is involved in morphine analgesia is also suggested by some recent data showing that an intracerebral injection of 5,6 dihydroxytryptamine (5,6-HT), which causes selective degeneration of 5HT neurons in the central nervous system (4), significantly reduces the effect of morphine in rats (19,58). A possible explanation is that the different findings with different lesions in the raphe nuclei may be the result of differences in distribution of 5HT neurons originating in or passing through these brain areas. As for other aspects of behavior (24,27,51), the nucleus medianus and the nucleus dorsalis may have a different regulatory influence on morphine analgesia. Although the integrity of the area in which the DR is localized is not particularly important for the effect of morphine, the 5HT neurons originating in this nucleus do appear to play a role in morphine analgesia, as indicated by the fact that electrical stimulation of this area markedly potentiates the effect of morphine in rats (45). Exploration of the possible anatomical and functional connections between the two raphe nuclei might be of great help in building up a more appropriate interpretation of these results.

In agreement with histochemical studies indicating there are no direct serotonergic connections between the nucleus raphe medianus and the spinal cord (14,16), the spinal 5HT content was not affected in animals lesioned in the MR, suggesting that spinal 5HT is not directly involved in the reduction of morphine analgesia observed in MR-lesioned rats. However, some involvement of spinal 5HT in the effect of morphine is

suggested by recent experiments (40) in which electrolytic lesions were placed in the nucleus raphe magnus,
which projects mainly, if not exclusively, to the
spinal cord (14,16). A very good correlation was
found between the extension of raphe magnus lesions
and reduction of morphine analgesia.

The descending 5HT neurons have recently been suggested as having an important role in morphine analgesia on the basis of experiments using 5,6-HT (58) or
examining changes in 5HT metabolism in the spinal cord
following morphine treatment (48). Most data, therefore, are compatible with the hypothesis that various
components of the serotonergic system can influence
the activity of morphine at several levels in the
central nervous system.

We have recently attempted to explore the possibility that 5HT might be involved in the activity of
other analgesics. In our first experiments (43) we
found that only the effect of morphine was reduced in
animals with MR lesions, while other drugs such as
meperidine, methadone, propoxyphene, and codeine were
not affected. In these experiments we used a single
dose of the various compounds and the effect was
evaluated only at 30 min after the drug administration.
In more recent studies using various doses and plotting
a more complete time course of the analgesic effect of
the compounds, we found that the MR lesion reduces not
only the effect of morphine, but also that of etorphine,
heroin, pethidine, methadone, and pentazocine, suggesting that 5HT may play a more general role in the
analgesic effect than that indicated by previous
experiments. Table 8 shows the effect of some representative doses of analgesics in animals with lesions
of the nucleus raphe medianus. That brain 5HT could
be involved in the effect of morphine, etorphine,
pethidine, and pentazocine has been recently suggested
by Sewell and Spencer (47) in studies with mice.

In conclusion, although the exact nature and level
of the interaction remain to be established, the bulk
of available data suggests that various components of
the 5HT system may be involved in the analgesic effect
of morphine. In appropriate conditions, it appears
possible to demonstrate that 5HT might have a more
general part in narcotic activity than that suggested

TABLE 8. The effect of various analgesics in rats lesioned in the nucleus raphe medianus (MR)

Treatment	Dose (mg/kg s.c.)	Analgesic index ± S.E.			
		30'	60'	90'	120'
Sham-operated					
morphine HCl	2.5(a)	0.49 ± 0.10	0.75 ± 0.16	0.70 ± 0.12	0.14 ± 0.11
heroin HCl	0.5	0.72 ± 0.10	0.60 ± 0.12	0.38 ± 0.10	0.12 ± 0.11
etorphine HCl	0.002	1.00 ± 0.00	0.92 ± 0.08	0.54 ± 0.09	0.07 ± 0.04
pethidine HCl	15.0	0.55 ± 0.15	0.76 ± 0.13	0.63 ± 0.20	0.41 ± 0.19
methadone HCl	4.0(a)	0.95 ± 0.06	0.96 ± 0.04	0.91 ± 0.10	0.83 ± 0.17
pentazocine lactate	15(a)	0.47 ± 0.15	0.75 ± 0.17	0.68 ± 0.18	0.38 ± 0.18
MR-lesioned					
morphine HCl	2.5(a)	0.14 ± 0.05 ***	0.14 ± 0.02 **	0.02 ± 0.01 ***	0.01 ± 0.01
heroin HCl	0.5	0.41 ± 0.11 *	0.16 ± 0.05 **	0.07 ± 0.04 ***	0.08 ± 0.05
etorphine HCl	0.002	0.95 ± 0.05	0.46 ± 0.11 ***	0.06 ± 0.03 ***	0.02 ± 0.02
pethidine HCl	15.0	0.12 ± 0.05 *	0.20 ± 0.07	0.06 ± 0.04 ***	0.03 ± 0.03 ***
methadone HCl	4.0(a)	0.92 ± 0.08	1.00 ± 0.00	0.44 ± 0.07 *	0.20 ± 0.08 ***
pentazocine lactate	15(a)	0.09 ± 0.04	0.06 ± 0.01	0.09 ± 0.05	0.08 ± 0.03

Analgesic index was calculated according to Cox et al. (10)
Analgesia was measured by the tail compression test (44)
Each figure is the mean ± S.E. of six animals
(a) calculated as base

* $p < 0.05$
** $p < 0.02$ compared with sham-operated (Student's t test)
*** $p < 0.01$

by studies with morphine. The data obtained with
narcotics appear to be in general agreement with
various reports (3,30) suggesting that serotonin might
constitute one of those systems which regulate the
transmission and/or perception of painful stimuli in
the central nervous system.

REFERENCES

1. Adler, M., Kostowski, W., Recchia, M., and Samanin,
    R. (1975): Eur.J.Pharmacol., 32: 39-44.
2. Aghajanian, G.K., Kuhar, M.J., and Roth, R.H.,
    (1973): Brain Res., 54: 85-101.
3. Akil, H., and Mayer, D.J. (1972): Brain Res., 44:
    692-697.
4. Baumgarten, H.G., Björklund, A., Lachenmayer, L.,
    Nobin, A., and Stenevi, U. (1971): Acta Physiol.
    Scand., 84: Suppl.373: 1-15.
5. Blane, G.F., Boura, A.L.A., Fitzgerald, A.E., and
    Lister, R.E. (1967): Br.J.Pharmacol.Chemother.,
    30: 11-22.
6. Bläsig, J., Reinhold, K., and Herz, A. (1973):
    Psychopharmacologia, 31: 111-119.
7. Bray, G.A. (1960): Anal.Biochem., 1: 279-285.
8. Buxbaum, D.M., Yarbrough, G.G., and Carter, M.E.
    (1973): J.Pharmacol.Exp.Ther., 185: 317-327.
9. Ciofalo, F.R. (1974): J.Pharmacol.Exp.Ther.,
    189: 83-89.
10. Cox, B.M., Ginsbug, M., and Osman, O.H. (1968):
    Br.J.Pharmacol.Chemother.,33: 245-256.
11. Curzon, G., and Green, A.R. (1970): Br.J.Pharmacol.
    39: 653-655.
12. Curzon, G., Joseph, M.H., and Knott, P.J. (1972):
    J.Neurochem., 19: 1967-1974.
13. Dahlström,A., and Fuxe, K. (1964): Acta Physiol.
    Scand., 62: suppl.232: 1-55.
14. Dahlström, A., and Fuxe, K. (1965): Acta Physiol.
    Scand., 64: suppl.247: 7-36.
15. Fennessy, M.R., and Lee, J.R. (1970): J.Pharm.
    Pharmacol., 22: 930-935.
16. Fuxe, K. (1965): Acta Physiol.Scand., 64: suppl.247
    37-85.
17. Garau, L., Mulas, M.L., and Pepeu, G. (1975):
    Neuropharmacology, 14: 259-263.

18. Garcia Leme, J., and Rocha y Silva, M. (1961): J.Pharm.Pharmacol., 13: 734-742.
19. Genovese, E., Zonta, N., and Mantegazza, P. (1973): Psychopharmacologia, 32: 359-364.
20. Goodlet, I., and Sugrue, M.F. (1974): Eur.J. Pharmacol., 29: 241-248.
21. Görlitz, B.-D., and Frey, H.H. (1972): Eur.J. Pharmacol., 20: 171-180.
22. Grahame-Smith, D.G. (1971): J.Neurochem., 18: 1053-1066.
23. Gray, E.G., and Whittaker, V.P. (1962): J.Anat., 96: 79-88.
24. Gumulka, W., Samanin, R., Valzelli, L., and Consolo, S. (1971): J.Neurochem., 18: 533-535.
25. Haubrich, D.R., and Blake, D.E. (1973): Biochem. Pharmacol., 22: 2753-2759.
26. Ho, I.K., Lu, S.E., Stolman, S., Loh, H.H., and Way, E.L. (1972): J.Pharmacol. Exp. Ther., 182: 155-165.
27. Jacobs, B.L., Wise, W.D., and Taylor, K.M. (1974): Brain Res., 79: 353-361.
28. Knapp, S., and Mandell, A.J. (1972): Life Sci., 11: pt.1, 761-771.
29. Koe, B.K., and Weissman, A. (1966): J. Pharmacol. Exp. Ther., 154: 499-516.
30. Liebeskind, J.C., Guilbaud, G., Besson, J.-M.,and Oliveras, J.-L. (1973): Brain Res., 50: 441-446.
31. Lorens, S.A., and Guldberg, H.C. (1974): Brain Res., 78: 45-56.
32. Lorens, S.A., and Yunger, L.M. (1974): Pharmacol. Biochem. Behav., 2: 215-221.
33. Lovenberg, W., Jequier, E., and Sjoerdsma, A. (1968): Adv. Pharmacol., 6A: 21-36.
34. Lowry, O.H., Rosebrough, N.J., Farr, A.L., and Randall, R.J. (1951): J.Biol.Chem., 193: 265-275.
35. Major, C.T., and Pleuvry, B.J. (1971): Br.J. Pharmacol., 42: 512-521.
36. Maruyama, Y., Hayashi, G., Smits, S.E., and Takemori, A.E. (1971): J.Pharmacol.Exp.Ther., 178: 20-29.
37. Moffat, J.A., and Jhamandas, K. (1976): Eur.J. Pharmacol., 36: 289-297.
38. Papeschi, R., Theiss, P., and Herz, A. (1975): Eur.J.Pharmacol., 34: 253-261.

39. Pérez-Cruet, J., Thoa, N.B., and Ng, L.K.Y. (1975): Life Sci., 17: 349-362.

40. Proudiff, H.K., and Anderson, E.G. (1975): Brain. Res., 98: 612-618.

41. Reinhold, K., Bläsig, J., and Herz, A. (1973): Naunyn-Schmiedebergs Arch.Pharmacol., 278:69-80.

42. Samanin, R., and Bernasconi, S. (1972): Psychopharmacologia, 25: 175-182.

43. Samanin, R., Ghezzi, D., Mauron, C., and Valzelli, L. (1973): Psychopharmacologia, 33: 365-368.

44. Samanin, R., Gumulka, W., and Valzelli, L. (1970): Eur.J.Pharmacol., 10: 339-343.

45. Samanin, R.,and Valzelli, L. (1971): Eur.J. Pharmacol., 16: 298-302.

46. Schneider, J.A. (1954): Proc.Soc.Exp.Biol.Med., 87: 614-615.

47. Sewell, R.D.E., and Spencer, P.S.J. (1975): Psychopharmacologia, 42: 67-71.

48. Shiomi, H., Murakami, H., and Takagi, H. (1974): Jap.J.Pharmacol., 24: suppl.87, abs.130.

49. Sigg, E.B., Caprio, G., and Schneider, J.A. (1958): Proc.Soc.Exp.Biol.Med., 97: 97-100.

50. Sparkes, C.G., and Spencer, P.S.J. (1971): Br.J. Pharmacol., 42: 230-241.

51. Srebro, B., and Lorens, S.A. (1975): Brain Res., 89: 303-325.

52. Tagliamonte, A., Tagliamonte, P., Pérez-Cruet, J., Stern, S., and Gessa, G.L. (1971): J.Pharmacol. Exp.Ther., 177: 475-480.

53. Takagi, H., Takashima, T., and Kimura, K. (1964): Arch.Int.Pharmacodyn.Ther., 149: 484-492.

54. Tenen, S.S. (1968): Psychopharmacologia, 12:278-285.

55. Tilson, H.A., and Rech, R.H. (1974): Psychopharmacologia, 35: 45-60.

56. Tripod, J., and Gross, F. (1957): Helv.Physiol. Pharmacol.Acta., 15: 105-118.

57. Verri, R.A., Graeff, F.G., and Corrado, A.P. (1968): Int.J.Neuropharmacol., 7: 283-292.

58. Vogt, M. (1974): J.Physiol.(Lond.), 236: 483-498.

59. Way, E.L., Loh, H.H., and Shen, F.H. (1968): Science, 162: 1290-1292.

60. Way, E.L.,and Shen,F.H. (1971): In: Narcotic Drugs. Biochemical Pharmacology, edited by D.H.Clouet, pp.229-253. Plenum Press, New York.

61. Yarbrough, G.G., Buxbaum, D.M., and Sanders-Bush,
    E. (1973): J.Pharmacol.Exp.Ther., 185: 328-335.

Factors Affecting the Action of Narcotics, edited by
M.L. Adler, L. Manara, and R. Samanin.
Raven Press, New York©1978.

Dietary Effects on Analgesic Drug Potency

L.D.Lytle, L.Phebus, L. A. Fisher, and R.B.Messing

Massachusetts Institute of Technology
(Present address: Dept. of Psychology, University of
California, Santa Barbara, California 93106, U.S.A.)

INTRODUCTION

Recent experiments conducted in a number of
laboratories now suggest that certain aspects of brain
composition (and ultimately brain function) may be
altered by the quality or quantity of food eaten by
animals or humans. The diet-induced changes in brain
function appear to involve alterations in the ability
of cells to communicate with one another vis à vis the
release of neurotransmitter compounds. In most cases,
those compounds currently thought to be neurotransmitters in the brain are low-molecular-weight substances
that are direct metabolites of amino acids (serotonin,
norepinephrine, dopamine, epinephrine, and histamine),
or are amino acids themselves (gamma-aminobutyric
acid, glycine, aspartate); in other cases, some neurotransmitters are synthesized from substrate precursor
compounds derived from a variety of metabolic pathways
(acetylcholine) (44). It now seems clear that
restrictions in the intake of amino acids or other
compounds that are precursors for brain neurotransmitters, or that are neurotransmitters themselves, will
substantially reduce transmitter biosynthesis and,
possibly, release (67). Many of the neurotransmitters
whose synthesis depends on adequate dietary sources
of precursor compounds also play important roles in a
variety of physiological and behavioral responses;
moreover, the physiological and behavioral potency of
many pharmacological agents depends at least in part on
their relative abilities to alter the metabolic fates
of these compounds.

In this paper, we will review evidence that brain

543

serotonin-containing neurons may normally mediate the
sensitivity and/or reactivitiy of animals to noxious
stimuli, as well as mediate the analgesic effects of
various drugs, including the opiate and non-opiate
analgesics. This discussion will include a review of
evidence that the concentrations of serotonin in brain
neurons may depend on the availability of its indispensable amino acid precursor, tryptophan, and a description of an animal model that may have possible utility
for understanding how diet-induced changes in brain
neurochemistry might be important for normal and drug-
mediated responses to painful stimuli.

BRAIN SEROTONIN AND THE RESPONSE TO PAINFUL STIMULI

Anatomical Localization and Metabolism of Serotonin
Neurotransmitters. Significant concentrations of
serotonin are found in a variety of peripheral tissues,
including the enterochromaffin cells of the gastro-
intestinal tract, the parenchymal cells of the pineal
gland (where serotonin is a precursor compound in the
synthesis of the hormone melatonin), blood platelets,
the terminals of sympathetic nerves innervating the
pineal gland, and in the mast cells of some mammals(5).
Serotonin probably does not function as a neurotransmitter compound in most of these peripheral
tissues.

Serotonin-containing neurons are found predominantly
in the central nervous system; although these cells are
not visualized particularly well by histochemical
fluorescence methods, it seems clear that virtually
all of the serotonin neuronal cell bodies are localized
in the midline raphe nuclei of the medulla and pons(6).
These cell bodies give rise to fibers with large
numbers of collaterals that descend in the spinal cord
to innervate gray matter, or that ascend in the medial
forebrain bundle and terminate in many diencephalic and
telencephalic brain regions, including the hypothalamus
septal nuclei, striatum, and cortex (64).

Brain neurons that utilize serotonin as a neurotransmitter appear to contain all of the precursors
and enzymes necessary for its synthesis and catabolism
(Fig. 1). The initial step in the synthesis of

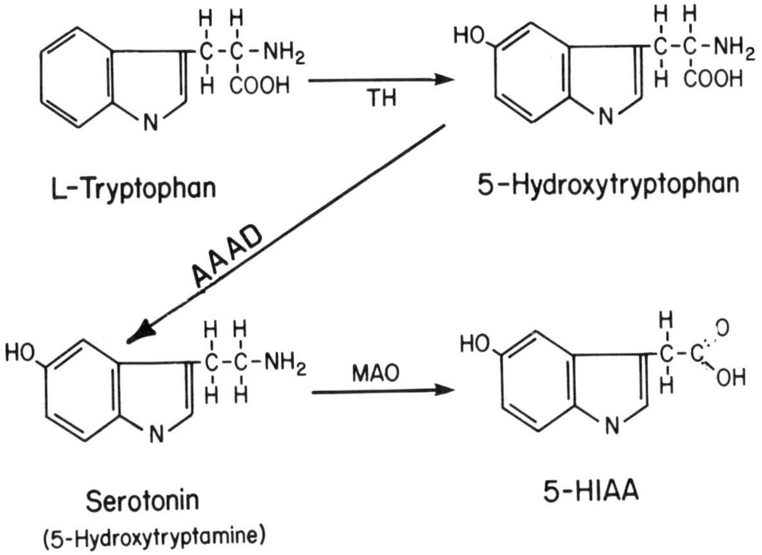

FIG. 1. The synthesis and catabolism of brain serotonin.
The essential amino acid tryptophan is 5-hydroxylated
in a reaction catalyzed by the enzyme tryptophan
hydroxylase (TH). The resultant product, 5-hydroxy-
tryptophan, is then decarboxylated by the enzyme
aromatic 1-amino acid decarboxylase (AAAD) to form the
neurotransmitter serotonin. Once released and taken
back up into the presynaptic neuron, serotonin molecules are deaminated and oxidized by monoamine oxidase
(MAO) to form the inactive metabolite, 5-hydroxy-
indoleacetic acid (5-HIAA).

serotonin involves the 5-hydroxylation of the amino
acid tryptophan in a reaction catalyzed by the enzyme
tryptophan hydroxylase, to form the corresponding
amino acid 5-hydroxytryptophan. 5-Hydroxytryptophan
is normally rapidly decarboxylated by the enzyme
aromatic 1-amino acid decarboxylase to form serotonin
(5-hydroxytryptamine). Serotonin molecules, most
probably stored intracellularly in more than one pool,
are released into brain synapses following electrical
stimulation of the neuron (2). Some of these molecules
are then taken up again by the presynaptic neuron,

where they are deaminated and oxidized by the enzyme monoamine oxidase to form an inactive metabolite, 5-hydroxyindole-acetic acid (5-HIAA). Other molecules that are released interact with receptors.

Tryptophan is an indispensable amino acid that cannot be synthesized de novo by most mammals; molecules of the amino acid available to brain thus originate only from the lysis of body proteins, or from circulating tryptophan derived from the diet or from small tissue pools of the amino acid (67). The amount of tryptophan available to brain tissue appears to be an important rate-limiting factor in the control of brain serotonin biosynthesis, inasmuch as the enzyme tryptophan hydroxylase does not appear normally to be saturated in vivo with its substrate (42), and because there appears to be little control of synthetic enzyme activity by end-product inhibition (22). Moreover, several lines of evidence show a direct relationship between brain tryptophan concentrations and the rate of serotonin biosynthesis: 1) injections of relatively small doses of tryptophan that increase plasma and brain concentrations of the amino acid (to an extent similar to that normally occurring diurnally)increase brain serotonin synthesis (18); 2) many drugs (amphetamine, lithium,dibutyryl cyclic AMP, reserpine) and other manipulations (electroconvulsive shock, exposure to hot ambient temperatures) that increase brain tryptophan concentrations also increase brain serotonin synthesis (12); and 3) various neutral amino acids (para-chlorophenylalanine phenylalanine, valine, leucine) that compete with tryptophan for transport into the brain from the plasma decrease brain tryptophan concentrations and suppress serotonin synthesis (47,67).

Since all tryptophan molecules available for serotonin biosynthesis ultimately derive from the diet, it is not too surprising that the quality of food consumed by mammals has been shown to influence brain serotonin synthesis: 1) animals chronically fed artificial or natural diets containing abnormally low concentrations of tryptophan have decreased concentrations of the amino acid in plasma and brain, and reductions in the concentrations of brain serotonin; 2) animals fed a high-carbohydrate, protein-free meal,

or injected with relatively low doses of insulin,have
increased plasma and brain concentrations of
tryptophan and brain serotonin; and 3) animals fed
artificial amino acid diets which increase the ratio
of plasma tryptophan relative to the concentrations
of other large neutral amino acids (tyrosine, valine,
leucine, isoleucine, and phenylalanine) that compete
with tryptophan for transport into the brain, have
increased brain tryptophan and serotonin levels (20,
68). Although other control mechanisms /such as the
rate at which tryptophan is transported intracellularly into nerves (45)7 may also be important for the
regulation of brain serotonin concentrations, possible
dietary influences on these processes have not yet
been studied in any detail.

Brain Serotoninergic Role in the Response to Painful
Stimuli. Surgical or pharmacological manipulations
that modify brain serotonin concentrations are also
associated with changes in the response to painful
stimuli. In an initial experiment testing this possible interrelationship, Tenen (61) found that animals
injected with para-chlorophenylalanine, a drug that
decreases brain serotonin concentrations by reducing
the levels of brain tryptophan and by inhibiting irreversibly the enzyme tryptophan hydroxylase (36),
showed hyperalgesic responses to presentations of
electric shock. The drug-induced reductions in brain
serotonin, and the increased sensitivity and/or
reactivity of para-chlorophenylalanine treated rats
to electroshock could be restored to normal by administration of 5-hydroxytryptophan (21,61). Somewhat
surprisingly, normal animals injected with tryptophan
or 5-hydroxytryptophan do not show any significant
changes in their responses to noxious stimuli, even
though the brains of these animals have been found to
contain supra-normal concentrations of serotonin as a
result of these pharmacological manipulations(30,35,43,
61). However, these drug treatments may not always
increase functionally releasable pools of brain
serotonin, even though overall levels of the neurotransmitter are elevated in brain. Compatible with
this view are the observations that drugs such as
fluoxetine (Lilly 110140), which increase synaptic
concentrations of serotonin by blocking its reuptake

into presynaptic neurons (47,48), or quipazine, a
putative serotonin receptor agonist (57), produce
analgesia by increasing the probability of serotoninergic neurotransmission at the synaptic or receptor
level. Hence, the available evidence based on
pharmacological studies supports the hypothesis that
reductions in brain serotoninergic neurotransmission
are associated with increased sensitivity and/or
reactivity to painful stimuli, whereas increases in
serotoninergic neurotransmission in brain are related
to analgesia. However, other interpretations of these
data are also possible (35).

Based on the results of the pharmacological studies
described previously, it might be anticipated that
brain lesions that destroy serotoninergic nerves should
produce hyperalgesia, whereas electrical stimulation
of these neurons might induce analgesia. Although the
results of these studies are not unambiguous, the data
obtained from experiments examining the effects of
lesions or stimulation of brain serotonin-containing
neurons are generally compatible with this hypothesis.
For example, Harvey and his coworkers (29,31,32,40,41)
have found that electrolytic lesions aimed at brain
regions containing the axons or terminals of serotonin
nerves generally produce hyperalgesic responses in
rodents; injections of the serotonin amino acid
precursor 5-hydroxytryptophan reverse the hyperalgesia
seen in these brain-lesioned animals (32,40). It is
interesting to note that the efficacy of this 5-hydro-
xytryptophan reversal apparently depends on its
decarboxylation to serotonin in neurons that normally
contain the catecholaminergic neurotransmitters
dopamine, norepinephrine, or epinephrine (68,71).
Somewhat surprisingly, animals with lesions aimed at
serotonin nerve cell bodies in raphe nuclei have
comparable reductions in forebrain concentrations of
the neurotransmitter, but do not show any changes in
their responses to noxious stimuli (31,34,50). The
reasons for these discrepancies are not immediately
clear; however, all brain lesions aimed at serotonin
neurons regardless of whether or not they are placed
in regions containing cell bodies, axons, or terminals,
also destroy other types of neurotransmitter-contain-
ing cells. Hence, these differences may result from

interactive changes between serotoninergic nerves and
these other cells.

In general, the results of most of the lesion
experiments suggest that an <u>ascending</u> serotoninergic
brain system normally mediates the response to painful stimuli; however, results obtained from studies
in which various raphe nuclei have been stimulated
electrically suggest that a <u>descending</u> system (with
serotonin cell bodies localized in the posterior raphe
nuclei and axons descending in the spinal cord to innervate gray matter) may also be involved in the pain
response. Electrical stimulation throughout the midbrain ventral or periaqueductal gray matter generally
produces analgesia (3,38,39,46); similarly, electrical
stimulation of the nucleus raphe dorsalis in cats (49)
or the nucleus raphe magnus in rats (52), also induces
analgesia. This stimulation-induced analgesia can be
blocked in animals pretreated with para-chlorophenylalanine, and can be enhanced in animals treated with
5-hydroxytryptophan (3,4). The finding that lesions
of the dorsolateral funiculus of the spinal cord, an
area through which descending serotoninergic nerves
project, prevent stimulation-induced analgesia (38),
and the fact that the microiontophoretic application
of serotonin in the spinal cord inhibits the electrophysiological responses of neurons to noxious stimuli
(53), also lend indirect support to the hypothesis
that a descending serotoninergic system mediates responses to pain.

   <u>Brain Serotonin and Morphine Analgesia</u>. The
results of most, but not all (9,11,31,54), pharmacological experiments suggest that brain serotonin
neurons may alter the analgesic potency of morphine
and other opiate narcotics. For example, morphine
analgesia is attenuated in rodents pretreated with
para-chlorophenylalanine, and can be restored to
normal levels in these animals if they are then
injected with 5-hydroxytryptophan (26,61,63). Furthermore, injections of a variety of drugs /5,6-dihydroxy-
tryptamine (25,65), para-chloroamphetamine (60,63),
or fenfluramine (14)/ that permanently destroy or
deplete brain and spinal serotonin, also attenuate the
analgesia associated with morphine. Similarly, drugs
thought to block serotonin receptors (methysergide,

cinanserin, or cyproheptadine) also antagonize the
analgesia induced by morphine (26,27). It should be
noted that many of the pharmacological treatments shown
to be effective in altering morphine analgesia have
little or no effects on the sensitivity or reactivity
to noxious stimuli when they are given alone; hence, it
is possible that certain sets of serotoninergic nerves
in the brain and spinal cord might mediate the normal
response to noxious stimuli, whereas different sets
of nerves containing this neurotransmitter might be
involved in mediating the effects of analgesic drugs.

It has also been found that some, but not all (7,9,
31), brain lesions that destroy serotoninergic nerves
are also effective in reducing morphine analgesia.
Initial experiments showed that midbrain raphe lesions
were effective in attenuating morphine analgesia (37,
50,55,56,58,59,70). Although subsequent experiments
found little if any change in morphine analgesia following other raphe nuclei lesions that also produced
large reductions in forebrain concentrations of
serotonin (7,9), more recent studies have shown that
the most critical brain serotonin region necessary for
normal opiate analgesia involves the nucleus raphe
medianus, a cell body area that sends ascending
serotonin fibers and terminals into forebrain limbic
structures such as the amygdala and hippocampus (1).
In addition to the possible involvement of ascending
brain serotoninergic nerves in morphine analgesia,some
evidence also suggests that descending, spinal cord
serotoninergic neurons may also be critical for these
effects. In one study, intraventricular injections of
the serotonin neurotoxic drug 5,6-dihydroxytryptamine
were found to reduce morphine analgesia in rats (65).
This reduction in drug potency was accompanied by
rather large decreases in the concentrations of spinal
cord, but not brain, serotonin. In another study, the
analgesic effects of morphine have been shown to depend
at least in part on the integrity of descending
serotoninergic nerves in the spinal cord dorsolateral
funiculus (38).

Hence, the available evidence suggests that both
ascending and descending brain and spinal cord
serotoninergic neurons, whose cell bodies are localized
in the raphe nuclei of the pons and medulla,are

important for normal responses to painful stimuli,
and may also mediate analgesia induced by morphine or
electrical stimulation.

DIET-INDUCED CHANGES IN BRAIN SEROTONIN : RESPONSE TO PAINFUL STIMULI

Low-Tryptophan Diets and Brain Serotonin. Earlier
work in other laboratories had shown that the brains
of rats or mice fed a tryptophan-deficient natural or
synthetic diet for long periods of time contained 40-
50% less serotonin than did the brains of well-nourish-
ed, control animals (8,13,23,24,62,72). Conversely,
animals fed diets supplemented with greater-than-
normal amounts of tryptophan typically had increased
concentrations of brain serotonin (27,66). Thus, these
previous studies demonstrated clearly that the amount
of tryptophan consumed by animals produced parallel
changes in the concentrations of brain serotonin.

In more recent experiments, Fernstrom and Wurtman
(17,19) have presented evidence describing some of the
possible mechanisms by which these diet-induced changes
in the brain neurotransmitter are accomplished. In
their studies, young rats were fed a tryptophan-
deficient, low-protein, corn-based diet, or a casein-
based control diet that contained sufficient amounts
of protein and tryptophan adequate for normal growth
and health. Plasma and brain concentrations of tryptophan, and brain concentrations of serotonin and
5-hydroxyindoleacetic acid were all reduced in animals
that had been eating the corn-based diet for at least
2 weeks. The corn diet-induced reductions in these
compounds are apparently related to the fact that the
diet contained inadequate amounts of tryptophan, rather
than due to the low protein nature of the diet: control
groups of animals fed a corn diet supplemented with
tryptophan, or groups of animals fed a low-protein
casein diet, have near-normal concentrations of plasma
and brain tryptophan, and brain 5-hydroxyindoles(17,47).
Other experiments also support the hypothesis that the
neurochemical changes seen in animals fed the corn
diet are related to the inadequate amounts of
tryptophan, and not protein, in the diet. For example,
animals fed the corn or the casein diet for 6 weeks

and then injected with various doses of tryptophan
have brain 5-hydroxyindole concentrations that are
elevated to approximately the same extent, regardless
of the type of food eaten prior to the injection (16).
The rates at which corn or casein-fed animals
synthesize 5-hydroxytryptophan from tryptophan loads
are also identical (33). Hence, it seems likely that
the decreased concentrations of serotonin in the brains
of animals fed the corn diet are due to the inadequate
concentrations of the precursor amino acid tryptophan
available for serotonin biosynthesis, and are not due
to diet-induced reductions in the abilities of these
animals to synthesize serotonin when they are given
adequate amounts of the substrate amino acid.

Diet-Induced Changes in the Response to Painful
Stimuli. If the relationship between brain serotonin
levels and changes in the response thresholds of
animals to painful stimuli seen in previous studies
utilizing pharmacological or surgical manipulations of
serotonin are real, and not merely chance correlations,
then it should be possible to demonstrate changes in
pain sensitivity or reactivity in animals receiving
nutritional manipulations of brain serotonin. To test
this hypothesis, we fed groups of animals the corn-
or casein-based diets and tested them for their
behavioral responses to presentations of electric
shocks at various time intervals after institution of
the diets (43). Electroshock response thresholds
were determined for each animal using the flinch-jump
response method of Evans (15). The shock intensity
necessary to elicit a jump response in animals fed the
casein control diet was fairly constant over the entire
14 weeks testing period; in contrast, animals fed the
tryptophan-poor corn diet showed jump response thresholds approximately half those of the control groups
after they had consumed the corn diet for at least 2
weeks. Thereafter, the hyperalgesic responses of these
animals were consistently lower as long as they
continued to eat the corn diet (Fig.2). The change in
electroshock sensitivity seen in the corn-fed animals
is correlated temporally with the effects of the diet
on brain serotonin concentrations, inasmuch as it
takes approximately 2 weeks before brain serotonin is
reduced significantly below control values in the corn-

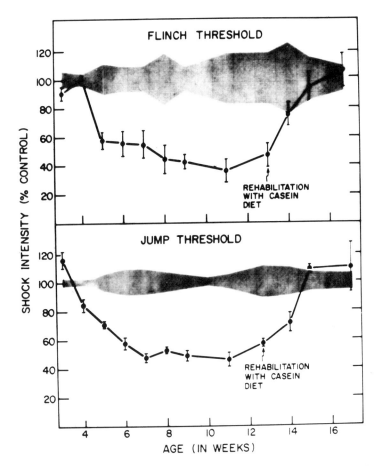

FIG. 2. Animals were placed on tryptophan-deficient corn diets (closed circles, solid lines) or on amino acid balanced casein control diets (shaded areas) beginning at week 3 after birth. After 10 weeks on the corn diet, rats were rehabilitated by feeding them the 18 percent casein diet (beginning at week 13 after birth). All values are the percentages (means ± S.E.) of the shock intensities in the controls for eliciting the flinch or the jump response. /Reprinted from Lytle, Messing, Fisher and Phebus (43),with permission/.

fed rats (Lytle,Pilistine and Phebus,in preparation).
    After some of the animals had consumed the casein- or corn-based diets for 10 weeks, we offered half of

the corn-fed rats the casein control diet that contained adequate concentrations of amino acids and protein.
The jump response thresholds of the animals rehabilitated with the casein diet returned to normal values
within 2 weeks (Fig.2). Again, the behavioral rehabilitation produced by this manipulation correlated
temporally with a return to normal of brain tryptophan
and serotonin concentrations.

Since the corn diet is deficient in both tryptophan
and protein, whereas the casein control diet contains
adequate amounts of both, it was not possible to tell
from the results of this initial experiment whether the
behavioral and neurochemical changes were due to differences in the tryptophan content of the diet, or
whether they were due to differences in their relative
protein concentrations. To examine these possibilities,
we switched rats previously fed the corn diet for 9
weeks to a similar diet that was supplemented with
amounts of tryptophan equivalent to those consumed by
animals eating the casein control diet (47). Just as
the casein rehabilitation had reversed the behavioral
and neurochemical changes induced by the corn diet in
the previous experiment, the jump response thresholds
and brain serotonin concentrations of the animals fed
the tryptophan-supplemented, corn-based diet also
returned to normal values within 4 weeks (Table 1).
These data indicate that the behavioral and biochemical
changes seen in corn-fed animals were most probably
related to the inadequate tryptophan, and not the
deficient protein, content of this particular diet.

The results of other experiments lend support to
the hypothesis that the behavioral and neurochemical
changes seen in animals eating the corn-based diet are
related to its depressing effects on brain serotonin
biosynthesis due to the diet-induced deficiencies in
amino acid substrate availability.   Animals fed the
corn-based diet for 6 weeks, and then injected with
various single replacement doses of tryptophan show
dose-related increases in jump response thresholds. In
contrast, animals fed the casein control diet and then
injected with the same doses of tryptophan showed no
changes in their behavioral responses to the electroshock (43) (Table 2).
The acute, amino acid-induced reversal of the hyper-

TABLE 1. Effects of different diets on brain 5-hydroxy-indoles and on the jump threshold to electro-shock

Diet	Jump Threshold (mA)	Brain 5-HT (µg/g)	Brain 5-HIAA (µg/g)
Casein	.88 ± .06	.44 ± .01	.50 ± .01
Corn	.41 ± .01*	.27 ± .01*	.21 ± .01*
Corn + Tryptophan	.73 ± .04^{ns}	.46 ± .01^{ns}	.48 ± .03^{ns}

Weanling albino rats were given access to a tryptophan-poor corn diet or to an 18% casein control diet beginning at 21 days of age. Nine weeks later, half of the corn-fed rats were given access to the corn diet supplemented with l-tryptophan (.16%, dry weight). Four weeks later, rats were tested for their responses to electric shock or were killed for biochemical assays.

All values are the means ± S.E. (six rats per group).

* P < .001 compared to casein-fed control groups;

^{ns}not statistically different from casein-fed control group. /From Messing et al. (47)7.

algesia seen in corn-fed rats appears to be related to the specific effects of tryptophan on brain serotonin, inasmuch as other amino acids (such as l-dopa or lysine) have no effects on brain serotonin or on the jump response thresholds of animals fed either of the 2 diets (43).

Diet-Induced Changes in the Potencies of Drugs that Alter the Response to Painful Stimuli. Since a number of drugs that produce analgesia or hyperalgesia appear to do so by altering serotoninergic neurotransmission, we next determined the extent to which the behavioral potency of these drugs might be altered in animals consuming the corn diet (47). As in some of the

TABLE 2. Effects of l-tryptophan injections on electroshock sensitivity in rats consuming the casein or corn diets

Tryptophan Dose	Shock Sensitivity (mA)	
	Casein Diet	Corn Diet
Vehicle	.85 ± .05	.43 ± .02°
62.5 mg/kg	.95 ± .04	.54 ± .06
125 mg/kg	.78 ± .06	.69 ± .02*
250 mg/kg	.88 ± .04	.63 ± .04*

Different groups of animals were fed a tryptophan-deficient corn diet or a casein control diet for 6 weeks, and then were injected with the vehicle or various doses of l-tryptophan. Jump responses to presentations of electric shock were determined 1 hr after the injection.
All values are the means ± S.E. (eight rats per group).

* P < .01 compared to vehicle injected group;

° P < .001 compared to vehicle injected, casein control group. /From Lytle et al.(43)7

previous experiments, different groups of animals were fed the corn or casein diets for 6 weeks, and then were injected with the tryptophan hydroxylase inhibitor para-chlorophenylalanine, the serotonin uptake blocking drug fluoxetine, or the opiate narcotic morphine; some of the animals were killed for biochemical assays, and others were tested for their responses to electric shock. The casein-fed animals treated with para-chlorophenylalanine had decreased concentrations of brain 5-hydroxyindoles, and were hyperalgesic to the electroshock presentations (Tables 3 and 4).
This drug also produced comparable reductions in the levels of brain 5-hydroxyindoles and increases in the pain sensitivities of the corn-fed animals, relative to their own vehicle-injected control baseline values. Injections of fluoxetine, on the other hand,

TABLE 3. Effects of various drugs on the jump
thresholds of rats fed casein or corn diets

Drug	Jump Threshold (mA)	
	Casein	Corn
Para-chlorophenylalanine		
Vehicle	.70 ± .05	.33 ± .05°°°
150 mg/kg	.34 ± .04***	.18 ± .06*
Fluoxetine		
Vehicle	.63 ± .03	.32 ± .02°°°
10 mg/kg	.82 ± .08*	.51 ± .02***
Morphine		
Vehicle	.64 ± .03	.32 ± .02°°°
5 mg/kg	.96 ± .06***	.37 ± .03^{ns}

Different groups of animals were fed a tryptophan-
deficient corn diet or a casein control diet for at
least 6 weeks prior to testing, and then were injected
with para-chlorophenylalanine or the pH 10 H_2O vehicle
intraperitoneally 48 hr before the test. Fluoxetine
or the H_2O vehicle was administered 1 hr before testing. Morphine sulfate or the H_2O vehicle was administered subcutaneously .5 hr prior to the test.

All values are the means ± S.E. (eight rats per group).

* $P < .05$;   *** $P < .01$; ^{ns} not statistically different
from appropriate vehicle injected control group.
°°° $P < .01$ compared to vehicle-injected, casein control
group.

significantly increased the jump response thresholds of
both the casein- and the corn-fed rats. This drug-
induced analgesia was correlated with small but
significant reductions in the concentrations of brain
5-hydroxyindoleacetic acid in the casein-fed group,
but not in the animals eating the corn diet.
In contrast to the consistent analgesic potency of
fluoxetine seen in either of the 2 diet groups, the

TABLE 4. Effects of various drugs on brain tryptophan and 5-hydroxyindole levels in rats fed casein or corn

Treatment		Brain Concentration (µg/g)		
		Tryptophan	5-HT	5-HIAA
pCPA				
Casein	Vehicle	3.82 ± .30	.44 ± .01	.40 ± .03
	150 mg/kg	2.26 ± .25**	.17 ± .02***	.08 ± .01***
Corn	Vehicle	1.79 ± .64°	.26 ± .03°°°	.15 ± .03°°°
	150 mg/kg	1.72 ± .25°	.07 ± .01***	.04 ± .01***
Fluoxetine				
Casein	Vehicle	3.82 ± .30	.44 ± .01	.40 ± .03
	10 mg/kg	4.25 ± .34	.43 ± .01	.32 ± .01*
Corn	Vehicle	1.79 ± .64°	.26 ± .03°°°	.15 ± .03°°°
	10 mg/kg	2.67 ± .51	.34 ± .04	.19 ± .04°°
Morphine				
Casein	Vehicle	5.03 ± .45	.31 ± .01	.38 ± .01
	5 mg/kg	5.32 ± .34	.30 ± .01	.41 ± .01
Corn	Vehicle	3.33 ± .31°°	.25 ± .01°°	.29 ± .02°°
	5 mg/kg	3.48 ± .32°	.25 ± .01°°	.30 ± .02°

Different groups of animals were fed a tryptophan-deficient corn diet or a casein control diet for at least 6 weeks prior to testing and then were injected with p-chloro-phenylalanine, fluoxetine, morphine or their vehicles. Animals were killed at the times described in Table 3. All values are the means ± S.E.(six rats per group). *p < .05; ** p < .01; ***p < .001 compared with appropriate vehicle-injected control group. °p < .05; °°p < .01; °°°p < .001 compared with vehicle-injected, casein control group.

analgesic effects of morphine, seen in animals fed
the casein diet, were completely absent in the corn-
fed rats. The morphine injections produced no observable changes in the concentrations of brain tryptophan
or 5-hydroxyindoles, a finding generally consistent
with the results of other laboratories using comparable
doses of the drug (28,51). However, it should be noted
that larger doses of morphine have been shown to
increase the rate of serotonin biosynthesis, by an as-
yet-to-be-identified mechanism (51). Preliminary
evidence (Phebus, Fisher and Lytle , in preparation)
indicates that the reduced behavioral potency of
morphine seen in the corn-fed animals may not be
characteristic of the effects of the diet on other
narcotic analgesics, inasmuch as the analgesic potencies of meperidine and codeine appear to be potentiated
in corn-fed rats.

CONCLUSIONS

A growing body of evidence now indicates that brain
and spinal cord nerves that use serotonin as their
neurotransmitter are most probably involved in mediat-
mediating normal and drug-induced responses to nociceptive stimuli; however, it would be presumptuous to
assume at this stage that these sets of neurons are
the only ones, or even that they are the most important
cells for maintaining the integrity of responses necessary to protect the organism from injury and harm.
Certainly other brain and peripheral neurotransmitters
are also involved in the sensitivity or reactivity to
painful stimuli; however, their precise roles remain to
be worked out in detail.

The data show clearly that the type or the amount of
food eaten by animals can have important effects on
brain function, behavior, and drug potency; yet it is
still too early to assess with any precision how
comparable changes in dietary quality or quantity might
alter human brain function and behavior. Thus far, we
have only been able to study one experimental dietary
model in any detail; it would be of interest to know,
for example, whether some of the more acute, diet-
related alterations in brain neurotransmitters might
also produce predictable changes in normal or drug-

induced behaviors. Moreover, we are not at all certain
whether all of the observed dietary effects on behavior
and drug potency are due solely to changes in brain
serotoninergic neurotransmisssion. For example, it is
well known that animals chronically malnourished have
an impaired ability to metabolize a rather wide variety
of drugs (10). Although it is possible that the
altered potency of some of the hyperalgesic or
analgesic drugs seen in animals consuming the corn-
based diets in our studies might be related in part to
changes in the relative abilities of these animals to
metabolize drugs, it is not intuitively obvious that
this hypothesis can easily account for all of the data.
However, this possibility is presently under investigation in our laboratory. Certainly it is safe to assume
at this point that the old adage, "you are what you
eat", may have some empirical credence after all.

ACKNOWLEDGMENTS

Some of the studies reported in this paper were supported by grants from the W.T. Grant Foundation and the
Eli Lilly Co., and by grants MH-25075 and AM-14228
from the National Institutes of Health. L.D.L. holds
an Alfred P. Sloan Foundation Fellowship in neurosciences and L.A.F. holds a National Science Foundation
Fellowship. The authors are grateful to Mrs. Louise
Kittredge for her assistance in the preparation of the
manuscript.

REFERENCES

1. Adler, M., Kostowski, W., Recchia, M., and Samanin,
     R. (1975): Eur.J.Pharmacol., 32: 39-44.
2. Aghajanian, G.K., Rosecrans, J.A., and Sheard, M.H.
     (1966): Science, 156: 402-403.
3. Akil, H., and Liebeskind, J.C. (1975): Brain Res.,
     94: 279-296.
4. Akil, H., and Mayer, D.J. (1972): Brain Res., 44:
     692-697.
5. Axelrod, J. (1974): Science, 184: 1341-1348.
6. Bjorklund, A., Falck, B., and Owman, C. (1972): In:
     The Thyroid and Biogenic Amines, edited by J.E.
     Rall, and I.J.Kopin, pp.318-368, North Holland,

Amsterdam.

7. Blasig, J., Reinhold, K., and Herz, A. (1973): Psychopharmacologia, 31: 111-119.
8. Boullin, D.J. (1963): Psychopharmacologia, 5: 8-38.
9. Buxbaum, D.M., Yarbrough, G.G., and Carter, M.E. (1973): J.Pharmacol.Exp.Ther., 185: 317-327.
10. Campbell, T.C., and Hayes, J.R. (1974): Pharmacol. Rev., 26: 171-197.
11. Cheney, D.L., and Goldstein, A. (1971): J.Pharmacol. Exp.Ther., 177: 309-315.
12. Costa, E., and Meek, J.L. (1974): Annu.Rev. Pharmacol., 14: 491-511.
13. Culley, W.J., Saunders, R.N., Mertz, E.T., and Jolly, D.H. (1963): Proc.Soc.Exp.Biol.Med., 113: 645-648.
14. Duncan, C., and Spencer, P.S.J. (1973): J.Pharm. Pharmacol., 25: 124P-125P.
15. Evans, W.O. (1961): Psychopharmacologia, 2: 318-325.
16. Fernstrom, J.D., and Hirsch, M.J. (1975): Life Sci., 17: 455-464.
17. Fernstrom, J.D., and Wurtman, R.J. (1971): Nature New Biol., 234: 62-64.
18. Fernstrom, J.D., and Wurtman, R.J.(1971): Science, 173: 149-152.
19. Fernstrom, J.D., and Wurtman, R.J. (1974): In: Advances in Psychopharmacology: Serotonin New Vistas, edited by E.Costa, G.L. Gessa, and M. Sandler, pp.133-142. Raven Press, New York.
20. Fernstrom, J.D., and Wurtman, R.J.(1974): Scientific Amer., 230: 84-91.
21. Fibiger, H.C., Mertz, P.H., and Campbell, B.A. (1972): Physiol.Behav., 8: 259-263.
22. Gal, E.M. (1974): In:Aromatic Amino Acids in Brain, Ciba Fnd., pp.343-359, Elsevier, Amsterdam.
23. Gal, E.M., and Dewes , P.A. (1962): Proc.Soc.Exp. Biol.Med., 110: 368-371.
24. Gal, E.M., Dewes, P.A., and Barraclough, C.A. (1962): Biochem.Pharmacol., 8: 32-37.
25. Genovese, E., Zonta, N.Z., and Mantegazza, P.(1973): Psychopharmacologia, 32: 359-364.
26. Gorlitz, B.-D., and Frey, H.H. (1972): Eur.J. Pharmacol., 20: 171-180.

27. Green, H., Greenberg, S.M., Erickson, R.W., Sawyer, J.L., and Ellison, T. (1962): J.Pharmacol.Exp.Ther. 136: 174-178.

28. Harris, L.S. (1970): Fed.Proc., 29: 28-31.

29. Harvey, J.A., and Lints, C.E. (1965): Science, 148: 250-252.

30. Harvey, J.A., and Lints, C.E. (1971): J.Comp. Physiol.Psychol., 74: 28-36.

31. Harvey, J.A., Schlosberg, A.J., and Yunger, L.M. (1975):Fed.Proc., 34: 1796- 1801.

32. Harvey, J.A., and Yunger, L.M. (1973): In: Serotonin and Behavior, edited by J.Barchas, and E.Usdin, pp.179-190. Academic Press, New York.

33. Hirsch, M.J., and Fernstrom, J.D.(1976): Fed.Proc., 35: 241.

34. Hole, K., and Lorens, S.A. (1975): Pharmacol. Biochem.Behav., 3: 95-102.

35. Hole, K., and Marsden, C.A. (1975): Pharmacol. Biochem.Behav., 3: 307-309.

36. Koe, K.B., and Weissman,A. (1966): J.Pharmacol.Exp. Ther., 154: 499-516.

37. Kostowski, W., Giacalone, E., Garattini, S., and Valzelli, L. (1968): Eur.J.Pharmacol., 4: 371-378.

38. Liebeskind, J.C., Giesler, G.J., and Urca, G. (1976) In: Sensory Function of the Skin in Primates,with Special Reference to Man, edited by Y.Zotterman, Pergamon Press, Oxford, in press.

39. Liebeskind, J.C., Mayer, D.J., and Akil, H. (1974): Adv.Neurol., 4: 261-268.

40. Lints, C.E., and Harvey, J.A. (1969):J.Comp.Physiol. Psychol., 67: 23-31.

41. Lorens, S.A., Sorensen, J.P., and Harvey, J.A. (1970): J.Comp.Physiol.Psychol., 75: 284-290.

42. Lovenberg, W., Jequier, E., and Sjoerdsma, A.(1968): Adv.Pharmacol., 6A: 21-36.

43. Lytle, L.D., Messing, R.B., Fisher , L., and Phebus, L. (1975): Science, 190: 692-694.

44. Lytle, L.D., and Wurtman, R.J. (1976): In: Dahlem Workshop on Hormone and Antihormone Action, edited by J. Clark, J.Wolff, A.Levitski, and W.Klee, Dahlem Konferenzen, Berlin,in press

45. Mandell, A.J., and Knapp, S.(1975): In: Chemical Tools in Catecholamine Research II, edited by

O.Almgren, A.Carlsson, and J.Engel, pp.9-16,
North Holland, Amsterdam.

46. Mayer, D.J., and Liebeskind, J.C. (1974): Brain Res.
    68: 73-93.

47. Messing, R.B., Fisher, L.A., Phebus, L., and Lytle,
    L.D. (1976): Life Sci., 18: 707-714.

48. Messing, R.B., Phebus, L., Fisher, L.A., and Lytle,
    L.D. (1975): Psychopharmacol.Commun., 1: 511-521.

49. Oliveras, J., Besson, J.M., Builbaud, G.W,and
    Liebeskind, J.C. (1974): Exp.Brain Res., 20: 32-44.

50. Pepeu, G., Garau, L., and Mulas, M.L. (1974): In:
    Advances in Psychopharmacology: Serotonin New
    Vistas, edited by E.Costa, G.L.Gessa, and M.Sandler
    pp.247-252. Raven Press, New York.

51. Perez-Cruet, J., Thoa, N.B., and Ng, L.K.Y. (1975):
    Life Sci., 17: 349-362.

52. Proudfit, H.K., and Anderson, E.G. (1975): Brain
    Res., 98: 612-618.

53. Randic, M., and Yu, H. (1975): Neurosci.Abstr., 1:
    151.

54. Reinhold, K., Blasig, J., and Herz, A. (1973):
    Arch.Pharmacol., 278: 69-76.

55. Samanin, R., Bendotti, C., Ghezzi, D., and Mauron,
    C. (1974):Proc.IX Congress Int.Neuropharmacol.
    Paris, in press

56. Samanin, R., and Bernasconi, S. (1972):
    Psychopharmacologia, 33: 365-373.

57. Samanin, R., Bernasconi, S., and Quattrone, A.
    (1976):Psychopharmacologia, 46: 219-222.

58. Samanin, R., Ghezzi, D., Mauron, C., and Valzelli,
    L. (1973):Psychopharmacologia, 33: 365-368.

59. Samanin, R., Gumulka, W., and Valzelli, L. (1973):
    Eur.J.Pharmacol., 10: 339-348.

60. Takemori, A.E., Tulunay, F.C., and Yano, I. (1975):
    Life Sci., 17: 21-28.

61. Tenen, S.S. (1968): Psychopharmacologia, 12: 278-
    285.

62. Thomas, R.G., and Wysor, W.G. (1967): Proc.Soc.Exp.
    Biol.Med., 126: 374-380.

63. Tulunay, F.C., Yano, I., and Takemori, A.E. (1976):
    Eur.J.Pharmacol., 35: 285-292.

64. Ungerstedt, U. (1971): Acta Physiol.Scand., 367:
    1-48.

65. Vogt, M. (1974): J.Physiol.(Lond.), 236:483-498.
66. Wang, A.L., Harwalkar, V.H., and Waisman, H.A. (1962): Arch.Biochem.Biophys., 96: 181-184.
67. Wurtman, R.J. (1974): In: Frontiers in Neurology and Neuroscience Research, edited by P.Seeman, and G.M. Brown, pp.16-25. University of Toronto Press, Toronto.
68. Wurtman, R.J., and Fernstrom, J.D. (1974): In: The Neurosciences: Third Study Program, edited by F.O.Schmitt, and F.G. Worden, pp.685-693. M.I.T. Press, Cambridge.
69. Yaksh, T.L., DuChateau, J.C., and Rudy, T.A.(1976): Brain Res., 104: 367-372.
70. York, J.L., and Maynert, E.W. (1973): Pharmacologist 15: 242.
71. Yunger, L.M., and Harvey, J.A. (1976): J.Pharmacol. Exp.Ther., 196: 307-315.
72. Zbinden, G., Pletscher, A., and Studer, A. (1958): Z.Ges.Exp.Med., 129: 615-620.

Factors Affecting the Action of Narcotics, edited by
M.L. Adler, L. Manara, and R. Samanin.
Raven Press, New York © 1978.

Parallels Between the Neuromodulator Mechanisms of
Stimulation Analgesia and Morphine Analgesia

A. Akil, S.J. Watson, R.B. Holman and J.D. Barchas

Department of Psychiatry and Behavioral Sciences
Stanford University School of Medicine
Stanford, California 94305
U.S.A.

STIMULATION ANALGESIA AND ITS RELATION TO MORPHINE

In the last few years, the phenomenon of stimulation-produced analgesia (SPA) has been widely explored employing behavioral, electrophysiological, pharmacological, and clinical tools. Aside from its intrinsic value in understanding CNS modulation of noxious input, and its clinical effectiveness in relieving chronic intractable human pain, SPA has shed light on the possible mechanisms of narcotic action. This paper will focus on the role of various neuromodulators in the production and maintenance of SPA, and will stress the parallels to and differences from the neurotransmitter modulation of opiate analgesia.

There are several salient features of analgesia produced by electrical stimulation of the brain. The pain inhibition thus obtained is as potent as a large dose of morphine; it is highly selective, leaving other sensory-motor modalities largely unaltered (31, 35). Its analgesic effects outlast the duration of stimulation by seconds to hours, and its effectiveness has been established in several species (30,34) including man (45, 46, 47). Early in the study of SPA, we were struck with some of the similarities between SPA and narcotic analgesia (5). This has led to specific comparisons of the two types of pain inhibition, resulting in our suggestion of an endogenous pain inhibitory system which can be activated by either electrical stimulation or morphine (6, 35). Before focusing on the role of specific neurotransmitters in this pain inhibitory system, it may be worthwhile point out both the similarities and differences between the two methods of pain control.

Both SPA and morphine analgesia can be obtained

565

from a mesial system surrounding the rostral aspect of the fourth ventricle, the aqueduct and the third ventricle (22, 28, 40, 44, 51, 53, 54, 58).Both types of analgesia can modulate spinally mediated withdrawal reflexes such as the tail flick of the rodents, which are difficult to block by other means. Both morphine and SPA are particularly effective for visceral pain in man and animals (19, 46, 47). More importantly,SPA exhibits two of the most characteristic phenomena associated with narcotics: tolerance and reversal by narcotic antagonists. However, unlike the case with narcotics, both the naloxone-antagonism and the tolerance are partial and highly variable between animals. Mayer and Hayes (33) have reported that tolerance develops upon repeated stimulation, with recovery occurring after several weeks. Further, they demonstrated cross-tolerance between SPA and morphine.Akil et al. (5,6), demonstrated blockade of SPA in the rat by naloxone. Furthermore, we have also reversed SPA in man with small doses of naloxone (8), and have demonstrated some electrophysiological correlates of naloxone blockade in the cat (7). However, the nature and magnitude of the naloxone effect differs from that seen with narcotics. While some animals and human patients exhibit rapid and reliable blockade, others respond to naloxone with little change. The possible reasons for this variability will be discussed below. However, SPA remains one of the few non-narcotic phenomena to be altered by 'pure' antagonists.

Based on the above findings, we suggested that pain blockade by SPA occurs via an active mechanism,rather than the mere interruption of pain input. Recent advances in the field of narcotic research have uncovered the existence of endogenous morphine-like peptides, the enkephalins (25,26,27). We have, therefore, hypothesized that these endogenous peptides may function as modulators in the pain inhibitory system, and that SPA results from their activation or release (2,6). If this were the case, the study of the role of neurotransmitters in SPA and in narcotics would be very instrumental in understanding the nature and connectivity of the enkephalin system.

WHY SIMILARITIES AND DIFFERENCES?

It must be stated here that this is a case of circumstantial evidence. Ideally, we should establish that SPA results from the selective activation of the enkephalin-containing neurons, and that morphine analgesia results from the activation of the enkephalin receptors (also known as opiate receptor).Subsequently,

we could employ morphine and SPA for manipulating the
endogenous systems and studying its interactions with
other neurotransmitters. In fact, we have achieved
the first important step in that direction. We have
recently established that SPA is accompained by a
significant rise in the level of brain opiate-like
peptides (9). However , we have yet to correlate this
rise more directly with the production of analgesia.

Still, reviewing the evidence on SPA and neuromodulators may allow us to make guesses about the organization of pain inhibitory systems in the brain. The
similarities to morphine should be revealing. However,
even if SPA and morphine do, in fact, activate the
same system, we would expect differences in their
neurochemical and pharmacological interactions.

It must be recalled that most of the studies on
morphine and monoamines were carried out using systemic morphine injections. These would presumably
recruit opiate sensitive systems, both analgetic and
non-analgetic. The neurochemical interactions with
other systems are, therefore, likely to be very
complex, and their manifestations highly dependent on
the test systems chosen. On the other hand, SPA is
elicited from a well-localized brain region. Any
pharmacological or neurochemical manipulations would
have to affect the particular system being activated
if they are to alter SPA. It would, therefore, be
more appropriate to compare the role of neuromodulators
on SPA and on morphine microinjected at the same brain
site, and employing the same pain tests. Few such
studies currently exist.

Even under the circumstances outlined above, we
would still expect to see discrepancies in the transmitter modulation of SPA and narcotics.   While
narcotics are thought to activate opiate receptors
directly, SPA is thought to do so only indirectly, by
releasing endogenous opiate factors. Furthermore, in
some sites and at certain stimulation parameters, we
might expect to bypass the opiate receptor and directly
activate the postreceptor responses. This may partially explain the variability in the tolerance and
naloxone effect, and the incomplete nature of these
phenomena. It may also lead us to expect some significant differences in the effects of various neurotransmitters on SPA and narcotic analgesia.

INTERACTIONS OF SPA WITH SPECIFIC NEUROMODULATORS

The work on the role of neurotransmitters in
morphine analgesia is too extensive to review here.
We will, therefore, confine ourselves to reviewing the

SPA-related data, while broadly outlining the thrust
of the narcotic literature.

Obviously, the main common modulator shared by
morphine and SPA are the enkephalins. As mentioned
above, SPA raises the level of these peptides (9)
while narcotics would activate the receptor.But little
remains known about the nature of the enkephalin
system, and whether it actually qualifies as a 'neurotransmitter'. The other neurotransmitter systems
which have been examined in relation to SPA have been
the monoamines, to be reviewed below.

SPA AND SEROTONIN

There is a good deal of consistency in the literature relating to the role of 5-HT in both SPA and
morphine analgesia. Further, there is good evidence
that serotonergic mechanisms are involved in pain
responsiveness under nonanalgetic conditions. Several
investigators, employing the flinch-jump method, have
demonstrated that depletion of 5-HT either by pCPA or
by lesioning leads to hyperresponsivity to painful
input (21, 52). Furthermore, long-term consumption of
tryptophan-poor diet leads to a reduction in brain
levels of 5-HT and to hyperalgesia, while pretreatment
with a serotonin uptake inhibitor yields analgesia(36).
It is, therefore, crucial to attempt to differentiate
the effects of 5-HT modifiers on baseline from their
effects on the analgesic potency of SPA or narcotics.

Ascending 5-HT Systems

Since SPA is primarily obtained in the vicinity of
dorsal raphe, one of our earliest studies was to administer pCPA in doses that had little effect on baseline
responsiveness, and study changes in SPA (3,4). Whenever the electrode site was in the immediate vicinity
of dorsal raphe, SPA was blocked by pCPA treatment.
However, analgesia could be obtained in sites distant
from raphe, and was then impervious to pCPA treatment.
The pCPA effect was reversible by 5-HTP pretreatment,
and 5-HTP alone produces a potentiation of SPA (3).
Similarly, in the cat, Guilbaud, Besson, Oliveras, and
Liebeskind (20) have found that analgetic stimulation
inhibits spinal cord interneurons; in their hands,LSD,
an agent known to inhibit firing of 5-HT neurons (1)
blocked the SPA effects when it derived from raphe
sites, but not when it derived from stimulation elsewhere in midbrain. Yunger, Harvey, and Lorens (61),
found that pCPA does not alter hot-plate analgesia
from lateral hypothalamic sites. This may be due to
the possibility that such analgesia bypasses the 5-HT

link.   Further, hypothalamic analgesia differs in
several ways from periaqueductal gray analgesia (c.f.
discussion in Akil and Liebeskind (3).

Neurochemically, SPA obtained from ventral central
gray leads to profound changes in levels and utilization of brain serotonin (Akil, Holman and Barchas,
unpublished data). Animals were subjected to 30 min
of analgesia-inducing electrical stimulation in the
central grey and sacrificed immediately. The region
of the electrode (near dorsal raphe), the terminal
areas (hypothalamus, caudate, septal area), and the
area caudal to the electrode (medulla-pons) were assayed for 5-HT and 5-HIAA levels, using the procedure
of Holman, Angwin, and Barchas (24).
Table I shows the significant rise in 5-HIAA in all
regions, and the decline in 5-HT in the dorsal raphe
region-suggesting an increased utilization of serotonin
with SPA.

TABLE   I

Effect of SPA on Levels of 5HT and 5HIAA ($\mu g/g$) in Various
Brain Regions

AREA	CONTROL		SPA		SPA/CONTROL	
MEDULLA-PONS	5HT :	0.42+0.05	5HT:	0.41+0.02	99%	NS
	5HIAA :	0.41+0.05	5HIAA:	0.53+0.03	130%	p<0.05
MIDBRAIN	5HT :	0.61+0.04	5HT:	0.44+0.04	72%	p<0.01
	5HIAA :	0.45+0.05	5HIAA:	0.68+0.07	152%	p<0.025
HYPOTH.-CAUDATE	5HT :	0.48+0.02	5HT:	0.44+0.05	92%	NS
SEPTUM	5HIAA :	0.56+0.01	5HIAA:	0.92+0.16	163%	p<0.05

Descending   5-HT-Systems

There is ample evidence that excellent analgesia can
be obtained by stimulation of the bulbar raphe system
(38, 39, 43).   This is of particular interest since
Basbaum, Marley, and O'Keefe (10) have reported that
discrete lesions of dorsolateral funiculus of the
spinal cord block stimulation-produced analgesia.This
pathway is thought to contain the 5-HT axons deriving
from the bulbar raphe system (16).   It, therefore,
appears that both ascending and descending serotonergic
systems may be critical links in SPA, especially when
analgesia results from stimulation near the raphe
system.

Parallels to Morphine

The study that comes the closest to the ideal direct comparison between SPA and morphine was carried out by Yaksh and co-workers (60). These investigators employed morphine microinjections in the periaqueductal grey (sites identical to SPA loci) and demonstrated their reversal by the 5-HT blockers, methylsergide and cinanserin. However, the study did not examine the effect of these drugs in morphine-sensitive sites outside the periaqueductal grey. It is interesting that Yaksh, Duchateau, and Rudy (60) report that local injection of methylsergide does not result in similar blockade of morphine analgesia. These authors also speculate as to the importance of both ascending and descending 5-HT systems in analgesia.

Numerous studies have implicated 5-HT in general and the dorsal raphe in particular in narcotic analgesia. Lesions of midbrain raphe reduce morphine analgesia (49) while electrical stimulation of the dorsal raphe enhances morphine analgesia (50). Inhibition of 5-HT synthesis by pCPA (52) or destruction of 5-HT neurons by 5,6-dihydroxytryptamine (18), also lead to blockade of the antinociceptive effect of morphine.

The descending 5-HT system has been extensively studied by Anderson and his co-workers and implicated in morphine and stimulation analgesia. Proudfit and Anderson (41, 42) have shown that lesions of the bulbospinal serotonergic pathway blocks morphine analgesia. Repkin et al. (43) report that morphine administration augments the presumed presynaptic inhibition of sensory input in primary afferents, and that this effect can be blocked by cinanserin. Finally, Vogt (57) has demonstrated that 5,6-dihydroxytryptamine injection causes severe loss in spinal 5-HT, while brain 5-HT remains relatively unchanged. She also demonstrated a blockade of morphine analgesia by DMT, thus implicating the spinal 5-HT system in narcotic analgesia.

In sum, both SPA and morphine analgesia appear dependent on scrotonin integrity, and both ascending and descending 5-HT systems appear to facilitate these analgesias. The relative importance of the two systems may be, in part, dependent on the pain response under study. For example, a spinally mediated pain response may exhibit more dependence on the descending 5-HT system than a supraspinal response. It is conceivable that the bulbar 5-HT system modulates the sensory aspects of pain input at the first synapse, while the ascending 5-HT system might mediate the polysynaptic and possibly emotional response to pain in limbic structures. The direct interactions between

these two systems, and their connections to enkephalins
and opiate receptors remain to be determined.

CATECHOLAMINES AND SPA

Anatomical Evidence

As mentioned earlier, both SPA and morphine analgesia
share a common anatomical substrate , a mesial system
from fourth to third ventricle, via the aqueduct. These
regions coincide in part with the dorsal periventricular bundle (DBP), the catecholaminergic system recently
described by Lindvall and Björklund (32). Therefore,
we have directly investigated the possible role of this
pathway in SPA (58). Each animal was implanted with
two stimulating electrodes , one aimed at the DBP, the
other laterally. After testing for analgesia, the
animals were sacrificed and the relation of electrode
tip of CA structures established, employing the glyoxy-
lic acid histochemical technique of Watson and Barchas
(59). When the midbrain-thalamic extent of the bundle
was thus   mapped, a strong positive correlation
emerged between proximity to this catecholamine bundle
and analgetic potency.   Sites which were clearly
distant from the dorsal periventricular bundle rarely
produced any signs of pain inhibition. It should be
noted that both catecholamines, dopamine and noradrenaline, are intertwined within this system, and the
DA cell bodies are widely distributed and begin in
central grey at the level of dorsal raphe (c.f. Fig. 1).

Pharmacological Evidence

A series of pharmacological manipulations employing
synthesis inhibitors, potentiation with precursors,
receptor blockers and stimulants   were carried out to
examine the role of catecholamines in SPA (3).   Typically, depletion of both catecholamines (TBZ, AMPT)
leads to blockade of SPA as obtained from central grey.
Further examination of the dopaminergic system employing a receptor blocker (haloperidol), a receptor
stimulant (apomorphine), and the precursor(L-DOPA),
confirmed the notion that DA activation facilitates
SPA, and its blockade interferes with SPA. On the
other hand, selective depletion of noradrenaline using
disulfiram led to a potentiation of SPA. Further, a
combination of AMPT and L-DOPA leads, at a particular
time, to a rise in DA levels while NA levels remain
depressed. This is correlated with a significant
enhancement in SPA. We therefore concluded that the
dopaminergic system facilitates SPA elicited from central grey, while the noradrenergic system inhibits it.

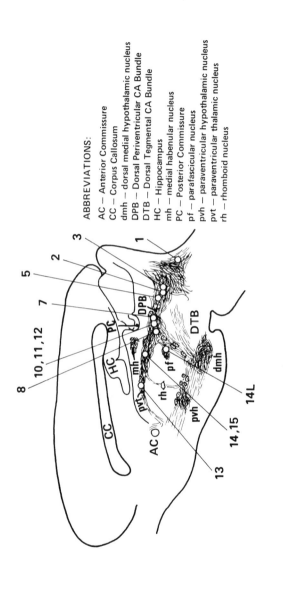

ABBREVIATIONS:

AC — Anterior Commissure
CC — Corpus Callosum
dmh — dorsal medial hypothalamic nucleus
DPB — Dorsal Periventricular CA Bundle
DTB — Dorsal Tegmental CA Bundle
HC — Hippocampus
mh — medial habenular nucleus
PC — Posterior Commissure
pf — parafascicular nucleus
pvh — paraventricular hypothalamic nucleus
pvt — paraventricular thalamic nucleus
rh — rhomboid nucleus

FIG. 1   Schematic diagram of the dorsal periventricular bundle with
analgesia producing electrode sites.

There is little known about the potential differential roles of ascending and descending noradrenergic systems.

Neurochemical Evidence

Preliminary data from our laboratory indicates that SPA is accompanied by significant changes in catecholamine levels. Rats were tested for SPA, and once the ideal parameters were selected, they were stimulated for 30 minutes immediately prior to sacrifice. The brains were dissected into the area surrounding the electrode, the CA terminal regions (caudate, hypothalamus, septum), and the CA cell regions (medulla-pons). Table 2 indicates that levels of NE were significantly decreased in the region of the electrode and in regions caudal to the electrode site. Similar effects were seen in the DA system. While the turnover or utilization rates of catecholamines remain to be determined, it is clear that these neurotransmitters are dramatically altered during SPA. Their specific relations to the production of analgesia, its maintenance, and the development of tolerance remain to be worked out.

TABLE   II

Effect of SPA on Levels of NA (μg/g) in Various Brain Regions

	CONTROLS	SPA	SPA / CONTROL	
MEDULLA-PONS	0.64+0.06	0.45+0.03	70%	p <0.025
MIDBRAIN-THALAMUS	0.61+0.03	0.45+0.05	77%	p < 0.05
HYPOTH.-CAUDATE SEPTUM	1.18+0.04	1.05+0.06	82%	NS

Parallels of Morphine

The literature on morphine and catecholamines abounds in contradictions and evidence abounds both for and against the pattern of evidence suggested for SPA. The interactions between morphine and dopamine are particularly confusing. While some authors have shown facilitation of morphine analgesia by dopamine (14,17, 37, 48), others have demonstrated the opposite effect (15,55,56).

On the other hand, the noradrenergic role in morphine analgesia is somewhat less controversial, though far from clear-cut. Several investigators have failed to find an effect of noradrenergic-altering agents on morphine analgesia (c.f. 55). However, there is also some evidence that noradrenaline does antagonize morphine analgesia— as it does SPA. Korf, Bunney, and

T A B L E   III

Parallels Between SPA and Morphine Analgesia

5HT MECHANISMS	1. Facilitation by ascending 5HT system: SPA (4,20); morphine analgesia (49, 60).
	2. Facilitation by descending 5HT: SPA (10,38,39,43) ; morphine (43, 57).
CA MECHANISMS	1. Involvement of dorsal periventricular bundle in SPA (58). Involvement of a similar anatomical system in morphine.
	2. DA facilitates SPA (3) DA facilitates morphine analgesia for some (14, 17, 37, 48) and inhibits it in the hands of others (55).
	3. NE inhibits SPA (3) and morphine analgesia (11). Morphine blocks locus coereleus cells (29) and its analgetic effects are enhanced by β-adrenergic agents (13).
PHENOMENOLOGICAL	1. Pain inhibition spinal withdrawal reflexes.
	2. Inhibition of visceral pain responses (31, 46).
	3. Tolerance and cross-tolerance between SPA and morphine (33).
	4. Reversal by naloxone (5,6,7).
ANATOMICAL	1. SPA and morphine in periaqueductal periventricular regions (40,44,46,58).
PRESUMED MECHANISM OF ACTION	1. SPA increases enkephalin levels (9) morphine presumably activates the enkephalin receptors.

Aghajanian (29) have reported that low doses of morphine cause complete and selective inhibition of locus coereleus cell firing, an effect reversible by naloxone. Cicero, Meyer, and Smithloff (13) have described the antinociceptive activity of α-adrenergic blocking agents and their ability to enhance morphine-induced analgesia. Finally, Calcutt, Doggett, and Spencer (11) and Calcutt, Handley, Sparkes and Spencer (12) have applied noradrenaline directly via intraventricular cannulas and blocked the anti-nociceptive effects of morphine.

The above is good suggestive evidence for an inverse relation between noradrenergic activity and narcotic analgesia. While this is congruent with our SPA data, direct comparisons employing morphine microinjections in specific midbrain sites remain lacking.

CONCLUSION

It is apparent from the above evidence that both SPA and narcotic analgesia are active phenomena resulting from the complex interplay of several neurotransmitter systems. Probably, pain responsiveness at any given moment is determined by the integration of facilitory and inhibitory mechanisms, centripetal and centrifugal. However, the inhibitory mechanisms can be modified separately, as demonstrated by the various pharmacological manipulations which do not alter baseline pain responsiveness but produce dramatic changes in the potencies of SPA and morphine analgesia. This is congruent with the notion that analgesia has its own anatomical, electrophysiological and neurochemical substrates, possibly a system(s) which has evolved to modulate the basic sensory interactions involved in transmission of noxious input. It is tempting to speculate that substance P is primarily involved in pain transmission (c.f. 23), while the enkephalins play a critical role in pain inhibition. It is obvious from the above review that the monoamines are intimately involved in the pain inhibitory system, with 5-HT facilitating it, and NE probably inhibiting it (c.f. Table III for summary). However, it is also likely that cholinergic, gabergic, substance P, and other neuromodulator systems interact with these peptides. The task ahead is to determine the specific relations between the enkephalins and other neurotransmitters in the modulation of pain. We need to establish which modulators are essential to analgesia and which are only its secondary repercussions. This must await the detailed anatomical study of the endogenous opiate-like factors, and the elucidation of their physiological role as possible neurotransmitters or neuromodulators.

ACKNOWLEDGEMENTS

This research was supported by NIMH Program Grant, MH 23861 and PHS Grant 5, ROI DA O12O7. H. Akil is currently supported by National Institutes of Health Fellowship, NS O2336, and Alfred P. Sloan Research Fellowship in Neurophysiology, BR-1609. JDB holds Research Scientist Development Award, MH 24161.

REFERENCES

1.Aghajanian, G.K., Haigler, H.J., and Bloom, F.E. (1972) : Life Sci., 11 (Part I) 615-622.
2.Akil, H. (1977): In: Neuroregulators and Psychiatric Disorders, edited by E. Usdin, D.A. Hamburg, and J. D. Barchas, Oxford Press, Oxford.
3.Akil, H., and Liebeskind, J.C. (1975) : Brain Res. 94 : 279-296.
4.Akil, H.,and Mayer,D.J. (1972) : Brain Res. 44 : 692.
5.Akil, H., Mayer, D.J., and Liebeskind, J.D. (1972): C.R. Acad. Sci. (Paris) 274:3603.
6.Akil, H. Mayer, D.J. and Liebeskind,J.D. (1976) : Science , 191 : 961.
7.Akil, H. and Richardson, D.E. (1974) : Society for Neurosciences.
8.Akil, H. and Richardson, D.E. : In preparation.
9.Akil, H., Watson, S.J., and Barchas, J.D. (1976) : Society for Neurosciences.
10.Basbaum, A.I., Marley, N., and O'Keefe, J. (1975): In : First World Congress on Pain. 268.
11.Calcutt, C.R., Doggett, N.S., and Spencer, P.S.J. (1971) : Psychopharmacologia,21 : 111-117.
12.Calcutt, C.R., Handley, S.L., Sparkes, C.G., and Spencer, P.S.J. (1973) : In : Agonist and Antagonist Actions of Narcotic Analgesic Drugs, edited by H.W. Kosterlitz, H.O.J. Collier, and J.E.Villereal, pp. 176-191, University Park Press, Baltimore.
13.Cicero, T.J., Meyer,E.R., and Smithloff, B.R. (1974): J. Pharmacol. Exp. Ther , 189 : 72.
14.Contreras, E., Quijada, L., and Tamayo, L. (1973) : Psychopharmacologia ,28 : 319.
15.Contreras, E., and Tamayo, L. (1966) : Arch. Int. Pharmacodyn. Ther., 160 : 312.
16.Dahlström, A., and Fuxe, K. (1965) : Acta Physiol. Scand. , 64, Suppl. 247 : 5.
17.Dewey, W.L., Harris, L.S., Howes, J.F., and Nuite, J.A. (1970) : J. Pharmacol. Exp. Ther. , 175 : 435.
18.Genovese, E., Zonta, N., and Mantegazza, P. (1973): Psychopharmacologia, 32 : 359.
19.Giesler, G.J., and Liebeskind, J.C. (1976) : Pain, 2:43.
20.Guilbaud, G., Besson, J.M., Oliveras, J.L., and

Liebeskind, J.C. (1973) : Brain Res., 61 : 417 - 422.

21. Harvey, J.A., and Lints, C.E. (1971) : J. Comp. Physiol. Psychol. , 74 : 28-36.

22. Herz, A., Albus, K., Metys, J., Schubert, P., and Teschemacher, H. (1970) : Neuropharmacology , 9 : 539.

23. Hökfelt, T., Kellerth, J.O., Nillsson, G., and Pernow, B. (1975) : Science , 190 : 889.

24. Holman, R.B., Angwin, P., and Barchas, J.D. (1976): Neuroscience, 1:147.

25. Hughes, J. (1975) : Brain Res., 88 : 295.

26. Hughes, J. (1975) : In : Opiate Receptor Mechanisms edited by S. Snyder and S. Matthysse,Neurosci.Res. Progr. Bull., 13 : 55.

27. Hughes, J., Smith, T.W., Kosterlitz, H.W., Fothergill, L.A., Morgan, B.A., and Morris, H.R. (1975) : Nature (Lond.), 258 : 577.

28. Jacquet, Y.F., and Lajtha, A. (1973) : Science , 182 : 490.

29. Korf, J., Bunney, B.S., and Aghajanian, G.K.(1974): Europ. J. Pharmacol. 25 : 165.

30. Liebeskind, J.C., Guilbaud, G., Besson, J.-M., and Oliveras, J.-L. (1973) : Brain Res., 50 : 441.

31. Liebeskind, J.C., Mayer, D.J., and Akil, H.(1974) : In: Advances in Neurology, vol. 4, edited by J.J. Bonica, Pain, p. 261, Raven Press, New York.

32. Lindvall, P., and Björklund, A. (1974) : Acta Physiol. Scand. Supplementum, 412: 1.

33. Mayer, D.J., and Hayes, R. (1975) : Science, 188: 941.

34. Mayer, D.J., and Liebeskind, J.C. (1974) : Brain Res., 68 : 73.

35. Mayer, D.J., Wolfle, T.L., Akil, H., Carder, B., and Liebeskind, J.C. (1971) : Science, 174:1351.

36. Messing, R.B., Phebus, L.E., Fisher, L.A., and Lytle, L.D. (1975) : Psychopharmacol. Commun., 1: 511-521.

37. Nakamura, K., Kuntzman, R., Maggio, A.C., Augulis, V., and Conney, A.H. (1973) : Psychopharmacologia, 31 : 177.

38. Oleson, T.D., and Liebeskind, J.C. (1975) : Physiologist, 18 : 338.

39. Oliveras, J.L., Redjemi, F., Guilbaud, G., and Besson, J.M. (1975) : Pain , 1 : 139.

40. Pert, A., and Yaksh, T. (1974) : Brain Res., 80 : 135.

41. Proudfit,H.K., and Anderson, E.G. (1974) : Pharmacologist, 16 : 203.

42. Proudfit, H.K., and Anderson, E.G. (1974) : Brain Res. , 65 : 542.

43. Repkin, A.H., Proudfit, H.K., and Anderson, E.G. (1974) : Pharmacologist, 16 : 203.
44. Rhodes, D.L., and Liebeskind, J.C. (1974) : Society for Neurosciences ,392.
45. Richardson, D.E., and Akil, H. (1973) : Annual Meeting of the American Association of Neurological Surgery.
46. Richardson, D.E., and Akil, H. (1977): J. Neurosurg. 47:178.
47. Richardson, D.E., and Akil, H. (1977):J.Neurosurg., 47:184.
48. Saarnivara, L. (1969) : Ann. Med. Exp. Biol. Fenn. 47 : 103.
49. Samanin R., Gumulka, W., and Valzelli, L. (1970) : Eur. J. Pharmacol., 10 : 339.
50. Samanin, R., and Valzelli, L. (1971) : Eur. J. Pharmacol., 16 : 298.
51. Sharpe, L.G., Garnett, J., and Cicero, T.J. (1974): Behav. Biol., 11 : 303.
52. Tenen, S.S. (1968) : Psychopharmacologia, 12 : 278.
53. Teschemacher, H.J., Schubert, P., and Herz, A. (1973) : Neuropharmacology, 12 : 123.
54. Tsou, K., and Jang, C.S. (1964) : Scientia Sinica, 13 : 1099.
55. Tulunay, F.C., Yano, I., and Takemori, A.E. (1976): Eur. J. Pharmacol., 35 : 285-292.
56. VanderWende, C., and Spoerlein, M.T. (1973): Res. Commun. Chem. Path. Pharmacol. , 5 : 35.
57. Vogt, M. (1974) : J. Physiol. (Lond) , 236 : 483.
58. Watson, S.J., Akil, H., and Barchas, J.D. (1977) : Brain Res., 130:335.
59. Watson, S.J., and Barchas, J.D. (1975) : Psycho-pharmacol. Comm. , 1 : 523 - 531.
60. Yaksh, T.L., Duchateau, J.C., and Rudy, T.A. (1976): Brain Res. 104 : 367-372.
61. Yunger, L.M., Harvey, J.A., and Lorens, S.A.(1973): Physiol. Behav.,10 : 909-913.

Factors Affecting the Action of Narcotics, edited by
M.L. Adler, L. Manara, and R. Samanin.
Raven Press, New York©1978.

Monoaminergic Control of Lamina V Interneurons Activity

G.Benelli

Zambon S.p.A. Research Laboratories, Bresso-Milan,
Italy

INTRODUCTION

After the discovery of the laminar organization of
the spinal cord (28), many efforts were made to clarify
the functional role of the different laminae. Great
attention was devoted to the interneurons of the lamina
V because it was found that they are involved in the
transmission of peripheral nociceptive afferentation
towards superior nervous centers (2,17,37,40). It has
been demonstrated that lamina V interneurons receive
excitatory inputs mainly from small cutaneous and
visceral afferent fibres, i.e., the fibres which are
thought to carry the painful afferentation (6,7,8,21,
25,26,32,39).
A powerful descending inhibitory control is known
to be exerted by some encephalic centers on the afferent input at dorsal spinal level. After the
demonstration by Carlsson et al.(13) of descending
catecholamine containing fibres which form a dense
network particularly in the dorsal horn of the spinal
cord, an inhibitory action of catecholamine precursors
and catecholamines on neuronal activity of the spinal
cord was described (3,4,18,19). Inhibition of the firing of lamina V cells was obtained by Liebeskind et al.
(24) stimulating the periaqueductal gray matter and
Guilbaud et al. (20) have shown that the inhibition of
lamina V interneurons achieved by stimulating the
dorsal raphe nucleus was abolished by administration of
lysergic acid diethylamide (LSD), a serotonin
antagonist. Besson et al.(9) have demonstrated that
the brain stem exerts a potent inhibitory influence on
the same type of nerve cells. Moreover, Takagi et al.

579

(34) have found that dihydroxyphenylalanine (L-DOPA) inhibits the activity of lamina V cells both in intact and spinalized rabbits.

Because of these physiological properties the lamina V interneurons were chosen for studying the effects of various narcotic analgesics on the transmission of nociceptive messages.

Evidence in the literature suggests that morphine may produce analgesia acting on a monoaminergic inhibitory pathway. p-Chlorophenylalanine, a tryptophan hydroxylase inhibitor, and reserpine, which depletes catecholamines from the storage vesicles, antagonize morphine analgesia (33,35,36,38). Moreover, Samanin et al. (29) and Proudfit and Anderson (27) have demonstrated that lesion of raphe serotoninergic neurons decreases the analgesic effect of morphine. On the other hand, Akil and Mayer (1) reported that electrical stimulation of the raphe is followed by analgesia, and Samanin and Valzelli (30) demonstrated that the same procedure enhances morphine analgesia. Satoh and Takagi (31) suggested that morphine produces an activation of the descending inhibitory catecholaminergic pathways; however, other authors (6,10,14,22,23) demonstrated that various narcotic analgesics depress lamina V interneuron activity in acutely spinalized animals too. Morphine (2 mg/kg) in cats inhibits by about 50% the activation of lumbar lamina V interneurons provoked by painful pinch of the skin or by supramaximal electrical stimulation of afferent fibres of the hindlimb nerves (5,23). In the same experimental conditions, even stronger activity is shown by the pyrrylethanolamine derivative, viminol, a new synthetic compound with marked central analgesic properties (14,16). The administration of naloxone, a specific morphine antagonist, immediately reversed the inhibitory action both of morphine and viminol (15). In a recent paper Takagi et al. (34) also reported a depression of lamina V interneuron activity in acutely spinalized rabbits treated with morphine.

The aim of the present work was to clarify the action of two catecholamine precursors, L-DOPA and 5-hydroxytryptophan (5-HTP), and a dopaminergic drug, apomorphine, on the discharge of lamina V interneurons provoked by peripheral nociceptive stimulation in

spinalized cats. We also investigated whether morphine
may act by interfering with a monoaminergic mechanism
at spinal level.

METHODS

The experiments were performed in unanesthetized
cats, spinalized in C_1 and immobilized with gallamine
triethiodide. Laminectomy was made from L_4 to L_7
segments. Hindlimb peroneal, sural and tibial nerves
were isolated and placed on platinum stimulating
electrodes. Spinal cord and hindlimb nerves were
covered by warm paraffin oil.
   Temperature and systemic blood pressure were continuously monitored. Electrophysiological, topographic
and histological methods were employed for lamina V
interneuron identification.
Recordings of single lamina V interneuron discharges,
due to electrical supramaximal stimulation of one
peripheral nerve, were obtained by the conventional
microelectrode technique. The responses of single
lamina V cell to 128 stimuli, carried out at a frequency of 0.8-1 cycle/sec, were averaged as post-stimulus
histograms by means of a Hewlett-Packard analyzer and
photographed on an oscilloscope screen or transferred
to paper. The solutions of the drugs were injected
intravenously.

RESULTS

Effects of L-DOPA and Apomorphine Administration on
Lamina V Interneuron Activity

Fig.1 represents an example of the depressive action
of L-DOPA (10 mg/kg) on the activation of a lamina V
cell provoked by electrical stimulation of the peroneal
nerve in the spinalized cat. This inhibitory action
reached a maximum in 15-20 minutes. Spontaneous
recovering was observed 40-50 minutes after injection
of the drug (15 experiments). Our results are in
agreement with those obtained by Takagi et al. (34)
who have recently demonstrated the depressive action of
20 mg/kg of L-DOPA on bradykinin induced activation of
lamina V interneurons in both intact and spinalized

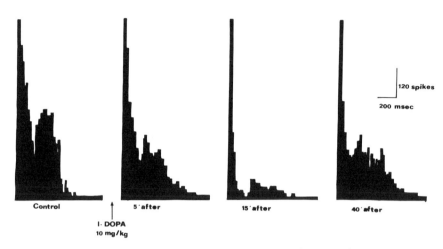

FIG. 1. Inhibitory effect of L-DOPA (10 mg/kg) on the
activity of a lamina V interneuron. Note the spontaneous recovery of control activity 40 minutes after
injection of the drug.

rabbits.

It was of interest to investigate whether a direct
stimulation of postsynaptic dopamine receptors by
apomorphine was able to mimic the action of L-DOPA.
The experiments performed demonstrated that the activity of a lamina V interneuron was also depressed by the
administration of apomorphine (500 μg/kg). The maximum
drug action at this   dose was reached in 30 minutes
and full spontaneous recovery of control activity in
about 60 minutes (4 experiments).

The specificity of the action of both L-DOPA and
apomorphine on a supposed dopaminergic receptor at
spinal level was controlled by pretreating the animals
with specific receptor blocking agents, such as
haloperidol and phenoxybenzamine.

Panel A of Fig. 2 shows the protective action of
pretreatment with haloperidol (500 μg/kg) which
antagonizes the inhibitory action of L-DOPA (10 mg/kg).
Panel B shows the control activity of the same nerve
cell 90 minutes after haloperidol injection; subsequent

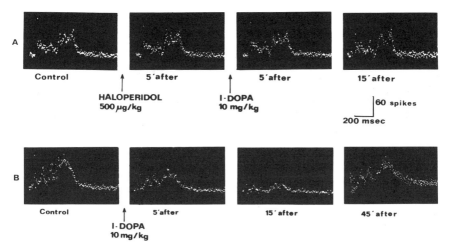

FIG. 2. Panel A : protective action of haloperidol
(500 µg/kg) against the inhibitory action of L-DOPA.
Panel B : recovery of the depressive action on the same
interneurons by L-DOPA (10 mg/kg), administered 90
minutes after haloperidol.

administration of L-DOPA again produces an inhibitory
effect.   Complete recovery of neuronal activity is seen
45 minutes later (7 experiments).   Similar results were
obtained with phenoxybenzamine pretreatment (2 mg/kg)
(6 experiments).

The antagonism of haloperidol on the depressive
activity of apomorphine was also tested.   We demonstrated that after a pretreatment with haloperidol
(500 µg/kg), apomorphine (500 µg/kg) does not inhibit
lamina V interneuron activity.   The depressive action
of apomorphine was restored about 2 hours after
haloperidol administration (6 experiments).

The influence of naloxone (50-100 µg/kg) on the
depression of lamina V interneurons provoked by L-DOPA
and apomorphine was then examined; the experiments
clearly demonstrated that naloxone is not able to
reverse, as it does for morphine, the depression provoked by L-DOPA (3 experiments) and apomorphine (3
experiments).

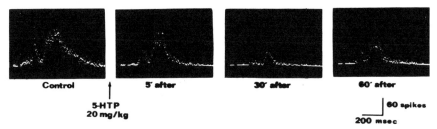

FIG. 3. Inhibitory effect of 5-HTP (20 mg/kg) on the
activity of a lamina V interneuron. Note the spontaneous recovery of control activity 60 minutes after
injection of the drug.

Effects of 5-HTP Administration on Lamina V Interneuron
Activity

To our knowledge no reports exist in the literature
about 5-HTP action on lamina V cells. In Fig.3 it can
be seen that an intravenous injection of 5-HTP (20 mg/
kg) is followed 5 minutes later by a reduction of
neuronal activity. After 30 minutes the reduction was
more pronounced. Spontaneous recovery of the original
cell activity was found 60-70 minutes later (9 experiments).

Experiments were performed to check the specificity
of the action of 5-HTP on a supposed serotoninergic
receptor by pretreating the animals with serotonin
blocking agents, such as cyproheptadine and LSD. Our
results demonstrated that cyproheptadine (2 mg/kg, 3
experiments) and LSD (1 µg/kg, 3 experiments) suppressed the inhibition of lamina V interneurons induced by
5-HTP.

We also tested the action of naloxone on the depression of lamina V interneuron firing provoked by 5-HTP
but it did not antagonize the action of 5-HTP (3
experiments).

Since haloperidol (500 µg/kg) antagonized the
depressive action of 5-HTP on lamina V interneuron
activity (Fig.4) it seems likely that the effect of

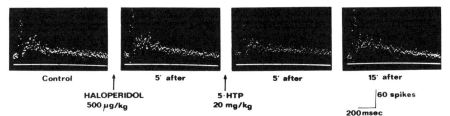

FIG. 4. Protective influence of haloperidol (500 µg/kg) on a lamina V interneuron against the depressive action of 5-HTP.

5-HTP is mediated by a dopaminergic mechanism.

Effects of Morphine Administration on Lamina V Interneuron Activity

   Beside a descending inhibitory pathway Brown et al. (11,12) postulated the existence of a segmental inhibitory system at the spinal level. In a previous paper (5) we also suggested that narcotic analgesics may act by activating a local segmental inhibitory mechanism.
   To investigate whether catecholamines are involved in the function of this system, we tested the action of haloperidol on the inhibition of the lamina V interneuron activity provoked by morphine (9 experiments). A pretreatment with haloperidol (500 µg/kg) fully protected the discharge of lamina V interneurons from the inhibitory influence of 2 mg/kg of morphine (Fig.5, panel A). The action of morphine was recovered 80 minutes after haloperidol injection (Fig.5, panel B).

CONCLUDING REMARKS

   Evidence has been obtained suggesting that monoamine precursors (L-DOPA and 5-HTP) and a dopamine receptor stimulating agent (apomorphine) may depress the firing of lamina V cells by activating a segmental inhibitory

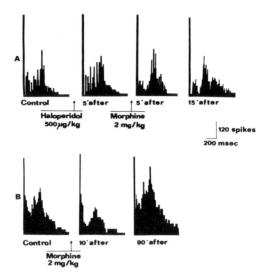

FIG. 5. Panel A : protective action of haloperidol
(500 µg/kg) against the depressive action of morphine.
Panel B : recovery of the inhibitory properties of
morphine administered 90 minutes after haloperidol.

system. Since haloperidol blocks the inhibitory
action of 5-HTP, it seems likely that 5-HTP acts on
lamina V cells through a dopaminergic mechanism.

Morphine produces effects similar to those of
L-DOPA, 5-HTP and apomorphine; moreover, its inhibitory
action is blocked by haloperidol. This suggests that
the depressive effect of morphine on lamina V interneurons may be mediated by dopamine or serotonin. The
fact that naloxone antagonizes morphine activity on
lamina V interneurons but fails to reduce the inhibitory influence of L-DOPA, apomorphine, and 5-HTP on
the same cells suggests that morphine may interact
with specific receptors responsible for the segmental
inhibitory system activation.

On the basis of these previous results, it does not
seem unrealistic to postulate that morphine, dopamino-
mimetic and serotoninergic drugs may have specific
effects acting not only at different levels, but also
interacting with specific, distinct receptors
responsible for an effective modulating influence on

the painful afference transmission.

REFERENCES

1. Akil, H., and Mayer, D.J. (1972): Brain Res., 44: 692-697.
2. Albe-Fessard, D., Levante, A., and Lamour, Y.(1974): Brain Res., 65: 503-509.
3. Andén, N.E., Jukes, M.G.M., and Lundberg, A. (1966): Acta Physiol.Scand., 67: 387-397.
4. Andén, N.E., Jukes, M.G.M., Lundberg, A., and Vyklicky, L. (1966): Acta Physiol.Scand., 67: 373-386.
5. Benelli, G. (1976): Riv. Farmacol. Terapia, 7: 395-404.

6. Benelli, G., Besson, J.M., and Della Bella, D. (1975): Communication at the 1st World Congress of International Association for Study of Pain, Florence (Italy), Sept.5-8.
7. Benelli, G., Besson, J.M., Guilbaud, G., and Lombard, M.C. (1974): J.Physiol.(Paris), 69: 221A.
8. Besson, J.M., Conseiller, C., Hamann, K.F., and Maillard, M.C. (1972): J.Physiol.(Lond.), 221: 189-205.
9. Besson, J.M., Guilbaud, G., and Le Bars, D. (1975): J.Physiol.(Lond.), 248: 725-739.
10. Besson, J.M., Wyon-Maillard, M.C., Benoist, J.M., Conseiller, C., and Hamann, K.F. (1973): J.Pharmacol.Exp.Ther., 187: 239-245.
11. Brown, A.G., Hamann, W.C., and Martin, H.F. (1974): Adv.Neurol., 4: 253 -259.
12. Brown, A.G., Kirk, E.J., and Martin, H.F. (1973): J.Physiol.(Lond.), 230: 689-705.
13. Carlsson, A., Falck, B., Fuxe, K., and Hillarp, N.A. (1964): Acta Physiol.Scand., 60: 112-119.
14. Della Bella, D., Benelli, G., and Besson, J.M. (1975): Life Sci., 17: 73 -74.
15. Della Bella, D., Benelli, G., and Sassi, A. (1976): Pharmacol.Res.Commun., 8: 111-126.
16. Della Bella, D., Ferrari, V., Frigeni, V., and Lualdi, P. (1973): Nature New Biol., 241: 282-284.
17. Dilly, P.N., Wall, P.D., and Webster, K.E. (1968): Exp.Neurol., 21: 550-562.

18. Engberg, I., Lundberg, A., and Ryall, R.W. (1968):
    Acta Physiol.Scand., 72: 115-122.
19. Engberg, I., Lundberg, A., and Ryall, R.W. (1968):
    Acta Physiol.Scand., 72: 123-133.
20. Guilbaud, G., Besson, J.M., Oliveras, J.L., and
    Liebeskind, J.C. (1973): Brain Res., 61: 417-422.
21. Hillman, P., and Wall, P.D. (1969): Exp.Brain Res.,
    9: 284-306.
22. Kitahata, L.M., Kosaka, Y., Taub, A., Bonikos, K.,
    and Hoffert, M. (1974): Anesthesiology, 41: 39-48.
23. Le Bars, D., Guilbaud, G., Jurna, I., and Besson, J.
    M. (1975): Communication at the 1st World Congress
    of International Association for Study of Pain,
    Florence (Italy) September 5-8.
24. Liebeskind, J.C., Guilbaud, G., Besson, J.M., and
    Oliveras, J.L. (1973): Brain Res., 50: 441-446.
25. Pomeranz, B., Wall, P.D., and Weber, W.V. (1968):
    J.Physiol.(Lond.), 199: 511-532.
26. Price, D.D., and Wagman, I.H. (1970): Exp.Neurol.,
    29: 383-399.
27. Proudfit, H.K., and Anderson, E.G. (1974):
    Pharmacologist, 16: 203.
28. Rexed, B. (1952): J.Comp. Neurol.,96: 415-495.
29. Samanin, R., Gumulka, W., and Valzelli, L. (1970):
    Eur.J.Pharmacol., 10: 339-343.
30. Samanin, R., and Valzelli, L. (1971): Eur.J.
    Pharmacol., 16: 298-302.
31. Satoh, M.,and Takagi, H. (1971): Eur.J.Pharmacol.,
    14: 60-65.
32. Selzer, M., and Spencer, W.A. (1969): Brain Res.,
    14: 331-348.
33. Sigg, E.B., Caprio, G., and Schneider, J.A. (1958):
    Proc.Soc.Exp.Biol.Med., 97: 97-100.
34. Takagi, H.,Doi, T., and Kawasaki, K. (1975): Life
    Sci., 17: 67-72.
35. Takagi, H., Takashima, T., and Kimura, K. (1964):
    Arch.Int.Pharmacodyn.Ther., 149: 484-492.
36. Tenen, S.S.(1968): Psychopharmacologia, 12:278-285.
37. Trevino, D.L., Coulter, J.D., and Willis, W.D.
    (1973): J.Neurophysiol., 36:750-761.
38. Vogt, M. (1974): J.Physiol.(Lond.), 236: 484-498.
39. Wall, P.D. (1967): J.Physiol.(Lond.),188: 403-423.
40. Willis, W.D.,Trevino, D.L., Coulter,J.D., and Maunz,
    R.A. (1974):J.Neurophysiol., 37: 358-372.

5. ENVIRONMENTAL AND

PATHOLOGICAL CONDITIONS,

DRUG INTERACTIONS

Factors Affecting the Action of Narcotics, edited by
M.L. Adler, L. Manara, and R. Samanin.
Raven Press, New York©1978.

Environmental Concomitants: Introduction to the Topic

L. Valzelli

Istituto di Ricerche Farmacologiche "Mario Negri",
    Via Eritrea 62 - 20157 Milano, Italy

Variability in response to drug treatment often
makes it difficult to evaluate the therapeutic efficacy of psychotropic drugs and to utilize them most effectively in clinical practice. Over the past 30 years
such variability led to a still growing and rather
confusing body of knowledge relating to such issues as
environment, personality characteristics, attitude,
expectations and related concepts, all described as
capable of influencing drug response.

The results expected after the administration of
psychoactive compounds often appear to be modified by
many more unforeseen factors than are usually found in
studying such drugs as hypotensives, antiarrhythmics,
or antibiotics. Furthermore, many so-called "non-drug"
factors are extremely elusive in their nature and
rather difficult to rank in an unequivocal way.

Pharmacology is classically associated with a number
of factors which can modify a drug effect and these
can be listed as follows : 1) age, 2) body weight,
3) sex, 4) route and time of administration, 5) rate
of inactivation and excretion, 6) tolerance, 7) biochemical and physiological state, 8) pathologic state,
9) genetic factors, 10) drug interactions and mixtures
and 11) environment (8). Clinicians, on the other
hand (13) call attention to another series of factors
responsible for a psychotropic drug effect such as 1)
physiological characteristics of the drug, 2) dose
and   route of drug administration,   3) target
symptoms,   4) ego strength, 5) environment, 6)
personality characteristics, 7) expectation of the
patients and 8) expectations of the therapist. Some
more recent issues such as 9) social-interpersonal

variables, 10) race and 11) psychiatric variables (15) might perhaps be added. However, aside from some relatively elementary areas of overlap, such as the route of drug administration and the pathologic state or target symptoms, the two lists are quite different, having in common only the environmental concept. The differences can be attributed, in part, to the fact that the pharmacologist's list reflects results primarily obtained in animal experiments while the clinical list includes those observations made in human subjects. In fact, according to the first principle formulated by Fisher (9) on this matter "the more the response system being measured involves cortical processes such as awareness, consciousness, and subjective feelings, the greater will be the role of nonspecific factors influencing drug response", and it should be noted that such cortical processes constitute the principal brain activities with which one is concerned when dealing with human beings.

In the field of neuropsychopharmacology, this situation could represent a very dangerous gap between the experiments conducted in animals and the outcome observed in patients after psychoactive drug administration, unless the huge amount of data collected over the past twenty years demonstrates that the environment, social setting and previous experiences in animals are capable of modifying both their behavior and their response to drugs. This would allow the animal experiments to be of relevance in experimental neuropsychopharmacology for the assessment of some variables which can modify the action of psychoactive drugs.

Since morphine belongs to the broad family of psychoactive drugs, the above general considerations can be applied to these studies as well. Morphine is known to have a wide spectrum of pharmacological actions which are essentially believed to depend on the involvement of brain structures. The highly standardized conditions under which animal experiments are usually carried out may, at least to a certain extent, overshadow the effect that internal and external environment can exert upon morphine activity.

Under the heading of "internal environment" come the manifold variables which characterize and differentiate species from species on the emotional,metabolic and endocrine levels; and, within the same species,strain from strain. Thus, just as dextroamphetamine had been shown to act in a markedly different way according to the strain of mice in which it was injected (5,6) morphine too was shown to have a differential effect upon motor activity and analgesia according to the strain of mice used (14). This finding suggests that differences in the internal environment, as genetically predetermined or consequent to a spontaneous or experimentally induced modification, can result in changes of drug activity, morphine being included among such drugs.

Still following this line, external environment and its physical properties (heat, light, noise) or socio-emotional characteristics (housing, sensory deprivation or isolation, crowding) can induce physical (body temperature, sleep cycle, circadian rhythm) or emotional (behavioral alterations) changes as well. For example, it has been shown that reserpine (10) and dextroamphetamine (6) are modified in their activity by changes in the room temperature at which experimental animals are maintained. Variations in morphine activity result from alterations in environmental temperature (3). In addition, morphine analgesia and dependence are modified by social isolation or aggregation in animals (1,2,4,11).

Since norepinephrine, dopamine and serotonin, as well as other neurochemicals are involved in synaptic transmission in the brain, these endogenous chemicals have also been implicated in the mechanism of action of several psychoactive drugs including morphine. An important consideration is that both physical and socio-emotional components of the environment, as well as differences in the strains, may involve a number of neurochemical diversities at the brain level (6,7, 10,12,16,17) by which the activity of morphine can be modulated .

REFERENCES

1. Adler, M.W., Bendotti, C., Ghezzi, D., Samanin, R. and Valzelli, L. (1975): Psychopharmacologia, 41: 15-18.

2. Adler, M.W., Mauron, C., Samanin, R., and
   Valzelli, L. (1975): Psychopharmacologia,41:11-14.
3. Cochin, J. this volume
4. De Feudis, F.V., Somoza, E., and De Feudis, P.A.
   this volume
5. Dolfini, E., Garattini, S., and Valzelli, L.(1969):
   Eur.J.Pharmacol., 7: 220-223.
6. Dolfini, E., Garattini, S., and Valzelli, L.(1969):
   J.Pharm.Pharmacol., 21: 871-872.
7. Ebel, A., Hermetet, J.C., and Mandel, P. (1973):
   Nature(New Biol.), 242: 56-58.
8. Fingl, E., and Woodbury, D.M. (1965): in: The
   Pharmacological Basis of Therapeutics, edited by
   L.S. Goodman, and A. Gilman, 3rd.ed., pp.1-3.
   Mac Millan, New York.
9. Fisher, S. (1970): In: Clinical Handbook of Psychopharmacology, edited by A. Di Mascio, and R.I.
   Shader, pp.17-39. Science House Publ., New York.
10.Garattini, S., and Valzelli, L. (1958): Science,
   128: 1278-1279.
11.Katz, D.M., and Steinberg, H. (1972): In:
   Biochemical and Pharmacological Aspects of
   Dependence and Reports on Marihuana Research,
   edited by H.M.Van Praag, F. De Erven, and N.V.Bohn
   pp. 46-61, Haarlem, Netherlands.
12.Kempf, E., Greilsamer, J., Mack, G., and Mandel, P.
   (1974): Nature(Lond.), 247: 483-485.
13.Malitz, S. (1963): In: Specific and Non-Specific
   Factors in Psychopharmacology, edited by M.Rinkel,
   pp.141-148. Philosophical Library Inc., New York.
14.Oliverio, A., and Castellano, C. (1974):
   Psychopharmacologia, 39: 13-22.
15.Overall, J.E., Hollister, L.E., Kimbell, I. and
   Shelton, J. (1969): Arch.Gen.Psychiatry,21: 89-94.
16.Valzelli, L. (1973): Psychopharmacologia, 31: 305-
   320.
17.Valzelli, L., and Garattini, S. (1972):
   Neuropharmacology, 11: 17-22.

Factors Affecting the Action of Narcotics, edited by
M.L. Adler, L. Manara, and R. Samanin.
Raven Press, New York©1978.

Social and Other Influences on Morphine
Action in Rodents

Hannah Steinberg

Department of Pharmacology,
University College London,
Gower Street
London, W.C.1 England

INTRODUCTION

It has long been known that the manifest effects of
psychoactive drugs on behavior partly depend on the
past and present circumstances of the recipient, and
opiates are no exception. Even so, and despite the
importance of this group of drugs, drug-environment
interactions appear to have been studied rather less than
one might expect, possibly because the drugs are so
powerful that their primary pharmacological actions are
assumed to override all else.

This paper deals only with opiate experiments on the
behavior of rodents, though it is hoped that implications for man will emerge. Both 'acute' and 'chronic'
opiate effects will be considered, the second mostly
in the context of drug dependence.

Environmental factors which can affect morphine
action may be classified and discussed according to
different schemes (15,30,41). I shall distinguish and
limit myself to aspects of three main kinds of factor,
chosen partly because they are especially relevant to
research work with which I have myself been associated
and partly because they seem to be implicitly or
explicitly involved in most animal behavior experiments.
1. Characteristics of the physical environment
where morphine experiments are carried out (these are
sometimes designated 'extrinsic' or 'external' environmental factors). 2. Characteristics of the experimental subjects (sometimes called 'intrinsic' or
'internal' environmental factors, but there is much
overlap with the previous category). I shall consider
in particular animals' previous histories of drug
administration and of housing (social isolation or
grouping). 3. Social competition and its effects on

595

morphine reactions. Again, this overlaps with the previous two categories.

Section 1 is intended as a reminder of a now widely recognized phenomenon; section 2 is mainly about published results of experiments done in this laboratory, and also reviews literature from various other laboratories, including that of our hosts at this symposium; and section 3 describes a method for studying social competition and some preliminary findings and ideas.

1. Characteristics of the Physical Environment where Morphine Experiments are Carried out

That laboratory rats can be very sensitive to places, and especially to changes in their accustomed environment and routines can be demonstrated by various means, most simply perhaps by monitoring losses in body weight (Fig. 1) (35). Abrupt loss of body weight is also, as it has turned out, one of the most reliable consequences of withdrawing morphine from addicted rats (21). The far-reaching bodily effects which environmental factors can sometimes have, are interestingly illustrated by McArthur et al. (24) : a measure of basic metabolic activity, the incorporation of radioactivity in liver protein from labelled amino acids, was found to discriminate between mice which were taken from their cages in different orders.

As for opiates and environments, some of the earlier studies have been reviewed by Steinberg et al. (33). A classical experiment is that of Thompson and Ostlund (37) who showed that it is easier to readdict rats in the experimental environment in which they originally became dependent on morphine than in a different one. Wikler and Pescor (42) have reported similar findings on withdrawal : if morphine dependent rats were deprived of the drug, they showed more symptoms of withdrawal ('wet dog shakes') in environments where they had previously spent periods in a state of withdrawal, than in environments where they had access to a drug which relieved withdrawal symptoms. These and more recent and elaborate studies of this kind have become part of a lively literature which discusses addiction and especially tolerance (8, 19, 29, 30) in terms of learning, conditioning, reinforcement, extinction and so forth. There is now little reason to doubt that previous and present environmental cues can have a crucial role at probably every stage of opiate dependence.

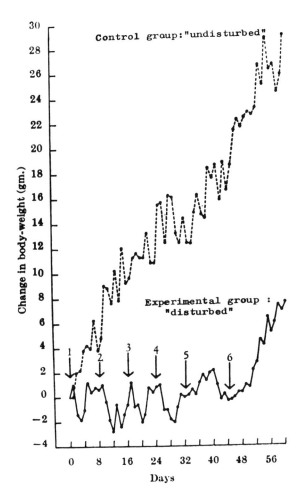

FIG. 1. Arrest of gain in weight in rats subjected to environmental changes

The control group remained undisturbed in the colony room throughout. The experimental group had successively the following treatments : 1 , transfer to another room; 2 , change in the form of diet; 3 , segregation from cage mates; 4 , daily oral injections; 5 , daily change of cage; 6,"recovery", that is, no further alterations in the environment were made. The arrows indicate when each kind of treatment began. Weight changes are expressed as mean gains or losses from the mean body weight of each group at the beginning of the experiment (35).

2. Characteristics of the Experimental Subjects

Influences such as age, sex, species and strain, circadian and other rhythms, and ambient temperature(9) are increasingly being recognized as important and in need of being controlled or allowed for in some other way. The results are still too divergent for clear generalizations to be made, and it seems likely that many of the effects are "situation dependent" rather than robust. Nozaki et al. (25), for example, after briefly reviewing earlier literature,compared reactions to morphine in rats of different ages. They found that growth rates were inhibited in older but not in younger rats by 3 weeks'administration of increasing doses of morphine. Loss in body weight after morphine withdrawal was not affected by the animals' ages. Analgesic effects of morphine measured by reactions to footshock were greater in 12-week-old than in 4- or 7-week old rats. Analgesic effects were, however, reduced in all groups with repeated administration of morphine, though this tolerance to the drug developed more quickly in young rats than in older rats, both with a fixed dose and with an "equipotent" dose regime. Age, therefore, seemed to lead to a complex pattern of interaction with morphine; it would also have been interesting to study animals older than Nozaki et al.'s oldest group which was only 12 weeks old.

Previous drug history can be of particular relevance to current concerns about "escalation" or "stepping stone" theories in man, as well as having inherent scientific interest. Most addicts have a history of multiple drug use, though evidence for causal relationships or of a progression up a scale of increasingly dangerous drugs, is mostly indirect. It is possible that mainly social factors such as fashion convenient availability of particular drugs or group membership are primary. However, animals are an obvious source of information about any clear pharmacological progression, and it is perhaps mainly the laboriousness of such experiments that is responsible for their relative scarcity.

Several years ago my colleagues and I attempted to examine such possible relationships in some detail(36). Rats had made available to them solutions of alcohol, amylobarbitone, chlordiazepoxide, or dexamphetamine during the daily 7-hour drinking period to which they had previously become accustomed. A pattern of two days of "forced" trials alternating with one day of "choice" trials was adopted for altogether 46 days.Most of the drug solutions were consumed in substantial amounts, at least during the earlier trials (Fig. 2),

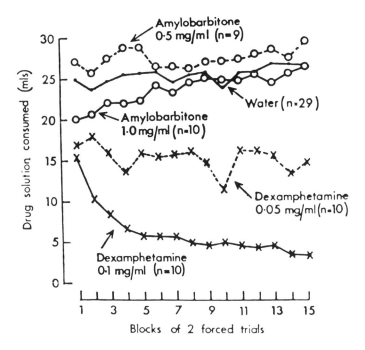

FIG. 2.   Consumption of different drug solutions by
rats during forced trials

It can be seen that, although most of the solutions
were consumed in substantial amounts, there is a
progressively increasing rejection of dexamphetamine,
particularly of the stronger solution. The intake of
the amylobarbitone solutions did not differ greatly
from that of water. (36).

though there was no clear evidence of dependence, in the
sense that substantially more than 50% of the daily
fluid intake was,in choice trials, consumed as drug
solution . Next, the rats were given access to morphine
solutions, using a similar cycle of two "forced" trials
interspersed by a single "choice" trial, as has been
described elsewhere (21). It was found that the rats
which had been exposed to solutions of different drugs
learnt to drink morphine solutions at more or less the
same rate as did water controls (Fig. 3 & 4).   Thus,
previous experience of other drugs, which has so often
been regarded as preliminary to addiction to "hard"
opiates, failed to influence the development of morphine

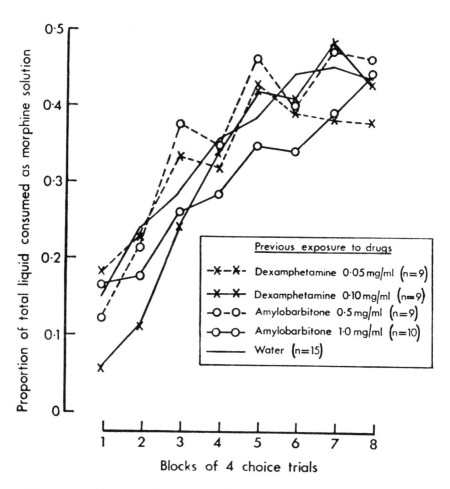

FIG. 3. Failure of ingested solutions of dexamphetamine and amylobarbitone to influence the subsequent development of dependence on morphine

The different drug solutions had been made available on choice and forced trials for a total of 46 days, after which morphine solution was made available on a similar regime (36).

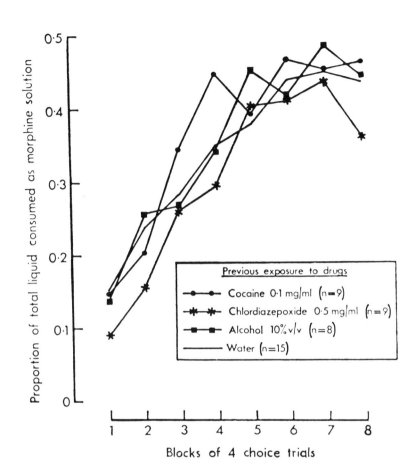

FIG. 4. Failure of ingested solutions of cocaine, chlordiazepoxide or alcohol to influence the subsequent development of dependence on morphine

For details of the procedure see Fig. 3 (36).

dependence, at any rate in the particular conditions of these experiments. Dexamphetamine was the only exceptional drug, especially in the larger dose used, it seemed to become progressively more aversive during the 46 days (Fig. 2); this aversion seemed to transfer, for a time, to morphine self-administration, so that less morphine solution was drunk to begin with (Fig. 3) which illustrates once again how experience and learning can affect the development of dependence. Without further experiments it is, however, not possible to identify the precise cues for what was learnt.

Various drugs have, of course, been shown capable of influencing morphine reactions in other ways as is illustrated by the considerable literature on tolerance and antagonists (8), methadone (22,23) and some recent experiments with lithium by Tomkiewicz and Steinberg (39) (Fig. 5).

I now come to a factor in animals' experience which in the nature of things affects them all, but which is often not made explicit: housing conditions, and in particular being housed singly as compared with being housed in groups, both before and while being tested.

For many purposes, including morphine self-administration experiments, it is convenient to house animals singly, so that for example, individual liquid and food consumption can readily be determined. For other purposes, such as single administration experiments where sleeping times or activity are to be measured, housing animals in groups is easier, cheaper, and more usual. Sometimes animals' housing is changed from one kind of condition to the other, and little seems to be done about any consequences.

The precise definitions and implications of terms such as "isolation" and "grouping" and of related terms such as "crowding" or "aggregation", are more complex than might at first appear. This is illustrated by experiments reported by Bell et al. (7). Groups of 1 to 32 mice were housed for 75 days in cages of a constant size so that group size and crowding were correlated, and were compared with similar groups which were housed in cages where the floor space varied with group size, so that the bigger the group the more space it had. Maze exploration was found to be less, the bigger the group in which the animal had been housed, regardless of crowding. Wheel activity depended both on group size and degree of crowding: in the crowded groups, activity generally decreased as group size increased; in the groups where cage space increased in proportion to group size, activity decreased up to group size 16 and then increased with further increases in group size. Physiological reactions also were variously affected.

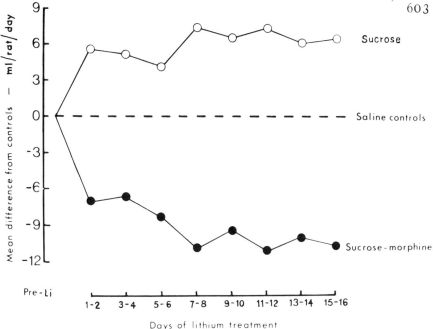

FIG. 5.   Reduction by lithium of morphine consumption

Addicted rats which were given daily choices between
solutions of, ●,10% sucrose + 0.5 mg ml^{-1} morphine
hydrochloride (sucrose-morphine), and,○, 10% sucrose
alone (sucrose), were injected daily with either 13 ml
kg^{-1} of isotonic saline or with 2 mmol kg^{-1} of LiCl
(n= 7 per group). Lithium-treated rats reduced their
consumption of sucrose-morphine from 23 ml d^{-1} to an
average of 15 ml d^{-1} (saline controls increased theirs
slightly), and increased their intake of sucrose. The
results are represented as mean differences from the
controls (saline controls) (39).

Body weight increased regardless of treatment group. Mean
brain weights and mean pituitary weights increased with increasing group and cage size; in the "crowded" groups
mean brain weights decreased with increasing group size,
but mean pituitary weights were a curvilinear function
of group size, with the lightest weights in a group of
16 mice. Mean adrenal weights did not differ among
treatment groups. Living in larger groups, whether
crowded or not, was accompained by reduced concentrations

of brain protein and nucleic acids, but the rate of intracellular synthesis of RNA and protein by DNA was
more dependent on the size of the living space.

Thus, in undrugged animals, housing conditions seemed
to lead to a remarkably complex pattern of behavioral
and physiological effects, and it is difficult to
discern any underlying common factor; "stress" has
sometimes been invoked, and terms such as "isolation
stress" have been used (26); but both isolation and
group housing and especially crowding, have at some time
been demonstrated to be stressful by different investigators. It is tempting to suggest a continuum which
follows an inverted u-shaped curve with total social
isolation (no visual, auditory, olfactory, etc. contact
with other animals) at one extreme, via "aggregation"
(groups of whatever size housed in cages which provide
an adequate amount of living space per animal), to
crowding (animals housed together in little space), at
the other extreme, but the evidence is far from being
incontrovertible (see reference 14 for an interesting
investigation of population density in rats and alcohol
consumption; cf. also reference 11).

Several investigations have been concerned with the
effects of individual or social housing on toxic effects
of opiates.

Spoerlein (32) has briefly reported that the
toxicity of morphine, when measured by LD50's, increased
if mice were kept in groups, as compared with mice kept
in isolation. Vedernikov (40) placed mice in groups
of 10 in small cages, and compared LD50's for morphine
with those for mice which were isolated in larger cages,
but he found no significant differences. Davis and
Brister (10) housed mice for 7-10 days in conventional
plastic boxes, 20-25 mice to a box. The mice were then injected and placed either singly or in groups of 5 into
small steel cages.   Group housed mice had significantly
lower LD50's for morphine, and this was also true when
pethidine or methadone were given. A feature of the
procedure was that checks for deaths were made at 4
hourly intervals and among grouped mice any that died
were replaced by fresh untreated mice so that group
size was maintained.

The isolated mice, therefore, seem more resistant to
large doses of drugs. With responses such as sleep,
prolonged social isolation also seems to make animals
more resistant to hypnotics. Baumel et al. (5,6) have
reported that the sleep induced by a single dose of
hexobarbitone in male mice, was much shorter in animals
which had been socially deprived for various periods,
than in group housed controls. Physiological and biochemical changes in these isolated mice were also noted.

For example, the drug-metabolizing activity of hepatic microsomes was increased, and drug concentrations on awakening in these animals were higher than in controls. Isolated male mice became aggressive, but this did not correlate with reduced responses to a barbiturate.

Effects of short and long-term isolation and grouping on various reactions to morphine in rats have been reported by Katz and Steinberg (16,17,18) and Katz(15). For 39 days after weaning, rats were either grouped, 12 per cage, in standard large cages, or housed singly in standard small cages. Food and water were available ad lib., and the animals were not handled. Several tests were then carried out with morphine. One of them involved self-administration in the drinking water(20, 21). The rate at which morphine dependence developed was found not to differ significantly between the two types of rat; grouped rats voluntarily drank a slightly higher proportion of their total liquid intake in the form of morphine solution, than the isolated rats, but differences over 66 days' drinking were not significant. Similarly, when body weights changes following withdrawal of morphine were determined, both isolated and grouped rats lost about the same amount of weight as compared with saline controls, and then resumed gaining weight. Hence differences in housing seemed to have had no effect on factors involved in the self administration of morphine.

From experiments with another kind of set-up, Ricci-Gamalero(27) has however reported that in a social situation (grouped-housed rats tested in pairs), abstinence reactions from morphine and effect of morphine on tolerant rats were more marked than in singly tested rats.

Y-maze activity under the influence of single doses of morphine in the investigations described by Katz and Steinberg behaved differently, moreover. Pilot experiments with group-housed female hooded rats led to clear dose response curves. The smallest dose left one kind of activity (number of entries) into the arms of the Y unaffected, but increased another (number of rears).With progressively greater doses, both kinds of activity decreased as one would expect. When male grouped and isolated rats were tested with a dose which had been clearly depressant in the pilot experiments, the activity of grouped rats in terms of entries duly decreased, but that of isolated rats, if anything increased. There was no difference between the corresponding saline controls. With the other measure of activity, rears, the picture was similar except that with morphine the isolated rats, though significantly more active than the corresponding grouped rats, did not quite reach the level of the isolated saline controls.

This resistance to a normally depressant dose, however disappeared and isolated animals became responsive to the drug, if they underwent a short period of social housing immediately before being injected and tested.   Thus the effect of long-term isolation was abolished and could be considered unstable or "labile". The converse was not true. The previously grouped animals were isolated for a short time before being injected with morphine and tested, but this did not make them react like isolated animals. It therefore seems that the conditions prevailing at the time of actual testing and shortly before, were by themselves not sufficient to change test behavior.

Adler et al. (1) studied morphine dependence in differentially housed rats (singly or in groups of 4) for 11 - 12 weeks and found no difference in the development of dependence between grouped and isolated rats (15,17). Most signs of abstinence following naloxone-precipitated withdrawal did not discriminate between grouped and isolated rats either, but the isolated rats showed less jumping and less diarrhea than grouped rats. This suggested a lesser degree of dependence in isolated animals and/or a possibly greater resistance to naloxone. What has been said applied, remarkably, to all isolated rats, regardless of whether they became muricidal (about 35% did) or not. Examples of the sensitivity of isolated rats to substances other than centrally active drugs occur in Balazs et al. (3) and Bauer and Bauer (5).

Pain thresholds to morphine in grouped and isolated animals have been studied by several investigators. Katz and Steinberg (17,18) and Katz (15) have reported a small but significant difference in that, with a "struggle response" to a tail-press procedure,isolated rats showed an enhanced response to 2 doses of morphine, as compared with grouped animals.
Adler et al. (2) were unable to detect any difference in morphine pain thresholds due to prolonged differential housing. They assessed analgesia by two methods, tail compression and a hot plate, and housing was either single or in groups of four for 7-9 weeks before pain tests. They used Wistar rats, which were fully mature, as compared with Katz' rats which were 26 days old at the beginning of the experiment. Moreover, Adler et al's rats were transferred to clean cages twice weekly during the later period of isolation or grouping. Katz' rats were not handled throughout. How far these and other differences in detailed procedure are sufficient to account for the discrepancies in the experimental results, can only be determined by further research.

More recently still, however De Feudis et al. (13), (see also 12) have reported the effects of 10-13 weeks differential housing, that is, isolation vs. aggregation, 24 per cage, on morphine-induced analgesic responses to pain, using mice and a hot-plate method. Isolated mice gave an enhanced response to morphine as compared with aggregated mice, which is similar to the findings reported by Katz and Steinberg (17, 18) and Katz (15).

Thus two sets of results at least agree over the effects of aggregation vs. isolation on morphine and reactions to painful stimuli,despite the use of different pain tests, different species of animal and different details of procedure; the importance of housing for tests of analgesia therefore cannot be disregarded. Yet few published reports seem to mention it, and it may be that to do so should become mandatory.

The influence that social factors such as isolation and group housing can have on some responses to morphine and in particular the "restorative" effect of even a brief period of social living on isolated rats, naturally lead to questions about the kind of social life that these animals can have in laboratory conditions. One way of approaching this, is through the creation of small social groups, in which competition for a single source of reward can be evoked and measured, and "social dominance hierarchies" can be determined.

3. Social Competition

Tomkiewicz (38) in this laboratory has developed a quantitative method for studying social rank and "hierarchies" in groups of four rats. A water spout in a specially designed hood is so arranged that only one rat can drink from it at a time. If the rats are thirsty, they compete vigorously for the spout, and the time which individual rats spend in control of the spout can be measured; the rat which consistently spends the longest time in control of the spout, is considered to be the most dominant, and the rat which spends the least time, is considered the least dominant. After some two weeks, a distinct hierarchy usually emerges which remains in force for long periods of time, though it can temporarily be disrupted by, for example, repeated doses of amylobarbitone (34).

Preliminary findings (by Tomkiewicz, personal communication) using a morphine self-administration (drinking) procedure, with the rats singly housed and in other respects also similar to the procedure already described (21), suggest that the extent to which rats

became addicted to morphine was influenced by their
previous status in the hierarchy.For example, the
rats which had been second in the hierarchy, seemed
most readily to become addicted to morphine, possibly,
one might conjecture, because they were subject to
the most stress. In other pilot experiments, rats were
again induced to form stable water hierarchies, were
next made dependent on morphine by the drinking method
as before while housed singly, but were then reunited
with their former cage mates and allowed to compete
for solutions of morphine. In these circumstances the
rats formed new dominance hierarchies which were
different from the original pre-addiction ones. Eventually these new "morphine' hierarchies become stable,
and the status of individual rats appeared to be
inversely related to their previous morphine consumption
when singly housed: the more addicted a rat had
previously been, the less vigorously did it appear to
compete for morphine. Since, the social hierarchies,
once they are established, tend to be clear cut
and robust, they can be used as baseline behavior.
Withdrawal reactions and re-addiction can be studied
by this kind of method, and it is possible that these
reactions will turn out to develop more quickly and
more intensely in the context of social competition,
than when animals are tested one at a time. Comparisons
between competition for morphine and for alcohol
solutions, are also being carried out (31).

This work is still very much in the "in progress"
stage, and the preliminary results are mainly intended
to illustrate the potential of the method. Perhaps
one might add that, working with grouped and competing
animals, can be particularly stimulating also for the
experimenters.

CONCLUSIONS

The influences which have been the subject of this
paper are of a kind often described as "non specific",
"non drug" or "milieu" factors (28). In man they
tend to be closely linked with "placebo" effects :
sometimes it is thought appropriate to substract these
effects from the total manifest changes in behavior
produced by the drug, in order to arrive at the "true"
drug effect.

The parallel in animals is to substract the saline
from the drug results, or to make other allowance for
them. There are circumstances where this may be
helpful and may, indeed, for many reasons be the best
that can be done. Usually, however, the situation
is more complex. Some non specific factors can be

manipulated so as to lead to marked modifications of the drug effect in their own right; others may be so intertwined with the "true" drug effect that they cannot be distinguished from it.

In planning experiments one should probably try to identify as many relevant factors as possible, so as to be able to hold them constant or to arrange appropriate controls. When one interprets the results of experiments, the "factors" are probably best regarded as contributing to the basis of individual differences in the reactions of different animals, and sometimes also in the practices of different experimenters, who produce conflicting results by apparently similar procedures.

One of the most important aims of the use of psychoactive drugs, is to optimize wanted effects in relation to unwanted ones. An understanding, however rudimentary, of the environmental and other factors which influence drug action, could be a powerful step along this road.

ACKNOWLEDGEMENTS

I thank Mr. Malcom East, Drs. David Katz & E.A.B. Sykes, Mr. Michal Tomkiewicz, the Medical Research Council and the Foundations Fund for Research in Psychiatry for help.

REFERENCES

1. Adler, M.W., Bendotti, C., Ghezzi D., Samanin R., and Valzelli L. (1975) : Psychopharmacologia, 41: 15-18.
2. Adler, M.W., Mauron, C., Samanin R., and Valzelli, L. (1975) : Psychopharmacologia, 41 : 11-14.
3. Balazs, T., Murphy, J.B., Grice, H.C. (1962) : J. Pharm. Pharmacol., 14 : 750-755.
4. Bauer, E.R., and Bauer, F.S. (1969) : Physiol. Behav., 4 : 435-437.
5. Baumel, I., Defeo, J.J., and Lal, H. (1969) : Psychopharmacologia, 15 : 153-158.
6. Baumel, I., Defeo, J.J., and Lal, H. (1970) : Psychopharmacologia, 18 : 320-324.
7. Bell, R.W., Miller, C.E., and Ordy, J.M. (1971) : J. comp. physiol. Psychol. 75 : 258-263.
8. Cochin, J. (1970) : Fed. Proc. 29 : 19-27.
9. Cochin, J. (1977) :This Volume.
10. Davis, W.M., and Brister, C.C. (1971) : J. Pharm. Pharmacol., 23 : 882-884.
11. Deatherage, G. (1972) : Physiol. Behav., 9 : 55-57.

12. DeFeudis, F.V. (1975) : In :Current Developments in Psychopharmacology, Vol. 1, edited by Essman, W.B. and Valzelli L., pp. 143-201. Spectrum Publ.,New York.
13. DeFeudis, F.V., De Feudis, P.A., and Somoza, E. (1976): Psychopharmacology, 49:117-118.
14. Heminway, D.A., and Furumoto, L. (1972): Q.J.Stud. Alc., 33 : 794-799.
15. Katz, D.M. (1976) : Ph. D. Thesis.
16. Katz, D.M., and Steinberg, H. (1970) : Nature, 228: 469-471.
17. Katz, D.M., and Steinberg, H. (1972) : In: Biochemical and Pharmacological Aspects of Dependence and Reports on Marihuana Research, edited by H.M. Van Praag, pp. 46-61. De Erven F. Bohn, N.V. Haarlem.
18. Katz, D.M., and Steinberg H. (1972) : In : Drug Addiction. Vol. 2. Clinical and Socio-legal Aspects edited by J.M. Singh, L.H. Miller, and H. Lal, pp. 85-97. Futura Pub. Co., New York.
19. Kornetsky, C. (1976): Pharmacology. Drugs Affecting Behaviour, Wiley, New York.
20. Kumar, R., Steinberg, H., and Stolerman, I.P. (1968) : Nature, 218 : 564-565.
21. Kumar, R., Steinberg, H., and Stolerman, I.P. (1969): In : Scientific Basis of Drug Dependence, edited by H. Steinberg, pp. 209-220. Churchill, London.
22. Kumar, R., and Stolerman, I.P. (1972) : J. Comp. Physiol. Psychol., 78: 457-465.
23. Kumar, R., Stolerman, I.P., and Steinberg, H. (1973) : In : Agonists and Antagonist Actions of Narcotic Analgesic Drugs, edited by H.W.Kosterlitz, H.O.J. Collier, and J.E. Villareal, Br. Pharmacol. Soc. pp. 255-265. MacMillan Press Ltd., London.
24. McArtur, J.N., Dawkins, P.D., and Smith, M.J.H. (1971) : Nature, 229 : 66.
25. Nozaki, M., Akera, T.,Cheng-Yi L., and Brody, T.M. (1975): J. Pharmacol. Exp. Ther., 192: 506-512.
26. Parker, L.F., and Radow, B.L. (1974) : Physiol. Behav., 12 : 1-3.
27. Ricci-Gamalero, S. (1974) : Pharmacol.Res.Commun., 6 : 559-563.
28. Rickels, K. (1968) : Non-Specific Factors in Drug Therapy. Charles C. Thomas, Illinois.
29. Schwartz, A.S., and Marchok, P.L. (1976) : Psychopharmacology, 47 :149-152.
30. Siegel, S. (1975) : J. Comp. Physiol. Psychol., 89: 498-506.
31. Sinclair, J.D., Adkins, J., and Walker, S. (1973) : Nature, 246 : 425-427.
32. Spoerlein,M.T. (1968) : Pharmacologist, 10 : 104.

33. Steinberg, H., Kumar, R., Kemp, I., and Bartley,H. (1968) : In : Adolescent Drug Dependence, edited by C.W.M. Wilson, pp. 29-40. Pergamon, Oxford.
34. Steinberg, H., and Tomkiewicz, M. (1973) : In : Psychopharmacology, Sexual Disorders and Drug Abuse, edited by T.A. Ban et al., pp. 343-353. North Holland, Amsterdam.
35. Steinberg, H., and Watson, R.H.J. (1960) : Nature, 185 : 615-616.
36. Stolerman, I.P., Kumar, R., and Steinberg, H. (1971) : Psychopharmacologia, 20 : 321-336.
37. Thompson, T., and Ostlund, W. (1965) : J. Comp. Physiol. Psychol., 59 : 388-392.
38. Tomkiewicz, M. (1972) : Br. J. Pharmacol., 44: 351.
39. Tomkiewicz, M., and Steinberg, H. (1974) : Nature , 252 : 227-229.
40. Vedernikov, Y.P. (1970) : Psychopharmacologia , 17: 283-288.
41. Weeks, J.R. (1975) : Fed. Proc., 34 : 1755-1758.
42. Wikler ,A., and Pescor, F.T. (1967) : Psycho-pharmacologia, 10 : 255-284.

Factors Affecting the Action of Narcotics, edited by
M.L. Adler, L. Manara, and R. Samanin.
Raven Press, New York©1978.

Environmental Model for Drug Addiction : Studies
on the Binding of Dihydromorphine and Morphine to
Synaptic Particles of the Brains of
Differentially Housed Mice

De Feudis, F.V., Somoza, E., De Feudis, P.A.,Pugnaire,
M.P.*, Orensanz Munoz, L.M.**, Gonzalez Portal, C.***,
Ibanez, A.E.***,and Bonnet, K.A.[1]

Departamento de Investigacion, Centro Nacional "Ramón
y Cajal" and Facultad de Medicina, Universidad
Autonoma, Madrid, Spain
[1] Department of Psychiatry, New York University
    Medical Center, New York,N.Y., U.S.A.

INTRODUCTION

The etiologies of excessive drug use and addiction
(i.e., tolerance, physical dependence and compulsive
craving for the drug) in man, likely include elements
of "social isolation", depression, and mild despair.
A person who might feel helpless in controlling the
causative factors in his <u>external</u> environment might
attempt to modify his perception by using drugs to
alter his <u>internal</u> environment (21,22,23). A model
system for drug addiction has now been constructed
which relates changes in external environment to cerebral subcellular structure. Differentially-housed
male mice have been used to characterize the cerebral
chemical and structural changes which appear to be
associated with changes in the actions and subcellular
"binding" of certain centrally-active (addictive)drugs.
The changes in cerebral chemistry, pharmacology and
morphology and in behavior produced by environmental

----
* Summer fellow from McGill University
** Summer fellow from Universidad Complutense de Madrid
*** Medical Student; Facultad de Medicina,Universidad
    Autonoma de Madrid.

impoverishment of mice have been well documented (10, 20,35,37).

Previous studies have indicated that environmental impoverishment (isolation-rearing) of mice increased the "binding" (retention) of two psycho-active agents, d-amphetamine and Li$^+$, to cerebral synaptic particles (8,10,13) . It was suggested that a change in the number of macromolecular "binding" sites for these ligands might have been caused by the environmental change (10,11). In accord with the theory of "denervation supersensitivity" (5), the decreased sensory input received by "isolated" animals could alter drug receptors and thereby increase drug sensitivity.

Other studies have revealed that central stimulants (e.g., d-amphetamine) are metabolized less rapidly (13,14) and that central depressants (e.g., hexobarbital) are metabolized more rapidly by "isolated" mice (4, 26) than by their "grouped" counterparts. Other in vivo experiments have shown that "grouped" mice are more tolerant than "isolated" mice to d-amphetamine (39), and that injections of d-amphetamine elicited a more pronounced stereotypy in socially-deprived rats than in controls (28). However, the duration of hexobarbital-induced narcosis was shorter in "isolated" mice (3,4,26), indicating a reduced sensitivity to barbiturates. These findings should be contrasted with those of Yanai and Ginsburg (40) which revealed that individual housing of mice increased their susceptibility to chronic ethanol treatment. Other studies have revealed that treatment with the antimanic agent, Li$^+$, caused an increase in pyruvate carbon atom entry into the brain that was selective to "isolated" mice (16). d-Amphetamine treatments produced an opposite effect on cerebral energy metabolism (decreased glucose carbon atom entry into brain) which was also selective to the "isolated" mice (17,18).

These studies have revealed that isolation-rearing of mice can lead to marked alterations in the actions and metabolic dispositions of centrally-active agents, some of which (e.g., ethanol, d-amphetamine) could be addictive. Previous findings have also indicated that "long-term" isolation increased the sensitivity of hooded rats to morphine-induced analgesia (25). In more recent studies no differences in either pain thresholds or in responses to morphine-induced analgesia were found between "grouped" and "isolated" rats of another strain (2), but differential housing did alter the abstinence syndrome in morphine-dependent rats that had been previously subjected to long-term isolation (1).

The present studies were aimed at determining the effects of environmental impoverishment on the central actions of addictive narcotic analgesics. Studies were conducted using both morphine and dihydromorphine. Analgesic responses to acute morphine injections, the entry of injected ^{3}H-dihydromorphine (^{3}H-DHM) into brain regions, and the "binding" of ^{3}H-DHM and ^{3}H-morphine to synaptic particles were compared in male Swiss albino mice that had been differentially housed for 4 to 13 weeks. DHM is chemically and pharmacologically similar to morphine (29).

Hot-Plate Testing for Acute Analgesic Responses to Morphine

Spoerlein (33) reported a difference in the acute LD$_{50}$ of morphine between mice tested under "isolated" vs "aggregated" conditions, but this finding was not confirmed (36). More recently, Davis and Brister (6) found that the lethality due to injected morphine-SO$_4$ and other narcotic analgesics in male mice could be significantly enhanced by subjecting the animals to "short-term" aggregation. However, chronically isolated rats, whether developing muricidal behavior or not, did not differ from controls in their thresholds to pain or in their tail compression or hot-plate responses to morphine-induced analgesia (2).

In the present study, analgesic responses to acute morphine-HCl treatments were monitored in male Swiss albino mice that had been subjected to "long-term" (10 to 13 wks) differential housing (see DeFeudis(7) for the method of differential housing). Analgesic responses were determined using a hot-plate which was maintained at 57°C (19,27). Latencies of the animal's responses before and at various times after morphine injection; i.e., the times that elapsed from their initial placement on the hot-plate until they either licked their paws or jumped from the plate, were

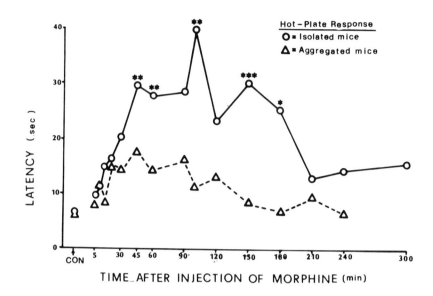

FIG. 1. <u>Latencies of responses of differentially housed</u>
<u>mice to a hot-plate maintained at 57°C.</u> Mean values;
5 mice in all cases; *, ** and *** indicate $p \cong 0.05$
$p < 0.05$ and $p < 0.01$ by comparison of these values
with corresponding values for "aggregated" mice
(Student's <u>t</u>-test; two-tailed)

recorded. Figure 1 shows that "isolated" mice displayed less sensitivity to pain than their "aggregated"
counterparts after injection of morphine.

Another series of experiments confirmed this effect
of isolation. Litters of Swiss albino mice, received
at 16 days of age with nursing dams (Blue Spruce Farms,
Altamont, New York), were maintained in intact litters
for one week under standard colony conditions. At 23
days of age animals were separated from the dams and
placed in groups of fifteen ("grouped") in transparent
plastic cages (19.0 x 11.5 x 28.0 cm) or "isolated"
in opaque cages (of the same size) placed in a quiet,
dimly-lighted room. All animals were maintained on
the same light-dark cycle (light from 7:00 a.m. to
7:00 p.m.) at ambient temperature with food and water
available <u>ad libitum.</u> After twelve weeks, animals

from both rearing conditions were tested for "nociception" on a hot-plate maintained at 45°C. Each
animal was placed on the hot-plate and the occurrence
of four response types (1,abduction of front or rear
paw; 2, licking of paws; 3, tetany of paws; and 4,
vertical jumping) were recorded throughout a 30-sec
test period. Latencies to first response were determined.

TABLE 1. Latencies of first responses to a hot-plate
of Swiss albino mice reared from weaning for twelve
weeks under conditions of "isolation" or "aggregation":
effects of morphine

Time after morphine (min)	Latency (sec)	
	Aggregated mice	Isolated mice
0	8.23 ± 0.79	5.96 ± 0.93^c
10	12.59 ± 2.06^a	12.77 ± 1.33^b
30	13.11 ± 2.56^a	13.63 ± 1.52^b
60	7.08 ± 0.26	$13.02 \pm 2.01^{b,d}$
90	5.23 ± 0.50^b	$11.00 \pm 1.65^{b,d}$
120	4.53 ± 0.41^b	7.99 ± 0.95^d
180	3.96 ± 0.29^b	6.34 ± 0.93^c
225	4.72 ± 0.72^b	5.72 ± 0.77
300	3.27 ± 0.23^b	5.06 ± 0.65^d

The hot-plate was kept at 45°C. All animals received
20 mg/kg morphine-SO$_4$,i.p.; data from 12 animals (6
male plus 6 female) in all cases; Means $\pm$ S.E.M.;
[a] and [b] indicate $p < 0.05$ and $p < 0.01$, respectively,
for differences between these values and that for pre-
injection latency within each group;
[c] and [d] indicate $p < 0.05$ and $p < 0.01$, respectively, by
comparison of these values with corresponding values
for "aggregated" mice (data of K.A. Bonnet, 1976,
unpublished).

Results indicated that isolation-reared mice had a significantly shorter latency to first response on the initial hot-plate test, when compared to "aggregated" mice (Table 1). Ten minutes after injection of morphine-SO_4 both groups of animals were significantly analgesic, and reached nearly identical response latencies. Thus, the net increase in latency in the "isolated" mice caused by morphine-SO_4 was significantly greater than in their "aggregated" counterparts ($p < 0.01$). Analgesia persisted for at least 30 min in "aggregated" mice, then declined to pre-injection latency by about 60 min. "Isolated" mice maintained the same level of analgesia for at least 60 min, and declined to pre-injection latency only after 2–3 hr, with no further change occurring by five hr post-injection. "Aggregated" mice, however, developed a progressive hypersensitivity (as evidenced by shortened latencies) by 90 min post-injection that persisted to at least 5 hours post-injection. These studies provided evidence that differences in the housing conditions of mice can influence their analgesic responses to morphine.

Entry of Injected ^{3}H-DHM into Regions of the CNS

Thirty minutes after subcutaneous injection of a "tracer" amount of ^{3}H-DHM (0.2 μCi/g; 4.4 n-moles/kg), significantly more label was found in the hippocampi, pons-medullae and spinal cords of "aggregated" mice than in their "isolated" counterparts, whereas no change occurred in the cerebral cortex (Table 2). In view of the latter finding, it is not quite clear whether such changes reflect differences in basal metabolic rate and in drug disposition, which appear to exist between "isolated" and "aggregated" mice (10,38).

Studies on the Binding of ^{3}H-Dihydromorphine (^{3}H-DHM) to Cerebral Synaptic Particles

The subcellular method of DeFeudis et al.(12) was used; all incubations were carried out in darkness. Studies with ^{3}H-DHM (1.4×10^{-9} $\underline{M}$ or 1.1×10^{-8} $\underline{M}$), in bicarbonate-buffered medium containing physiological concentrations of Na^+ and other ions, indicated that significantly more label was bound to synaptosome-

TABLE 2. Incorporation of subcutaneously-administered ^{3}H-dihydromorphine into four CNS regions of differen - tially housed mice

Region	^{3}H-dihydromorphine	
	mole($\times 10^{15}$)/g wet wt	mole($\times 10^{15}$)/mg protein
Isolated mice		
Cerebral cortex	255 ± 30 (9)	1.99 ± 0.23 (9)
Hippocampus	117 ± 8 (9)[a]	0.88 ± 0.04 (9)[a]
Pons-medulla	154 ± 6 (9)[b]	1.32 ± 0.05 (9)[b]
Spinal cord	207 ± 12 (9)[c]	1.99 ± 0.05 (9)[c]
Aggregated mice		
Cerebral cortex	231 ± 32 (9)	1.80 ± 0.19 (9)
Hippocampus	149 ± 16 (9)	1.07 ± 0.08 (9)
Pons-medulla	212 ± 19 (9)	1.73 ± 0.12 (9)
Spinal cord	307 ± 52 (9)	3.10 ± 0.07 (9)

Male Swiss albino mice were housed either singly ("isolated") or in groups of 24 ("aggregated") from the age of 25 days for 10 weeks.
All mice were killed by decapitation 30 min after injection of ^{3}H-dihydromorphine (0.2 µCi/g; 4.4 n-moles/kg). Means $\pm$ S.E.M.; numbers of determinations in parentheses;
[a,b] and [c] indicate, respectively, $p \cong 0.05$, $p < 0.01$ and $p < 0.001$, for comparisons of these values with cor-responding values for "aggregated" mice (Student's $\underline{t}$-test; two tailed).

---

enriched (P_2) fractions prepared from whole forebrain (rostral to inferior colliculi; excluding cerebellum) and cerebral cortices of "isolated" mice than to identically-prepared fractions of "aggregated" mice (see Tables 3 and 4). Since such changes were significant only when the data were expressed as mole ^{3}H-DHM/mg protein, they could be accounted for by the smaller amount of protein present in synaptosomal

TABLE 3. Binding of ^{3}H-dihydromorphine to synaptosome-enriched fractions of the brains of differentially housed mice

Parameter	Isolated mice	Aggregated mice
f-mole of ^{3}H-DHM bound/mg protein	65.4 ± 1.1[a] (27)	62.3 ± 0.9 (26)
$\dfrac{\text{dpm } ^3\text{H/g P}_2}{\text{dpm } ^3\text{H/g S}_2}$	4.61 ± 0.05 (27)	4.71 ± 0.06 (26)
p-mole of ^{3}H-DHM/g P$_2$ (corrected for sucrose space)	23.1 ± 0.31 (27)	23.4 ± 0.39 (26)

Male Swiss albino mice were differentially housed from 34-36 days of age for 4-5 weeks. Synaptosome-enriched P$_2$ fractions were prepared from 20-volume sucrose homogenates of whole forebrain by the method of DeFeudis et al. (12) and incubated at 0°C, 10 min, with 1.4×10^{-9} M ^{3}H-dihydromorphine in bicarbonate-buffered medium. Means $\pm$ S.E.M.; numbers of determinations in parentheses; [a] indicates that this value differed significantly ($p < 0.05$) from the corresponding value for "aggregated" mice (Student's t-test; two tailed).

fractions of the "isolated" mice (Table 4; see also 9, 15). Lineweaver-Burk plots of the binding of ^{3}H-DHM revealed no significant differences in K_B and B_{max} values between whole forebrain P$_2$ fractions of "isolated" and "aggregated" mice; $K_B = 7.4$ nM and $B_{max} = 91$ p-mole/g P$_2$ fraction (see Fig. 2). Particles possessed only about one-third the binding capacity (B_{max}) but about a four-fold greater affinity (K_B) for DHM than for morphine (see the following section "Studies on the Binding of ^{3}H-Morphine"), when

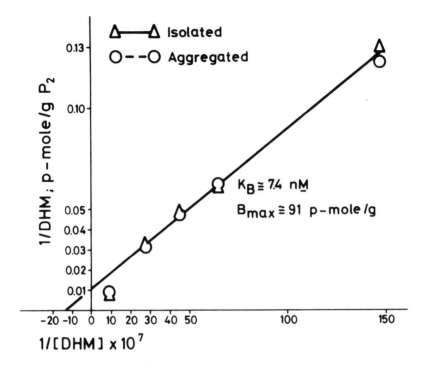

FIG. 2. Lineweaver-Burk plot of the binding of ^{3}H-dihydromorphine to synaptosome-enriched fractions of the brains of differentially housed mice. No difference existed between "isolated" and "aggregated" mice; K_B and B_{max} are indicated

experiments were conducted using a similar concentration range of drug. Interestingly, the potent opiate antagonist, naloxone (2.5×10^{-4} and 2.5×10^{-5} $\underline{M}$), caused some inhibition of the binding of ^{3}H-DHM (1.1×10^{-8} $\underline{M}$) to whole brain synaptosomal fractions of "isolated" mice, whereas it had no effect on those prepared from "aggregated" mice (Tables 5 and 6). This naloxone-displaceable fraction of total DHM binding in "isolated" mice was not present in particles prepared from "aggregated" mice and could represent an environmentally-induced increase in number of "free" opiate sites.

TABLE 4. Binding of ^{3}H-dihydromorphine to synaptosome-enriched fractions of three brain regions of differentially housed mice.

Condition of mice	Brain region	f-mole ^{3}H-DHM/ mg protein	mg protein/ g pellet	p-mole ^{3}H-DHM/ g P_2 (Uncorrected)	$\dfrac{\text{dpm } ^3\text{H/g } P_2}{\text{dpm } ^3\text{H/g } S_2}$
Isolated	cerebral cortex	44.9 ± 1.0 (18)[a]	90.5 ± 1.3 (18)[a]	4.05 ± 0.07 (18)	3.3 ± 0.05 (18)
Aggregated	cerebral cortex	41.2 ± 0.7 (17)	97.5 ± 2.2 (17)	4.00 ± 0.10 (18)	3.2 ± 0.07 (17)
Isolated	cerebellum	101.2 ± 4.0 (16)	70.2 ± 1.4 (17)	7.07 ± 0.23 (17)	5.6 ± 0.2 (17)
Aggregated	cerebellum	97.3 ± 5.6 (18)	77.9 ± 3.4 (18)	7.30 ± 0.23 (18)	5.9 ± 0.3 (18)
Isolated	brain stem	47.0 ± 0.6 (18)	78.0 ± 1.0 (18)[b]	3.65 ± 0.03 (18)[b]	2.9 ± 0.03 (17)[b]
Aggregated	brain stem	47.6 ± 0.7 (17)	83.4 ± 0.9 (17)	3.96 ± 0.04 (17)	3.2 ± 0.05 (17)

Mice were differentially housed at age 34-36 days for 6-7 weeks. Fractions were prepared by the method of DeFeudis et al. (12) using 30-volume sucrose homogenates for cerebellum and 10-volume sucrose homogenates for cerebral cortex and whole brain stem; tissues from four mice were pooled for each region. The concentration of ^{3}H-DHM in the medium was 1.4 x 10^{-9} M. Means ± S.E.M.; numbers of determinations in parentheses; a and b indicate $p < 0.01$ and $p < 0.001$, respectively, by comparison with "aggregated" mice (Student's t-test; two-tailed).

TABLE 5. Binding of ^{3}H-dihydromorphine to synaptosome-enriched fractions of the brains of differentially housed mice; effect of naloxone

Concentration of naloxone ($\underline{M}$)	^{3}H-DHM; p-mole/g P$_2$ (corrected for sucrose space)
Isolated mice	
0	78.3 ± 4.1 (9)[b]
2.5 x 10^{-4}	66.3 ± 4.3 (6)[a]
2.5 x 10^{-5}	67.9 ± 2.0 (6)[a]
2.5 x 10^{-6}	84.5 ± 3.2 (6)[c]
All values combined	74.7 ± 2.3 (27)[d]
Aggregated mice	
0	67.1 ± 3.9 (9)
2.5 x 10^{-4}	60.4 ± 2.4 (6)
2.5 x 10^{-5}	66.7 ± 1.3 (6)
2.5 x 10^{-6}	62.4 ± 7.7 (6)
All values combined	64.5 ± 2.2 (27)

Male Swiss albino mice were differentially housed from the age of 25 days for 7 weeks. The concentration of ^{3}H-DHM in the medium was 1.1 x 10^{-8} $\underline{M}$. Means ± S.E.M.; numbers of determinations in parentheses; [a] indicates $p < 0.05$ by comparison with the control (no drug) value for "isolated" mice. [b], [c] and [d] indicate, respectively, $p < 0.05$, $p < 0.02$, and $p < 0.001$ by comparison of these values with corresponding values for "aggregated" mice (Student's $\underline{t}$-test; one-tailed). Note that two differences exist: 1) More drug was bound to particles of "isolated" mice in the absence of naloxone; 2) Naloxone decreased the binding of ^{3}H-DHM only to particles of the "isolated" mice.

TABLE 6. Binding of ^{3}H-dihydromorphine to synaptosome-enriched fractions of the brains of differentially housed mice; effects of naloxone

Concentration of naloxone ($\underline{M}$)	^{3}H-dihydromorphine	
	p-mole/mg protein	$\dfrac{\text{dpm/g pellet}}{\text{dpm/g supernatant}}$
Isolated mice		
0	0.29 ± 0.01 (9)[a]	2.26 ± 0.08 (9)[a]
2.5×10^{-4}	0.23 ± 0.01 (6)	2.04 ± 0.07 (6)
2.5×10^{-5}	0.26 ± 0.02 (6)	2.07 ± 0.04 (6)
2.5×10^{-6}	0.29 ± 0.01 (6)[a]	2.39 ± 0.06 (6)[c]
All values combined	0.269 ± 0.007 (27)[b]	2.199 ± 0.042 (27)
Aggregated mice		
0	0.26 ± 0.008 (9)	2.05 ± 0.07 (9)
2.5×10^{-4}	0.22 ± 0.01 (6)	1.92 ± 0.04 (6)
2.5×10^{-5}	0.25 ± 0.006 (6)	2.05 ± 0.02 (6)
2.5×10^{-6}	0.26 ± 0.009 (9)	2.07 ± 0.002 (4)
All values combined	0.248 ± 0.005 (25)	2.019 ± 0.028 (25)

Male Swiss albino mice, 25 days of age, were subjected to differential housing for 7 weeks. P_2 fractions were exposed to ^{3}H-DHM (1.1×10^{-8} $\underline{M}$) for 10 min at 0°C. Means $\pm$ S.E.M.;
numbers of determinations in parentheses;
a, b and c indicate, respectively, $p < 0.05$, $p < 0.01$ and $p < 0.001$ when these values are compared with corresponding values for "aggregated" mice (Student's $\underline{t}$-test; one-tailed).

Studies with Discontinuous Sucrose Gradients

Using discontinuous sucrose gradients (method of DeFeudis et al.(15), it was shown that slightly more ^{3}H-DHM was bound to synaptic particles of the brains of "isolated" mice only when data were expressed in mole ^{3}H-DHM/mg protein. However, this difference was not significant for the sums of fractions Nos. 4-31 (1780 $\pm$ 270 (8) for "isolated" vs 1660 $\pm$ 127 (6) for "aggregated"; means $\pm$ S.D., no. of determinations in parentheses; $p > 0.2$) or for any individual fraction of the gradients (see Fig.3). Since expression of the data in terms of mole ^{3}H-DHM/fraction, as with the above data expressed as mole ^{3}H-DHM/g pellet or as pellet/supernatant fluid distribution ratios, revealed no differences, it appears likely that the same total number of ^{3}H-DHM binding sites existed in both populations of mice and that the difference in synaptic protein is not related directly to these sites.

For these studies, 10-volume 0.32 $\underline{M}$ sucrose homogenates of the combined cerebral cortices of two mice were represented in each sample. After centrifuging 2.0 ml portions of homogenates at 1.000 x g for 10 min at 0°C, 1.0 ml of the resultant supernatant fractions (S_1) was mixed with 1.0 ml of bicarbonate-buffered solution containing 1.17×10^{-9} $\underline{M}$ of ^{3}H-DHM. Portions (1.2 ml) of the resultant mixtures were layered onto the gradients and centrifuged for 60 min at 53.000 x g. Gradients were fractionated by puncturing the bottoms of the tubes and perfusing a solution of 2.0 $\underline{M}$ sucrose through these punctures. Perhaps further studies on ^{3}H-DHM binding should be undertaken using Na$^+$ -free media since it has been shown that Na$^+$ decreases the binding of agonists to opiate receptors (31,32).

Studies on the Binding of ^{3}H-Morphine

The methods employed in these studies were identical to those used for studies of ^{3}H- DHM binding (see above), except that experiments were conducted with Na$^+$ -free, TRIS-buffered medium (pH 7.5; 50 m$\underline{M}$). The binding of ^{3}H-morphine (1 /n-^{3}H/ morphine; Radiochemical Centre, Amersham, England; 27 $\underline{Ci}$/m-mole) was studied over a concentration range of 1 to 10 n$\underline{M}$.

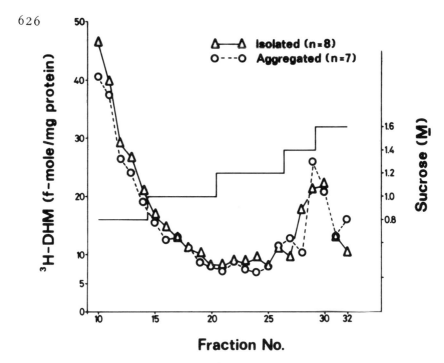

FIG. 3 A

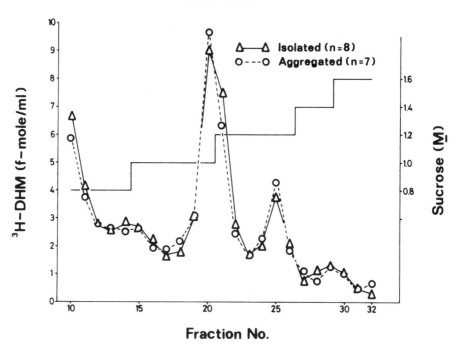

FIG. 3 B

Legend to FIG. 3. Profiles of the binding of ^{3}H-
dihydromorphine (DHM) to gradient fractionated
"synaptosomal-mitochondrial" (S_1) fractions of the
brains of differentially housed mice
Data are expressed as mole DHM/mg protein (A) and as
mole DHM/ml of fraction collected (B). Sucrose
molarities of the gradients are indicated; fractions
are numbered from top to bottom of the tubes. No
significant differences existed between values for
"isolated" and "aggregated" mice. The final concentration of ^{3}H-DHM at which incubation was carried out was
5.85 x 10 $^{-10}$ M.

Lineweaver-Burk plots revealed that K_B and B_{max} values
for the binding of ^{3}H-morphine to P_2 particles of
"isolated" and "aggregated" mice were not significantly
different; combined values for all mice were : K_B =
27.0 nM; B_{max} = 282 p-moles/g P_2 fraction (least
squares regression analyses; 4 drug concentrations;
6 to 9 values per drug concentration). Studies with
discontinuous sucrose gradients revealed no differences
between P_2 fractions prepared from the cerebral
cortices of "isolated" and "aggregated" mice. As with
^{3}H-DHM, major bands were localized at the 1.0:1.2 M
interface and above the 1.2:1.4 M sucrose interface
(see Fig. 3b)

GENERAL CONCLUSIONS

The data presented herein, together with previous
findings, suggest that an animal's social (external)
environment can play a significant role in mediating
the central effects of potentially-addictive agents.
Both the metabolic dispositions and the direct central
effects of drugs which alter behavior may be modified
by environmental changes. The finding that environmental modification altered the binding of such agents
to cerebral synaptic particles has provided evidence
for an environmental basis for drug addiction.
Environmental impoverishment, by altering the cerebral
structure of mice, thus increases their susceptibility
to addictive agents. Alterations in the effective

numbers of opiate receptor sites caused by environmental modification could provide a basis for solving
problems of opiate tolerance and dependence in man.
These changes would be of a relatively long-term nature
and would require rather long periods of environmental
stress for their initiation. Variations in the
central concentration of the endogenous "morphine-
like" substance, "enkephalin" (24,30,34), could be
involved in the mediation of such changes.

ACKNOWLEDGEMENTS

This study was supported in part by Centro Nacional
"Ramón y Cajal" de la Seguridad Social and Fundacion
Juan March. Thanks are due to Srta. Maria Francisca
Moya and Srta. Amparo Latorre for technical assistance.

REFERENCES

1. Adler, M.W., Bendotti, C., Ghezzi, D., Samanin, R.
    and Valzelli, L. (1975): Psychopharmacologia,
    41: 15.
2. Adler, M.W., Mauron, C., Samanin, R. and Valzelli,
    L. (1975): Psychopharmacologia, 41: 11.
3. Baumel, I.,   DeFeo, J. and Lal, H. (1969):
    Psychopharmacologia, 15: 153.
4. Baumel, I., DeFeo, J. and Lal, H. (1970):
    Psychopharmacologia, 18: 320.
5. Cannon, W.B. and Rosenblueth, A. (1949): The
    Supersensitivity of Denervated Structures.
    MacMillan, New York.
6. Davis, W.M. and Brister, C.C. (1971): J. Pharm.
    Pharmacol. 23: 882.
7. DeFeudis, F.V. (1971): Life Sci. 10: pt. 2, 1187.
8. DeFeudis, F.V. (1972): Brain Res., 43: 686.
9. DeFeudis, F.V. (1972): Experientia, 28: 1427.
10. DeFeudis, F.V. (1975): In: Current Developments in
    Psychopharmacology, Vol. 1, edited by W.B. Essman
    and L. Valzelli, p. 144, Spectrum Publ., New York.
11. DeFeudis, F.V. (1976): In: Proc. of the Fourth
    World Congress on Psychiatric Surgery, Madrid,
    Sept. 7-10, 1975 (in press).
12. DeFeudis, F.V., Balfagon, G., Sagarra, M.R.de.,
    Madtes, P., Somoza, E. and Gervas-Camacho, J.

(1975): Exp. Neurol., 49: 497.
13. DeFeudis, F.V. and Marks, J.H. (1973): Experientia, 29: 1518.
14. DeFeudis, F.V. and Marks, J.H. (1973): Biol. Psychiatr., 6: 85.
15. DeFeudis, F.V., Ojeda, A., Madtes, P. and DeFeudis, P.A. (1975): Naturwissenschaften, 62: 585.
16. DeFeudis, F.V. and Paolino, R.M. (1972): Experientia, 28: 309.
17. DeFeudis, F.V., Paolino, R.M. and DeFeudis, P.A. (1972): In: Fifth International Congress of Pharmacology, San Francisco, abst. n. 318, p.53.
18. DeFeudis, P.A., Paolino, R.M. and DeFeudis, F.V. (1975): Psychopharmacologia, 45: 167.
19. Eddy, N.B. and Leimbach, D. (1953): J. Pharmacol. Exp. Ther., 107: 385. (Cited by Reinis).
20. Essman, W.B. (1972): In: Sleep and the Maturing Nervous System, edited by C.D. Clemente, D.P. Purpura and F.E. Mayer, p. 99, Academic Press, New York.
21. Freedman, D.X. (1968): Federal Probation, June issue.
22. Freedman, D.X. (1970): Postgrad. Med., 47: 110.
23. Freedman, D.X. (1970): Postgrad. Med., 47: 150.
24. Hughes, J. (1975): Brain Res., 88: 295.
25. Katz, D.M. and Steinberg, H. (1972): In: Biochemical and Pharmacological Aspects of Dependence and Reports on Marihuana Research, edited by H.M. van Praag, F. De Erven, and N.V. Bohn, p. 46, Haarlem, Bohn.
26. Lal, H., DeFeo, J.J., Pitterman, A., Patel, G., and Baumel, I. (1972): In: Drug Addiction: Experimental Pharmacology, Vol. 1, p. 255, Futura Publ., Mount Kisco, New York.
27. Reinis, S. (1975): Arch. Int. Pharmacodyn. Ther., 215: 222.
28. Sahakian, B.J., Robbins, T.W., Morgan, M.J. and Iversen, S.D. (1975): Brain Res., 84: 195.
29. Scrafani, J.T. and Clouet, D.H. (1971): In: Narcotic Drugs: Biochemical Pharmacology, edited by D.H. Clouet, p. 137, Plenum Press, New York.
30. Simantov, R., Kuhar, M.J., Pasternak, G.W. and Snyder, S.H. (1976): Brain Res., 106: 189.

31. Simon, E.J. and Groth, J. (1975): Proc. Nat. Acad. Sci., 72: 2404.
32. Snyder, S.H., Pert, C.B. and Pasternak, G.W. (1974): Ann. Int. Med., 81: 534.
33. Spoerlein, M.T. (1968): Pharmacologist, 10: 172. (Cited by Davis and Brister, 1971).
34. Terenius, L. and Wahlstrom, A. (1975): Life. Sci., 16: 1759.
35. Valzelli, L. (1973): Psychopharmacologia, 31: 305.
36. Vedernikov, Y.P. (1970): Psychopharmacologia, 17: 283 (Cited by Davis and Brister, 1971).
37. Welch, A.S. and Welch, B.L. (1971): In: The Physiology of Aggression and Defeat, edited by B.E. Eleftheriou and J.P. Scott, p. 91, Plenum Press, New York.
38. Welch, B.L. (1965): In: Symp. on Medical Aspects of Stress in the Military Climate, edited by D. Mck Rioch, p. 39, U.S. Government Printing Office, Washington, D.C.
39. Welch, B.L. and Welch, A.S. (1973): In: Current Concepts in Amphetamine Abuse, edited by E.H. Ellinwood Jr. and S. Cohen, p. 107, U.S. Government Printing Office, Washington, D.C.
40. Yanai, J. and Ginsburg, B.E. (1976): Psychopharmacologia, 46: 185.

Factors Affecting the Action of Narcotics, edited by
M.L. Adler, L. Manara, and R. Samanin.
Raven Press, New York©1978.

Ambient Temperature and Morphine Action

Joseph Cochin, Carl Rosow, and
Joel Miller

Department of Pharmacology
Boston University School of Medicine
80 East Concord Street
Boston, Massachusetts 02118, U.S.A.

Body temperature change has been recognized as a
morphine effect for over a hundred years, but few investigators have studied it in a systematic fashion.
We became interested in this particular effect for
several reasons: 1. Some of morphine's body temperature
effects have been demonstrated to be centrally mediated,
susceptible to specific blockage by opiate antagonists,
and altered by chronic administration. 2. A few of
our preliminary experiments indicated that temperature
changes occurred at doses barely detectable with analgesic assays, and temperature measurements were made
with relative freedom from observer bias. 3. We wished
to compare temperature effects with data already obtained for analgesia and locomotor activity in the mouse.
It is clear that body temperature is the product of
many interacting physiologic processes and environmental
variables. A drug which interferes with thermoregulation
need not cause any change in body temperature. The
latter depends upon the degree of thermal stress to
which the animal is subjected and the integrity of its
compensatory mechanisms. Theoretically morphine could
be acting peripherally on heat production and heat loss
mechanisms or centrally at hypothalamic centers such as
the preoptic nucleus. For instance, morphine has been
shown to decrease metabolic heat production in mice,
rabbits, and dogs (9). It also affects various heat
loss mechanisms directly such as vasodilatation and
panting. There is little evidence, however, that
morphine actually changes body temperature through a
direct action on any peripheral site. In practice, it
is difficult to predict what a given dose of morphine
will do to body temperature in any particular species,
since its effect depends on the species to which the
drug is administered. Table 1 shows the effects of

631

morphine on temperature in various species reported in the literature.

TABLE 1.   Species Variation in Body Temperature Effect of Morphine

Increase/Decrease	Increase	Decrease
RAT	CAT	DOG
MOUSE	COW	RABBIT
GUINEA PIG	GOAT	PRIMATE
	HORSE	BIRD

Several studies in rats show that low doses of morphine produce hyperthermia while high doses produce hypo-thermia (3). It is often mentioned that the temperature effect is biphasic, that is , a depressant or hypo-thermic phase may be followed by an excitant or hyper-thermic phase. This is especially true in rodents. Hermann (5) showed that the threshold for this change after subcutaneous injection was about 30 mg/kg. This sort of response is not specific for morphine (under appropriate conditions nicotine can produce the same sort of temperature changes) (8).

In the middle and late 1960's much progress was made in elucidating CNS thermoregulatory mechanisms, and morphine was frequently used as a tool in these studies. Foster et al. (1) showed that the quaternary N-methyl derivative of morphine has no effect in the rat when given systematically but produces hypothermia after intrahypothalamic injection. Lotti and Lomax (10,11) showed that morphine produces hypothermia in the rat after intravenous injection or administration directly into the anterior preoptic nucleus. They further demonstrated that intravenous morphine could be antago-nized by intracerebral doses of nalorphine which were far too small to be effective systematically. Lotti showed that in cases where morphine produces a biphasic temperature response, nalorphine antagonizes only the hypothermic phase. In fact, the hyperthermia is fre-quently enhanced in the presence of antagonists. Not only are these two responses differentially susceptible to antagonist blockade, but recent studies indicate that they may be mediated by different sets of neuro-transmitters (2,4,12,14).

There have been few studies of tolerance to the

temperature effects of morphine. In the rabbit, repeated
injections cause attenuation of the hypothermic response. In primates and rats, chronic treament not
only attenuates the drop in temperature, but it
produces a progressively increasing hyperthermia.
Gunne (3) showed that measurement of latency to the peak
of the hyperthermic response is a good indicator of
tolerance in rats, and that it parallels analgesic
tolerance as measured with the hot plate. Finally,
Lomax et al. (7) showed that concomitant intracerebral
administration of morphine and nalorphine blocks the
development of acute tolerance to both analgesic and
hypothermic effects.
    In our preliminary studies in mice, we noted that
the stress of repeated handling caused variations in
baseline body temperature, so our subsequent experiments
were done with a specially designed rubber restraining
collar. Temperatures were measured using an indwelling
rectal thermistor probe. Animals were acclimated in the
chamber for two hours, baseline temperatures were then
recorded, and water or morphine (5,10, or 20 mg/kg) was
injected subcutaneously. Temperature changes were
recorded every 30 minutes for 3 hours. Body temperature
changed only in the morphine groups; but the magnitude
and direction of the changes seemed to vary unpredictably.
We learned later that malfunctioning of our laboratory
air-conditioning system had allowed room temperature
to vary from 21 to 27.5°C during our series of experiments. An animal's actual body temperature at the
time it experienced maximal change from baseline was
correlated with the room temperature measured
simultaneously. Morphine caused an increase in body
temperature when the room was 24°C or warmer and a decrease when the room was less than 24°C. We reproduced
these results by running the experiment in a small
temperature-controlled chamber which consisted of a
coil of copper tubing sandwiched between two steel
cylinders. Cold or hot water pumped through the coil
kept the chamber temperature at 20° or 30°C. The
results confirmed those of our first experiments. Body
temperature and ambient temperature were significantly
correlated (P < .01) in the morphine group.
    The literature in this field contains many contradictory
findings which may be due to careful but arbitrary
control of ambient temperature. That is, two experiments performed at different ambient temperatures may
give opposite results. As far as we know there has
been only one other study of the influence of ambient
temperature on morphine temperature response : Paolino
and Bernard (13) showed that morphine given to rats
caused hypothermia at 5°C and hyperthermia at 32°.

Morphine appears to be altering the relationship between environmental and body temperature by interfering with the animal's capacity to thermoregulate.

Our major series of experiments was designed to test the effects of a wide range of morphine doses at several ambient temperatures. We developed a new type of animal restraint which holds a mouse by the tail and allows it to shiver, groom and posture normally. At the same time we set up a larger temperature-controlled chamber which utilized a wiring harness and multiple switching system to facilitate temperature measurements on 30 or more animals simultaneously. We first established that our new restraint did not impair thermoregulation. Animals injected with water and monitored for 4 1/2 hours showed minimal changes in temperature. The animals were tested weekly for ten weeks at 20 and 30° C. There was no significant change in body temperature on any day, from week to week, or from one ambient temperature to another. In another experiment we established that acute drug effects were not influenced by body weight, age, or prior exposure to the testing apparatus (Fig. 1).

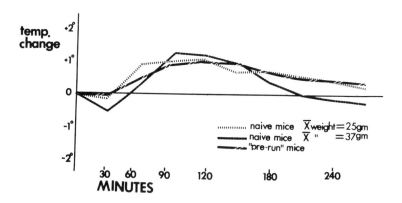

FIG. 1. Effect of a single 10 mg/kg morphine injection to mice in a 20°C ambient temperature. Results are shown for older (37 g), and younger (25 g) animals, and for animals experienced with this procedure ("Pre-run") and inexperienced (naive).

We then measured the effects of 2.5, 10, 40 and 160 mg/kg of morphine at ambient temperatures of 20,25 and 30°C. Temperatures outside of this range proved lethal to many of the animals and thus chronic studies were restricted to 20-30°C. Figure 2 shows the effects of these four morphine doses on naive animals at 20,25, and 30°C. The increase in both hypothermia and hyperthermia is dose related at 25°C. However, at the higher and lower ambient temperatures, the dose-response relationships are partially obscured.

When the dose of morphine is held constant, the effect in a naive animal at 20°C ambient is primarily hypothermia; at 30°C, hyperthermia; and at 25°C, a biphasic response is seen.

Figure 3 shows the effects of 40 mg/kg morphine sulfate at the three ambient temperatures. The effects of the interaction of the drug and temperature are evident.

It would be an oversimplification to say that morphine renders mice poikilothermic, since the drug produces temperature changes in environments close to the thermal neutral point. Neverthless, this temperature range (20-30°C)represents no stress at all to an untreated mouse. Mice injected with water but not morphine are able to hold their body temperature fairly constant for a number of hours at both 20° and 30°C. Even with a dose of 2.5 mg/kg, a dose at which no analgesic effect can be detected on the hot plate, body temperature clearly becomes more susceptible to environmental stresses (Figure 4).

For our studies of tolerance animals were given two injections of morphine daily and tested at weekly intervals. Figure 5 illustrates the development of tolerance to 40 mg/kg at two different ambient temperatures over a six week period. The disappearance of the hypothermic response and the augmentation of the hyperthermia is evident. The trend is toward increasing hyperthermia. After eight weeks of chronic morphine administration (not shown in Figure 5), the hyperthermia began to diminish as well.

At the conclusion of the experiment, after nine weeks of morphine injections, all animals were tested with 160 mg/kg (Figure 6). The changes produced by chronic morphine dosage were reversed by the high dose test, an indication that these changes were in fact tolerance.

There is another interesting change which occurs with chronic administration. Naive mice given a high dose of morphine return to baseline temperatures in 4-5 hours. After 14 injections (one week) they are no longer able to make this adjustment. Over subsequent weeks of testing, body temperatures at the end of the 4 1/2-hour experiment more closely approximated control readings.

This phenomenon could be some cumulative or toxic effect of morphine to which tolerance developed only slowly.

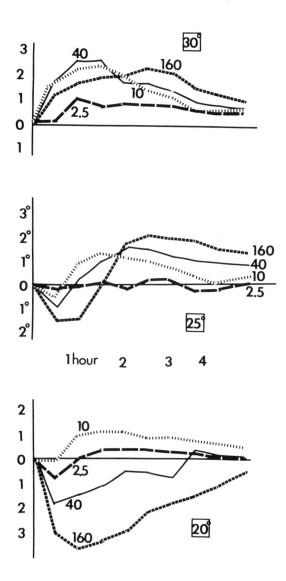

FIG. 2. Acute effect of morphine on mouse rectal temperature at three different ambient temperatures (30°, 25°, 20°C). At each ambient temperature, separate groups of mice were given 2.5, 10, 40 or 160 mg/kg morphine sulfate.

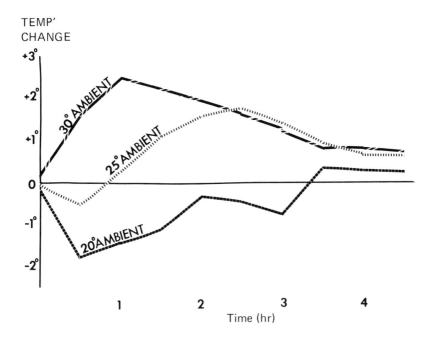

FIG 3. Mouse rectal temperature change after 40 mg/
kg morphine sulfate at 20°, 25°, or 30° C ambient
temperature.

In another group of experiments, we examined the
lethal effects of morphine and temperature stress using the method of Litchfield and Wilcoxon (6).Morphine
LD50's were determined in naive mice at various ambient
temperatures. As expected, even moderate heat or cold
stress markedly reduces the acute morphine LD50. In
order to evaluate the effect of chronic administration
in the interaction between morphine and temperature
stress, LD50's were determined using mice pretreated
with 14 injections (one week) of either 40 or 80 mg/kg
of morphine. The lethal interaction of morphine and
temperature stress appears to be unaffected by one
week of morphine pretreatment.
    We are now undertaking a series of experiments to
clarify these observations. It is not suprising to us
that tolerance to the lethal interaction of morphine
and stressfully high or low temperatures develops
slowly, if at all. Many of the papers published in the
early part of this century were attempts to demonstrate
tolerance to the lethal effects of morphine, and most
showed that such tolerance was extremely difficult to

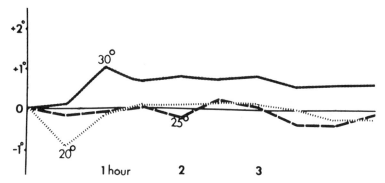

FIG. 4.   Effect of 2.5 mg/kg morphine sulfate on
mouse rectal temperature in ambient temperatures of
20°, 25°,and 30°C.

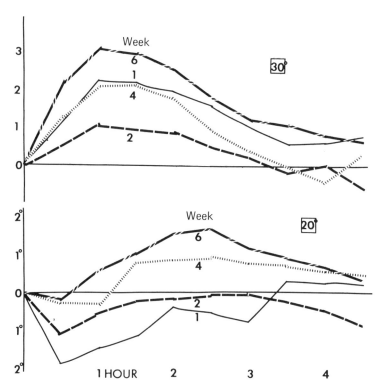

FIG. 5.   Mouse rectal temperature effect of chronic
administration of 40 mg/kg morphine sulfate twice daily.
Results are shown for tests done on weeks 1,2,4 and
6 at ambient temperatures of 20° and 30°C.

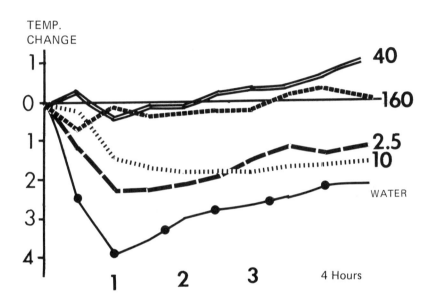

FIG. 6.   Tolerance to the temperature effect of a 160 mg/kg morphine sulfate test dose after nine weeks of pretreatment.   Pretreatment consisted of twice-daily injections of morphine sulfate 2.5, 10 , 40 or 160 mg/kg.   Control group was injected twice daily with water.

demonstrate, especially in rodents.

In summary, this work is the beginning of an in-depth evaluation of the effect of one element of the environment, namely, ambient temperature, on a response to morphine. We originally chose body temperature as the response to be measured for reasons that were not associated with investigations of the interaction of environment and morphine. We had been looking at body temperature as a sensitive measure of drug effect, tolerance and dependence. Although body temperature is a sensitive measure of drug effect, it may be extremely sensitive to the complicated interaction with environment.

Other morphine responses, locomotor activity, for instance, may demonstrate a complex interaction with ambient temperature, and this may explain many of the puzzling and seemingly contradictory results reported in the literature.

ACKNOWLEDGEMENT

This work was supported in part by Research Grants #R 01-DA-00016 and P 01-DA-00257 from the National Institute on Drug Abuse.

REFERENCES

1. Foster, R.S., Jenden, D.J., and Lomax, P. (1967) : J. Pharmacol. Exp. Ther., 157 : 185.
2. Fuller, R.W., and Baker, J.C. (1974) : Res. Commun. Chem. Pathol. Pharmacol., 8 : 715.
3. Gunne, L.M. (1960) : Arch. Int. Pharmacodyn. Ther., 129 : 416.
4. Haubrich, D.R., and Blake, D.E. (1971) : Life Sci., 10 : 175.
5. Hermann, J.B. (1942) : J. Pharmacol. Exp. Ther., 76: 309.
6. Litchfield, J.T.,Jr., and Wilcoxon, F. (1949) : J. Pharmacol. Exp. Ther. , 96 : 99.
7. Lomax, P., and Kirkpatrick, W.E.(1967):Med.Pharmacol. Exp., 16 : 165.
8. Lomax, P., and Knox, G.V. (1973) : In : The Pharmacology of Thermoregulation edited by E.Schoenbaum and P. Lomax, p. 146, Karger Press, Basle.
9. Lotti, V.J. (1973) : In : The Pharmacology of Thermoregulation edited by E. Schoenbaum and

P. Lomax, p. 382, Karger Press, Basle.
10. Lotti,V.J., Lomax, P., and George, R. (1965) : J.
    Pharmacol. Exp. Ther., 150 : 135.
11. Lotti,V.J., Lomax, P., and George, R. (1965) : J.
    Pharmacol. Exp. Ther., 150 : 420.
12. Oka, T., Nozaki, M., and Hosoya, E. (1972) : J.
    Pharmacol. Exp. Ther., 180 : 136.
13. Paolini, R.M., and Bernard, B.K. (1968) : Life Sci.
    7 : 857.
14. Warwick, R.O., Blake, D.E., Miya, T.S. and Bousquet,
    W.F. (1973) : Res. Commun. Chem. Pathol. Pharmacol.
    6 : 19.

Factors Affecting the Action of Narcotics, edited by
M.L. Adler, L. Manara, and R. Samanin.
Raven Press, New York ©1978.

Influence of Environmental Stimuli Associated with Narcotic Administration on Narcotic Actions and Dependence

H. Lal, S. Miksic, and R. Drawbaugh

Department of Pharmacology and Toxicology
and
Department of Psychology, University of Rhode Island
Kingston, RI 02881, U.S.A.

INTRODUCTION

It has now become evident that environments intimately associated with the administration and resulting pharmacological actions of narcotic drugs are important in determining the future actions and potential of these drugs.   Such environments are also believed to be determining factors in acquisition and maintenance of drug-seeking behavior, as well as relapse to drug abuse (22, 27, 40).   The environment can influence drug action in many ways.   This paper is devoted to the consideration of environments as conditional stimuli.

As early as the first part of this century, workers in Pavlov's laboratory observed (34) that salient environmental events routinely paired with morphine injections gradually became effective themselves in eliciting salivation and vomiting in dogs.   Those observations of Pavlov were subsequently replicated and confirmed by others (1, 7, 14, 43).

In the past decade interest has been renewed in the study of environmental contingencies which interact with drug actions.   This interest was stimulated by a constantly escalating problem of drug abuse and inadequacies of present treatment methods.   Some of the recent studies concerning conditional aspects of environments related to narcotic drugs will be reviewed in this paper.   Similar studies with barbiturates

643

(36) and CNS stimulants (18) have been described
elsewhere, and others were reviewed at a **symposium**
(40).

Administration of narcotic drugs produces a variety
of physiological changes in the body.   Certain
environmental events termed conditional stimuli (CS)
acquire a property of eliciting those drug-like actions by themselves when systematically paired with
the drug-elicited physiological and psychological
changes.   Thereafter, previously neutral environments
do not remain neutral, but begin to produce pharmacological actions of narcotics without actual administration of a drug.   This phenomenon has been termed
"conditioning of drug action".

ACUTE ACTIONS OF NARCOTICS

Hyperthermia

Narcotic drugs produce a bipasic effect on rectal
temperature.   A very short-lived hypothermia, initially produced, is followed by pronounced hyperthermia which lasts for the duration of the drug action.
High doses produce only hypothermia, as is illustrated
in Fig. 1.   The initial hypothermia can be detected
only if morphine is injected intravenously, as shown
in Table 1, or given intracerebrally as described by
Lotti et al. (26).   After chronic administration,
only the hyperthermic action of narcotics can be
detected, as is shown in Fig.2.   Also, tolerance does
not develop to the hyperthermic action of narcotics.
Inspecting the data in Fig. 3, we see that a constant
dose of morphine produces similar hyperthermia after
a single dose, or after multiple administrations.
Only the time of onset of hyperthermia is reduced by
chronic administration.

Because of a lack of tolerance to the hyperthermic
action of morphine, it offers an excellent opportunity
for using a large number of repeated injections, which
are necessary for pairings with specific environmental
events in conditioning experiments.   In our research,
either a bell sound, a tone, or anise odor was paired
with each morphine injection. These stimuli were found
neutral before **pairing.** In other words, they did
not cause hyperthermia when presented to naive rats,

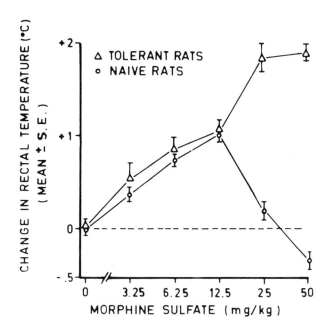

FIG. 1. Dose-response curve for morphine's effects
on rectal temperature in naive and morphine tolerant
rats   Temperature responses to morphine were recorded at one hour following injection.   Each dose was
administered to different groups, each consisting of
9-18 rats.   Morphine-induced hyperthermia was
statistically significant in tolerant subjects for all
doses tested (p < 0.01).   Naive rats showed significantly lower temperatures when compared with tolerant
rats at 25 and 50 mg/kg.

or rats in which morphine was administered without
systematic pairings with these stimuli.   For example
data summarized in Table 2 show that the bell sound,
as well as handling, did not produce any change in the
rectal temperature of rats previously treated with
two daily injections of morphine sulfate for 15 days.
The rectal temperature before the bell sound was lower

TABLE 1. Acute action of morphine, injected intravenously, on rectal temperature in the rat

Dose, Morphine mg/kg	N[1]	Pre-injection Temperature	Temperature change (°C) Mean ± S.E.		
			Saline	Morphine-induced Hypothermia[2]	Morphine-induced hyperthermia[3]
2.5	4	37.80 ±0.20	+ 0.12 ± 0.04	- 0.22 ± 0.02 (8 ± 2)	+ 0.90 ± 0.25 (70 ± 20)
10.0	3	37.27 ±0.39	+ 0.03 ± 0.03	- 0.43 ± 0.19 (41 ± 14)	+ 0.97 ± 0.28 (116 ± 4)
20.0	2	37.50 ±0.20	+ 0.08 ± 0.23	- 2.25 ± 0.75 (105 ± 5)	not achieved (> 120)

1 Number of observations

2 Maximal magnitude of hypothermia observed following morphine. Number in parentheses indicates the time after morphine (Mean ± S.E., minutes) when maximal effect occurred.

3. Maximal magnitude of hyperthermia observed following morphine. Number in parentheses indicates the time after morphine (Mean ± S.E., minutes) when maximal effect occurred.

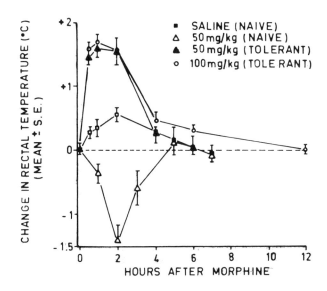

FIG. 2.   Time course of morphine's effect on rectal
temperature in naive and morphine-tolerant rats
Each group consisted of 9-18 rats.   In tolerant
subjects both 50 and 100 mg/kg produced hyperthermia
significantly different ($p < 0.01$ at 0.5, 1 and 2 hrs)
from that induced by saline, while 50 mg/kg in naive
subjects produced a significant hypothermia ($p < 0.05$
at 1 hr; $p < 0.01$ at 2 hrs).

TABLE 2.   Elicitation of morphine hyperthermia by a
            conditional bell sound

Pairing Condition	Test Condition	Pre-Exposure Temperature	Change after Exposure	P
Morphine	Handling	37.3 ± 0.03	−0.10	N.S.
	Bell Sound	37.3 ± 0.05	−0.01	N.S.
Morphine/ Bell Sound	Handling Bell Sound	37.3 ± 0.07 37.2 ± 0.04	+0.05 +0.82	N.S. 0.05

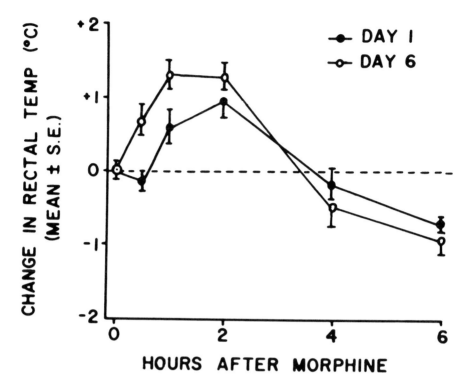

FIG. 3.   Effect of morphine (20 mg/kg) on rectal
temperature in 10 rats treated daily for six days
The hyperthermic responses produced at .5 hr and 1 hr.
on day 6 are significantly greater than those
recorded on day 1 ($p < 0.01$, $p < 0.05$, respectively).

----

than usual, which is an indicator of narcotic
withdrawal (11).   Handling itself did not cause any
hyperthermia in rats for whom the bell sound was
paired with each morphine injection.   However,
exposure to the bell sound alone elicited a hyperthermia of 0.83° C.   This magnitude of hyperthermia was
equal to that produced by an injection of morphine
sulfate at doses of 5-15 mg/kg in similarly treated
rats as is shown in Fig. 1.   This experiment has
been replicated (8, 9, 23, 37).

   From the above experiments it can be concluded that
an environmental event such as an auditory stimulus,
which is neutral in itself, can acquire properties of

a CS when it is systematically paired with morphine injections. The CS-induced hyperthermia is seen only in animals exposed to the bell sound paired with each morphine injection. When naive rats are exposed to the bell sound, no significant change in rectal temperature is seen. No significant hyperthermic response is seen in a group of rats exposed to an equal number of bell presentations given at random intervals on days when morphine injections are being given or in another group injected with morphine without any exposure to the bell stimulus.

In another experiment (31) a tone was used as an environmental event paired with each morphine injection. Rectal temperature of a group of rats was measured daily for 5 days, 30 min after handling which included a saline injection. Following these 5 days, all rats were injected daily with one i.p. dose (20 mg/kg) of morphine sulfate. Immediately following this injection the rats were taken into a sound-attenuated chamber where they were exposed to a tone for 2 hr (conditioning trial) on trial 8,10,14,23 and 61, rectal temperature was measured both before the morphine injection and 30 min after the initiation of tone. On trial 19, 28, and 68, only saline was injected before the tone, and temperature was measured 30 min after tone initiation. From trial 75 onward, morphine injections were discontinued and only saline injections preceded the tone (extinction trials). Before conditioning, as shown in Fig. 4, handling and saline injection produced some hypothermia. After conditioning, each morphine injection caused hyperthermia in all rats. Following the conditioning period a saline injection paired with tone also elicited hyperthermia. This CS-elicited hyperthermia was extinguished in 7 extinction trials. All of these effects were statistically significant.

In order to establish that the CS property of mimicking a morphine action is not limited to auditory stimuli, we also tested an olfactory stimulus for its "conditionability" with respect to morphine hyperthermia (23). Rats were exposed to systematic pairings of anise odor and injections of morphine sulfate (10 mg/kg). The odor exposure was begun 5 min before

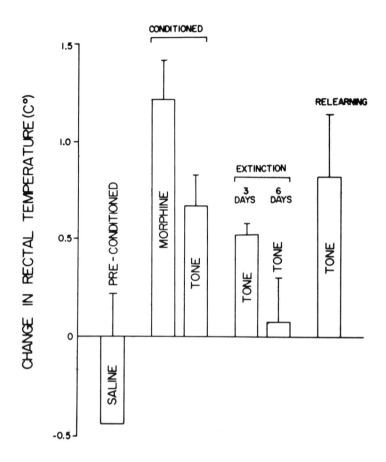

FIG. 4.   Effect of morphine and a conditional
auditory stimulus on rectal temperature of rats
Data are expressed as Mean (± S.E.) of 5 subjects.
A pre-conditioning treatment of handling and a saline
injection caused some hypothermia.   During conditioning and prior to the relearning test morphine
injections were paired with tone.   During extinction
trials tone was presented without a morphine injection.
  Adapted from Miksic et al. (**31**).

and continued until 25 min after, each injection.
The CS effect was measured after 13, 24, and 35
pairings, as described above.   Data summarized in
Table 3 show that exposure of these subjects to anise
odor alone elicited conditional hyperthermia, as did
morphine injections in the other test trials.
Again, the anise odor itself was neutral in naive rats
or rats in which it was not previously paired with
morphine injections.

TABLE 3.   Elicitation of hyperthermia by an olfactory
            conditioned stimulus

	Rectal Temperature (°C), Mean + S.E.		
	Pre-CS	Post-CS	Change
No treatment	37.3 + 0.06	37.4 + 0.07	+ 0.03
Anise odor	37.4 + 0.07	38.2 + 0.08	+ 0.78

Hyperglycemia and Elevation of Striatal Homovanillic Acid

We have recently begun studies on the measurement
of morphine induced biochemical changes which are
susceptible to conditional alteration by an environmental stimulus.   In the experiments completed to
date, we have employed an environmental event paired
with each morphine injection.   As described before,
each injection of morphine sulfate was paired with
a 30 min exposure to anise odor.   After 40 pairings
the rats were exposed to anise odor alone and
sacrificed for the biochemical measures.   Data summarized in Table 4 show serum glucose levels of
various groups of rats. As is seen, hyperglycemia in a
morphine-elicited action to which rapid tolerance is
developed.   A single dose of morphine caused a 40%
increase in blood glucose, but after 5 injections of

morphine, doses up to 80 mg/kg were ineffective.

TABLE 4.   Effect of a conditional stimulus and morphine injections on serum glucose in the rat

Experimental Group	Treatment	Serum Glucose (mg/100 ml)
Naive Rats	Saline	99 ± 4
	Morphine sulfate 20 mg/kg	140 ± 5
Tolerant Rats	Morphine sulfate	
	20 mg/kg	98 ± 8
	80 mg/kg	104 ± 11
	160 mg/kg	122 ± 9
Conditioned Rats	Handling	102 ± 3
	Anise Odor	120 ± 6

A dose of 160 mg/kg was required to cause a 25% increase in serum glucose. It is also seen that there was approximately a 20% increase in blood glucose after exposure to anise odor in rats for whom anise odor was paired with each morphine injection for 40 trials.   To our knowledge this is the first evidence that a biochemical action of morphine can be conditioned.   Following our success with hyperglycemia we extended our studies to the conditioning of morphine-elicited elevation of homovanillic acid (HVA).   It is seen that morphine sulfate increases striatal HVA at a dose of 10 mg/kg (Table 5). The significance of this action has been previously discussed (16, 25).   To determine the "conditionability" of morphine-elicited HVA, morphine injections were paired with anise odor as described before. After a sufficient number of pairings, the action of anise odor itself was tested.   As seen from data given in Table 5, exposure to anise odor elicited elevation of striatal HVA, a metabolite of brain dopamine.   These data are similar to those recently reported by Perez-Cruet (35), who used a bell sound paired with methadone injection.

TABLE 5.   Effectiveness of olfactory conditional
            stimulus in eliciting elevation of striatal
            homovanillic acid

Experimental Groups	Treatment		Striated HVA µg/g
	Drug	mg/kg	
Naive rats	Saline	–	0.45 ± 0.03
	Morphine	10 mg/kg	0.73 ± 0.05
		100 mg/kg	0.85 ± 0.08
Conditioned Rats	Handling	–	0.45 ± 0.01
	Anise odor	–	0.59 ± 0.03

CONDITIONING OF CHRONIC ACTIONS OF NARCOTICS

Reduction of Withdrawal Signs

One of the important actions of narcotic drugs is alleviation of narcotic withdrawal signs which provides a relatively withdrawal-free state.   It was suggested (37) that stimuli which regularly accompany the withdrawal-blocking action of narcotics may gradually acquire conditional properties of producing such blockade without the actual administration of a narcotic.   We tested this hypothesis systematically by pairing well-defined environmental stimuli with morphine injections which unconditionally eliminate narcotic withdrawal signs.

Auditory Stimuli

We have completed several experiments in which hypothermia induced by morphine withdrawal was

alleviated by a CS consisting of a bell sound.
In these experiments rats were given two equally
spaced injections of morphine sulfate daily, each
injection being paired with a bell-produced auditory
stimulus of 1-min duration (for procedural details,
see Drawbaugh and Lal (9)). The morphine dose was
increased gradually to 100-mg/kg injections.   The CS
effect on rectal temperature was measured during
withdrawal from morphine.   The data from 8 different
experiments are summarized in Table 6.

TABLE 6.   Effectiveness of a conditional stimulus in
alleviating morphine withdrawal hypothermia
in eight experiments[1]

| Replications | Rectal Temperature (°C) mean ± S.E.[2] | | |
	Pre-CS	Post-CS	Change
1	37.40 ± 0.09	38.06 ± 0.06	0.69 ± 0.14
2	37.00 ± 0.08	38.04 ± 0.06	1.00 ± 0.11
3	37.39 ± 0.09	38.06 ± 0.04	0.70 ± 0.07
4	37.23 ± 0.06	38.17 ± 0.08	0.93 ± 0.13
5	37.18 ± 0.09	38.11 ± 0.16	0.93 ± 0.14
6	37.31 ± 0.03	38.03 ± 0.08	0.82 ± 0.08
7	37.11 ± 0.07	37.87 ± 0.08	0.76 ± 0.10
8	37.12 ± 0.10	37.84 ± 0.09	0.76 ± 0.14

[1] In each experiment   rats were made morphine-
dependent.   The temperature was measured at 24 hr
of withdrawal.   After Pre-CS measurement, they were
exposed to the CS of bell sound and, 30 min later,
a second measurement was taken.

[2] Based on 6 rats per group.

After withdrawal hypothermia was measured in each rat,
all subjects were exposed to either the auditory CS, a
morphine injection, or no treatment.   The withdrawal

hypothermia was reversed by either the CS or morphine. The morphine injection also produced a characteristic hyperthermia. The CS-induced alleviation of withdrawal hypothermia was seen only in animals which were previously exposed to the pairing of the bell sound with morphine injections. When naive rats were exposed to the auditory stimulus no change in rectal temperatures was seen. Also, a group of rats exposed to an equal number of random bell sound presentations on the days of morphine treatment, as well as another group made morphine-dependent with no exposure to bell sound, did not show any reversal of withdrawal hypothermia in response to the auditory stimulus during withdrawal testing.

The periodic occurrence of "wet-dog"-like body shakes is a characteristic sign of morphine withdrawal in experimental animals (11). Recently, a tone was used as a CS to reduce such withdrawal shakes (32). In these experiments, i.v. injections of morphine were paired with a tone. After several pairings, the tone acquired CS properties and was able to significantly reduce body shakes. These data are illustrated in Table 7.

TABLE 7. Reduction of Morphine-Withdrawal Shakes by a Conditional Stimulus and a Morphine Injection

Test Treatment	N[1]	Withdrawal Shakes % Change
None	40	+ 14 ± 6
Conditional Tone	52	− 32 ± 3
Morphine (15 mg/kg)	38	− 82 ± 3

[1]Number of observations.

Recently, Tye and Iverson (42) also found that a tone paired with morphine injections was able to relieve

inhibition of operant responding during morphine
withdrawal.   This observation was somewhat similar
to that reported by Thompson and Schuster (41) in
addicted monkeys.

Olfactory Stimulus

Earlier we discussed the finding that a CS of
anise odor is effective in eliciting morphine action
in a variety of situations. Because of its effectiveness in other situations, we selected this as a
conditional stimulus to reduce withdrawal signs in
morphine-dependent rats.   These rats were allowed
to experience 12 hr of withdrawal, then they were
placed in glass jars containing anise odor.   After
remaining in the jar for 5 min, while experiencing
withdrawal, the rats were removed one by one, injected
with morphine, and returned to the environment
containing anise odor where they remained for another
25 min.   After each morphine-anise pairing the rats
were returned to their home cages.   Following a
predetermined number of such pairings, all rats were
tested for CS effects of anise odor.   As expected,
a test exposure to anise odor reduced all signs of
withdrawal.   Anise odor was not effective in rats
not previously exposed to morphine-anise pairings,
or in other groups where the exposure was at random.
The alleviation of withdrawal hypothermia and
withdrawal shakes, as seen in this experiment, is
important because these signs are easily quantified
and objectively measurable (11).

Social Stimuli

Aggression is a socially relevant behavior which
is seen in a variety of animal species undergoing
narcotic withdrawal (15).   This aggression has been
considered a valid animal analogue of socio-pathic
behavior often observed in heroin addicts.   As
narcotic drugs are known to reduce aggressive
behaviors in naive and morphine-withdrawn animals.
(20), the effectiveness of social stimuli as a CS
for elicitation of the anti-aggressive action of

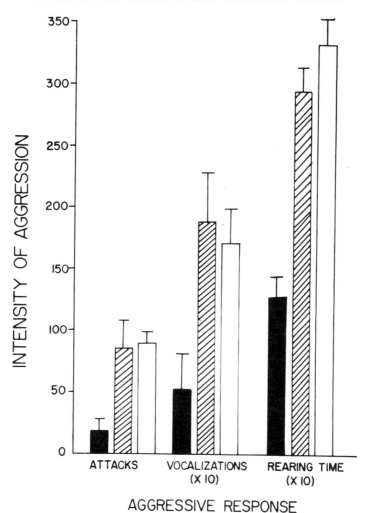

FIG. 5. <u>Aggressive behavior of rats made morphine</u>
<u>dependent and withdrawn 72 hr before measurement</u>
Attacks are number of approaches resulting in attacks
and/or bites. Vocalizations are number of occurrences.
Rearing time is duration in seconds of a 60-min
measurement period. Data are mean ± S.E., based on 5
groups for each treatment. Solid bars show data of
conditioned rats for whom each morphine injection was
paired with 30 min of grouping. The hatched bar
represents data of socially isolated subjects. The
open bars show data of rats housed continuously in
groups of four. Adapted from Miksic et al. (30).

narcotics was investigated (30).

In this experiment, rats were injected with morphine sulfate in the presence of other rats. At the time of morphine injection the rats were placed together for 30 min. After 40 pairings the rats were allowed to experience spontaneous withdrawal for 72 hr and were then tested for response to the social CS. The results are summarized in Figure 5. Without any treatment, as expected from previous experiments (24), all rats showed withdrawal aggression. The intensity of aggression in two control groups was similar. The rats which were constantly grouped during the pre-withdrawal period did not differ from those socially isolated and similarly handled. However, rats which were grouped only for the 30 min during which they received drug injections showed far less aggression when subsequently grouped. This is seen consistently in every measure of aggression including vocalization, rearing posture, attacks, and bites.

Induction of Psychologically Perceived Stimuli

Narcotic-Induced Discriminable Stimuli

A property of narcotic analgesics which is intimately related to abuse liability is the euphoria typically produced by these drugs (for discussion, see Lal (17)). There is insufficient parametric data to define clearly narcotic euphoria. It is considered to be a CNS-mediated action subjectively perceived as a feeling of "unusual well-being" that is incommensurate with the objective reality of the situation. Another property of this euphoria is the production of an obsessive drug-seeking behavior (or drive state) requiring periodic or continuous administration of a drug to produce pleasure and avoid deprivation discomfort. According to Eddy et al. (10) "this mental state is the most powerful of all the factors involved in chronic intoxication with psychotropic drugs: with certain types of drugs it may be the only factor involved, even in most intense craving and perpetuation of compulsive abuse".

It has often been postulated that the environments in which narcotic euphoria is experienced gradually become a critical factor in the continuous abuse of narcotics, and also in promoting the well-known relapse of ex-addicts to heroin abuse (22, 27, 43). A likely explanation of these observations can be provided if experimental data can be found to show that the environment can acquire a CS property of aliciting morphine euphoria.   However, experimental demonstration of euphoria elicited by a CS is difficult because an objective measure of such a euphoric action in laboratory animals has not been available.

Recently, it was shown that narcotics produce discriminable stimuli (DS) which can control discrimination behavior in laboratory animals (3, 5, 12, 38, 39).   In these experiments, rats were trained to perform one of two different responses, the selection of which was based entirely upon pretreatment with either a narcotic or the drug vehicle.   Following sufficient training, the rats reliably discriminate narcotics from non-narcotic analgesics or other drugs (13, 21).   It was subsequently proposed (3, 5, 12, 38, 39) that the DS thus produced reflect a specific action of narcotics which is subjectively perceived, and may, therefore, provide an indirect measure of narcotic euphoria.   This suggestion was based upon several lines of evidence (for review, see 6, 21). DS associated with narcotics generalize to all narcotics, but not to any non-narcotic drug (2, 4, 13).   Narcotic antagonists block and reverse the DS produced by narcotics (4, 13).The DS are not produced by peripheral actions of narcotics (3,12) and they are not mimicked by non-narcotic psychoactive drugs (13). Also, tolerance develops to the narcotic DS (29, 39), but it is of far lower order than tolerance to analgesia.   The narcotic DS can be perceived even when analgesia is reduced to subthreshold level by tolerance development (29).   With these data available, we undertook to investigate "conditionability" of the morphine DS in order to provide additional information on the role of environment in elicitation of morphine euphoria. (28).

We trained rats to press one lever after they were

injected with morphine, and an alternate lever when
injected with saline, as described before (12, 13).
Once adequately trained, these rats reliably demonstrated morphine-saline discrimination by pressing either
the morphine-appropriate or saline-appropriate lever
on the test days.   Here, when they were injected
with either morphine, methadone, or fentanyl, they
emitted the morphine-appropriate response.   Likewise,
they selected the saline-appropriate lever when
injected with any of the non-narcotic drugs (for
details, see 21) or when exposed to an olfactory
environmental stimulus consisting of anise odor.
All rats were then given systematic exposures to
morphine-anise pairing.   Twice a day they were injected with morphine, and each injection was paired
with 30-min exposure to anise odor as described above.
During those pairings, they were not allowed any
experience in the behavioral chambers where they were
originally trained.   After a predetermined number of
pairings, each rat was tested for morphine-saline
lever selection after a pre-test exposure either to
anise odor alone, or to no odor and no injection of
morphine.   As described in Fig. 6, these rats
emitted morphine-appropriate responses after exposure
to anise odor, thus suggesting a CS property of anise
odor in eliciting a morphine-associated DS.
The acquisition of a conditional discrimination of the
morphine stimulus depended upon the number of pairings
administered.   Complete acquisition (100% of
subjects responding on the morphine-appropriate lever
after exposure) was accomplished after 45 pairings of
anise odor with morphine injections.   These data
provide an original laboratory demonstration to show
that environments in which morphine injections are
allowed to elicit a subjectively perceived stimulus
acquire a conditional property of eliciting subjective
effects of narcotics without actual drug injection.

Secondary Reinforcing Property

Morphine administration has been shown to act as a
primary reinforcer for both dependent and naive
animals.   It is also known that a stimulus, when

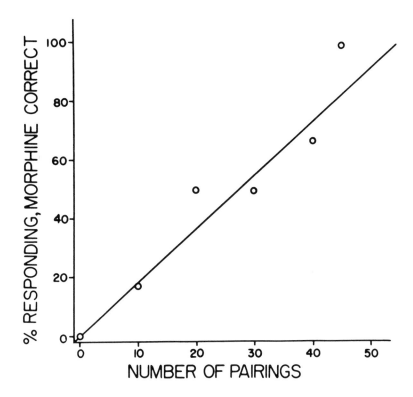

FIG. 6. Selection of morphine-appropriate lever by discrimination trained subjects following exposure to anise odor and a saline injection, as a function of pre-trial anise odor-morphine pairings   Each point represents the proportion of total subjects tested who responded on the drug-appropriate lever (21).

repeatedly paired with a primary reinforcer, can acquire some of the motivational properties of that reinforcer and therefore can be designated as a secondary reinforcer.   Since we have already established that stimuli paired with morphine injections come to be conditional stimuli for morphine-like actions, we employed this approach to determine if our stimuli had acquired properties of a secondary reinforcer.   In the first experiment we measured lever

pressing for a previously established CS for morphine-
dependent rats.   We found that the bell sound used as
the CS was aversive to all rats irrespective of
whether they were previously conditioned to it or not.
Apparently the loudly ringing bell in a closed chamber
was so aversive that secondary reinforcing properties,
if any, were masked.   We than employed a Y-maze and
a soft tone as the secondary reinforcer.   Rats were
trained to run to one arm of the maze for morphine
injections paired with a tone.   After the correct
response was well established, extinction trials were
run.   During extinction, half of the subjects
received neither morphine nor tone as a consequence of
a correct response, while the other half received the
tone but no morphine.   The rats receiving the tone
during extinction required significantly more trials
to reach the extinction criteria than those rats not
receiving tone presentations.   Extinction with the
tone also facilitated relearning of the maze response.
These data support the view that a stimulus accompanying morphine administration acquired the properties
of a secondary reinforcer (33).

MECHANISMS OF ENVIRONMENTAL INTERACTION

Conditional Stimulus Effects

As illustrated in previous sections, environmental
events consistently paired with the actions of
narcotic drugs acquire certain pharmacological
properties of those drugs in the form of conditional
stimuli.   Thereafter, as conditional stimuli, they
usually elicit physiological changes resembling the
drug action, although effects counter to the drug
action may also result (36).   These physiological
changes then interact with the acute action of drug
and may alter the characteristics of its actions.

Role of Biogenic Amines

The biological mechanisms underlying the elicitation of physiological effects by drug-related
conditional stimuli have not been fully investigated.

It is likely that prior to the behavioral observation of final drug action certain neuropathways are stimulated or inhibited.   To pinpoint these pathways we employed conventional stimulators and inhibitors of well-known neurotransmitter actions.   Each of those drugs was injected before an injection of morphine sulfate or application of a conditional stimulus which had earlier been shown effective in eliciting hyperthermia resembling a similar action of morphine. Following pretreatment with a ganglionic blocking agent (mecamylamine) an alpha-adrenergic blocking agent (phenoxybenzamine), a dopaminergic blocking drug (haloperidol), or an anticholinergic drug (benztropine) the action of the CS was blocked.   A blocker of serotonin receptors (cyproheptadine) or a blocker of beta-adrenergic receptors (propranolol) was ineffective in blocking the CS action.   In contrast, the hyperthermic action of morphine was blocked by pretreatment with mecamylamine, phenoxybenzamine, and cyproheptadine, but not by haloperidol, benztropine, or propranolol.   These data were recently reported and discussed in greater detail (9).

It is clear that morphine-induced hyperthermia is produced through activation of a neural network which inclused alpha-adrenergic and serotonergic receptors.   The CS elicited hyperthermia involved stimulation of alpha-adrenergic receptors and dopaminergic receptors.

Role of Endorphins

Endorphin is a name given to the naturally occurring substances which mimic many actions of narcotic drugs.   The presence of these substances in mammalian brain has been reported by many workers (for review, see 19).   One likely mechanism for the elicitation of CS effect is the release of an endorphin which produces a morphine-like action.   At present, direct methods to measure the release of endorphin are not available.   It is known, however, that the actions of the endorphins are blocked by naloxone, a specific narcotic antagonist.   We took advantage of this property of endorphins in order to study the interactions between a morphine-related CS and naloxone, both tested in the absence of any endogenously injected narcotics.   It was found that CS-related hyperthermia (8, 23) and reduction of body shakes induced by morphine withdrawal Lal and Numan, to be published, were effectively blocked by naloxone in a dose-dependent manner.   Unless hitherto unknown, direct effects of naloxone in blocking hyperthermia and motor disorders can be shown, the only plausible interpretation of these data are that the CS acquires an ability to cause release of an endorphin during its pairing with morphine injections.   The release of this endorphin then causes morphine-like actions in the absence of a morphine injection.

SIGNIFICANCE IN RESEARCH AND CLINICAL PRACTICE

The significance of findings such as those reported above lies in many areas of research and clinical practice.   Some of them are outlined below.

Conditioning of Drug Effects

In psychology most conditioning studies are limited to the conditioning of physiological reflexes and autonomic responses.   New studies with drugs open a novel field of investigation that consists of conditioning of drug actions.   Since drug actions differ in several respects from the naturally occurring physiological responses, study of their conditioning may reveal new conditioning principles and their applications in many disease states.

Narcotic Abuse

Biological reasons for continuous narcotic abuse are not fully understood.   Once the initial behavior of drug seeking is acquired, its continuation depends upon several factors.   Among them are included several environmental factors.   The data reviewed in this paper show that certain environments associated with drug administration become established as conditional stimuli.   Thereafter, the availability of such environments as CS promotes resistence to extinction of drug-seeking behavior at times when the actual drug is not available. This can also be the basis for the effectiveness of placebo in the narcotic abusers.

The other reason for continuous abuse of a narcotic drug is that it is the only method available to avoid withdrawal sickness. The demonstration that a CS in the environment can reduce intensity of withdrawal sickness suggests that it can be usefully employed in the treatment of narcotic dependence. Use of actual narcotics for this purpose will be expected to perpetuate the neuropathology of dependence. At the same time, the above data also suggest that, for long-lasting, effective therapy, counter-conditioning of the environmental CS must be included in a total therapeutic approach.

Our work has shown that the social environment of a narcotic abuser can act as a conditional stimulus. This finding explains the fact that many rehabilitation centers find it advantageous to employ ex-addicts to participate in the treatment process. Here the ex-addicts may serve as CS to which extinction is produced during therapy.

Psychosomatic Diseases

The strong conditioning components seen with morphine dependence and withdrawal may also be present in many other illnesses. The results from such studies offer a new approach to investigation of psychosomatic illness. The conditioning of neurochemical processes are particularly interesting in this respect.

Treatment of Pain

We presented data to show that the environmental stimuli once associated with injections of a narcotic may be able to release endogenous morphine-like substances. Although analgesic properties of these substances are not yet known, it is likely that their release can be employed to produce analgesia. In this way a non-drug procedure to control pain may be found.

ACKNOWLEDGEMENTS

The research reported in this paper was supported
by Grant DA 00418 from National Institute of Drug
Abuse, Dept. of Health, Education and Welfare and a
Public Health Service Fellowship 1F31-DA 05069.
We thank Mrs. Elda Pellerin for secretarial assistance

REFERENCES

1. Collins, K., and Tatum, A. (1925): Am. J. Physiol.
74: 14.
2. Colpaert, F.C. (1977): Life Sci., 16: 717-728.
3. Colpaert, F.C., Lal, H., Niemegeers, C.J.E., and
Janssen, P.A.J. (1975): Life Sci., 16: 705-716.
4. Colpaert, F.C., Niemegeers, C.J.E., and Janssen,
P.A.J. (1976): J. Pharmacol. Exp. Ther., 197:
180-187.
5. Colpaert, F.C., Niemegeers, C.J.E., and Janssen,
P.A.J. (1976): Psychopharmacologia, 46: 169-177.
6. Colpaert, F.C., Niemegeers, C.J.E., and Janssen,
P.A.J. (1976): Arch. Int. Pharmacodyn. Ther.,
220: 329-332.
7. Crisler, G. (1930): Am. J. Physiol., 84: 553.
8. Drawbaugh, R., and Lal, H. (1974): Nature, 247:
65-67.
9. Drawbaugh, R., and Lal, H. (1976):Neuropharmacology
15: 375-378.
10. Eddy, N.B., Hallech, H., Isabell, H., and
Seevers, M.H. (1970): In: Drug Abuse, Data and
Debate, edited by P.H. Blaeky. Thomas
Springfield.
11. Gianutsos, G., Drawbaugh, R., Hynes , M., and Lal,
H.(1975):In:Methods in Narcotic Research, edited
by S.Ehrenpreis and A. Neidel,pp.293-310, Marcel
Dekker, New York.
12. Gianutsos,G., and Lal, H. (1975):
Psychopharmacologia,41: 267-270.
13. Gianutsos,G.,and Lal,H.(1976):Life Sci.,19:91-98.
14. Kleitman, N., and Crisler, G. (1927): Am.J.
Physiol., 79: 571.

15. Lal, H. (1975): In: <u>Methods in Narcotic Research</u>, edited by S. Ehrenpreis, and E.I. Neidel, pp. 149-171, Marcel Dekker, New York.

16. Lal, H. (1975): <u>Life Sci.</u>, 17: 483-496.

17. Lal, H. (1976): In: <u>Synthetic Antidiarrheal Drugs</u>, edited by W. Van Bever, and H. Lal, pp. 235-250. Marcel Dekker, New York.

18. Lal, H., DeFeo, J., Pitterman, A., Patel, G., and Baumel, I. (1972): In: <u>Drug Addiction-Experimental Pharmacology</u>, edited by J. Singh, L. Miller, and H. Lal, pp. 255-268. Future Publishing Co., Mount Kisko, New York.

19. Lal, H., and Ehrenpries, S. (1977): In: <u>Drug Abuse, Clinical and Basic Aspects</u>, edited by S.N. Pradlan, and S. Datta. Mosby, St. Louis, Mo. in press.

20. Lal, H., Gianutsos, G., and Puri, S. (1975): <u>Life Sci.</u>, 17: 29-34.

21. Lal, H., Gianutsos, G., and Miksic, S. (1977): In: <u>Discriminative Stimulus Properties of Drugs</u>, edited by H. Lal, pp.23-47. Plenum Press, New York.

22. Lal, H., Miksic, S., Drawbaugh, R., Numan, R., and Smith, N. (1976): <u>Pav. J. Biol. Sci.</u>, 11: 251-262.

23. Lal, H., Miksic, S., and Smith, N. (1976): <u>Life Sci.</u>, 18: 971-976.

24. Lal, H., O'Brian, J., and Puri, S.K. (1971): <u>Psychopharmacologia</u>, 22: 217-223.

25. Lal, H., Puri, S., and Volicer, L. (1976): In: <u>Tissue Responses to Addictive Drugs</u>, edited by D. Ford, and D. Clouet.pp. 187-207, Spectrum, New York.

26. Lotti, V.J., Lomax, P., and George, R. (1965): <u>J. Pharmacol. Exp. Ther.</u>, 150: 135-139.

27. Lynch, J., Fertziger, A., Teitelbaum, H., Cullen, J., and Gantt, W. (1973): <u>Conditional Reflex</u>, 8: 211-223.

28. Miksic, S., and Lal, H. (1976): <u>Psychopharmacol. Commun.</u>, 2: 357-367.

29. Miksic, S., and Lal, H. (1977): submitted for publication to <u>Psychopharmacology</u>.

30. Miksic, S., Smith, N., and Lal, H. (1976): <u>Psychopharmacology</u> 48: 115-117.

31. Miksic, S., Smith, N., Numan, R., and Lal, H. (1975): Neuropsychobiology, 1: 277-283.
32. Numan, R., Smith, N., and Lal, H. (1976): Psychopharmacol. Comm. 1: 295-303.
33. Numan, R., Banerjee, U., Smith, N., and Lal, H. (1976): Pharmacol. Biochem. Behav., 5: 395-399.
34. Pavlov, I.P. (1927): Conditioned Reflexes. Translated by C. Anrep, Oxford University Press, New York.
35. Perez-Cruet, J. (1976): Pav. J. Biol. Sci., in press.
36. Roffman, M., and Lal, H. (1974): J. Pharmacol. Exp. Ther., 191: 358-369.
37. Roffman, M., Reddy, C., and Lal, H. (1973): Psychopharmacologia, 29: 197-201.
38. Rosecrans, J.A., Goodloe, M.H., Bennet, G.J., and Hirschorn, I.D. (1973): Eur. J. Pharmacol., 21: 252-256.
39. Shannon, H.E., and Holtzman, S.G. (1976): J. Pharmacol. Exp. Ther., 198: 54-65.
40. Thompson, T., and Pickens, R. (1972): Stimulus Properties of Drugs, Appleton-Century-Crofts, New York.
41. Thompson, T., and Schuster, C.R. (1964): Psychopharmacologia, 5: 87-94.
42. Tye, N., and Iverson, S. (1975): Nature, 255: 416-418.
43. Wikler, A. (1973): Arch. Gen. Psychiat., 28: 611-616.

Factors Affecting the Action of Narcotics, edited by
M.L. Adler, L. Manara, and R. Samanin.
Raven Press, New York©1978.

Cerebral Hypoxia and Opiate Actions

H.S. Bachelard

Department of Biochemistry
University of Bath, U.K.

In this paper, the effects of hypoxia on cerebral biochemical function will be reviewed and an indication given as to which of these may be expected to affect reactions at the opiate receptor.

HYPOXIA AND ENERGY METABOLISM

Until recently, it seemed almost self-evident that the functional and behavioral responses to cerebral hypoxia were due to an energy deficit, as in anoxia and ischemia. Any serious deprivation of oxygen would inevitably lead to a failure of energy production, which seemed sufficient to explain the changed EEG, the drowsiness, coma and ultimate death which can ensue in severe hypoxia.

The classical biochemical picture of ischemia, illustrated by Lowry and his co-workers (21), showed a rapid decrease in cerebral concentrations of the carbohydrate stores, glucose and glycogen, with a concomitant increase in lactate (Fig. 1a). At the same time, concentrations of ATP and creatine phosphate fell, while those of ADP and AMP rose (Fig. 1b). This pattern of events is seen also in cerebral anoxia, but not in cerebral hypoxia, especially if the hypoxia is controlled at a level which produces changes in the EEG and causes drowsy behavior, but which is not sufficiently severe to cause any perceptible decrease in the overall respiration rate of the brain. It is now known, from a large number of studies on a variety of mammalian species (see 2 for review), that mild controlled hypoxia causes the changes in glycolytic intermediates,increased use of glucose and increase production of lactate similar to those of Fig. 1a,without any perceptible effect on respiration or on the concentrations of the energy phosphates seen in ischemia or anoxia (Fig. 1b). This increased glycolysis, in the absence of changes in respiration or the energy state, is seen in mild hypoglycemia as well as in hypoxia, and is apparently as true of localized regions of the brain as of the whole brain (15).

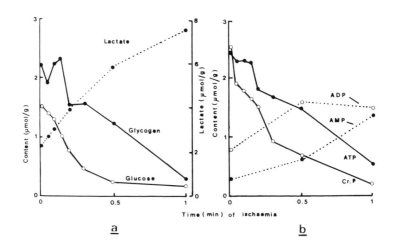

FIG. 1.   Effects of ischemia on a. glycolytic intermediates b. energy phosphates, of mouse brain
in vivo. (21).

TABLE 1. Conditions affecting cerebral glycolysis without detectable effects on adenine nucleotide levels.

CONDITION	OBSERVED ACTION	EFFECT ON GLYCOLYSIS
Barbiturate	Post-syn potential	Inhibits
Halothane	Post-syn potential	Inhibits
Amphetamine	Amine re-uptake	Stimulates
Methionine sulphoximine	Inh. synthesis of glutamine	Inhibits?
Allylglycine	Inh. synthesis of GABA	Inhibits?
Mild Hypoglycaemia	Behavioral	No change?
Mild Hypoxia	Behavioral	Stimulates

It should be noted that all of these conditions are
likely to affect the EEG.

The concept of changes in behavior and in the physiological state of the brain (indicated by the EEG and by the acidosis caused by increased glycolytic production of lactate) in the absence of any detectable energy deficit is becoming well established from studies on the effects of various centrally active drugs (Table 1).

The normal respired oxygen content of 20% of the air inhaled can be reduced to about 10% in mammals without causing any marked physiological or behavioral change although cerebral blood flow and glycolysis are increased. Below 10% (the concentration usually studied is from 5 to 7%), there is a pronounced increase in glycolysis but no change in respiration(Table 2). It is only when the oxygen content of the inhaled air falls to below 5% that real changes in energy metabolism or cellular damage are observed.

TABLE 2. Effects of arterial hypoxia on cerebral metabolism in vivo.

SPECIES	O_2 used	% CHANGE OBSERVED	
		Glucose Used	Lactate Produced
Man	+ 3	+ 28	+ 365
Dog	-	+140	+ 400

Data from A/V difference studies (7,13).

The increased glycolytic rate in mild hypoxia results from activation of regulatory enzymes of the glycolytic pathway, i.e. hexokinase, phosphofructokinase and pyruvate kinase (4,14) (Norberg and Siesjö personal communication), but the mechanism of the activation (Fig. 2) has not been elucidated. In these studies also there was no change in concentrations of adenine nucleotides.

It should be noted that while the "energy state" (based on estimation of concentrations of intermediates) is unchanged, this does not necessarily imply that there has been no effect on the turnover rate of any of these intermediates. If, for example, a decrease in ATP production occurred to the same extent as a decrease in its utilization, the amount present would remain the same though the turnover rate had fallen. We have no direct evidence on this, but the indirect evidence

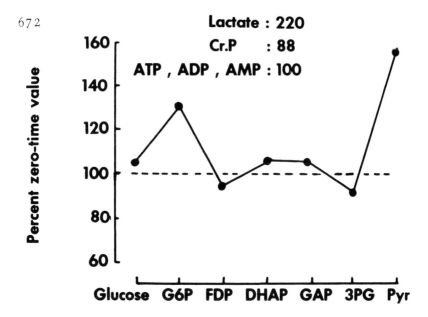

FIG. 2. Effects of mild arterial hypoxia on intermediates of cerebral glycolysis (4).

suggests that the turnover rate is not affected by mild
hypoxia. A slower rate of production of ATP should be
expected to be associated with a slower rate of respiration. A slower rate of ATP utilization would be
likely to be reflected by a change in cation distribution, since cation pumping is the major ATP-consuming
process in the brain. As described below, there seems
to be no real change in the distribution of Na^+ and K^+
in mild hypoxia, although the situation is not abso-
lutely clear.

The acidosis which occurs in vivo has been shown to
be associated with a change in the distribution of Na^+
and K^+ (22,23) but this change seems to occur only in
severe hypoxia when an energy deficit is clearly present. Inhalation of 7% O_2 (which causes increased
glycolysis but no change in respiration) has been shown
not to affect cation distribution (24). It is not as
easy to correlate these functions in vivo as it is in
vitro. Swanson (28) studied the effects in cerebral
cortex slices of severe hypoxia on cations and energy
phosphates and found an impaired distribution of
cations under conditions where the metabolism of ATP
and creatine phosphate appeared normal. We have no
clear indication of the situation in mild hypoxia. From
the studies that have been performed, however, it seems
reasonable to conclude that mild hypoxia causes no
marked change in cation distribution, whereas severe

hypoxia does. Further investigation is needed on any effect on calcium, which is so intimately involved in neurotransmission.

HYPOXIA AND NEUROTRANSMISSION

TABLE 3. The effects of mild hypoxia on cerebral amines and amino acids.

COMPOUND	% CHANGE IN CONCENTRATION
Dopamine	- 15
Serotonin	- 50
GABA	+ 21
NH_3	+230

Animals (rats and rabbits) were exposed to mild hypoxia for 30 min (11, 30).

Mild arterial hypoxia produces a slight but significant effect on the cerebral amines considered to function as neurotransmitters (Table 3) but the effects on the amino acids are less. Formation of aromatic amines in the brain occurs by processes which use molecular oxygen directly; the aromatic amino acid hydroxylases involved in their formation are far more sensitive to lowered oxygen than is the process of respiration (Table 4). The K_m values for the hydroxylases (of the order of 0.5 to 1 mM) are not far below the calculated tissue concentration of 2 mM (19). So these hydroxylases do seem very likely to be vulnerable to limited availability of oxygen. Since the amines occur in very low concentrations in those areas of the brain where they are believed to function (1), even a slight decrease in rates of formation could have profound consequences in electrical activity and on behavior.

The formation of cyclic AMP is increasingly invoked as being associated with neurotransmission, especially that mediated by catecholamines (10). Hypoxia exerts interesting effects on cyclic AMP and on the enzyme which forms it (Table 5). Thus, mild hypoxia produces an increase in adenyl cyclase activity and in cyclic AMP under conditions when ATP is unchanged, whereas more severe hypoxia gives the opposite effect - a fall both in enzyme activity and its product.

TABLE 4. Oxygen requirements for cerebral respiration and aromatic amine formation.

PROCESS	K_m (mM-O_2)
Mitochondrial respiration	0.0001
Tyrosine hydroxylation	0.5
Tryptophan hydroxylation	1.0

Data from Fisher & Kaufman (16); Kaufman, (19) ; Clark, et al. (6).

TABLE 5. Hypoxia, cyclic AMP and adenyl cyclase activity

ARTERIAL OXYGEN %	CYCLIC AMP (nmol/g)	ADENYL CYCLASE (mU/g)	ATP (μmol/g)
13.5	3.2	25.2	2.3
6	4.0	31.1	2.5
4	6.1*	46.3*	2.2
2.5	1.5*	12.9*	1.7*

* $P < 0.05$

Data from dog cerebral cortex (5).

So, in assessing the functional consequences of hypoxia in the brain, we should distinguish between mild hypoxia (for convenience, from 5 to 7% O_2) and severe hypoxia (0 to 4% O_2). From the foregoing, it seems reasonable to think of mild hypoxia as being associated with behavioral changes, effects on the EEG and on adenyl cyclase activity, but without effects on energy metabolism or necessarily on monovalent cation distribution. On the other hand, severe hypoxia more clearly causes an energy deficit, a changed cation distribution, and morphological damage (Table 6).

It seems important to keep these distinctions in mind

TABLE 6. Guide to cerebral effects of mild and severe hypoxia.

CRITERION	MILD HYPOXIA $(4-7\% \ O_2)$	SEVERE HYPOXIA $(0-4\% \ O_2)$
Behavior	Drowsiness	Coma
Acidosis (lactate)	Marked	Marked
Adenyl cyclase	Increased	Decreased
Cyclic AMP	Increased	Decreased
ATP, CP	No change	Decreased
Na^+, K^+ distribution	No change?	Marked change
Amino acids	Little change	Marked change
Aromatic amines	Slight loss	Marked loss
Morphology	Swelling of cells?	Mitochondria lost

when speculating on the possible effects of hypoxia on opiate actions since the energy deficit and cell damage in severe hypoxia may serve to cloud the issue. It is possible that lowered oxygen acts as a signal to the brain which responds in a way unrelated to the mechanisms of oxidative metabolism (2, 20). This has only recently been conjectured and seems worth following up.

HYPOXIA AND OPIATE ACTIONS

We have at least three main areas where mild hypoxia provokes a clear biochemical reaction: glycolysis, adenyl cyclase activity, and the formation of biogenic amines. More severe hypoxia shows effects also on energy metabolism, amino acid metabolism, and cation pumping (Table 6). We can therefore speculate on whether any of these is likely to affect actions of opiates with their receptors.

Glycolysis and Energy Metabolism

Morphine is known to decrease cerebral glycolysis presumably at the phosphofructokinase stage (12) and, when used as an analgesic in surgery, to depress the respiratory centers of the brainstem. It is possible, therefore, that the increased glycolysis and acidosis

which occurs in hypoxia could modify these cerebral
responses to the opiate. The effects on the respiratory
centers are thought (17) to involve adrenergic and
serotonergic processes discussed below.

Cyclic AMP

There is an accumulating recognition of the role of
the biogenic amines in morphine analgesia, which is
lessened if serotonin synthesis is inhibited (29), but
this role is considered to be secondary to the role
played by cyclic AMP (8).

Narcotic agents such as morphine inhibit the
prostaglandin-dependent adenyl cyclase activities of
cultured brain cells (9, 25). Not only does morphine
decrease the concentrations of cyclic AMP as a result
of this inhibition but it also increases that of cyclic
GMP (18). Dopamine, noradrenaline and adrenergic
agonists have similar effects to morphine in causing
depolarization and in decreasing cyclic AMP concentrations (31) and it was suggested that these agents are
acting on the cation permeability properties of the cell
membrane.

If the reactivity of the morphine receptor is
functionally coupled to the actions of cyclic AMP and
the catecholamines, it is very likely to be modified by
hypoxia, which, as discussed above, affects the metabolism
of these compounds. Since morphine decreases cyclic
AMP and mild hypoxia increases it, one might expect the
sensitivity of this system to morphine to be lessened
by mild hypoxia. In contrast, severe hypoxia, which
decreases cyclic AMP, could have the opposite effect in
increasing sensitivity to morphine.

Monovalent Cations

Sodium has been shown to increase the number of
opiate antagonist binding sites (26). If the opiate
receptor is on the outside of the cell membrane, it is
likely to react to extracellular concentrations of Na^+.
The data of Fig. 3 show the binding of both agonist and
antagonist to be very sensitive to change in $/\overline{Na}^+/$ at
its intracellular concentration of about 40 mM, but
quite insensitive to extracellular concentrations (about
130 nM). The extracellular concentration of Na^+ would
have to change drastically to affect binding of opiates
to the receptor. This seems unlikely to occur in mild
or severe hypoxia.

TENTATIVE CONCLUSION

The above arguments suggest that the biochemical
effects of mild hypoxia (increased cyclic AMP, decreased

catecholamines, and increased glycolysis) would all
tend to act in the same direction, which would to be
lessen the sensitivity of the brain to morphine. As
far as I am aware, there is no direct evidence on this
but it is subject to experimental investigation. For
those interested in hypoxia and the need to compare
published values for oxygen concentrations expressed in
various units, a nomogram for that purpose has been
published (3).

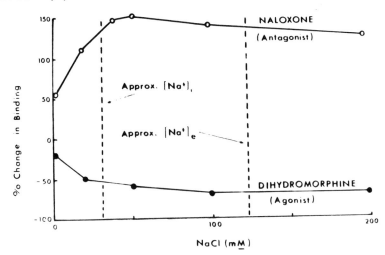

FIG. 3. Effects of Na$^+$ on opiate agonist and antagonist binding
(27).

REFERENCES

1. Bachelard, H.S. (1974). Brain Biochemistry,Chapman &
   Hall, London.
2. Bachelard, H.S. (1976) In : Biochemistry of Neurological Disorder, Chapter 5, pp.228-277, edited by
   A.N. Davison , Blackwell Scientific Publications,
   Oxford.
3. Bachelard, H.S. (1976):Clin. Sci. Mol. Med.,51 :
   203-204.
4. Bachelard, H.S.,Lewis, L.D., Pontén, U. and Siesjö,
   B.K. (1974) : J. Neurochem. , 22 : 395-401.
5. Benzi, G., and Villa,R.F. (1975) : J.Neurol.Neurosurg.
   Psychiatry ,34 :77-83.
6. Clark, J.B., Nicklas, W.J. and Degn, H. (1976) :
   J. Neurochem. , 26 : 409-411.
7. Cohen, P.J. (1971) : In : Ion Homeostasis of the
   Brain, edited by B.K. Siesjö, and S.C. Sørensen,
   pp. 417-423, Munksgaard, Copenhagen.
8. Collier, H.O.J., Francis, D.L., McDonald-Gibson,W.

J., Roy, A.C., and Saeed, S.A. (1975) : Life Sci., 17: 85-90.

9. Collier, H.O.J., and Roy, A.C. (1974) : Nature,248: 24-27.
10. Daly, J. (1975) : In : Handbook of Psychopharmacology edited by L.L. Iversen, S.D. Iversen, S.H. Snyder, vol.5:pp.47-130, Plenum Press, New York.
11. Davis, J.N., and Carlsson, A. (1973) : J.Neurochem. 21: 783-790.
12. Dodge, P.W., and Takemori, A.E. (1972) : Biochem. Pharmacol., 21 :287-294.
13. Drewes, L.R. and Gilboe, D.D. (1973) : J.Biol.Chem. 218: 2489-2496.
14. Duffy, T.E., Nelson, S.R., and Lowry, O.H. (1972): J. Neurochem.,19: 959-977.
15. Ferrendelli, J.A. (1975) : In : The Working Brain, edited by D. Ingvar and D. Lassen, Munksgaard, Copenhagen.
16. Fisher, D.B., and Kaufman, S. (1972) : J.Neurochem. 19 :1359-1365.
17. Floréz, J., Delgado, G., and Armyo, J.A. (1972) : Psychopharmacologia,24: 258-274.
18. Gillis, R., Traber, J., and Hamprecht, B. (1975) : Nature,256 : 57-59.
19. Kaufman, S. (1974) : In : CIBA Foundation Symposium No. 22, pp. 85-108, Elsevier, Amsterdam.
20. Lowry, O.H. (1975) : In:Brain Work, edited by P.H. Ingvar and N.A. Lassen, pp. 48-63, Munksgaard, Copenhagen.
21. Lowry, O.H., Passonneau, J.V., Hasselberger, F.X. and Schulz, D.W. (1964) : J. Biol. Chem.,239: 18-30.
22. Meyer, J.S., Gotoh, F., Ebihara, S., and Tomita,M. (1965) : Neurology,(Minneap.),15: 892-901.
23. Meyer, J.S., Kanda, T., Shinohara, Y., and Fukuuchi, Y. (1971) : Neurology,(Minneap.), 21: 889-895.
24. Portnoy, H.D., Thomas, L.M., and Gurdjian, E.S. (1964) : Neurology,(Minneap.),14 : 324-337.
25. Sharma, S.K., Nirenberg, M., and Klee, W.A. (1975): Proc. Natl. Acad. Sci., USA,72 : 590-594.
26. Snyder, S.H. (1975) : Neurosci. Res. Program. Bull. 13: 137-140.
27. Snyder, S.H., Pasternak, G.W., and Pert, C.B.(1975): In : Handbook of Psychopharmacology, edited by L.L. Iversen, S.D. Iversen and S.H. Snyder,vol.5 : pp. 329-360, Plenum Press, New York.
28. Swanson, P.D. (1969) : J. Neurochem.,16: 35-45
29. Takemori, A.E., Tulunay, F.C., and Yano, I. (1975): Life Sci.,17: 21-28.
30. Thorn,W., Grieshaber, Th. and Junge, H. (1973): Pflügers Arch. , 345 : 347-351.

31. Traber, J., Reiser, G., Fischer, K., and Hamprecht, B. (1975): FEBS Lett. 52 327-332.

Factors Affecting the Action of Narcotics, edited by
M.L. Adler, L. Manara, and R. Samanin.
Raven Press, New York © 1978.

Morphine Action in Myocardial Metabolopathies

Walter B. Essman

Queens College, of the City University of New York Flushing, N.Y., U.S.A.

INTRODUCTION

The clinical utility in the sedative and analgesic effects of morphine has warranted the continued use of this agent in a number of systemic disorders. One system to which the actions of morphine are particularly relevant both clinically and physiologically, comprises the elements of cardiovascular regulation. A number of limited studies have examined the biochemical and physiological effects of morphine upon constituents of the cardiovascular system, but such investigations have been limited in scope and have only rarely involved altered functional states upon which the effects of morphine have been superimposed.

Morphine, although shown to increase brain catecholamine synthesis, did not have similar effects upon the heart (33), and whereas brain catecholamine content was reduced by morphine (38), no comparable effect occurred in mouse heart. In the isolated rabbit heart an antagonistic effect between morphine and ouabain was demonstrated (43). The myocardial depressant effect of morphine has been attributed to its possible interference with calcium transport (36) and is enhanced by a calcium deficiency. A related finding in support of a calcium interdependency for morphine action, is that the analgesic effects of the narcotic are antagonized in mice given calcium (17). In studies of spontaneously beating, perfused heart, a reduction in calcium produced bradycardia, which was further enhanced by morphine. The prevention of calcium accumulation in the heart with ouabain, and the resulting tachyarrhythmia, may be attenuated by morphine (14,25,43).

A biphasic effect of morphine upon sinus rate has been reported in waking dogs; an immediate, brief sinus tachycardia was followed by a delayed, prolonged sinus bradycardia (40). A vagolytic as well as vagomimetic

681

effect of morphine was indicated; morphine increased vagal tone, preventing atropine-induced increases in sinus rate. The use of counterpulsation to assist circulation in dogs in cardiogenic shock, led to the appearance of stable ventricular arrhythmias. Morphine reduced or eliminated such arrhythmias (9). The possible action of morphine was attributed to its effect upon endogenous catecholamines (20,24), however, initial sinus tachycardia induced by morphine infusion, could not be blocked by β-blockade with propranolol (9). Intravenous morphine, in doses of 300 μg to 1 mg, induced a negative chronotropic effect upon the SA node of the dog. At the higher dose, an initial positive chronotropic effect was produced and this could be completely blocked by propranolol (3). This finding suggested that norepinephrine release may be effected at higher doses of morphine. Increased heart rate in the conscious dog after acute coronary occlusion, could be blocked by morphine, which also decreased the heart rate increase by 37% and improved marginal segment shortening by 40% (39).

In patients with coronary artery disease, morphine (2 mg/kg) produced a significant rise (53 and 68%, respectively) in left heart filling pressure and right heart filling pressure. Mean pulmonary arterial pressure was increased; heart rate and rate-pressure product (an indirect index of myocardial oxygen consumption) were decreased by morphine (21).

It is apparent from a consideration of the myocardial effects of morphine that differences may arise depending upon the nutritional status of the tissue, its endogenous biochemical disposition, and conditions that affect its rhythm and rate. There are several myocardial metabolopathies which relate in various ways to such influences upon the cardiac effects of morphine; it is our purpose here to illustrate three representative sources for altered myocardial metabolism and the effects of morphine upon these events.

MYOCARDIAL METABOLISM IN ALLOXAN DIABETES: EFFECTS OF MORPHINE

Diabetes mellitus, both as the clinical entity and under experimental conditions, serves as a stimulating basis upon which the status of the myocardium may be altered. The early mortality for myocardial infarction in diabetic subjects is notably greater than overall in hospital mortality (28), and there is also a higher incidence of shock, congestive heart failure, and painless infarction (2,26). Carbohydrate intoler-

ance is also a frequent accompaniment of acute myocardial infarction (4,19,35). There is a dual basis
for giving consideration to the action of morphine on
the diabetic myocardium; its previously implicated role
in cardiac rate and rhythm disturbances and its possible action as a hyperglycemic agent (8), indicate the
possible basis for an altered metabolic action upon
the diabetic myocardium. Inasmuch as the chemical
structure of morphine resembles both steroids and
epinephrine, it may relate to carbohydrate metabolism
similarly by increasing obligatory glyconogenic enzyme
activity or enhancing the gluconeogenesis pathway in
the liver. A single dose of morphine has been shown
to significantly increase the activity of liver glycose-
6-phosphatase and phosphoenolpyruvate carboxykinase,
and the effect was attributed to enzyme induction (41).

In our experiments, male Sprague-Dawley rats (~280g)
were given intravenous (caudal vein) injections of
either 75 mg/kg of alloxan dissolved in 0.9% NaCl, or
a control injection of an equivalent volume of NaCl.
The animals were maintained on ad libitum food and
water for 18 days, when blood samples, obtained by
venopuncture, were assayed for serum glucose by photo-
metric monitoring of spectral change upon reaction with
glucose oxidase, and insulin assays were performed
utilizing a standardized radioimmunoassay. Glucose
levels in the alloxan-treated rats were significantly
elevated (226.4 ± 32.5) as compared with the saline-
treated controls (107.7 ± 6.2). Insulin levels for
the diabetic rats were significantly lower (53.87±
3.75 μU/ml) than among euglycemic rats (100.87 ± 13.50
μU/ml).

Myocardial tissue obtained from hyperglycemic or
from control rats was incubated under physiological
conditions in a Tris-KCl-sucrose buffer for 45 or 80
minutes with either C^{14}-leucine (1.66 μCi/ml), C^{14}-
orotic acid (1.25 μCi/ml), or C^{14}-Acetyl CoA (1.0 μCi/
ml). Either 0.9% NaCl or morphine (10^{-7}, 10^{-6}, or
10^{-5} M) were added to the incubation mixture. The
reaction was stopped and either protein, RNA, or fatty
acids were precipitated and/or extracted, and the
tissue or fraction protein concentration was determined.
The solubilized fractions were counted in a liquid
scintillation counter and the specific activity of the
incorporated isotope was determined.

The synthesis of protein, RNA and fatty acids, as
determined for the normal myocardium, have been summarized in Figure 1. Protein synthesis was increased by
10% and 17% by morphine at concentrations of 10^{-7} and
10^{-6} M, respectively, but at the higher concentration
(10^{-5} M) myocardial protein synthesis was not affected.

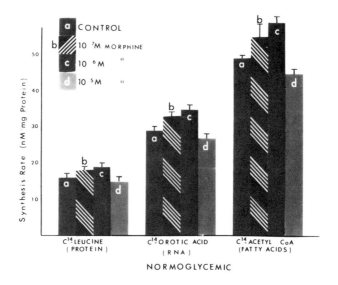

FIG. 1.   Mean (± S.D.) synthesis rate (n Moles/mg
protein) for protein, RNA, and fatty acids for normoglycemic rat myocardium: in vitro effects of morphine.

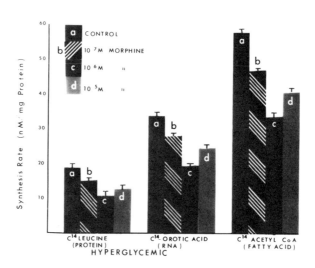

FIG. 2.   Mean (± S.D.) synthesis rate (n Moles/mg
protein) for protein, RNA, and fatty acids for hyperglycemic rat myocardium: in vitro effects of morphine

A similar pattern was observed for RNA and fatty acid
synthesis; morphine, at 10^{-7} M and 10^{-6} M, produced
changes of 17% and 24%, respectively (p< 0.02). At the
same concentrations of morphine, fatty acid synthesis
was altered by 12% and 21%, respectively (p<0.02). In
the diabetic myocardium, protein, RNA, and fatty acid
synthesis were decreased by morphine. Although as
compared with normoglycemic myocardium, there was a
somewhat higher control rate of protein (17%), RNA
(17%), and fatty acid (17%) synthesis in the diabetic
myocardium, synthesis generally was decreased at all
concentrations of morphine (Figure 2). Protein synthesis was maximally inhibited (40%) at 10^{-6} M morphine
in the diabetic myocardium, whereas the same general
relationship between concentration of morphine and
magnitude of inhibition was obtained for RNA and fatty
acid synthesis (i.e., greatest inhibition at 10^{-6} M
morphine, least inhibition with 10^{-5} M morphine).

Examination of the present data suggests that the
stimulation of protein, RNA, and fatty acid synthesis
occurs with morphine in the normal myocardium, with
maximal effect at 10^{-6} M morphine. In the diabetic
myocardium morphine also acts to inhibit the synthesis
of proteins, RNA, and fatty acids, maximally at a concentration of 10^{-6} M.

In order to examine specific myocardial sites at
which the in vitro effects of morphine might be acting
differentially, the tissue was fractionated by differential and density gradient methods, providing for a
nuclear, mitochondrial, and microsomal fraction. The
fractions were incubated and treated, as described
above. The results of the protein synthesis studies
in normal myocardium have been summarized in Table 1
and indicate that the increase in synthesis by morphine
is largely accounted for by the increases in the microsomal fraction. In Table 2 protein synthesis decrements
effected with morphine appear to be accounted for in
the nuclear and microsomal fractions, where significantly reduced leucine incorporation into proteins
occurred.

An examination of RNA synthesis in subcellular
fractions from normal and diabetic myocardial tissue
was carried out by assessing the in vitro incorporation of C^{14}-orotic acid into the nuclear fraction
derived from differential centrifugation; amino acid-
transfer RNA and nuclear ribosomes were removed by
resuspension in buffer with 0.0033 M $CaCl_2$, centrifuging, and removing the supernatant in which these were
contained. DNA was removed in the supernatant resulting from centrifugation (24 x 10^5 g min) of a stored
($2°C$ for 16 hr) mixture of the nuclear pellet in 19

TABLE 1. C^{14}-leucine incorporation into proteins of several subcellular fractions of normoglycemic rat myocardium: μ Moles/mg protein (S.E.)

Fraction	Control	Morphine		
		$10^{-7}M$	$10^{-6}M$	$10^{-5}M$
Nuclei	0.0842 (0.009)	0.0749 (0.003)	0.0867 (0.001)	0.1138[*] (0.002)
Mitochondria	0.2059 (0.003)	0.1394[*] (0.039)	0.1929 (0.001)	0.1141[*] (0.003)
Microsomes	0.0859 (0.024)	0.1106 (0.081)	0.3630[**] (0.089)	0.3811[**] (0.029)

[*] $p < 0.05$
[**] $p < 0.01$

TABLE 2. C^{14}-leucine incorporation into proteins of several subcellular fractions of hyperglycemic rat myocardium: μ Moles/mg protein (S.E.)

Fraction	Control	Morphine		
		$10^{-7}M$	$10^{-6}M$	$10^{-5}M$
Nulcei	0.3853 (0.001)	0.3856 (0.003)	0.2187[**] (0.021)	0.1720 (0.004)
Mitochondria	0.1086 (0.004)	0.1275 (0.006)	0.1115 (0.029)	0.1000 (0.009)
Microsomes	0.2094 (0.003)	0.1645[**] (0.005)	0.2347 (0.006)	0.1260[**] (0.004)

[**] $p < 0.01$

volumes of 1M NaCl solution. The resulting pellet was
resuspended and solubilized in scintillation fluid
with the resulting radioactivity representing 12-14%
of the RNA content of the original crude fraction.

In Table 3 the change in RNA synthesis in diabetic
myocardium has been summarized and the effects of morphine have been indicated. It is apparent that nuclear
RNA synthesis in the diabetic myocardium was markedly
increased and, at the lowest concentration of morphine,
was increased still further. RNA synthesis associated
with the mitochondrial and microsomal fractions this
relationship also held; although the magnitude of the
increased rate of RNA synthesis associated with hyperglycemia was reduced at increased concentrations of
morphine, RNA synthesis in this fraction still remained
significantly increased.

Fatty acid synthesis was determined by incubating
myocardial tissue fractions for 60 minutes, under a
constant stream of nitrogen, with C^{14}-acetyl-CoA in an
incubation medium containing non-labelled acetyl-co-
enzyme A, enzymes, and electrolytes. The free fatty
acids were saponified, acidified, and extracted with
pentane, which was evaporated from scintillation vials
overnight under nitrogen. Scintillation fluid was
added and the incorporated acetyl-CoA was determined
from counts. A summary of the effects of hyperglycemia
upon myocardial fatty acid synthesis and superimposed
morphine effects have been presented in Table 4. Mitochondrial and microsomal fatty acid synthesis, which
represent the largest pool for this event, were affected similarly by morphine; although microsomal synthesis
was stimulated in the diabetic myocardium, there was a
dose-related effect of morphine reducing the rate of
fatty acid synthesis. Mitochondrial fatty acid synthesis, decreased in the diabetic myocardium, was not
further altered by morphine.

TABLE 3. Per cent change in RNA synthesis in subcellular
fractions of myocardium from diabetic rats

Fraction	Control	Morphine		
		10^{-7}M	10^{-6}M	10^{-5}M
Nuclei	+351[**]	+415[**]	+214[**]	+51[*]
Mitochondria	-47[*]	-85[*]	-46[*]	-31
Microsomes	+45[*]	+49[*]	-35	-67[*]

[*]p < 0.05   [**]p < 0.01

TABLE 4. Per cent change in fatty acid synthesis in subcellular fractions of myocardium from diabetic rats

Fraction	Control	Morphine		
		$10^{-7}M$	$10^{-6}M$	$10^{-5}M$
Nuclei	+375**	+51*	+153**	+415**
Mitochondria	-49	-8	-46*	-31
Microsomes	+144**	+49*	-4	-69*

*p < 0.05
**p < 0.01

It is apparent that the action of morphine upon several major synthetic events in the rat myocardium in vitro may be affected by the in vivo status of carbohydrate metabolism in the animal. Altered carbo- hydrate metabolism, effected experimentally by β cell destruction with alloxan — decreased insulin and increased plasma glucose — causes morphine, which stimulates molecular synthesis in the normoglycemic myocardium, to inhibit molecular synthesis in the diabetic myocardium.

THE MYOCARDIUM IN HYPOTHYROIDISM: DEVELOPMENTAL METABOLIC EFFECTS OF MORPHINE

The relationship between thyroid function and myo- cardial metabolism represents a subject to which the effects of morphine appear relevant in several respects. Thyroid hormone has been shown to exert a number of effects upon myocardial metabolism; these include: an increase in myocardial oxygen metabolism (42), uncoupl- ing of oxidative phosphorylation (11,12), decreased myocardial glycogen concentration (10), an increase in free fatty acids and triglycerides and an increase in their mobilization (29), an increase in protein synthe- sis (34) and an increase in RNA (27). The reduction of thyroid hormone, as occurs in myxedema, is associated with reduced blood flow without congestive heart fail- ure (1) and, indeed, a reduction in thyroid hormone level has been used as a therapeutic adjunct to the treatment of congestive heart failure, intractable angina, recurrent atrial tachycardia or fibrillation. There are cardiac manifestations of hypothyroidism, however, and these include the possibility of cardiac

enlargement, hypertension, and left ventricular hyper-
trophy, and changes in the myocardial fibers including
loss of striations, vacuolizations, patchy fibrosis,
and mucopolysaccharide deposition. With those changes
characterizing the hypothyroid state, some source for
a difference in the effects of morphine upon myocardial
metabolism is presented. Indeed, one would expect that
with hypothyroidism, myocardial metabolism should be
generally reduced. There is one aspect of the interrelationship between hypothyroidism and the myocardial
effects of morphine that remains to be clarified to a
much greater extent than apparent in the current literature; that is, the developmental course of myocardial
metabolism with congenital hypothyroidism and the
effects of morphine upon myocardial metabolism during
the normal course of development and in congenital
myxedema.

Pregnant rats were individually housed with ad
libitum food and water until the third trimester (day
14) when a 0.02% solution of propylthiouracil was
provided in water bottles to the experimental animals;
the control rats were continued with ad libitum tap
water. The drinking solutions were maintained throughout pregnancy and post-partum. Rats were killed at
either 1,4,6,11,14, or 18 days of age and the myocardial
tissue was incubated in vitro under physiological
conditions, as previously described, with either C^{14}-
leucine, C^{14}-orotic acid, or C^{14}-acetyl CoA, and their
rate of incorporation into proteins, RNA, and free
fatty acids, respectively, was determined, as described
above. For each condition, the incubations were carried
out with the addition of 0.09% NaCl or morphine in concentrations of either 10^{-7} M, 10^{-6} M, or 10^{-5} M.

Protein synthesis in the euthyroid myocardium did
not change appreciably over the first 18 days of age.
The rate of protein synthesis over the first four days
of age was not affected by morphine; however, between
7 and 18 days of age, as shown in Figure 3, the rate
of protein synthesis increased with age under morphine
treatment (10^{-7} M and 10^{-6} M). A similar effect
occurred at the higher concentration of morphine (10^{-5}
M) with a 50%, or more, increase in protein synthesis
after 14 days of age. Statistically significant
increases in protein synthesis in euthyroid myocardium
were brought about by morphine at concentrations of
10^{-6}M and 10^{-5}M at 7, 14, and 18 days of age ($p < 0.01$).
In myocardial tissue from myxedematous pups, a similar
developmental sequence of protein synthesis as noted
in controls was again in evidence; a peak in synthesis
rate occurred in both at 11 days of age. In the hypothyroid myocardium there was decreased protein synthesis

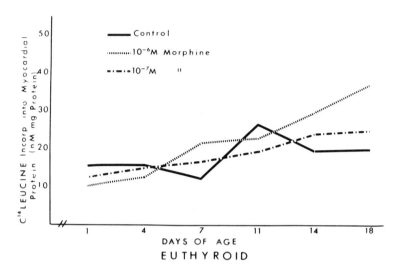

FIG. 3.   Protein synthesis (n Moles/mg protein) by
euthyroid rat myocardium as a function of age: <u>in vitro</u>
effects of morphine

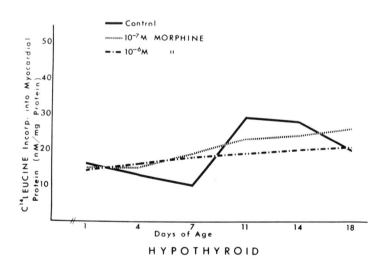

FIG. 4.   Protein synthesis (n Moles/mg protein) by
hypothyroid rat myocardium as a function of age:
<u>in vitro</u> effects of morphine

over the first 7 days (40%); this decrement did not
occur with morphine treatment (Figure 4), suggesting
that in the hypothyroid myocardium, unlike the euthyroid
tissue, protein synthesis was stimulated by morphine.
Between ages 11 and 18 days, protein synthesis in the
hypothyroid myocardium was depressed by morphine.
This was statistically significant at 11 and 14 days
of age at morphine concentrations of 10^{-7} M (22%;
$p < 0.02$), 10^{-6} M (33%, $p < 0.01$) and 10^{-5} M (14%,
$p < 0.05$). The rates of protein synthesis observed for
the myocardial tissue from 18-day-old rats was comparable to adult rates. Morphine-treated hypothyroid
myocardium did not exceed adult rates; however, morphine-treated euthyroid myocardium (18 days) did
exceed adult rates of protein synthesis by 50, 63, and
112%, respectively.

The increased rate of RNA synthesis with age did
not appreciable differ between the euthyroid and
hypothyroid myocardium, however the effects of morphine
did differ. Between 7 and 14 days of age morphine
increased euthyroid myocardial RNA synthesis. After
11 days of age, hypothyroid myocardial RNA synthesis
was suppressed by morphine. Although this effect was
consistent for all concentrations of morphine, the
general effect has been summarized in Figures 5 and 6.

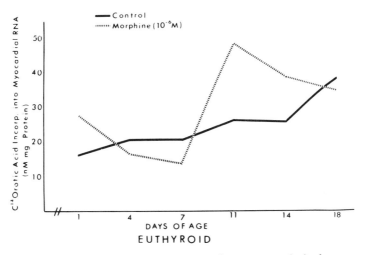

FIG. 5.   RNA synthesis (n Moles/mg protein) by euthyroid rat myocardium as a function of age: in vitro
effects of morphine.

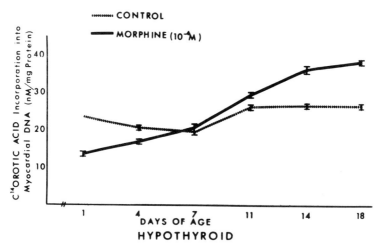

FIG. 6.   RNA synthesis (n Moles/mg protein) by euthyroid rat myocardium as a function of age: in vitro
effects of morphine.

Mitochondrial synthesis of fatty acids showed a
consistent pattern with age in both the euthyroid and
hypothyroid myocardium. Although the increase in
synthesis rate with age was slightly greater among
euthyroid rats (9.02 µMoles/mg protein/day) than for
the myocardial tissue from hypothyroid rates (6.64
µMoles/mg protein/day), morphine exerted a dose-
related increase in fatty acid synthesis of similar
magnitude for both conditions.
In contrast to what might be anticipated with a
reduced amount of thyroid hormone stimulation to the
myocardium, protein synthesis and RNA synthesis were
not reduced. The effects of morphine, however, did
appear to depend upon the thyroid-stimulated status
of the myocardium, particularly before 7 days of age
and after 11 days of age, where the effects differed.
Fatty acid synthesis was unaffected in the mitochondria
from hypothyroid myocardium and synthesis was stimulated normally by morphine.

METABOLIC EFFECTS OF MORPHINE UPON THE
HYPOMAGNESEMIC MYOCARDIUM

The interdependency of magnesium and myocardial
function has been established on several grounds. One

major issue is that potassium loss represents a major
factor in the susceptibility and pathogenesis of
cardiomyopathy, and the likelihood of potassium loss
is increased with magnesium deficiency. Cellular loss
of potassium in magnesium deficiency may be brought
about by a decreased maintenance of a concentration
gradient through decreased microsomal Mg-Na-K-ATPase
activity. This appears to be the case with hyper-
calcemia and its resultant cardiotoxicity, and inhibition of cardiotonic agents by Mg-dependent ATPase.
Digitalis toxicity is associated with myocardial Mg
loss (13) and such toxicity may be reversed by Mg
(32,37). Magnesium-deficient animals are also more
susceptible to the effects of cardiac glycosides (18).
Another possible basis for the maintenance of myocardial
potassium by Mg, resides in a potassium efflux through
the mitochondrion mediated by histone; K efflux and
mitochondrial swelling may be prevented by Mg (16,30).
Magnesium deficiency results in disruption of myocardial
mitochondria and efflux of potassium.

The rather consistent evidence that myocardial magnesium loss has also been associated,
as a dependent variable, with cardiomyopathies. Signi-
ficant loss of myocardial magnesium has been reported
with electrolyte-steroid cardiac necrosis (6). Myocardial magnesium loss in cardiac necrosis caused by
phosphate loading of parathyroidectomized animals or
with isoproterenol (22,23) was earlier and greater
than myocardial potassium loss. In clinical studies
the infarcted segment of tissue in an acute myocardial
infarction had approximately 26% less magnesium content
than a non-infarcted segment; the latter, however,
still had approximately 36% less magnesium than myocardium from patients without heart disease (15). An
extensive review of the interrelationship of magnesium
to ischemic heart disease has appeared (31), and some
of the clinical factors basic to hypomagnesemia and
their effect upon cardiolytic drugs has also been
considered (7).

The rather consistent evidence that myocardial
metabolism is altered in magnesium deficiency has
warranted consideration of the effects of morphine
upon this metabolopathy. Although a calcium-dependency
for morphine action has been indicated, little data
have been available for magnesium, which undoubtedly
is altered with changes in calcium availability. Myocardial protein and RNA synthesis might be expected
to decrease with hypomagnesemia, particularly in view
of the mitochondrial and microsomal effects of such a
deficiency state, as previously considered.

In our studies, male CF-Is strain mice, at 35 days
of age, were maintained on a low-magnesium test diet

(Nutritional Biochemicals) or a balanced diet of
Purina lab chow for 16 days. Food and water (double
glass-distilled) was provided ad libitum. One group
of Mg-deficient mice was place on an ad libitum Purina
lab chow diet with ad libitum tap water for two weeks.
Prior to the diet change, blood samples were obtained,
via the caudal vein, for Mg assay. The myocardial
tissue was removed, as were blood samples obtained
from the abdominal aorta. The latter were collected
in heparinized tubes containing NaF, and the plasma
was assayed for Mg concentration using atomic absorption spectroscopy. A similar assay was carried out
for extracts of fresh myocardium, and the remaining
tissue was utilized for in vitro studies of protein,
RNA, and fatty acid synthesis, as previously described,
at different concentrations of morphine.

Blood Mg levels among hypomagnesemic mice were
appreciably lower (2.37 ± 0.41 mg%) than for control
animals (3.20 ± 0.16 mg%), and after 14 days of a
normal diet, previously hypomagnesemic mice did show
increased blood levels (2.92 ± 0.19 mg%). Myocardial
Mg concentration was lower in the experimental mice
(14.21 ± 0.68 mEq/Kg), and hypomagnesemic mice, after
two weeks on a normal diet, did show increased myocardial Mg content (17.63 ± 0.56 mEq/Kg).

Protein synthesis by the hypomagnesemic myocardium
was reduced by 49%, and partial restoration of myocardial Mg with a normal diet failed to provide for
any increase in the depressed rate of synthesis, in
the normomagnesemic myocardium, morphine at all concentrations caused a significant decrease (p < 0.01) in
myocardial protein synthesis, whereas in the hypomagnesemic myocardium, morphine had no further effect
upon the already reduced rate of myocardial protein
synthesis. In the minimally hypomagnesemic myocardium
(Mg - deficient + normal diet), morphine increased
protein synthesis significantly (27%, p < 0.02) only at
the lowest concentration (10^{-7}M), whereas the increments
at higher concentrations (10% and 12%, respectively)
did not approximate statistical significance. These
data have been summarized in Figure 7. The changes in
protein synthesis observed in subcellular fractions
from magnesium-deficient myocardium and the effects of
morphine have been summarized in Table 5. Significant
effects were most notable in the mitochondrial fraction.

Whole hypomagnesemic myocardium as well as component
subcellular fractions thereof, showed significantly
reduced RNA synthesis. This effect, as well as the
in vitro effects of morphine, has been summarized in
Figure 8. The slightly hypomagnesemic myocardium from
the diet-supplemented mice, showed only a 13% reduction

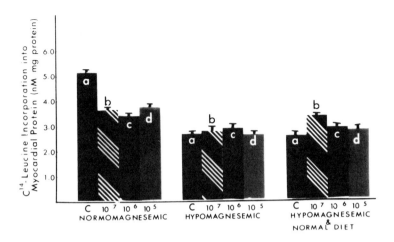

FIG. 7. Myocardial protein synthesis in hypomagnesemic states: effects of morphine.

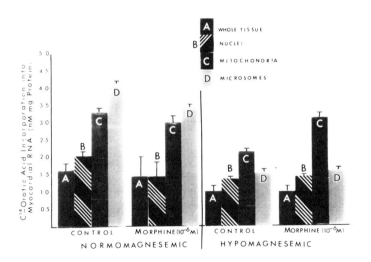

FIG. 8. Myocardial RNA synthesis in hypomagnesemia: effects of morphine.

TABLE 5.   Per cent change in protein synthesis in subcellular fractions of myocardium from magnesium deficient mice

Fraction	Control	Morphine		
		10^{-7}M	10^{-6}M	10^{-5}M
Nuclei	-24	-36^{*}	-26	-23
Mitochondria	$+37^{*}$	-62^{**}	$+65^{**}$	$+51^{**}$
Microsomes	-10	-26^{*}	$+23$	$+14$

* $p < 0.05$
** $p < 0.01$

TABLE 6.   Per cent change in RNA synthesis in subcellular fractions of myocardium from magnesium-deficient mice

Fraction	Control	Morphine		
		10^{-7}M	10^{-6}M	10^{-5}M
Nuclei	-34^{*}	$+9$	0	-16
Mitochondria	-35^{*}	$+99^{**}$	$+47^{**}$	-28
Microsomes	-63^{**}	-44^{*}	-54^{**}	-37^{*}

* $p < 0.05$
** $p < 0.01$

in RNA synthesis and approximately the same magnitude
of reduction in its subcellular fractions. Morphine
did not appreciably change RNA synthesis in the normomagnesemic myocardium or in its subcellular fractions,
at any of the concentrations utilized in the present
study.   In hypomagnesemic and partially hypomagnesemic
myocardium, morphine, at all concentrations, was without effect upon RNA synthesis, except for the mitochondrial fractions where the significant increments
summarized in Table 6 may be noted. The decreased RNA
synthesis associated with the microsomal fraction was
not dose-related.

The results of studies concerning mitochondrial and microsomal fatty acid synthesis in normomagnesemic and hypomagnesemic myocardium, and the effects thereupon of morphine have been summarized in Figure 9. Although fatty acid synthesis was not significantly altered by hypomagnesemia, the effects of morphine did differ. Mitochondrial fatty acid synthesis, while reduced by morphine in normomagnesemic myocardium (15, 42, and 34 per cent, respectively, at $10^{-7}M$, $10^{-6}M$, and $10^{-5}M$ morphine), was significantly increased by morphine in mitochondria from hypomagnesemic and partially hypomagnesemic myocardium. Microsomal fatty acid synthesis was unaffected by hypomagnesemia or by morphine.

It is apparent, therefore, that in the magnesium-deficient mouse myocardium, morphine had little direct effect on the already altered rates of protein and RNA synthesis. Fatty acid synthesis, which was not generally modified in the hypomagnesemic myocardium, was stimulated in mitochondria by morphine in contrast to the inhibition observed in mitochondria from normomagnesemic tissue.

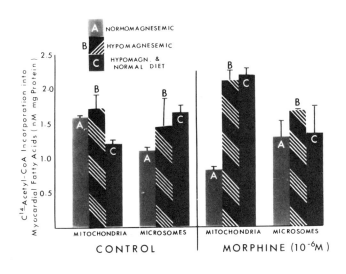

FIG. 9. Fatty acid synthesis in myocardial mitochondria and microsomes in hypomagnesemia: effects of morphine.

DISCUSSION

It is apparent from the foregoing data that a variety of myocardial metabolopathies that are characterized by alterations in the in vitro synthesis of several critical molecules, are capable of constituting different baselines upon which the in vitro effects of morphine occur. In the diabetic myocardium, morphine decreased molecular synthesis (particularly in mitochondrial and microsomal fractions) as compared with its stimulus to synthesis in the normoglycemic myocardium (particularly the microsomal fraction). These effects were not dose-dependent, and both peak stimulation (normoglycemic myocardium) and peak inhibition (diabetic myocardium) occurred with $10^{-6}M$ morphine. It would appear that those clinical applications for which morphine may be appropriate, at least in the normoglycemic state, could be affected differently in hyperglycemia if molecular synthesis is a functional corrollary of the myocardial alterations produced by morphine.

The developmental effects of morphine in hypothyroidism, point toward an interesting difference in molecular synthesis that separates the first 7 postnatal days from those between ages 11 and 18 days. The reduced molecular synthesis observed in the first 7 days in the hypothyroid myocardium could be reversed by morphine, and whereas morphine stimulated synthesis in euthyroid myocardium between 11 and 18 days of age, it inhibited synthesis at the same ages in hypothyroid myocardium. It is of interest to note that both thyroxine and hypomagnesemia cause an increased impairment of myocardial mitochondrial oxidative phosphorylation (5); one might, therefore, possibly anticipate opposite effects of hypothyroidism and hypomagnesemia, at least in mitochondria. Only for the first 11 days of age was mitochondrial fatty acid synthesis appreciably lower in the hypothyroid mitochondrial fraction; mitochondrial fatty acid synthesis in hypomagnesemic tissue was 9% higher than in normomagnesemic mitochondria. Although the comparison cannot be made directly, there is some indication that the metabolopathies of thyroid deficiency and hypomagnesemia may operate upon myocardial mitochondrial fatty acid synthesis in an opposite fashion. Morphine, however, increases fatty acid synthesis in mitochondria from both hypothyroid as well as hypomagnesemic myocardium. In contrast, normomagnesemic adult myocardial mitochondrial fatty acid synthesis inhibition and hypomagnesemic myocardial fatty acid synthesis stimulation by morphine, were dose-dependent.

It is apparent that the myocardial effects of morphine depend upon the nutritional and metabolic integrity of the myocardium. Changes that alter its synthetic machinery, either through limitations upon endogenous metabolic pathways or by causing structural and/or permeability changes in the membranes of subcellular organelles, appear consistently to alter the metabolic effects of morphine upon the myocardium.

ACKNOWLEDGEMENTS

The work described in this paper was supported in part by a grant from the Council for Tobacco Research, U.S.A. The author wishes to acknowledge the technical assistance of R. Rosenthal.

REFERENCES

1. Blumgart, H.L., Gargill, S.L., and Gilligan, D.R. (1930): J. Clin. Invest., 9: 91-106.
2. Bradley, R.F., and Schonfeld, A. (1962): Geriatrics, 17: 322-326.
3. Chiba, S. (1973): Arch.Int.Pharmacodyn.Ther., 206: 129-134.
4. Datey, K.K., and Nanda, N.C. (1967): N. Engl.J.Med. 276: 262-265.
5. Di Giorgio, J., Vitale, J.J. and Hellerstern, E.E. (1962): Biochem. J., 82: 184-187.
6. Du Ruisseau, J.P., and Mori, K. (1959): Br. J. Exp. Pathol., 40: 250-254
7. Essman, W.B.: In: Evaluation of New Drugs in Clinical Psychopharmacology, edited by Cassano, G.B., Edinter, Zürich, 1976 (in press).
8. Feldberg, W., and Gupta, K.P. (1974): J. Physiol. (Lond.), 238: 487-502.
9. Goīthi, J.J., Marquez, J., Castillo-Olivares, J.L., Avello, L.F., and Figurea, D. (1976): J.Cardiovasc.Sur., 17: 38-42.
10. Haugaard, N., and Hess, M.E. (1965): Pharmacol. Rev., 17: 27-69.
11. Hoch, F.L. (1962): Physiol. Rev., 42: 605-673.
12. Hoch, F.L. (1962): N. Engl.J.Med., 266: 446-454
13. Hochrein, H., Kuschke, H.J., Zaqqa, Q., and Fahl, E. (1967): Klin. Wochenschr., 45: 1093-1096
14. Holland, W.C., and Sekul, A.A. (1959): Am. J. Physiol., 197: 757-760.
15. Iseri, L.T., Alexander, L.C., McCarghey, R.S., Boyle, A.J., and Myers, G.B. (1952): Am. Heart J., 43: 215-227.
16. Johnson, C.J., Mauritsen, C.M., Starbuck, W.C., and Schwartz, A. (1967): Biochemistry, 6: 1121-1127.

17. Kakunaga, T., Kaneto, H., and Hano, K. (1966): J. Pharmacol. Exp. Ther., 153: 134-141
18. Kleiger, R.E., Seta, K., Vitale, J.J., and Lown, B. (1966): Am.J.Cardiol., 17: 520-527.
19. Kurt, T.L., Genton, E., Chidsey, C. III, Beck, P., and Sussman, K.E. (1973): Chest, 64: 21-25.
20. Lal, S., Savidge, R.S., and Chhabra, G.D. (1969): Lancet, 1: 379-381.
21. Lappas, D.G., Geha, D., Fischer, J.E., Laver, M.B., and Lowenstein, E. (1975): Anesthesiology, 42: 153-159.
22. Lehr, D. (1969): Ann. N.Y. Acad. Sci., 156: 344-378.
23. Lehr, D., Krukowski, M., and Colon, R. (1966): JAMA, 197: 105-112.
24. Lowenstein, E., Hallowell, P., Levine, F.A., Dagget, W.M., Austen, W.G., and Laver, M.B. (1969): N. Engl.J.Med., 281: 1389-1393
25. Lüllmann, H. and Holland, W. (1962): J. Pharmacol. Exp. Ther., 137: 186-192.
26. Margolis, J.R., Kannel, W.B., Feinleiv, M., Dawber, T.R., and McNamara, P.M. (1973): Am.J.Cardiol., 32: 1-7.
27. Norman, T.D. (1962): Progr.Cardiovasc.Dis., 4: 439-463.
28. Partamian, J.O., Bradley, R.F. (1965): N. Engl. J. Med., 273: 455-461.
29. Rich, C., Bierman, E.L., and Schwartz, I.L. (1959): J. Clin. Invest., 38: 275-278.
30. Schwartz, A. (1966): J. Biol. Chem., 241: 1122-1127
31. Seelig, M., and Heggtveit, H.A. (1974): Am. J. Clin.Nutr., 27: 59-79.
32. Seller, R.H., Neff, M.H., Mendelssohn, S., Kim, K. E., and Schwartz, C.D. (1970): Am.J.Cardiol., 25: 127.
33. Sheldon, M.I., Sorscher, S., Smith, C.B. (1975): J.Pharmacol.Exp.Ther., 193: 564-575.
34. Sokoloff, L., and Kaufman, S. (1961): J.Biol.Chem., 236: 795-803.
35. Soloff, L.A., and Schwartz, H. (1966): Lancet, 1: 449-452.
36. Sullivan, D.L., and Wong, K.C. (1973): Anesthesiology, 38: 550-556.
37. Szekely, P., and Wynne, N.A. (1951): Clin. Sci., 10: 241-247.
38. Takagi, H., and Narama, M. (1966): Jpn.J.Pharmacol. 16: 483-484.
39. Theroux, P., Ross, J. Jr., Franklin, D., Kemper, W.S., and Sasayama, S. (1976): Circulation, 53: 302-314.
40. Urthalei, F., Isobe, J.A., and James, T.N. (1975): Chest, 68: 222-228

41. Wang, S.C., Young, D., Au, K.S. (1974): <u>Biochem.</u>
    <u>Pharmacol.</u>, 23: 829-833.
42. Whaley, R.A., Hart, T.M., and Hlitgaard, H.M.
    (1959): <u>Am. J. Physiol.</u>, 196: 1258-1261.
43. Wong, K.C., Sullivan, S., Wetstome, D.L. (1975):
    <u>Anesth.Analg.</u>, 54: 787-791.

Factors Affecting the Action of Narcotics, edited by
M.L. Adler, L. Manara, and R. Samanin.
Raven Press, New York©1978.

The Effect of Neurological Diseases on Narcotic Actions

Philip L. Gildenberg[*] and Elizabeth A.M. Frost[**]

[*] Division of Neurosurgery,University of
Texas Medical School at Houston,
Texas, 77030 U.S.A.

[**] Department of Anesthesiology
Albert Einstein College of Medecine
Bronx, New York, 10461 U.S.A.

INTRODUCTION

On the surface, the preparation of a manuscript on the effect of neurological diseases on the action of narcotics seems like a rather reasonable task. After all, it is well known that patients with certain neurological diseases such as multiple sclerosis exhibit increased sensitivity to narcotics. It is equally apparent that mentally retarded patients have decreased sensitivity to narcotics and may require large doses. However, our extensive review of the literature revealed no concrete evidence for such truisms. Except perhaps for head injury, there have been few studies performed in neurological conditions using acceptable experimental models. There have been essentially no controlled narcotic studies in patients with those conditions for which we have no experimental model. Much of the relevant literature is anecdotal, reporting isolated observations on single or small groups of patients. Many impressions are conflicting.

It seemed that perhaps the anesthesia literature might be a storehouse of information, since the use of narcotics for premedication provides ample opportunity to study their effects in patients with a variety of diseases. Unfortunately, except for head trauma and conditions associated with increased intracranial pressure, the relevant anesthesia literature likewise contains little. Advice, such as not to use narcotics in certain conditions, is again also based on anecdote and isolated unfortunate experiences rather than controlled studies.

In this report we have considered not only the effect of neurological diseases on narcotic actions, but also

703

the reciprocal consideration, the effect of narcotics
in patients with neurological diseases.

Increased Intracranial Pressure and Trauma

Let us initially consider   the effects of narcotics
on conditions associated with increased intracranial
pressure, since we have more objective data concerning
these conditions than any other. As early as 1934
Munro (48) advocated, "It can be taken as a good
general rule : 'No morphine where increased intracranial
pressure is suspected". He admonished Russel (53) for
having stated just prior to that time, 'Morphine is
useful (in head injury)- and can apparently be given
without danger '. In 1935, Finesinger and Cobb (17)
documented that administration of morphine could result
in an increase in intracranial pressure, but in 1939
Gurdjian et al. (26) admitted that 'the reason for such
a rise is obscure '.

Meanwhile, the respiratory depressant effect of
morphine was reported by Dripps and Comroe (12) and
others. In a study in 1944, meperidine was given to 20
patients with various intracranial lesions. It was
noted that in 7 of the 20, the respiratory rate fell to
less than 12 per minute. Unfortunately, no measurement
was made of intracranial pressure. About the same time
Guttman (27) concluded that caution should be exerted
in the administration of narcotics to patients with
intracranial lesions. It was documented by Kepes (38)
in the 1950's that both morphine and meperidine given
to surgical patients with normal neurological function
caused a marked increase in cerebrospinal fluid pressure.
Swerdlow et al. (65) in 1955 wrote that the increased
intracranial pressure was 'no doubt associated...with
respiratory depression '.

Keats and Mithoefer (36) reported a well-controlled
study in which they demonstrated that the profound
decrease in alveolar ventilation and increase in
alveolar pCO_2 caused by narcotics could be correlated
with increased intracranial pressure. They plotted the
reciprocal narcotic induced changes in alveolar pCO_2
and intracranial pressure, and the prompt return toward
control levels with either hyperventilation or a
narcotic antagonist.   Other authors also noted that
such respiratory depression and consequent increased
intracranial pressure could be blocked or reversed by
narcotic antagonists (35, 36, 64). The increase in
intracranial pressure which can be correlated with increase in arterial pCO_2 (PaCo2) likewise can be prevented
or reversed by artificial ventilation, both experimentally (71) and clinically (19).

The respiratory depressant effect of narcotics is

primarily due to a central action on the medullary
respiratory center (19): rate decreases more than other
parameters. The depressed CO_2 response causes an increase in both alveolar and arterial pCO_2 (19,31). A
sudden increase in $PaCO_2$ leads to an increase in
cerebral vasodilation which, in turn, increases cerebral
blood flow, abruptly raising intracranial pressure.
Smith and Wollman (59) noted that cerebral blood flow
varied linearly with the $PaCO_2$ values between 20-60
torr. Although cerebral vasodilatation is directly
related to the hydrogen ion concentration, it is the
rapid diffusion of CO_2 which causes an abrupt shift
of ions and resultant sudden vasodilatation and increased intracranial pressure. If the $PaCO_2$ is
maintained at a constant level, the intracranial pressure does not increase, even though narcotics may be
administered. Narcotics alone have little direct
vasodilatory effect on the cerebrovascular system (59).
The increase in intracranial pressure is entirely due
to the respiratory depression. It has also been
reported that small doses of narcotics, such as fentanyl
as used in neuroleptanalgesia in combination with
tranquilizers, may (46) or may not (18) significantly
increase intracranial pressure.

Intracranial compliance, an index of the elasticity
within the cranium and spinal canal, is defined as the
ratio of change in intracranial pressure with a corresponding change in volume. With intracranial mass
lesions, compliance may decrease, in which case the
ability to compensate for increased intracranial blood
volume may diminish (44). Under these circumstances
even the slight cerebral vasodilatation which results
from a minor increase in $PaCO_2$, despite its remaining
within limits ordinarily considered normal, may
significantly increase intracranial pressure (23).

The rapid expanding mass of hematoma or edema
following trauma may cause significant sudden changes
in compliance. In addition, cerebral concussion causes
transient prolonged depression of the medullary respiratory center which may result in hypercarbia and a
resultant increase in intracranial pressure (32). This
can be compounded by a direct medullary injury such as
contusion, which might further depress respiration.
Similarly, edema or bleeding which frequently accompany
significant brain injury may cause increased intracranial pressure, which may further depress the medullary respiratory center (32). A vicious cycle may
ensue. Head injury may directly cause medullary depression. The resultant hypercarbia causes cerebral
vasodilatation which increases intracranial pressure.
Intracranial pressure also rises secondary to edema or
hematoma. Increased intracranial pressure produces

further medullary depression which, in turn, causes
additional hypercarbia with cerebral vasodilatation and
further increase in intracranial pressure. If the
additional respiratory depressant effect of a narcotic
is introduced into this cycle, the progressive downill
course is accelerated.

It has been demonstrated experimentally in cats that
narcotics in amounts which ordinarily produce no demonstrable respiratory depression can cause profound
medullary depression after even mild cerebral trauma
(32,50), so that tolerance to narcotics is significantly
lowered with even moderate head injury. However, drug
addiction and head injuries frequently coexist. A
patient in withdrawal may present with pulmonary edema
or upper airway obstruction. Administration of adequate
doses of narcotics is necessary to treat the withdrawal,
and respiration must be supported.

Narcotics should be avoided in patients with cervical
spinal cord injuries. Not only may pulmonary function
be impaired, but narcotics may precipitate shock in
patients who have interruption of sympathetic cardiovascular control (19).

Neurological Diseases

Patients with multiple sclerosis may have profound
respiratory depression or prolonged sedation from small
doses of a narcotic, evidenced by the albeit anectodal
report of four cases by Baskett and Armstrong (6). In
addition they observed that administration of narcotics
may cause an exacerbation of multiple sclerosis,although
it is not clear whether this results from the drug,
from the painful stressful situation for which the drug
was administered, or whether it is a coincidental exacerbation of the disease.

It has been reported (66) that usual doses of
morphine may cause sudden respiratory arrest or cyanosis
in patients with tabes dorsalis. This type of respiratory failure is described as a failure of automatic
respiration occurring during sleep when the patient
'forgets' to breathe. This same type of sleep-induced
apnea has been reported with other lesions involving
the cervical spinal cord (24,25,52,67), and also in
patients with cerebrovascular insufficiency.

Mentally retarded patients may require anesthesia
for procedures which ordinarily would be done with the
patient awake or under mild sedation. Consequently
they may receive narcotics as part of their premedication (9,11,37), or the narcotic may be used as part of
a balanced anesthetic technique. Generally the use of
narcotics in mental retardation or cerebral palsy
appears to be as safe as in the general population (9),

but no well-controlled study has been done. However, the rules for drug dosage by age and/or weight are not reliable in this group, particularly in hyperactive children. Although dosage schedules might be used as a guide, the usual amounts are frequently found to be ineffective (11,37) so that quite large doses of narcotics may be necessary. It is both frightening and amazing to see the tremendous individual variation in narcotic action in this heterogeneous group of patients.

Patients with cerebral palsy usually require sedation or general anesthesia for dental management. A combination of narcotics and tranquilizers has fre-quently been found beneficial for those patients with a great deal of anxiety or hostility. If the problem is primarily one of motor function without mental retardation, the dosage requirements do not appear to be unusual (51).

A special situation may exist when mental retardation is caused by phenylketonuria (34). The increased tissue phenylalanine, particularly if a monoamine oxidase inhibitor has been employed, may cause an idio-syncratic reaction to narcotics with increase in motor activity, increased heart rate, pallor, sweating, and agitation.

Anesthesia

Narcotics must be used with care when given as anesthetic premedication. Even patients who receive narcotic premedication for non-cerebral surgery of any kind generally have more respiratory depression on in-duction of even light anesthesia than patients who do not receive narcotics (13,20). An excellent review of the anesthetic implications of various syndromes, both neurological and others, includes references to the contraindication of narcotics in various diseases (33).

Age

There may be heightened sensitivity to narcotics at both extremes of age. Old patients, particularly with cerebral arteriosclerosis, may suffer an enhanced re-spiratory depressive effect on administration of narcotics (32,54). This is compounded by a decrease in respiratory reserve with decreased lung compliance and diminished functional residual capacity. Ordinarily, the aged compensate for hypercarbia by increasing the rate of respiration. However, narcotics especially depress the respiratory rate, which may rapidly lead to decompensation (19). This can be compounded when cerebral arteriosclerosis involves the respiratory center and the CO_2 response is compromised (19, 32). Aged patients who do require narcotics as premedication or for pain control, particularly if respiration is controlled or assisted, may be difficult to wean from the respirator at the conclusion of surgery.

Heightened sensitivity of newborns to morphine may result from higher concentration of drugs at the central site of activity (19,69), since the blood-brain barrier is still deficient in the neonate. Indeed, when morphine is administered to the mother, the central nervous system concentration may be higher in the fetus than in the mother (69), which may initially cause respiratory depression. However, the blood-brain barrier does not play as prominent a role in limiting the central nervous system access to some other narcotics, for instance, meperidine, so that it may not cause more respiratory depression in the newborn than in the adult. Also, the immature liver and kidneys may not yet be capable of efficiently detoxifying and excreting the narcotic so that the effect of a single dose may be prolonged. It may be necessary to withdraw the newborn child of a narcotic addict. These infants require large doses of narcotics very quickly at birth or they go into severe withdrawal with pulmonary edema. Usually they are fairly easily and sucessfully weaned from drugs in about seven days.

Alcohol

Narcotics are ordinarily contraindicated in patients with alcohol intoxication or delirium tremens. Both alcohol and narcotics are central depressants and may act synergistically to cause a profound or even fatal central respiratory depression (41). Cerebral edema frequently accompanies alcoholism with a resultant increase in intracranial pressure, and the contra-indication to the use of narcotics is the same when increased intracranial pressure is caused by alcoholism as in trauma. Additionally, alcoholics frequently have concomitant head trauma, which they may not remember, and may have hypoprothombinemia or even intravascular coagulopathy with increased bleeding tendency, so the incidence of unsuspected subdural hematoma is high in this group of patients.

Seizures

Although it has been demonstrated in the rat by Adler and his group (5, 60) that the narcotic withdrawal state is accompained by a decreased threshold to flurothyl seizures and that morphine has an anti-convulsant effect in that situation (4), there is a danger in the use of morphine in clinical epilepsy. Theoretically, the seizures might be enhanced by the reflex excitability of the spinal cord that results from narcotic administration (38). There is no firm clinical evidence that the administration of narcotics

helps to control seizures. Indeed, if the seizure is
due to an intracranial mass lesion, the narcotics may
further increase intracranial pressure or cause hypoxia
which may make the clinical situation worse.

Other Diseases

Diseases of organs outside the nervous system may
influence the action of narcotics on CNS function,
either directly or secondary to their effect on narcotic
metabolism. For instance, patients on dialysis with
end-state renal disease may have a dramatic and
potentially fatal depressant response to narcotics,
which may simply be due to the prolongation of the
half-life of the drug in chronic renal failure and the
gradual toxic accumulation of narcotic and its metabolites in the central nervous system (47).

Patients with hypothyroidism are hypersensitive to
the depressant effect of narcotics (19,32), whereas
patients with hyperthyroidism may have a decreased
sensitivity (18).

The deleterious effects of narcotics in certain
respiratory conditions may result in cerebral hypoxia.
Primary among these is chronic obstructive pulmonary
disease (32). The use of narcotics is generally
contraindicated in patients with asthma. Not only do
narcotics cause depression of the respiratory center
and decreased cough reflex, but the histamine-releasing
or cholinergic activity of the narcotic may have a
spastic effect on the bronchial musculature (19,32).
However, morphine may have a profound anxiety-allaying
effect in asthmatic patients with severe pain and may
be used in combination with aminophylline administration and/or respiratory support.

Nausea and vomiting may occur on administration of
narcotics, particularly morphine, by stimulation of
the medullary emetic center, especially in patients
without pain (32). In patients with depressed consciousness, this may lead to aspiration of stomach
contents and frequently to fatal pneumonitis.

Clinical Stereotactic Lesions

In addition to naturally occurring pathological
neurological lesions affecting the action of narcotics,
specific experimentally produced or clinically produced
lesions can also affect narcotic analgesia or narcotic
dependence.

It has become a recognized clinical procedure to
treat patients by making stereotactic lesions in the
thalamus when pain is intractable to any other means
of therapy (16,22,28,42,43,49,57,61,62,63). As early
as 1964 we had observed that after lesions were placed

in the thalamus of patients with intractable pain who
had become addicted to narcotics, the narcotics could
be abruptly discontinued without evidence of withdrawal symptoms, even though the lesions avoided
structures involving the control of emotions. This
observation was later confirmed by others (14). In
these patients stereotactic lesions were made at the
base of the thalamus extending into the intralaminar
area (61,63). The effects were on the physiologic
aspects of withdrawal, since no untoward psychological
changes were noted (16,57,61,63).

This is in contrast to the well-recognized phenomenon that psychosurgical procedures involving the limbic
system can abort the 'purposive' abstinence phenomena
(symptoms such as drug-seeking behavior under purpose-
ful control of the patient) (15,21,45,58,72,73), but
do not generally affect the physiologic or 'non-
purposive' phenomena (those phenomena involving physiologic, reflex, or autonomic activity not generally
under the patient's control) (68,72). It has been
suggested that the major effect on abrupt withdrawal
symptoms may be the result of mental depression,whereby
the limbic lesions temporarily decrease the patient's
reaction and awareness to symptoms in general, especially in the early stages when the acute withdrawal
symptoms are greatest.

Experimental Lesions

It has been verified that experimental lesions in
specific brain sites can affect many manifestations of
narcotic dependence. Areas of the medial thalamus have
been implicated in the action of narcotics by Wei et.
al. (70). Lesions in the centrum medianum and parafascicularis in the thalamus of the rat not only prevent
a drop in threshold to flurothyl seizures in withdrawal
(1,5,60) but may actually increase it. Centrum medianum,
parafascicularis, and limbic lesions modify certain
specific signs of abstinence in the rat. The particular
effects are dependent upon the site of chronicity of
the lesion (2).

Experimental lesions in the ventromedial hypothalamus
have been claimed by Kerr and Pozuelo (39,40) to lessen
the severity of the abstinence syndrome and to cause a
loss of tolerance to morphine. However, since the
lesions were acute, one must consider that changes in
blood-brain barrier might account for the apparent loss
of tolerance. The poor overall physical condition of
the animals also might have affected the physical expression of the withdrawal syndrome.

Other experimental lesions have been demonstrated to
affect the analgesic action of narcotics. Charpentier
(10) produced a series of lesions in the rat and studied

the alteration in the ability of morphine to modify the response to noxious stimuli. He concluded that the type of noxious stimulus determines the importance of a particular lesion.

Yeung et al. (74) noted that parafascicular or centrum medianum lesions in the rat had to involve more than 50% of these structures in order to cause an effect on morphine action. Thus, the inconsistent result of such lesions affecting the narcotic with-drawal syndrome in other studies might be because an insufficient portion of a specific nucleus or pathway had been destroyed.

Samanin and others (3,55,56) reported that lesions of the nucleus raphe medianus decreased the analgesic action of morphine, as tested by tail compression, hot plate, and electrical stimulation of the tail. In contrast, Blasig et al. (7) and Buxbaum et al. (8) reported that raphe lesions did not affect morphine analgesia. Adler et al. (3), however, identified a critical area in the midbrain (ventral) raphe nucleus. Lesions in this area markedly decreased the analgesic activity of morphine, while lesions in the dorsal raphe or the area between the two nuclei did not result in any change. They implicated the nucleus raphe medianus and the periaqueductal grey in the anti-nociceptive activity of morphine. Their results, in conjunction with the results of Samanin, suggest that analgesic properties and narcotic dependence are con-cerned with different areas of the brain, since bilateral lesions in the raphe nuclei had very little effect on the dependence to morphine or on the severity of with-drawal.

Other structures implicated in the antinociceptive action of narcotics include structures lining the floor of the fourth ventricle (29) and the periaqueductal grey (30).

CONCLUSION

Thus, we can appreciate that alteration of certain areas of the nervous system can cause profound changes in responsiveness to narcotics. One might anticipate that many neurological diseases, particularly degen-erative diseases, might cause naturally occurring lesions in areas involved in narcotic action. Knowl-edge of the altered activity to narcotics in such patients could be of considerable clinical significance and might lead to a better understanding of the action of narcotic agents. Certainly, the study of the effect of narcotics in patients with neurological disease has considerable potential reward. One would hope that researchers in this field would address themselves to the challenge of well-controlled, quantitative studies to answer many of the questions about how neurological disease may alter the action of narcotics.

ACKNOWLEDGEMENT

This work was supported in part by Grant ≠ DA 01498-03 from the National Institute of Drug Abuse.

REFERENCES

1. Adler, M.W. (1975) : In : Current Developments in Psychopharmacology, Spectrum, New York, in press.
2. Adler, M.W., and Gildenberg, P.L. (1976) In preparation.
3. Adler, M.W., Kostowski,W., and Samanin, R. (1975): Eur.J. Pharmacol. 32 : 39-44.
4. Adler, M.W., Lin, C.H., Keinath, S.H., Braverman, S., and Geller, E.B. (1976) : J. Pharmacol. Exp. Ther. (in press).
5. Adler, M.W., Smith, K.P., Lin, C., Tresky, R., and Gildenberg, P.L. (1974) : Psychopharmacologia 35: 243-247.
6. Baskett, P.J.E., and Armstrong, R. (1970) : Anaesthesia 25 : 397-401.
7. Blasig, J., Reinhold, K., and Hertz A. (1973): Psychopharmacologia 31 : 111-119.
8. Buxbaum, D.M., Yarbrough, G.G., and Carter, M.E. (1973) : J. Pharmacol. Exp. Ther. 185 : 317-327.
9. Castaldi C.R.(1961) : J. Dent. Child. 28 : 218-223.
10. Charpentier, J. (1967) : Psychopharmacologia 11 : 95-121.
11. Diamond, A.W., and Cochrane, D.F. (1976) : Anaesthesia 31 : 190-194.
12. Dripps, R.D., and Comroe, J.H. (1945) : Anesthesiology 6 : 462-468.
13. Eckenhoff, J.E.,and Helrich, M. (1958) : JAMA 167: 415-422.
14. Ervin, F.A. (1971) : Personal communication.
15. Faillace, L.W., Allen, R.P., McQueen, J.D., and Northrup, B. (1971) : Dis. Nerv. Syst. 32 : 171-175.
16. Fairman, D. (1966) : Confin. Neurol. 27 : 67-70.
17. Finesinger, J.E., and Cobb, S. (1935) : J. Pharmacol Exp. Ther. 53 : 1-33.
18. Fitch, W., Barker, J., and Jennett, W.B. (1969) : Br. J. Anaesth. 41 : 800-806.
19. Foldes, F.F., Swerdlow, M., and Siker, E.S. (1964): Narcotics and Narcotic Antagonists. Thomas, Springfield.
20. Foldes, F.F., Zeedick, F.J., and Koukal, L.R.(1957): Am. J. Med. Sci. 233 : 153-161.
21. Foltz, E.L., and White, L.E. (1968) : Int. J.Neurol. 6 : 353-373 .

22. Forster, D.M.C., Leksell, L., and Meyerson B.A. (1970): Presented at the Fifth International Symposium in Stereoencephalotomy. Freiburg, Germany.
23. Frost, E. A.M., and Gildenberg P.L. (1976) : Appl. Neurophysiol. (in press).
24. Gildenberg, P.L. (1969) : Cleveland Clinic Quarterly 36 : 783-788.
25. Gildenberg, P.L. (1974) : Clin. Neurosurg. 21 : 246-256.
26. Gurdjian, E.S., Webster, J.E., and Sprunk, C.J. (1939) : Arch. Neurol. Psychiat. 42 : 92-111.
27. Guttman, S.A. (1944) : JAMA 124 : 155-157.
28. Hecaen, H.,Talairach , J., David, M., and Dell,M.B. (1941) : Rev. Neurol. 81 : 917-931.
29. Herz, A., Albus, K., Metys, J., Schubert, P., and Teschemacher, H. (1970) : Neuropharmacology 9 : 539-551.
30. Jacquet, Y., and Lajtha, A. (1974) : Science 185: 1055-1057.
31. Jaffe, J.H., and Martin, W.R. (1975) : In : The Pharmacological Basis of Therapeutics (5th ed.) edited by Goodman, L.S. and Gilman A., pp. 245-283, MacMillan, New York.
32. Jeghers, H., and Brick, I.B. (1950):Med.Clin. North Am. 34 : 1761-1777.
33. Jones, A.P., and Pelton, D.A. (1976): Can. Anaesth. Soc. J. 23 : 207-226.
34. Jounela, A.J., and Kivimaki, T. (1973) : N. Engl.J. Med. 288 : 1411-1413.
35. Keats, A.S. (1954) : Fed. Proc. 13 : 374.
36. Keats, A.S., and Mithoefer, J.C. (1955) : Fed. Proc. 14 : 356.
37. Kennedy, J.B. Jr. (1961) : J. Oral Surg. 19 : 376-379.
38. Kepes, E.R. (1952) : Anesthesiology 13 : 281-286.
39. Kerr, F.W.L., and Pozuelo, J. (1971) : Fed. Proc. 30 : 375 Abs.
40. Kerr, F.W.L., and Pozuelo, J. (1971) : Mayo Clin. Proc. 46 : 653-665.
41. Leary, T. (1935) : N. Engl. J. Med. 212 : 216.
42. Mark, V.H., and Ervin, F.R. (1969) : In : Pain and the Neurosurgeon. edited by White, J.C. and Sweet, W.H., pp. 843-887, Thomas, Springfield.
43. Mark, V.H., Ervin, F.F., and Yakovlev, P.I. (1963): Arch. Neurol. 8 : 528-538.
44. Marmarou, A., Shulman, K., and LaMorgese, J.(1974): J. Neurosurg. 43 : 523-534.
45. Mason, T.H., and Hamby, W.B. (1948) : JAMA 136 : 1039-1040.
46. Miller, R., Tausk, H.C., and Stark, D.C.C. (1975): Can. Anaesth. Soc. J. 22: 502-508.

47. Mostert, J.W., Evers, J.L., Hobika, G.H., Moore, R.H., and Ambrus, J.L. (1971) : Brit. J. Anaesth. 43 : 1053-1059.
48. Munro, D. (1934) : N. Engl. J. Med. 210 : 287-294.
49. Orthner, H. (1966) : Conf. Neurol. 27 : 71-74.
50. Phillips, G. (1935) : Med. J. Australia 2 : 108-113.
51. Rosen, S., and Rosenstein, S.N. (1966) : J. Oral Ther. 3 : 194-202.
52. Rosomoff, H.L. (1969) : J. Neurosurg. 31 : 41-46.
53. Russell, W.R. (1932) : Brain 55 : 549-603.
54. Salter, W.T., and White, M.L. (1949) : Anesthesiology 10 : 553-561.
55. Samanin, R., and Bernasconi, S. (1972) : Psycho-pharmacologia 25 : 175-182.
56. Samanin, R., Ghezzi, D., Mauron, C., and Valzelli, L. (1973) : Psychopharmacologia 33 : 365-368.
57. Sano, K., Yoshioka, M., and Ogashiwa, M. (1966) : Conf. Neurol. 27 : 63-66.
58. Scarff, J.E. (1949) : Surg. Gynec. Obstet. 89 : 385-392.
59. Smith, A.L., and Wollman, H. (1972) : Anesthesiology 36 : 378-400.
60. Smith, K.P., Gildenberg, P.L., and Adler, M.W. (1971) : Fed. Proc. 30 : 277.
61. Spiegel, E.A., and Wycis, H.T. (1966): Conf. Neurol. 27 : 7-17.
62. Spiegel, E.A., Wycis, H.T., Szekely, E.G., and Gildenberg, P.L. (1966) : In : Pain edited by Knighton, R.S. and Dumke, P.R., pp. 503-517, Little Brown, Boston.
63. Spiegel, E.A., Wycis, H.T.,Szekely, E.G., Gildenberg, P.L., and Zanes,C. (1964) : J. Internat. Coll. Surg. 42 : 160-168.
64. Swerdlow, M. (1956) : Anaesthesia 11 : 149-155.
65. Swerdlow, M., Foldes, F.F., and Siker, E.S. (1955): Br. J. Anaesth. 27 : 244-249.
66. Taterka, H., and Pinéas, H. (1928) : Nervenarzt 1 : 543-547.
67. Tenicela, R., Rosomoff, H.L., and Feist, J. (1968): Anesthesiology 29 : 7-16.
68. Trafton, C.L., and Marques, P.R. (1971) : J. Comp. Physiol. Psych. 75 : 277-285.
69. Way, W.L., Costley, E.C., and Way, E.L. (1965) : Clin. Pharmacol. Ther. 6 : 454-461.
70. Wei, E., Sigel, S.S.R., Loh, H.H., and Way, E.L. (1975) : J. Pharmacol. Exp. Ther. 194 : 480-487.
71. Weitzner, S.W., McCoy, G.T., and Binder, L.S. (1963) : Anesthesiology 24 : 291-298.
72. Wikler, A. (1959) : Res. Publ. Ass. Res. Nerv. Ment. Dis. 37 : 334-355.
73. Wikler, A., Pescor. M.J., Kalbaugh, E.P., and

Angelucci, R.J. (1952) : Arch. Neurol. Psych. 67: 519-521.

74. Yeung, J.C., Yaksh,T.L., and Rudy, T.A. (1975) : Clin.Exp. Pharmacol. Physiol. 2 : 261-268.

Factors Affecting the Action of Narcotics, edited by
M.L. Adler, L. Manara, and R. Samanin.
Raven Press, New York©1978.

Effects of Drugs and Alcohol on Opiate
Disposition and Action

Mary Jeanne Kreek

The Rockefeller University
1230 York Avenue, New York, N.Y. 10021, U.S.A.

INTRODUCTION

It is estimated that there are now over 400,000
heroin addicts in the United States; over 85,000 are
receiving chronic methadone maintenance treatment. Also,
as medical science and technology have made advances
resulting in the prolongation of life in many patients
with terminal illnesses, increasing numbers of patients
with chronic pain are receiving narcotics for analgesia
over extended periods of time. Therefore, the problem
of the interaction of chronically administered narcotics
with other drugs and alcohol has assumed new and critical importance in clinical medicine. First, many
patients receiving narcotics regularly for the treatment of addiction or for the relief of pain require
other medications. Secondly, street heroin addicts,
and to a lesser extent patients on methadone maintenance treatment, may abuse a wide variety of drugs, especially tranquilizers, such as diazepam, and sedatives,
such as the barbiturates (15). Finally, and possibly
of greatest importance, alcohol is widely used socially
by all patient groups and is abused by many, including
large numbers of street addicts and those in treatment
(27).
In our early prospective studies of the first
patients treated with methadone, carried out from 1964-
1970, it was shown that at least 25% of patients maintained on methadone were also alcohol abusers, both
before and during methadone treatment, a finding subsequently confirmed by others in studies carried out
in different regions of the United States (3,8,22,24,25,
27,37,45). Furthermore, our studies showed that progressive, moderate to severe liver disease, is a serious
medical problem in the subgroup of methadone maintenance patients who also consume large amounts of alcohol
(24,25,27). Other studies have suggested that early

717

death from liver disease or its complications is a
frequent outcome in this group of patients (2). Alcohol
abuse is now recognized as the most common problem in
methadone maintenance patients and is the most frequent
reason for involuntary discharge of patients from
treatment (16). Concomitant alcohol and opiate abuse
now seems to be an increasing problem in adolescent as
well as adult drug abusers. However, effects of alcohol
on narcotic disposition and action in man, and the
mechanisms of action of such effects, have not been
defined, nor have specific clinical observations been
made to support the hypothesis of the existence of
alcohol-narcotic interactions.

Information concerning the effects of other drugs
and alcohol on opiate actions, particularly on the
development and maintenance of tolerance and dependence, is critical, both to gain insight into factors
affecting the development of addiction and to improve
care of patients receiving narcotics on a chronic
basis. Despite the importance and the magnitude of
potential clinical problems, only limited clinical
observations on the effects of other drugs and alcohol
on opiate action have been made. Even fewer studies
have been carried out to define the nature of any
clinically observed drug interactions. However, increasing numbers of animal studies now are being carried
out to look for and define possible drug interactions.

Various drugs and alcohol could alter opiate action,
either by effecting changes of opiate disposition which
could, in turn, alter the levels of drugs or active
metabolites available at critical receptors, or alternatively by effecting alterations of functional response
to opiates at receptor sites without altering their
disposition. The resultant effects of other drugs or
alcohol on opiate action could be additive, potentiating, synergistic or antagonistic. The primary focus of
this review will be on clinical studies of the effects
of various drugs and alcohol on opiate disposition
and action, with the inclusion of a few related animal
studies which have possible direct clinical applicability.

ANALYTICAL TECHNIQUES AND METHADONE METABOLISM IN MAN

After the initial early studies on opiate disposition of the 1950's, which relied primarily on chemical
and some radioisotope analytical techniques, few more
extensive studies were carried out until the last five
years, when sensitive, precise and specific assays were
developed by several laboratories to measure levels of

various narcotics and their metabolites in various
biological fluids and tissues. Gas chromatography,
mass spectrometry, high pressure liquid chromatography,
radioimmunoassay, and improved radioisotope and more
recently stable isotope techniques, have been employed
in these various assays.

With the development of these sensitive and specific
analytical procedures, it has become possible for the
first time to perform studies concerning the bioavaila-
bility, distribution, metabolism and pharmacokinetics
of narcotic drugs in man and in animal models. Using
techniques developed in our laboratory, we have carried
out clinical studies of three potential drug or alcohol
interactions in patients receiving chronic methadone
maintenance treatment for narcotic addiction (13,26,28,
29,30). Two additional recent sets of clinical studies
of potential drug interactions with opiates using new
analytical techniques, have been carried out by other
investigators in normal volunteer subjects receiving
meperidine or morphine (9,49).

After oral administration, methadone is essentially
completely absorbed and is promptly widely distributed
throughout the body. Therefore, peak plasma levels of
methadone are relatively low (usually less than 1 μg/ml),
even in patients receiving chronic daily maintenance
doses of 50-100 mg of methadone, and are very low (less
than 0.3 μg/ml) in rats receiving chronic daily methadone treatment of 5-10 mg/kg body weight (21,26,50 and
Kreek, Gutjahr and Korn, unpublished observations).
Methadone is metabolized primarily in the liver, where
it undergoes successive N-demethylations by the hepatic
microsomal drug metabolizing enzymes in the major pathway of biotransformation. After the first N-demethylations, cyclization occurs to form the major pyrrolidine
metabolite which has not been identified in peripheral
plasma, but which in man is excreted in urine in amounts
approximately equal to those of unchanged methadone.
Pyrrolidine is also the major excretory product in
feces. Some pyrrolidine may then be N-demethylated to
form a pyrroline metabolite, also excreted in urine and
feces in small amounts. Both the pyrrolidine and pyrroline metabolites may be hydroxylated (See Figure 1).
The pyrrolidine metabolite may also undergo spontaneous
oxidative degradation to form a pyrrolidone. Methadone
may also be metabolized by alternative minor pathways
resulting in the formation of hydroxymethadone, pyrrolidone and various methadol metabolites, of which only
the latter group have been shown to be pharmacologically
active as analgesics (See Figure 2). All of these
metabolites have been identified in urine by Dr. Hugh
Sullivan and colleagues, and the identity of most

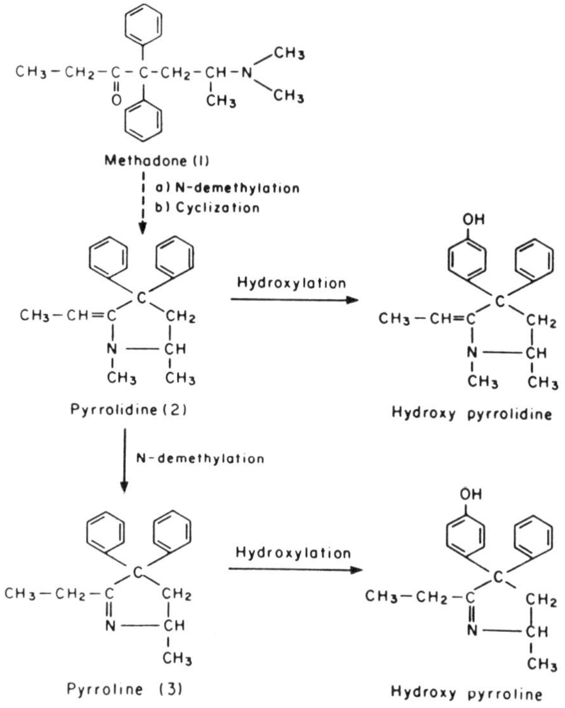

FIG. 1. Major pathways of methadone metabolism in man, based on compounds isolated from urine obtained from patients on methadone maintenance treatment (adapted from reference 51), and reprinted from <u>Heroin Dependency: Medical, Economic and Social Aspects</u>, edited by B. Stimmel, 1975, New York, with permission of the Stratton Intercontinental Medical Book Corp.).

confirmed by other laboratories (51).

In our laboratory, gas liquid chromatographic techniques have been developed for the quantitative analysis of methadone and its major pyrrolidine and the lesser pyrroline and pyrrolidone metabolites in plasma, urine, amniotic fluid, breast milk and, more recently, in feces (26,29,30,33). The lower limits of measurement of methadone and the pyrrolidine metabolite in plasma, urine and feces is 0.01 to 0.02 µg/ml (see Table 1).

In collaboration with Drs. Frank Field and David Bowen, chemical ionization mass spectrometric techniques for the qualitative analysis of several methadone metabolites including pyrrolidine, pyrroline, their

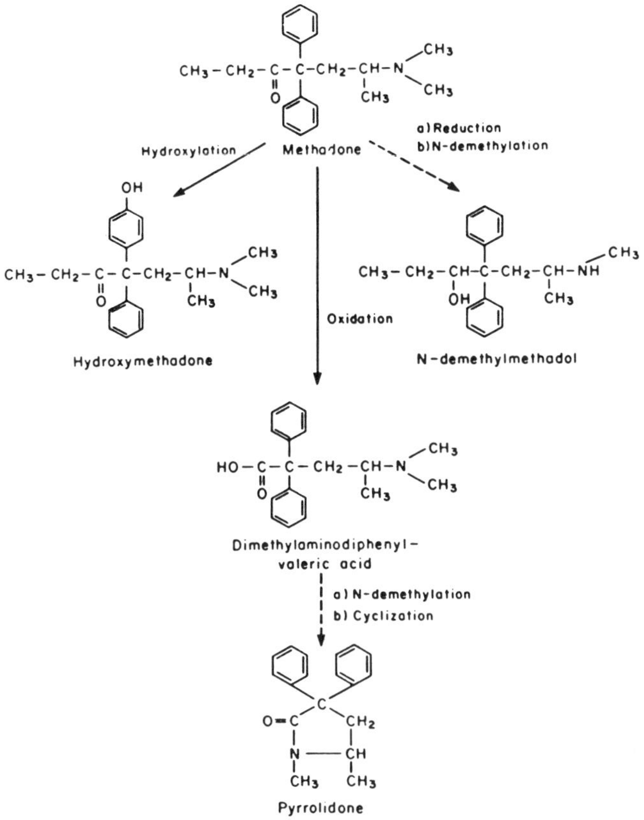

FIG. 2. Minor pathways of methadone metabolism in man, based on compounds isolated from urine obtained from patients on methadone maintenance treatment (adapted from reference 51, and reprinted from Heroin Dependency: Medical, Economic and Social Aspects, edited by B. Stimmel, 1975, New York, with permission of the Stratton Intercontinental Medical Book Corp.).

hydroxylated derivatives, hydroxy-methadone, pyrrolidone and the methadols, have been developed. Both direct probe and gas chromatographic introduction of samples to the mass spectrometer, have been used with ethylenediamine modified isobutane as the reactant gas, to increase sensitivity of detection in biological samples (7,29,33). Compounds can be identified by their gas chromatography retention times coupled with the mass of their protonated molecules, as determined by

TABLE 1. Quantitation of methadone and its pyrrolidine metabolite by gas liquid chromatography.

I. Methadone

	Plasma	Urine	Feces
Sensitivity	0.01 µg/ml	0.01 µg/ml	0.02 µg/ml
Precision	±3.3% S.D.	±2.6% S.D.	±6.0% S.D.

II. Pyrrolidine Metabolite

	Plasma	Urine	Feces
Sensitivity	N.D.[a]	0.01 µg/ml	0.02 µg/ml
Precision	N.D.	±6.6% S.D.	±8.1% S.D.

[a] N.D. = Not Detected

chemical ionization mass spectrometry. All of these techniques have been used in our studies of drug inter-actions with methadone to be discussed.

Also, in collaboration with Drs. Peter Klein and David Hachey of the Argonne National Laboratory, stable isotope technology has been modified and applied to studies of methadone disposition and pharmacokinetics in animals and in man. Stable isotope labeled methad-one, pentadeuteromethadone, has been synthesized by our group (19). Using the pentadeuteromethadone as an internal standard, a reverse isotope dilution method for the quantitation of methadone in biological samples has been developed (19). Isotope ratios of known or unknown amounts of unlabeled methadone and known amounts of stable labeled methadone, are measured using gas chromatography-chemical ionization mass spectrometry with a stable isotope ratiometer-multiple ion detection system. Dilution curves are constructed by graphing the logs of the differences in isotope ratios between the dilution standards and plasma or urine blanks, against the logs of the known mole ratios of unlabeled methadone to the stable labeled pentadeuteromethadone internal standard. Levels of methadone in plasma and urine down to 1 to 3 ng/ml can be measured using this more sensitive reverse isotope dilution technique.

Pentadeuteromethadone is now being used as a tracer in studies of methadone disposition and pharmacokinetics in animals and in man (31). Mole ratios of labeled and unlabeled methadone can be measured in plasma, as well

as in urine and feces, for at least nine days after a
single labeled dose is given to patients maintained on
methadone. Disappearance curves can be constructed
and kinetic measurements calculated. These various
stable isotope techniques will be used in some of our
future studies of drug interactions affecting narcotic
action.

DRUG INTERACTIONS IN PATIENTS RECEIVING METHADONE TREATMENT

We initially observed and then studied two types of
drug interactions in patients receiving methadone treatment. Both interactions resulted in the clinical
syndrome of narcotic abstinence (26,28).

Naloxone

First, a classical interaction of a narcotic agonist
and antagonist was observed when methadone and naloxone
were combined, 100 mg and 10 mg respectively, in a dose
form intended to prevent parenteral drug abuse of any
diverted medication (26). Based on animal studies, it
was assumed that only minimal, ineffective amounts of
naloxone would be absorbed, and thus the combined preparation would cause no untoward symptoms. Methadone
alone and the methadone-naloxone combination,were
administered in synthetic orange juice on a single-
blinded basis for two weeks to nine stabilized methadone maintenance patients (See Table 2). Two of the
nine patients developed severe symptoms of narcotic
withdrawal within thirty minutes after oral ingestion
of the combined medication. The symptoms included

TABLE 2. Naloxone - methadone interaction. Patients
studied to determine plasma levels of methadone after
methadone (100 mg) and methadone - naloxone (100 mg: 10
mg) administered orally[a].

Age (years)	Sex	Weight (kilos)	Previous Heroin Addiction (years)	Methadone Treatment (years)
27-50	6M 3F	65-84	3-23	1-5

[a] Data from reference 26

nausea, vomiting, anorexia, abdominal cramps, diarrhea, diaphoresis, pilocarpal erection, irritability, tremulousness and severe anxiety. These symptoms subsided after two to three hours, but returned each time the combined dose form was administered, for three and nine doses respectively. Three additional patients experienced milder withdrawal symptoms after each dose of combined preparation, but were able to tolerate the symptoms for the two week study period. Four patients experienced no symptoms during combined treatment. After three to fourteen days treatment with the methadone-naloxone combination and after fourteen days of methadone alone, plasma levels of methadone were determined at twenty-four hours (time zero), two, and six hours after an oral dose. No significant differences in plasma levels of methadone during treatment with the two dose forms were observed (26,30). Urine levels of methadone, the pyrrolidine metabolite and creatinine, were determined in single urine specimens obtained at twenty-four hours after the last study dose of each medication form. There was no significant difference in ratios of urinary concentrations of methadone to creatinine or of pyrrolidine to creatinine, during treatment with methadone alone or with the methadone-naloxone combination. The clinically observed drug interaction was therefore a central interaction at receptor sites between narcotic antagonist and agonist, without demonstrable changes in methadone disposition.

Rifampin

The second observed interaction of a second drug with methadone, occurred when the antituberculosis agent rifampin was added to chemotherapeutic regimens of patients maintained on methadone, who also had tuberculosis (28,29,30). Thirty patients in the Bellevue Chest Methadone Maintenance Program with far advanced tuberculosis, were treated with rifampin in addition to isoniazid, ethambutol and/or other agents (28). Twenty-one of these thirty patients developed mild, moderate or severe symptoms of narcotic withdrawal, within one to fourteen days after rifampin treatment was initiated. Withdrawal symptoms began each day six to eight hours after the combined methadone-rifampin treatment was given and increased in intensity until one to two hours after methadone was given on the following day. Mild symptoms included abdominal cramps, rhinorrhea, lacrimation, pilocarpal erection, yawning, irritability and restlessness and severe symptoms included nausea, vomiting, anorexia, chills, joint pains, insomnia, tremulousness and severe anxiety.

Seven of the twenty-one patients who developed narcotic withdrawal symptoms during combined methadone-rifampin treatment, experienced severe symptoms. In collaboration with Dr. Jane Garfield of the Bellevue Chest Service, New York University, six of these seven patients were further studied after obtaining informed consent, to determine the effects of rifampin on methadone metabolism (See Table 3). These patients were all males, ranging in age from 29 to 74 years and with a 6 to 30 year history of heroin addiction before entering methadone maintenance treatment. All six were also receiving isoniazid and/or ethambutol treatment. In addition to far advanced tuberculosis, one of these patients had adult onset diabetes requiring insulin treatment (#1); two were chronic abusers of alcohol with evidence of liver damage(#2 and #4); one had chronic persistent hepatitis(#5); one patient had idiopathic seizures unrelated to drug withdrawal and was receiving phenobarbital during the rifampin treatment study period, but not when off rifampin. Doses of methadone ranged from 30 to 90 mg per day and of rifampin from 600 to 900 mg per day. Each patient was studied both off and on rifampin treatment. Clinical histories and urine monitoring showed no evidence of polydrug abuse during these studies.

TABLE 3. Rifampin - methadone interaction. Patients studied to determine effects of rifampin on methadone metabolism [a]

Age (years)	Sex	Weight (kilos)	Previous Heroin Addiction (years)	Drugs	Rifampin Dose (mg/d)	Methadone Dose (mg/d)
29-74	6M	50-75	6-30	INH-#5 EMB-#4	600-900	30-90

INH = Isoniazid

EMB = Ethambutol

[a] Data from reference 28

Plasma levels of methadone were determined at twenty-four hours (time zero), three, six and again at twenty-four hours after receiving an oral daily dose of methadone with an without concomitant rifampin treatment. During rifampin treatment, plasma levels were consistently and significantly (p < 0.001) lower (33-68%) at each comparable time point, except when plasma levels were at the lower limit of detection (0.01 μg/ml) at twenty-four hours after a dose methadone, when off as well as when on rifampin (See Figure 3). However, inconsistent changes in plasma disappearance rates were observed. A more rapid plasma disappearance of methadone or shorter apparent half-life was observed in two patients (#3 and #6), in addition to the lowering of plasma levels of methadone during rifampin treatment. In patient #3, the apparent terminal plasma half-life of methadone was 30.8 hours off and 9.0 hours on rifampin; however, this patient was receiving phenobarbital during rifampin treatment only and this drug certainly may have accelerated plasma disappearance by enhancement of microsomal enzyme activity. In patient ≠ 6, the apparent terminal plasma half-life of methadone was 19.1 hours off and 13.8 hours on rifampin treatment. In three patients (#1, #2 and #4), plasma disappearance rates of methadone were not altered by rifampin and in one patient (#5), apparent plasma half-life was prolonged during rifampin treatment, despite a lowering of plasma levels of rifampin in each case.

Satisfactory twenty-four hour urine collections were obtained in four patients, both off and on rifampin treatment. In all four, urinary excretion of the major pyrrolidine metabolite increased during rifampin, with a mean 150% increase. Also, whereas usually less than 50% of a chronic daily oral dose of methadone is excreted in the urine, as the sum of unchanged methadone and the major pyrrolidine metabolite, during rifampin treatment, in two patients, more than 50% of the dose was excreted in urine as methadone plus pyrrolidine.

Satisfactory twenty-four hour fecal collections were obtained from two patients, both off and on rifampin. Less than 1 mg of unchanged methadone was excreted by this route, both during and off rifampin treatment. However, twenty-four hour fecal excretion of the pyrrolidine metabolite, increased markedly during rifampin treatment, from 7.6 to 31.8 mg in one and from 10.2 to 26.5 mg in the other (see Table 4) (29).

The three observed rifampin effects on methadone metabolism, a significant lowering of plasma levels of methadone coupled with an increased urinary and fecal excretion of pyrrolidine metabolite, might be solely due to an enhancement of hepatic microsomal drug

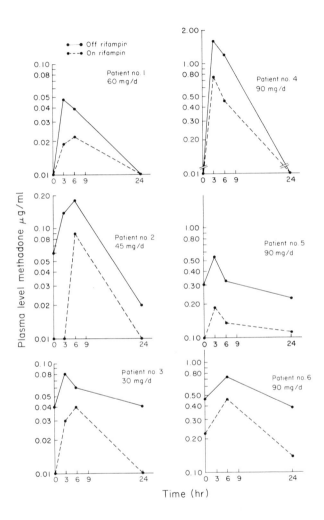

FIG. 3. Plasma disappearance of methadone shown by semilogarithmic plotting of plasma levels of methadone in individual patients studied off and on rifampin treatment (reprinted by permission from reference 28).

TABLE 4. Rifampin - methadone interaction: fecal
excretion of methadone and its pyrrolidine metabolite
off and on rifampin treatment

Patient	Methadone Dose (mg/d)	Rifampin Dose (mg/d)	Fecal Excretion in 24 Hours (mg)		
			Methadone	Pyrrolidine	Sum
A	60	---(off)	0.13	7.6	7.7
	60	600(on)	0.41	31.8	32.2
B	30	---(off)	0.63	10.2	10.8
	30	900(on)	0.44	26.5	26.9

metabolizing enzyme activities by rifampin, an effect
of this drug which has been previously demonstrated
(23,38,40). However, the inconsistent changes in
plasma disapperance rates, suggest that rifampin may
also alter methadone disposition in some other way.
The observed alterations of methadone action, that is,
the development of narcotic withdrawal symptoms during
rifampin treatment, is probably due to the abrupt
changes in methadone metabolism which were observed.
Alternatively, since it has recently been suggested in
animal studies by Gispen and colleagues that rifampin
may interfere with the development of tolerance to morphine, rifampin may have exerted its effect through
some central mechanism concerned with the maintenance
of tolerance or directly at a critical receptor (18).

ETHANOL AND OPIATES

The third clinical study, is the first of a sequence
of studies attempting to determine whether ethanol
causes any alterations of narcotic disposition or
central effects, which may result in altered narcotic
action, and conversely, whether narcotics may alter
ethanol action by dispositional or functional effects.
It has been suggested that ethanol may potentiate or
antagonize narcotic effects. It has also been suggested that chronic narcotic use may alter ethanol effects.
It has been shown in rats, that chronic ethanol

treatment results in enhanced hepatic microsomal N-demethylase activity after ethanol withdrawal, but decreased activity while ethanol is still present (35). It has also been suggested that alcohol and opiates may have similar effects, and also that each might modify the effects of abrupt withdrawal from the other (6,17,20,46,47). Several investigators have recently suggested a possible "commonality" between ethanol and narcotic effects, resulting from a postulated endogenous formation of similar or identical tetrahydroisoquinoline alkaloid compounds,from the condensation of endogenous or exogenous amines with aldehydes (4,5,10, 11,14,43,44,52). It is then postulated that these endogenous compounds, which also may be similar to narcotic alkaloids, may act at central sites to contribute to the development of tolerance, dependence and addiction to both ethanol and opiates. However, despite much provocative information,to date there is no direct clinical evidence or substantial direct animal data to substantiate this hypothesis.

In collaboration with Dr. Paul Cushman of St. Lukes Hospital and Dr. Enoch Gordis of Elmhurst General Hospital, a study was carried out in five stable chronic methadone patients whose regular use of alcohol was minimal, less than two drinks per week, to determine whether acute "social" use of alcohol alters methadone metabolism as reflected by plasma levels, and conversely, whether methadone alters alcohol metabolism as reflected by blood alcohol levels and disappearance rates (13). The patients ranged in age from 29 to 46 years; all were males who had been on methadone treatment from 1 to 6 years and were receiving 30 to 100 mg methadone daily (See Table 5).

TABLE 5. Ethanol-methadone interaction: patients studied to determine effects of ethanol on methadone metabolism and effects of methadone on ethanol metabolism [a]

Age (years)	Sex	Weight (kilos)	Methadone Treatment (years)	Methadone Dose (mg/d)	Other Drugs
24-46	5M	66-73	1-6	30-100	Methadone only in all 5

[a] Data from reference 13

There was no clinical or chemical evidence of polydrug
abuse during the study. Each patient was studied three
times.
     First, plasma levels of methadone were determined
after the usual dose of methadone alone. Then, plasma
levels of methadone and blood levels of ethanol were
determined before and for four hours after 90 ml of a
50% solution of ethanol were given, at one hour after
the last oral dose of methadone, to coincide with the
ascending part of the methadone plasma level curve.
Finally, plasma levels of methadone and blood levels of
ethanol, were determined before and for four hours
after a similar amount of ethanol was given, at twenty
to thirty-eight hours after the last oral dose of
methadone, a time when methadone levels are declining
very slowly. There were no significant differences in
plasma levels of methadone when ethanol was given one
hour after methadone, as compared with when methadone
was given alone (See Figure 4).

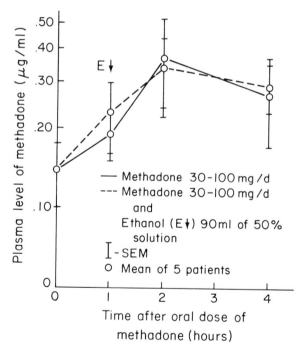

FIG. 4. Plasma levels of methadone in five stabilized
maintenance patients (not alcohol abusers) after oral
dose (30 to 100 mg) alone and after oral dose followed
in one hour by 90 ml of a 50% solution of ethanol;
determinations by gas liquid chromatography (13).

Also, when methadone was withheld until the completion
of the ethanol study, only the expected slight fall in
mean plasma methadone levels was observed.

Blood ethanol levels rose sharply in all patients
during both studies, reaching peak levels at 60 to 90
minutes. Blood ethanol disappearance rates were then
calculated from the straight lines fitted to the plasma
level points on the downward slope. The mean ethanol
disappearance rates when no methadone had been given
for 20 to 38 hours, were similar (0.23 ± 0.11 mg/100
ml/min) to the mean rates when methadone was given one
hour prior to ethanol administration (0.21 ± 0.09 mg/
100 ml/min). Thus, no significant acute interaction
between ethanol and methadone, as reflected by blood
disposition of each, was observed. Further studies of
such possible interactions in methadone maintenance
patients, who are also alcohol abusers, are in progress,
in addition to studies designed to examine the functional status of maintenance patients during acute and
chronic concomitant use of alcohol.

OTHER DRUG INTERACTIONS POSSIBLY AFFECTING OPIATE ACTIONS

Two other recent clinical studies of possible drug
interactions which could affect opiate actions, have
been carried out by other investigators, both using
normal volunteers as study subjects (9,49).

Aspirin

It has been suggested that aspirin, when combined
with codeine or morphine, may have synergistic activities. Brunk and colleagues carried out a study to
determine whether aspirin might decrease the normal
glucuronide conjugation of morphine and by doing so
cause higher blood levels of free morphine (9). Twelve
normal male volunteers, age 21 to 48, were treated with
aspirin (either 0.6 g or 1.2 g every 6 hours) for three
days. Approximately 10 mg of radiolabeled [14]C N-methyl
morphine was administered intravenously after 48 hours
of aspirin treatment. Free and conjugated plasma and
urine levels of morphine were determined using extraction techniques and radioactivity measurements. Similar
studies were carried out in the twelve subjects, following the administration of radiolabeled morphine alone,
without aspirin pretreatment.

Plasma free morphine levels were found to be lower
during aspirin treatment and glucuronide conjugated
morphine levels higher. Total cumulative radioactivity
in urine during aspirin treatment was unchanged, with

increased urine levels of free morphine and decreased levels of conjugated morphine. The N-demethylation of morphine, a minor pathway in man, was unchanged during aspirin treatment. Thus, aspirin did not inhibit glucuronidation of morphine and, in fact, plasma levels of free morphine were decreased by aspirin treatment. The investigators concluded that aspirin decreased the renal clearance of conjugated morphine.

Phenobarbital

Phenobarbital enhances a variety of microsomal enzyme activities including glucuronyl transferase and N-demethylases (12,34,39). Stambaugh carried out a study to determine if chronic phenobarbital treatment might alter the metabolism of a single dose of meperidine (49). Twelve medical student volunteers were treated for two weeks with either phenobarbital (100 mg/d) or placebo and then for two weeks with the other agent. After twelve days of pretreatment with placebo or with phenobarbital, a single 50 mg dose of meperidine was given intramuscularly. Serum levels of meperidine and cumulative 48 hour urinary excretion of unchanged meperidine and its normeperidine metabolite (togehter accounting for about 10-15% of the administered dose of meperidine), were determined using gas liquid chromatographic techniques.

Serum meperidine levels after a single dose were not altered by prior and concomitant treatment with phenobarbital. However, 48 hour cumulative urinary excretion of unchanged meperidine,was significantly reduced and that of normeperidine increased,during phenobarbital treatment. Thus, it was concluded that phenobarbital treatment altered the metabolism of meperidine by enhancing N-demethylation, but that serum levels following a single dose were not affected.

Several studies by various investigators on the effects of phenobarbital on narcotic disposition and action have been carried out in rats. Alvares and Kappas showed that pretreatment of rats with phenobarbital (75 mg/d i.p. for 3 days), increased N-demethylation of methadone by rat liver microsomes, which resulted in the increased formation of two then unidentified metabolites, detected by radioscanning of thin layer chromatograms (1). They also showed that four days pretreatment with phenobarbital, significantly reduced the duration of analgesic effects of acute doses of methadone (10 and 15 mg/kg body weight administered intraperitoneally).

Roerig and colleagues, later, studied the effect of phenobarbital on the biliary excretion of methadone in bile duct-cannulated rats. Animals were treated for

five days with phenobarbital (75 mg/kg i.p.) (42). Then
bile-duct fistulae were place surgically and, after
stabilization, a tracer dose of ^{14}C-methadone was
administered intravenously. Plasma and bile specimens
were obtained and radioactivity measured before and
after extraction and separation on thin layer chromatograms. Over the third minute period during which
plasma specimens were obtained, there were no differences in plasma radioactivity between the phenobarbital
treatment and control group. However, the total radioactivity recovered in bile during 90 minutes following
administration of radiolabeled morphine was significantly greater in the phenobarbital treated animals,
especially due to increased amounts of the second N-
demethylated product, pyrroline, and the hydroxylated
and conjugated metabolites. Similar studies carried
out by Roerig and colleagues on the effects of phenobarbital on morphine glucuronidation and biliary excretion in the rat, however, yielded curious, un-
explained opposite results (41).

We have carried out studies in rats first chronically
treated with methadone (5 mg/kg body weight) for two
weeks and then concomitantly treated with methadone
and phenobarbital (50 mg/kg body weight/d) for one
week (32). Control animals were treated with methadone
alone for three weeks. Blood specimens were obtained
at one hour after the last subcutaneous dose of methadone. Plasma levels of methadone, determined by
gas liquid chromatography, were significantly lower
in animals treated with phenobarbital concomitantly
(with a mean of 0.07 µg/ml, as compared with animals
treated with methadone alone with a mean of 0.24 µg/ml)
(See Figure 5). Animals similarly pretreated with
methadone and phenobarbital or methadone alone for
three weeks, were given a single dose of radiolabeled
^{14}C-methadone intravenously and then were given continued
treatment with methadone and phenobarbital, or methadone
alone, for eight additional days. Other animals were
treated with phenobarbital alone, or with saline and
received a single dose of radiolabeled methadone. All
urine and feces were collected for eight days and
cumulative excretion of radioactivity by each route
measured. No significant changes in urinary excretion
of total radioactivity from methadone were observed in
any group (See Figure 6). However, the cumulative
total radioactivity excreted in feces, was greater
during phenobarbital treatment, after a single dose of
methadone and during chronic methadone treatment. The
observed lowering of plasma methadone levels by

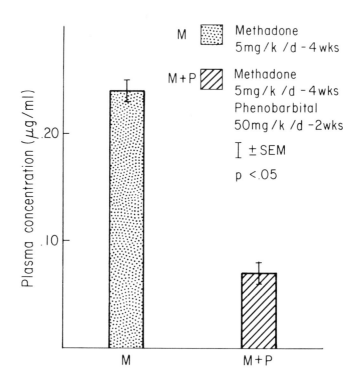

FIG. 5.   Plasma levels of methadone at one hour after
last subcutaneous dose in rats treated with methadone
alone (5 mg/kg/d, s.c., for 3 weeks), or with methadone
(5 mg/kg/d, s.c., for 3 weeks) and phenobarbital (50
mg/kg/d, s.c., for 1 week); determinations by gas
liquid chromatography (32).

phenobarbital during chronic methadone treatment, may
affect the action of that narcotic, just as action of
a single dose of methadone was shown to be reduced by
phenobarbital treatment.   Further studies are in progress
to explore that possibility.

Desipramine and Diazepam

Finally, the opposite type of drug interaction
affecting narcotic disposition and action in the rat
has been reported (36).   Pretreatment of rats with the

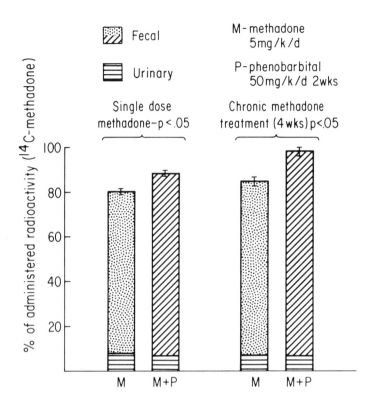

FIG. 6. Cumulative eight day urinary and fecal excretion of radioactivity from ^{14}C-2-methadone administered intravenously to rats during chronic treatment with methadone alone (5 mg/kg/d, s.c., for total of 4 weeks), or methadone (5 mg/kg/d, s.c., for total of 4 weeks) and phenobarbital (50 mg/kg/d, s.c., for total of 2 weeks); determinations by fecal homogenate oxiation and scintillation counting (32).

tricyclic antidepressant desipramine (20 mg/kg i.p.) one hour before the subcutaneous administration of methadone (5 mg/kg s.c.), increased the intensity and prolonged the duration of methadone analgesia, as determined by the hot plate method. Desipramine significantly reduced the effective analgesic dose of methadone and the lethal dose of methadone. When radiolabeled ^{14}C-methadone was given one hour after desipramine, increased brain uptake of ^{14}C and increased brain:

plasma ratios of radioactivity for three hours (as
compared with animals receiving methadone alone) were
observed. Using techniques for solvent extraction of
tissue homogenates and thin layer chromatography, it
was shown that desipramine pretreatment resulted in
increased amounts of unchanged methadone in liver.
Using liver microsomal preparations, it was shown that
desipramine inhibited the N-demethylation of methadone.
Thus, it was suggested that desipramine potentiated and
prolonged methadone analgesia by increasing brain concentrations of methadone and by inhibiting hepatic
microsomal metabolism of methadone. In another study,
Spaulding and colleagues have shown that diazepam
inhibits N-demethylation of methadone by liver microsomes and they have suggested that such an effect on
methadone disposition could enhance its effect in
humans when both drugs are taken (48).

CONCLUSIONS

These clinical and animal studies of the effects of
various drugs and alcohol on opiate disposition and
action, suggest that further studies using new specific,
sensitive analytical techniques are needed. An increased awareness of potential drug interactions should
improve clinical observations. Finally, at this time,
there is an especial need for the development of
improved technology to detect and measure quantitatively changes in opiate action, which might include
physical, functional, behavioral and emotional changes,
in man.   In the future, hopefully, correlations of
changes in drug disposition, any demonstrable changes
in endogenous opiate-like peptides or opiate receptors
and alterations in opiate action, will be able to be
made in studies carried out in animals and in man.

ACKNOWLEDGEMENTS

The author would like to acknowledge the expert
technical assistance in the laboratory of Mrs. Chai
Leng Gutjahr, Miss Holly Harte, Miss Laura Brown, Miss
Risa Korn, Mrs. Malgosia Hecht and Miss Leslie Steinberg
and in the preparation of this manuscript of Mr. Jay
Ruckel and Mr. Jeffrey Weinberg.
The author would also like to gratefully acknowledge
the research grants which made this work possible:
(DA-01138) from the National Institute of Drug Abuse
and (ODAS-84854) from the New York State Office of
Drug Abuse Services. The opinions expressed within are
not necessarily those of the Office.
Availability of clinical facilities at the Rockefeller

University were made possible by General Clinical
Research Center Grant (RR-00102) from the National
Institutes of Health.

BIBLIOGRAPHY

1. Alvares, A.P., and Kappas, A. (1972): J. Lab. Clin.
   Med., 79: 439
2. Baden, M.M. (1971): In: Methadone Maintenance,
   edited by S. Einstein, p. 143. Dekker Press, New
   York.
3. Bihari, B. (1974): Am. J. Drug Alc. Abuse, 2: 245
4. Blum, K., editor: Neurochemical and Behavioral
   Mechanisms of Alcohol and Opiate Dependence,
   Academic Press, New York, in press
5. Blum, K., Calhoun, W., Merritt, J., and Wallace,
   J.E. (1973): Nature, 242: 407
6. Blum, K., Wallace, J.E., Schwerter, H.A., and
   Eubanks, J.D. (1976): Experientia, 32: 79
7. Bowen, D.V., and Field, F.H. (1974): Organic Mass
   Spectrometry, 9: 195
8. Brown, B.S., Kozel, N.J., Meyers, M.B., and Dupont,
   R.L. (1973): Am. J. Psychiatry, 130: 599
9. Brunk, S.F., Delle, M., and Wilson, W.R. (1974):
   Clin. Pharmacol. Ther., 15: 283
10. Cohen, G., and Collins, M. (1970): Science, 167:
    1749
11. Cohen, G., Mytilineou , C., and Barrett, R.E.
    (1972): Science, 175: 1269
12. Conney, A.H. (1967): Pharmacol. Rev., 19: 317
13. Cushman, P., Kreek, M.J., and Gordis, E. (1976):
    (in preparation)
14. Davis, V.E., and Walsh, M.J. (1970): Science, 167:
    1005
15. DEA-NIDA (1975): Drug Enforcement Administration,
    National Institute of Drug Abuse, DAWN Statistical
    Report, December.
16. Gearing, F.R. (1970): Int. J. Addictions, 5: 517
17. Gelfand, R., and Amit, Z. (1976): Nature, 259: 415
18. Gispen, W.H., Krivoy, W., De Wied, D., and
    Zimmermann, E. (1975): Life Sci., 17: 247
19. Hachey, D.L., Kreek, M.J., and Mattson, D.H.:
    Proc. Second International Conference on Stable
    Isotopes, Argonne, Illinois, in press
20. Ho, A.K.S., Tsai, C.S., Chen, R.A. et al. (1975):
    Pharmacologist, 17: 197
21. Inturrisi, C.E., and Verebely, K. (1972): Clin.
    Pharmacol. Ther., 13: 633
22. Jackson, G.W., and Richman, A. (1973): Alcohol
    Health Res. World, 1: 25

23. Jezequel, A.M., Orlandi, F., and Tenconi, L.T. (1971): Gut, 12: 984
24. Kreek, M.J. (1973): JAMA, 223: 665
25. Kreek, M.J. (1973): Methadone Treatment Manual, U.S. Department of Justice (U.S.G.P.O.) ≠ 2700-00227, p. 85
26. Kreek, M.J. (1973): N.Y. State J. Med., 73: 2773
27. Kreek, M.J., Dodes, L., Kane, S., Knobler, J., and Martin, R. (1972): Ann. Intern. Med., 77: 598
28. Kreek, M.J., Garfield, J.W., Gutjahr, C.L., and Giusti, L.M. (1976): N. Engl. J. Med., 294: 1104
29. Kreek, M.J., Gutjahr, C.L., Bowen, D.V., and Field, F.H. (1977): Proc. of the Third National Drug Abuse Conference, New York, in press
30. Kreek, M.J., Gutjahr, C.L., Garfield, J.W., Bowen, D.V., and Field, F.H. (1977): Ann. N.Y. Acad.Sci., in press
31. Kreek, M.J., and Hachey, D.L. (1975): Clin. Res. 23: 571A
32. Kreek, M.J., Harte, E., Brown, L., Gutjahr, C.L., and Hecht, M. (1976):(in preparation)
33. Kreek, M.J., Schecter, A., Gutjahr, C.L., Bowen, D., Field, F., Queenan, J., and Merkatz, I. (1974): Am. J. Drug Alcohol Abuse, 1: 409
34. Kreek, M.J., and Sleisenger, M.H. (1968): Lancet, 2: 3
35. Liu, S.-J., Ramsey, R.K., and Fallon, H.J. (1975): Biochem. Pharmacol., 24: 369
36. Liu, S.-J., and Wang, R.I.H. (1975): J. Pharmacol. Exp. Ther., 195: 94
37. Maddux, J.F., and Elliott, B. (1975): Am. J. Drug Alcohol Abuse, 2: 245
38. Nitti, V., Ninni, A., Meola, G. et al. (1973): Chemotherapy, 19: 206
39. Remmer, H., and Merker, H.J. (1965): Ann. N.Y. Acad. Sci., 123: 79
40. Remmer, H., Schoene, B., and Fleischmann, R.A. (1973): Drug Metab. Dispos., 1: 224
41. Roerig, D.L., Hasegawa, A.T., Peterson, R.E., and Wang, R.I.H. (1974): Biochem. Pharmacol., 23: 1331
42. Roerig, D.L., Hasegawa, A.T., and Wang, R.I.H. (1975): Biochem. Pharmacol., 24: 355
43. Ross, D.H., Medina, M.A., and Cardenas, H.L. (1974): Science, 186: 63
44. Sandler, M., Carter, S.B., Hunter, K.R., and Stern, G.M. (1973): Nature, 241: 439
45. Schut, J., File, K., and Wohlmuth, T. (1973): Q. J. Studies on Alcohol, 34; 1356
46. Sinclair, J.D. (1974): Pharmacol. Biochem. Behav., 2: 409
47. Sinclair, J.D., Adkins, J., and Walker, S. (1973):

Nature, 246: 425
48. Spaulding, T.C., Minium, L., Kotake, A.N., and
    Takemori, A.E. (1974): Drug Metab. Dispos., 2: 458
49. Stambaugh, J.E. (1976): Hospital Practice, Special
    Report, January
50. Sullivan, H.R., and Blake, D.A. (1972): Res. Commun.
    Chem. Pathol. Pharmacol., 3: 467
51. Sullivan, H.R., and Due, S.L. (1973): J. Med. Chem.,
    16: 909
52. Tennyson, V.M., Cohen, G., Mytilineou, C., and
    Heikkila, R. (1973): Brain Res., 51: 161

Factors Affecting the Action of Narcotics, edited by
M.L. Adler, L. Manara, and R. Samanin.
Raven Press, New York©1978.

Effect of Propranolol on the Actions
of Narcotic Analgesics

Alan Cowan[1]

Department of Pharmacology, Reckitt & Colman,
Kingston-upon-Hull   HU8 7DS, England

INTRODUCTION

Interest in a possible interaction between propranolol and strong analgesics was recently stimulated by
reports from Grosz that this β-adrenoceptor antagonist
might be useful in the pharmacotherapy of heroin addiction (19,21,23). The proposition that pre- or post-
administration of propranolol can indeed modify certain
actions of narcotic analgesics in animals and man will
be reviewed in the present paper.

STUDIES WITH PROPRANOLOL IN THE TREATMENT
OF OPIATE ADDICTION

Grosz (19,20) was the first to claim that small
oral doses of propranolol blocked the euphoric action
of "street" heroin in out-patient addicts and attenuated drug craving in the post-withdrawal state. The
latter claim was confirmed to some extent by Lowenstein
(29) who observed that small doses of propranolol (20
mg four times daily) relieved a craving for pethidine
in one subject.
Grosz also reported the novel finding that pretreating heroin addicts with propranolol could cause a subsequent challenge with heroin or morphine to precipitate
a delayed yet protracted abstinence syndrome (21,22).
The implication from this work was that propranolol
(or a catabolite) could function as a long-acting
narcotic antagonist. Subsequent controlled trials,
however, have not supported this notion. Hollister
and Prusmack (26) found that propranolol had a slight
ameliorating effect on the withdrawal syndrome in
opiate-dependent patients undergoing detoxification

---

[1]Present address: Department of Pharmacology, Temple
University School of Medicine, Philadelphia,
Pennsylvania, U.S.A.

with methadone. This beneficial effect was not observed in patients with intense withdrawal syndromes. Jacob
et al. (27) also found that propranolol tended to
mitigate, rather than exacerbate, the self-rated opiate
withdrawal syndrome when patients were undergoing detoxification with methadone. Finally, Resnick et al.
(31) reported that propranolol neither relieved nor
precipitated opiate withdrawal when given in doses
ranging from 20-160 mg per day; moreover, propranolol
had no significant effect on heroin-induced euphoria.
    In summary, it would appear that attempts to verify
Grosz's description of propranolol as a clinical
opiate antagonist have been unsuccessful and therefore
use of such terminology is, on balance, premature.

ANIMAL STUDIES WITH PROPRANOLOL AND MORPHINE

    The interaction between propranolol and morphine in
animals has been studied in several pharmacological
tests since the former compound was first described in
1964 (2). The influence of propranolol on the antinociceptive effect of morphine has been the interaction most frequently investigated. Contreras et al.
(9) are alone in claiming that propranolol (5 mg/kg,
i.p.) significantly enhances the antinociceptive action
of morphine in the mouse hot-plate test. Two groups
have claimed that pretreating rodents with propranolol
(1-15 mg/kg, parenterally) significantly antagonizes
the antinociceptive effect of morphine. In both cases
the tail-flick test was employed; Heller et al. (25)
used mice in the hot water version of the test while
Shah et al. (35) used rats and a radiant heat stimulus.
    The majority of workers have found that propranolol,
when given by i.p., s.c. or intraventricular routes,
does not modify the antinociceptive effect of morphine
in mouse phenylquinone-writhing and hot-plate tests
(16), various mouse tail-flick tests (10,12,34,37), rat
paw-pressure and tail-pressure tests (10,17) and in the
rat hot-plate test (8,14). Finally, although the
balance of opinion is against a positive interaction
between propranolol and morphine, Tulunay et al. (38)
have recently reported that propranolol (but not
phenoxybenzamine) significantly increases the potency
of naloxone as a morphine antagonist in the mouse tail-
flick test. These authors found that the dose of
propranolol used (5 mg/kg, i.p.) did not alter the concentration of either morphine or naloxone in the mouse
brain 1 hr later. Clearly, this interesting three-way
interaction should also be quantified using additional
measures of agonist activity. This is particularly
necessary since, paradoxically, it has been claimed

that propranolol (2 mg/kg, i.p.) reduces binding of
tritiated naloxone to opiate receptors in whole mouse
brain within 30 min (6).

The prior injection of propranolol can influence
certain behavioral effects of morphine in animals. In
one study (3), the interaction was analyzed using rats
trained to press a lever on a VI 2-min schedule of
(liquid) reinforcement; that is, operant behavior was
reinforced with a drop of sweetened milk once every 2
min on the average. After stable base lines were
obtained, an auditory stimulus (lasting 4 min) was
introduced into the schedule and served as a fore-
warning of impending brief electric shock. Typically,
responding is suppressed when the sound is presented.
Whereas morphine (9 mg/kg, i.p.) reversed conditioned
suppression, the prior treatment of rats with racemic
propranolol (3 mg/kg, i.p.) attenuated this morphine
effect. In a second behavioral experiment, Black and
Grosz (3) provided further evidence of an interaction
between propranolol and morphine. Rats were trained
to press a lever to avoid receiving a brief, unsignalled
electric shock. Each response delayed the shock by
20 sec, but shocks were delivered every 5 sec if the
rat failed to respond. After morphine (9 mg/kg, i.p.),
the rats received more shocks; the response rate, however, was within control levels. Interestingly, pretreatment with d-propranolol (7 mg/kg, i.p.) diminished
the disruption of avoidance behavior caused by morphine.
A stereospecific effect was indicated since the same
dose of l-propranolol did not share this property
although it is curious that racemic propranolol (14
mg/kg, i.p.) was also without effect. In a recent
analysis of this interaction, Black et al. (4) found
that propranolol (i.p.) reduced the amount of unbound
^{14}C-morphine in blood plasma and certain brain areas.
When morphine was administered intraventricularly,
pretreatment with propranolol (presumably the d-isomer)
again diminished morphine-induced disruption of avoidance behavior. It was therefore concluded that the
interaction was not solely a consequence of reduced
morphine levels in the brain. That d-propranolol may
affect the passage of morphine out of the ventricular
system or that the membrane stabilization properties of
this compound prevent efficient uptake of morphine at
sites of action are points requiring further study.

Although propranolol can influence the actions of
morphine in operant situations, not all opiate-induced
behavioral effects are antagonized. For example, propranolol (2.5 mg/kg, i.p.) does not prevent the appearance of morphine-induced mania in cats (13). Also,when
propranolol (10 mg/kg, s.c.) is injected 10 min before

morphine (3-20 mg/kg, s.c.) into mice, and spontaneous locomotor activity is then quantified with an Animex monitor for 1 hr, the standard morphine dose-response line is not displaced to a significant extent (unpublished observation). This finding is in agreement with the report of Estler (15).

Both isomers of propranolol enhance the lethal effect of morphine in rats (41). This point is illustrated for the l-isomer in Fig. 1. When the sub-lethal dose of l-propranolol (25 mg/kg, i.p.) was injected 30 min after morphine, a dramatic increase in the frequency of death occurred with the higher doses of morphine. The dynamics of the interaction have yet to be clarified. From observation, it appears that propranolol potentiates the depressant effects of morphine.

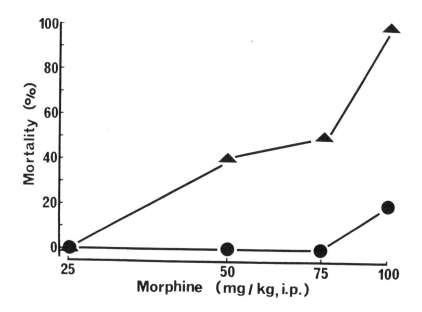

FIG. 1. Effect of l-propranolol hydrochloride on the lethality of morphine sulphate. Triangles represent experiments in which groups of 10 female rats received morphine followed 30 min later by l-propranolol (25 mg/kg, i.p.). Circles represent identical experiments but without treatment with propranolol. Reproduced with permission from Winter (41).

The influence of propranolol on animals receiving multiple doses of morphine has been evaluated in rodents and monkeys. Chipkin et al. (7) concluded that propranolol does not attenuate the naloxone-induced abstinence syndrome in rats. Results from the work of Harrigan and McCarthy (24) with monkeys gave no indication that propranolol might affect opiate-seeking behavior in man. Finally, Cowan and Macfarlane (10) monitored the naloxone-induced abstinence syndrome in monkeys receiving multiple s.c. injections of either saline + morphine (3 mg/kg) or propranolol (10 mg/kg) + morphine (3 mg/kg); the resulting abstinence syndromes were both of high intensity. The same workers found that propranolol (1-10 mg/kg, s.c.) neither precipitated abstinence syndromes in non-withdrawn, morphine-dependent monkeys nor modified the syndrome in 24-hr withdrawn, morphine-dependent monkeys. In contrast to the clinical findings of Grosz (21), subsequent injections of morphine did not intensify the withdrawal syndrome.

It was stated above that, in general, an acute dose of propranolol does not modify the antinociceptive effect of morphine in rodents. A different conclusion is reached, however, if multiple doses of propranolol are given prior to challenge with morphine (10). Thus, after 8 injections of dl-propranolol (30 mg/kg, s.c. twice daily for 4 days), mice were found to be tolerant to normally effective doses of morphine in the tail-flick test; moreover, when propranolol and morphine were administered concurrently, the morphine ED 50 value (on day 5) was twice as high as the ED 50 from a group of mice receiving multiple injections of morphine alone (Fig. 2). It is not known whether sufficient propranolol is present in the CNS of mice 17-18 hr after the course of injections to influence the receptor kinetics of morphine or whether multiple doses of propranolol induce a conformational change at opiate receptor sites such that they are no longer accessible to morphine. Results from a relevant study in which mice were used indicate that propranolol, at high concentrations, can interfere with the binding of morphine to subcellular fractions of brain in vitro (11).

When mice received 8 doses of d-propranolol, the isomer with practically no β-blocking properties (1), surprisingly large amounts of morphine were again required on day 5 during estimation of the antinociceptive ED 50 values (Fig. 3). It is therefore tempting to conclude that β-adrenoceptors play no part in the phenomenon. In contrast to the findings with d- and dl-propranolol, multiple dosing with practolol (30 mg/kg, s.c.), a β-sympatholytic agent which does not readily

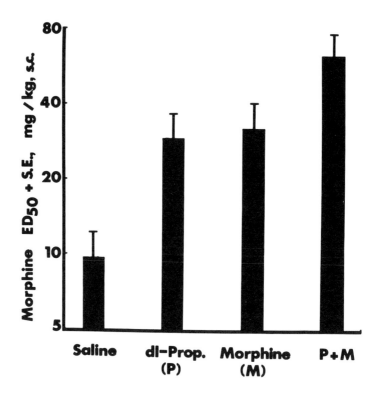

FIG. 2.   Effect of various pretreatments on the antinociceptive ED 50 of morphine in the mouse tail-flick
test.   Four groups of 45 mice were injected s.c. at
9.00 and 16.00 hr daily for 4 days with either saline,
dl-propranolol (P, 30 mg/kg), morphine (M, 70 mg/kg)
or P+M (same doses); the morphine ED 50 values were
estimated on day 5, 17-18 hr after the last injections.
Note that the ordinate is on a log scale.   Reproduced
with permission from Cowan and Macfarlane (10).

enter the brain (33), had no significant influence on
the ED 50 of morphine on day 5.   This result suggests
that the propranolol-morphine effect is centrally
mediated.

    The effect of the same multiple-dose schedule of
racemic propranolol has been studied against a second
agonist action of morphine i.e. hypothermia.   Thus,
when mice were pretreated with propranolol twice daily
for 4 days and then challenged with a dose of morphine
that invariably caused a large fall in esophageal

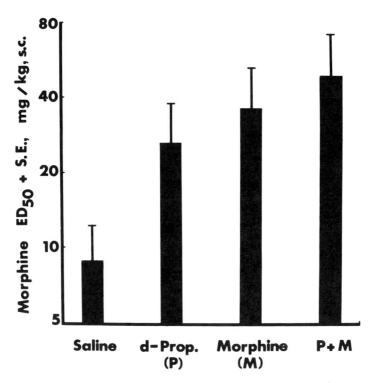

FIG. 3.   Effect of various pretreatments on the antinociceptive ED 50 of morphine in the mouse tail-flick
test.   Four groups of 45 mice were injected s.c. at
9.00 and 16.00 hr daily for 4 days with either saline,
d-propranolol (P, 30 mg/kg), morphine (M, 70 mg/kg) or
P+M (same doses); the morphine ED 50 values were
estimated on day 5, 17-18 hr after the last injections.
Reproduced with permission from Cowan and Macfarlane
(10).

temperature, it was found that the mean hypothermic
effect was significantly reduced and was only of the
same order as the saline control value (Fig. 4).   In
other words, mice receiving the propranolol pretreatment had again become tolerant to a normally effective
dose of morphine.   It is important to note that, in this
experiment, an acute dose of propranolol (30 mg/kg, s.c.)
caused marked hypothermia in mice pretreated with saline
(histogram e); furthermore, the same dose of propranolol induced a similar fall in temperature in mice

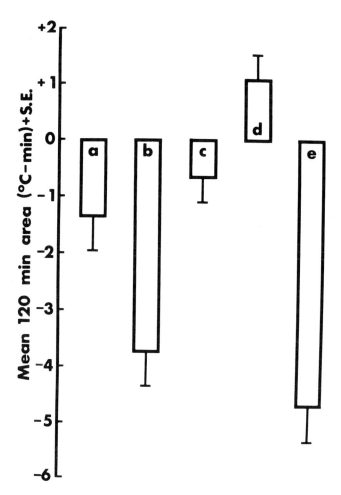

FIG. 4. Effect of various pretreatments on the hypothermic effect of morphine in mice. Five groups of
10-12 mice were injected s.c. at 9.00 and 17.00 hr
daily for 4 days with saline (histograms a, b and e),
dl-propranolol, 30 mg/kg (c) or morphine, 70 mg/kg (d).
On day 5, 19-20 hr after the last of the pretreatment
injections, intravenous injections of saline (a) or
morphine, 25 mg/kg (b, c and d) and s.c. injections of
dl-propranolol, 30 mg/kg (e) were given. Esophageal
temperatures were recorded immediately prior to drug
administration on day 5 and thereafter at 0.5 hr
intervals for 2 hr. Each histogram represents the
mean group area under the time-temperature curves of
individual mice (Cowan and Macfarlane, unpublished
observations).

pretreated with propranolol (data not shown). Thus, pretreating mice with propranolol greatly influences the magnitude of the hypothermic effect of a subsequent dose of morphine but not of a subsequent dose of propranolol. No information is currently available on the duration of this effect of propranolol.

PERSPECTIVE

Over the last decade, propranolol has been used as a psychotropic agent in the treatment of a surprisingly large number of conditions, for example, anxiety, schizophrenia, tremor, and the tension and depression accompanying withdrawal from alcohol or narcotic analgesics. A clear view on the role of propranolol as a psychotherapeutic agent in these states has yet to be established (18,28,39). Issues still to be resolved include the relative importance of the peripheral and possible central effects of propranolol; the significance of receptor blockade as opposed to membrane stabilization; and the contribution of pharmacologically active catabolites (32). The usefulness of propranolol in the pharmacotherapy of heroin addiction is a controversial issue since the interesting findings of the main proponent (Grosz) have not been confirmed by several other workers. From the few facts that are available on the nature of the propranolol-morphine interaction in man, it seems clear that propranolol does not influence the metabolism of the narcotic, at least in normal subjects (5).

An interpretation of propranolol-morphine interactions in neurochemical terms may soon be possible since the neuropharmacological profile of propranolol is gradually emerging. Thus, in rats, a large dose of propranolol (15-50 mg/kg, i.p.) a) increases the activity of striatal tyrosine hydroxylase (36), b) increases the level of 5-hydroxytryptamine and decreases the level of 5-hydroxyindoleacetic acid in the cerebral cortex, probably through inhibition of monoamine oxidase (30) and c) elevates the level of homovanillic acid in the olfactory tubercle, but not in the striatum, and increases the level of 3-methoxy-4-hydroxyphenylglycol in the remainder of the brain (40).

In view of the marked effects of repeated doses of propranolol on certain agonist actions of morphine in mice (vide supra), it may be worthwhile monitoring the neurochemical consequences of multiple injections of propranolol in future studies.

REFERENCES

1. Barrett, A.M., and Cullum, V.A. (1968): Br. J. Pharmacol., 34: 43
2. Black, J.W., Crowther, A.F., Shanks, R.G., Smith, L.H., and Dornhorst, A.C. (1964): Lancet, 1: 1080
3. Black, W.C., and Grosz, H.J. (1974): Brain Res., 65: 362
4. Black, W.C., McBride, W.J., and Grosz, H.J. (1975): Pharmacol. Biochem. Behav., 3: 701
5. Brunk, S.F., Delle, M., and Wilson, W.R. (1974): Clin. Pharmacol. Ther., 16: 1039
6. Charalampous, K.D., and Askew, W.E. (1974): Res. Commun. Chem. Pathol. Pharmacol., 8: 615
7. Chipkin, R.E., Dewey, W.L., Harris, L.S., and Lowenthal, W. (1975): Pharmacol. Biochem. Behav., 3: 843
8. Cicero, T.J. (1974): Arch. Int. Pharmacodyn. Ther., 208: 5
9. Contreras, E., Castillo, S., and Quijada, L. (1972): J. Pharm. Pharmacol., 24: 65
10. Cowan, A., and Macfarlane, I.R. (1975): Eur. J. Pharmacol., 34: 87
11. DeFeudis, F.V., and Grosz, H.J. (1972): Brain Res., 47: 510
12. Dewey, W.L., Harris, L.S., Howes, J.F., and Nuite, J.A. (1970): J. Pharmacol. Exp. Ther., 175: 435
13. Dhasmana, K.M., Dixit, K.S., Jaju, B.P., and Gupta, M.L. (1972): Psychopharmacologia, 24: 380
14. Eidelberg, E. (1976): Prog. Neurobiol., 6: 81
15. Estler, C.-J. (1973): Psychopharmacologia, 28: 261
16. Fennessy, M.R., and Lee, J.R. (1970): J. Pharm. Pharmacol., 22: 930
17. Görlitz, B.-D., and Frey, H.-H. (1972): Eur. J. Pharmacol., 20: 171
18. Greenblatt, D.J., and Shader, R.I. (1972): Curr. Ther. Res., 14: 615
19. Grosz, H.J. (1972): J. Indiana State Med. Assoc., 65: 505
20. Grosz, H.J. (1972): Lancet, 2: 564
21. Grosz, H.J. (1973): Lancet, 2: 612
22. Grosz, H.J. (1974): Ann. Int. Med., 80: 118
23. Grosz, H.J. (1975): In: Drug Dependence - Treatment and Treatment Evaluation, edited by H. Boström, T. Larsson, and N. Ljungstedt, p. 185. Almqvist and Wiksell, Stockholm.
24. Harrigan, S.E., and McCarthy, D.A. (1973): Pharmacologist, 15: 237
25. Heller, B., Saavedra, J.M., and Fischer, E. (1968): Experientia, 24: 804

26. Hollister, L.E., and Prusmack, J.J. (1974): Arch. Gen. Psychiatry, 31: 695

27. Jacob, R.G., Holmstrand, J., Eriksson, J.H., and Änggård, E. (1975): Psychopharmacologia, 41: 71

28. Jefferson, J.W. (1974): Arch. Gen. Psychiatry, 31: 681

29. Lowenstein, H. (1973): Lancet, 1: 559

30. Milmore, J.E., and Taylor, K.M. (1975): Life Sci., 17: 1843

31. Resnick, R.B., Kestenbaum, R.S., Schwartz, L.K., and Smith, A. (1976): Arch. Gen. Psychiatry, 33: 993

32. Saelens, D.A., Walle, T., Privitera, P.J., Knapp, D.R., and Gaffney, T. (1974): J. Pharmacol. Exp. Ther., 188: 86

33. Scales, B., and Cosgrove, M.B. (1970): J. Pharmacol. Exp. Ther., 175: 338

34. Sewell, R.D.E., and Spencer, P.S.J. (1975): Br. J. Pharmacol., 54: 256P

35. Shah, U.H., Jindal, M.N., Patel, V.K., and Kelkar, V.V. (1974): Arzneim. Forsch., 24: 1581

36. Sullivan, J.L., Segal, D.S., Kuczenski, R.T., and Mandell, A.J. (1972): Biol. Psychiatry, 4: 193

37. Takemori, A.E., Tulunay, F.C., and Yano, I. (1975): Life Sci., 17: 21

38. Tulunay, F.C., Yano, I., and Takemori, A.E. (1976): Eur. J. Pharmacol., 35: 285

39. Whitlock, F.A., and Price J. (1974): Drugs, 8: 109

40. Wiesel, F.A. (1976): Neurosci. Letters, 2: 35

41. Winter, J.C. (1974): Arch. Int. Pharmacodyn. Ther., 212: 195

6. PERSPECTIVES IN NARCOTIC

RESEARCH

Factors Affecting the Action of Narcotics, edited by
M.L. Adler, L. Manara, and R. Samanin.
Raven Press, New York©1978.

PERSPECTIVES IN NARCOTIC RESEARCH

ROUNDTABLE DISCUSSION

Chairman: Silvio Garattini
Reporter: Martin W. Adler

Panel: Joseph Cochin
                 E. Leong Way
                 Avram Goldstein
                 Hans Kosterlitz

The discussion was hosted by Dr. Garattini,
Director of the Mario Negri Institute for Pharmacological Research, who, after a brief introduction,
presented the panel with five questions for discussion.
The first issue dealt with problems of methodology and
included such items as the assessment of opioid activity and the meaning of the various tests utilized.
Dr. Kosterlitz opened the discussion by pointing out
that until a few years ago, the available opioid
compounds had a relatively simple spectrum of activity
and could be easily classified. In the past two or
three years, however, compounds had become available
which did not fit the usual pattern, e.g., agents with
antinociceptive activity that did not substitute for
morphine in dependent monkeys. In addition, there was
the opioid peptide explosion. Dr.Kosterlitz suggested
that no single assay is sufficient for the determination of opioid activity; rather, tests of various types
are necessary. He expressed the opinion that a
pharmacological assay is more reliable, as far as clas-
sification of compounds is concerned, than a binding
assay. In the latter, one only binds, but in a pharmacological assay one not only binds but activates the
"black box" behind the binding site. This distinction
is important since one can get binding, even stereo-

specific binding, in the absence of pharmacological
activity. Dr. Kosterlitz suggested that a combination of a binding assay plus one or two pharmacological
assays would be most appropriate. Although agreeing
with the others, Dr. Cochin proposed that one or more
pharmacological assays be carried out in the whole
animal. This idea was expanded upon by Dr. Adler who
suggested examining a broader spectrum of traditional
opioid action in the whole animal rather than merely
tests for analgesia. Dr. Goldstein added that naloxone
antagonism should be part of the definition of opioid
activity. All of the participants felt that naloxone
antagonism constituted a valuable criterion for opioid
activity at the present time, and Dr. Garattini cautioned that the antagonism should occur at reasonable
concentrations. Dr. Kosterlitz added that the antagonism should be stereospecific for either the + or -
isomer of naloxone. In concluding this discussion,
Dr. Way noted that the sequence and number of tests
conducted might be dictated, at least initially, by
the availability of the material under consideration.

The second question brought up the problem of
methodological approaches with regard to studies on
endorphin. Dr. Goldstein responded noting that we do
not yet really know the functions of the endorphin
systems, since showing an effect after the intracerebral administration of a drug is not tantamount to
demonstrating a physiological function. What should
one look for? He suggested that a first approach be
to determine whether naloxone itself has an effect;
that is, might it actually be blocking endogenous
systems? Naloxone does not appear to have much activity; however, the lack of activity may be due to
resistance of the endorphin system to naloxone blockade or to the possibility that the endorphin systems
are normally quiescent and are activated only under a
certain set of circumstances (e.g., some kind of
stress-induced or slow pain). Dr. Goldstein suggested
that the endorphin system might obtund chronic pain
without affecting perception of acute pain. Indeed,
this idea is reminiscent of what opiates do in the
clinical situation. Dr. Kosterlitz then pointed out
that although we normally only think of analgesia or
antinociception in regard to opiates, this effect is

only a small part of the spectrum of opiate actions.
Dr. Garattini commented that endorphins may be
involved   only with certain aspects of perception or
reaction to pain. He then asked whether there are any
distinct relationships between the endorphins and the
neurotransmitters. Dr. Kosterlitz replied that
current information indicates no correlation with any
particular transmitter and added that he would not be
surprised if the endorphins interacted with several
of the transmitters. Dr. Goldstein expressed the
feeling that one outcome of research with endorphins
would be a study of disturbances of endorphin synthesis, release, and metabolism consequent to the
administration of exogenous opiates. He suggested
that the prolonged abstinence syndrome described by
Dr. William Martin might be found to result from such
disturbances in the endorphin system. Dr. Way stated
that he is currently conducting research to determine
a possible biochemical basis for the prolonged abstinence syndrome.

An important point was raised from the floor by
Dr. Braude. She made a plea for some agreement in the
naming of the new endogenous peptides and ligands in
order to avoid the recent problems associated with the
naming of cannabinoids (i.e., Europeans use one system;
Americans, another). Although Dr. Goldstein said that
international rules are being followed for peptide
nomenclature, the members of the panel concurred that
Dr. Braude's point was well taken and great care must
be exercised in naming new compounds. Dr. Simon raised
raised yet another issue from the floor concerning
what happens in the "black box" after binding occurs.
An approach suggested by Dr. Adler was to examine some
of the factors discussed at this Symposium, e.g., age,
ambient temperature, strain, housing, disease states.
In seeing how the various systems in the whole animal
are affected by these factors, one may get some ideas
about the "black box". Dr. Hosoya then asked whether
administration of naloxone to a patient causes pain
and whether there is any endogenous substance that
antagonizes endorphin. Although considerable discussion ensued, the answers were highly speculative.
However, Dr. Cochin recalled that in early human
experiments with nalorphine, about 1/3 of the patients

had a peculiar response including a burning pain or
sensation. Finally, Dr. Herz said that since it has
been calculated that all receptors are occupied by
naloxone if a dose of 1 mg/kg is administered, higher
doses might result in some sort of a nonspecific
effect.

Raising the third question, Dr. Garattini stated
that in the pharmacological approach to the understanding of drug action, one adds a drug to learn the effect
on another drug by looking at the drug interactions.
Although this approach has been very useful, there may
be some problems to be considered in experiments
involving the interactions of two or more drugs.
What are the ways in which we can make these studies
more meaningful? Dr. Way responded that we, as
pharmacologists, must continually remind ourselves
that drugs have multiple effects. Because we choose a
drug for one particular action, we tend to forget its
other effects, particularly if we obtain the result
that we desire. Hypoxia, temperature, drug antagonism
or potentiation, and other factors must be taken into
consideration when dealing with more than one drug.
Drug distribution studies should be conducted to
ascertain that the second drug is not affecting the
distribution of the first drug, e.g., altering the
blood-brain barrier. Dr. Way added that it is essential to quantify and standardize the degree of tolerance or physical dependence produced and presented
examples to illustrate his point. Dr.Adler then suggested that there must be standardization : more than
the test itself the conditions under which the test is
performed must also be standardized. One must consider
too, that the second drug can alter those conditions,
e.g., a drug might alter body temperature or circadian
rhythm effects, thereby leading to false conclusions.
The apparatus used in the measurements should also be
standardized, e.g., size of chamber to look at escape
behavior. Several endpoints or signs are needed to
evaluate dependence, since one sign may be altered
while others remain unchanged. Dr. Way pointed out
that it was important to be aware of the shortcomings
of one's measurements with whatever tests are utilized.
Dr. Adler then stated that whether we are looking at
physical dependence or some other narcotic effect, it

must be realized that a drug can, in essence, alter
the conditions under which an animal is being tested,
if for example, it alters levels of biogenic amines
or body temperature.

In a comment from the floor, Dr. Manara cautioned
that in interpreting drug interaction studies, one
must be certain that one drug is not affecting the
availability of the other drug. In this regard, the
evaluation of negative data can be misleading.
Dr. Garattini noted that Dr. Sparber had pointed out
during the Symposium that the selection of a proper
experimental design can be critical for experiments
involving drug antagonism in distinguishing a pharmacological from a physiological antagonism. To determine the actual mechanism involved in the antagonism,
a large number of tests might be needed. Dr.Kreek
noted an existing need for multiple measurements for
drug dependence because the use of parameters such as
body temperature and body weight are not sufficient
with long-acting compounds. With respect to the term
"antagonism", Dr. Kosterlitz suggested that this word
be used only to mean antagonism at the receptor and
that another term, such as "reversal" be used to
indicate physiological antagonism. This suggestion was
disputed by Dr. Adler who noted that since the terms
"physiological antagonism" and "pharmacological
antagonism" are defined quite precisely and their use
is well ingrained in drug interaction literature,
there seemed to be no good reason to change the terminology.

Dr. Garattini posed the fourth question by asking
what can be said about treatment of addiction as a
result of this Symposium on Factors Affecting the
Actions of Narcotics? We must bear in mind that the
ultimate aim of what we are doing is to help patients.
Dr. Cochin opened the discussion by restating the issue
in somewhat different terms: what is the relevance of
this research to the real world? He broached the
subject by relating an incident which took place when
he was a medical student and teaching assistant in a
pharmacology laboratory. Having already decided to
study psychiatry, some of the sophomore medical
students were upset at having to learn pharmacology,
because it had "no relevance" for them as they were not

going to be using drugs. The year was 1951, just
before the advent of drugs for the treatment of psychiatric disorders. Since we cannot know ahead of
time the relevance of basic research, how can we
predict the consequences of basic research in practical
terms? Can we say, with any degree of certainty, that
the present breakthrough in opiate receptor research
and the isolation and characterization of the endogenous endorphins will lead to equally dramatic advances
in the therapy of addictive disorders? The only thing
we can state with certainty is that the data and hypothesis being generated will help us to comprehend the
mechanisms of tolerance and dependence and will
eventually lead to the development of new treatment
modalities and to understanding the whole process of
disease. Much of today's therapy stems from basic
research that was not aimed at new treatment modalities. As an example, Dr. Cochin pointed to the work of
Fraser and Isbell with methadone in man. Although
originally carried out for different purposes, the
research led to the use of methadone for detoxification
and, eventually, to methadone maintenance. He also
noted that present clinical studies on antagonist
treatment of addicts arose from basic research into the
pharmacology of dependence and the finding that pretreatment with an antagonist blocked any effects of a
subsequently administered narcotic. Dr. Goldstein
agreed with Dr.Cochin but felt that we can go further:
we can guarantee that the more information we gain, the
more practical uses will come from that information.
He cited a recent article by Comroe and Dripps (Science
192:105-111,1976) reporting the results of a five-year
study to assess the value of basic research in the
practical treatment of cardiovascular disease. The
results demonstrated the enormous impact of pure basic
research that had no clinical connection. Dr.Goldstein
then stated that from basic research we can undoubtedly
predict important outcomes for society in terms of
treatment of disease. Furthermore, the results of
opiate research could have much broader clinical implications than just in the area of heroin addiction. It
was obvious that the audience and the other members of
the panel supported the sentiments of Dr . Cochin and
Dr. Goldstein.

The last issue raised by Dr. Garattini pertained not
only to the narcotics field but to research in general.
He stated that when a number of people in research are
working on the same problem, it is a common occurrence
that some will develop similar ideas and draw similar
conclusions at the same time.   Because research is so
competitive, there is a tendency to publish fragmentary
results after only a few experiments.   He asked whether
there were any recommendations with regard to mini-
mizing the disadvantages of this publication problem.
Dr. Adler thought that a corollary problem was how to
make the scientific community aware of what is happen-
ing in a rapidly moving field.   He felt that in such
research, experiments reported in the literature may
not have to be as complete as in some other fields.
Even in this type of research, however, good scientific
methodology must be exercised, and the work should be
subject to peer review prior to publication.   In all
areas of research, there should be a feeling of respon-
sibility on the part of scientists not to publish
multiple reports of one experiment in several journals.
Dr. Adler suggested that one solution might be that
scientists attempt to instill such a philosophy in
their graduate students by setting the proper example.
Additionally, reviewers might be made aware of recently
submitted or published articles by the same investigators by requiring that authors submit such a list with
their manuscript.   On a related subject, Dr. Adler
asked how we can rapidly disseminate information to the
scientific community.   At the present time, most new
and exciting results are reported at Symposia or other
meetings.   Unfortunately, scientists not attending the
particular conference may wait for many months before
knowing the results reported at the meeting.   This
problem is especially true for the young investigator.
As a possibility, Dr. Adler suggested a journal or new
newsletter devoted to short summaries of meetings.
Perhaps these summaries could be published by organizations such as the American Association for the Advance-
ment of Science, since its publication Science has
worldwide distribution.   Dr. Goldstein said that he is
also concerned with the publication problem but pointed
out that scientists, like everyone else, do what is in
their own interest.   He said that we cannot appeal on

altruistic grounds alone and expect to get very far.
What is necessary, he proposed, is that those in
decision-making positions about grants, promotions, and
careers begin to look at quality of papers rather than
numbers. In fact, excessive numbers of papers should
be questioned. Dr. Goldstein also felt that many
scientists, particularly young ones, overestimate the
importance of rushing into publication. Accomplishments
are evaluated on the basis of years of work in a field,
the important thing being to work hard and long,
publish solid data, and not flit around from one project to another. Dr. Goldstein agreed that rapid communication of new information was important but saw no
clear way to accomplish it. Expressing a somewhat
contrary opinion, Dr. Simon said that he is not really
concerned with the proliferation of papers, even identical papers. He felt, as did Dr. Goldstein, that the
pressures to publish are too great. Dr. Simon expressed alarm at the fantastic rate with which new journals
are appearing. Regarding rapid communication of
reports from meetings, he suggested that arrangements
might be made with journal editors to publish quickly
the papers presented at the meetings. Finally, Dr.Way
thought that multiple publications had some redeeming
quality since different journals reach different
audiences.

Following a few additional comments from the floor,
Dr. Garattini formally called the meeting to a close
by expressing his opinion that the Symposium had been
a great success and had accomplished much. This feeling was obviously echoed by the participants.

                              Martin W. Adler

Author Index

Subject Index